PATHOPHYSIOLOGY
OF HEART DISEASE

*A Collaborative Project
of Medical Students and Faculty*

THIRD EDITION

PATHOPHYSIOLOGY OF HEART DISEASE

A Collaborative Project of Medical Students and Faculty

THIRD EDITION

EDITOR

Leonard S. Lilly, M.D.

Associate Professor of Medicine
Harvard Medical School
Chief, Brigham and Women's/Faulkner Cardiology
Cardiovascular Division
Brigham and Women's Hospital
Boston, Massachusetts

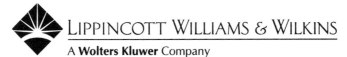

LIPPINCOTT WILLIAMS & WILKINS
A **Wolters Kluwer** Company
Philadelphia · Baltimore · New York · London
Buenos Aires · Hong Kong · Sydney · Tokyo

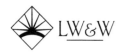 LW&W

Editor: Betty Sun
Managing Editor: Eric Branger
Marketing Manager: Aimee Sirmon
Project Editor: Christina Remsberg
Compositor: Graphic World
Printer: Courier-Kendallville

Printed in the United States of America

Library of Congress Cataloging-in-Publication Data

Pathophysiology of heart disease: a collaborative project of medical students and faculty / editor, Leonard S. Lilly.—3rd ed.
    p. cm.
  Includes bibliographical references and index.
  ISBN 0-7817-4027-4
    1. Heart—Pathophysiology. I. Lilly, Leonard S. II. Harvard Medical School.

  RC682.9 .P255 2003
  616.1'207—dc21

                        2002069426

The publishers have made every effort to trace the copyright holders for borrowed material. If they have inadvertently overlooked any, they will be pleased to make the necessary arrangements at the first opportunity.

To purchase additional copies of this book, call our customer service department at **(800) 638-3030** or fax orders to **(301) 824-7390**. International customers should call **(301) 714-2324**.

Visit Lippincott Williams & Wilkins on the Internet: http://www.lww.com. Lippincott Williams & Wilkins customer service representatives are available from 8:30 am to 6:00 pm, EST.

             04 05 06
       3 4 5 6 7 8 9 10

To Carolyn,

Jonathan, Rebecca,

Norma, and David Lilly

Foreword

It is axiomatic that when designing any product or service, the needs of the prospective user must receive primary consideration. Regrettably, this is rarely the case with medical textbooks, which play a vital role in the education of students, residents, fellows, practicing physicians, and paramedical professionals. A large majority of books are written for anyone who will read—or preferably buy—them. As a consequence they often provide a little for everyone but not enough for anyone. Many medical textbooks are reminiscent of the one-room schoolhouse, which included pupils ranging from the first to the twelfth grade. The need to deal with subject matter at enormously disparate levels of sophistication interfered with the educational process.

Medical educators appreciate that the needs of medical students exposed to a subject for the first time differ importantly from those of practicing physicians who wish to review an area learned previously or to be updated on new developments in a field with which they already have some familiarity. The lack of textbooks designed specifically for students leads faculty at schools around the country to spend countless hours preparing and duplicating voluminous lecture notes, and providing students with custom-designed "camels" (a camel is a cow created by a committee).

Pathophysiology of Heart Disease, a Collaborative Project of Harvard Medical Students and Faculty, represents a refreshing and innovative departure in the preparation of a medical text. Students, i.e., potential consumers, dissatisfied with currently available textbooks of cardiology made their needs clear. Fortunately, their pleas fell on receptive ears. Dr. Leonard Lilly, a respected cardiologist on the Harvard/ Brigham faculty, has played a leadership role in this project. He has brought together a group of talented Harvard Medical students and faculty who have collaborated closely to produce this fine introductory text *specifically* designed to meet the needs of medical students during their initial encounters with patients with heart disease. The text, tables, and illustrations are readily comprehensible to students. While *Pathophysiology of Heart Disease* is not meant to be encyclopedic or all-inclusive, it is remarkably thorough.

Quite appropriately, the first two editions of this fine book have been received enthusiastically, and *Pathophysiology of Heart Disease* is now a recommended text in many medical schools. It has been translated into other languages, has received two awards of excellence from the American Medical Writers Association, and has triggered several other student–faculty collaborative book projects.

Dr. Lilly and his colleagues—both faculty and students—have made a significant and unique contribution in preparing this important book. This third edition is not only an updated, but also an expanded version of the second edition. As such, it will prove to be even more valuable.

EUGENE BRAUNWALD, M.D.
Distinguished Hersey Professor of Medicine
Harvard Medical School
Faculty Dean for Academic Programs
Brigham and Women's Hospital,
and Massachusetts General Hospital
Boston, Massachusetts

Preface

This textbook is a comprehensive introduction to diseases of the cardiovascular system. Although excellent cardiology reference books are available, their encyclopedic content can overwhelm the beginning student. Therefore, this text was created to serve as a simplified bridge between courses in basic physiology and the care of patients in hospital wards and clinics. It is intended to help medical students and physicians-in-training form a solid foundation of knowledge of diseases of the heart and circulation, and is designed so that it can be read in its entirety during the one-month period usually allocated to courses in cardiovascular pathophysiology. Emphasis has been placed on the basic mechanisms by which cardiac illnesses develop to facilitate the later in-depth study of clinical diagnosis and therapy.

The original motivation for writing this book was the need for such a text voiced by our medical students as well as their desire to participate in its creation and direction. Consequently, the book's development is unusual in that it represents a close collaboration between Harvard medical students and cardiology faculty, who shared in the writing and editing of the manuscript. The goal of this pairing was to focus the subject matter on the needs of the students while providing the expertise of the faculty members. In this updated and rewritten third edition of *Pathophysiology of Heart Disease*, the collaborative effort has continued, between a new generation of medical students and our cardiovascular faculty.

The introductory chapters of the book review basic cardiac anatomy and physiology and describe the tools needed for understanding the clinical aspects of subsequent material. The main body of the text addresses the major groups of cardiovascular diseases. The chapters are designed and edited to be read in sequence but are sufficiently cross-referenced so that they can also be used out of order. The final chapter describes the major classes of cardiovascular drugs and explains the physiologic rationale for their uses.

It has been a great privilege for me to collaborate with the 65 talented, creative, and energetic students who have contributed to the first, second, and third editions of this book. Their enthusiasm and dedication have significantly facilitated the completion of each manuscript. I am also indebted to my faculty colleague coauthors for their time, their expertise, and their warm encouragement.

It has been a pleasure to work with the editorial and production staffs of our publisher, Lippincott Williams & Wilkins. In particular, I thank Betty Sun, Eric Branger, Christina Remsberg, Aimee Sirmon and their associates for their skill and enthusiastic participation in bringing this edition to completion.

A project of this magnitude could not be undertaken without the support and patience of my family, especially my wife Carolyn, and for that I am very grateful.

On behalf of the contributors, I hope that this book enhances your understanding of cardiovascular diseases and that you find this learning path an enjoyable one!

LEONARD S. LILLY, M.D.
Boston, Massachusetts

Contributors

Student Contributors

Yi-Bin Chen (M.D., '02)

George S.M. Dyer (M.D., '02)

Mark Friedberg (M.D., '03)

Mary Beth Gordon (M.D., '03)

Anurag Gupta (M.D., '02)

Jennifer E. Ho (M.D., '03)

Rajeev Malhotra (M.D., '04)

Chiadi E. Ndumele (M.D., '03)

Patrick Yachimski (M.D., '02)

Faculty Contributors

Elliott M. Antman, M.D.
Associate Professor of Medicine, Harvard
Medical School
Director, Samuel A. Levine Cardiac Unit,
Brigham and Women's Hospital
Boston, Massachusetts

Eugene Braunwald, M.D. *(Foreword)*
Distinguished Hersey Professor of Medicine,
Harvard Medical School
Faculty Dean for Academic Programs at
Brigham and Women's Hospital and
Massachusetts General Hospital
Boston, Massachusetts

Patricia Challender Come, M.D.
Associate Professor of Medicine, Harvard
Medical School
Cardiologist, Harvard Vanguard Medical
Associates
Associate Physician, Brigham and Women's
Hospital
Senior Physician, Beth Israel Deaconess
Medical Center
Boston, Massachusetts

Mark A. Creager, M.D.
Associate Professor of Medicine, Harvard
Medical School
Director, Vascular Center and Simon C.
Fireman Scholar in Cardiovascular Medicine,
Brigham and Women's Hospital
Boston, Massachusetts

G. William Dec, M.D.
Associate Professor of Medicine, Harvard
Medical School
Medical Director, Heart Failure and Cardiac
Transplantation Program, and Clinical Director,
Cardiology Section, Massachusetts General
Hospital
Boston, Massachusetts

Elazer Edelman, M.D., PhD
Thomas D. and Virginia W. Cabot Professor of
Health Sciences and Technology, Massachusetts
Institute of Technology
Associate Professor of Medicine, Harvard
Medical School
Associate Physician, Brigham and Women's
Hospital
Boston, Massachusetts

Michael A. Fifer, M.D.
Associate Professor of Medicine, Harvard
Medical School
Director, Coronary Care Unit, Massachusetts
General Hospital
Boston, Massachusetts

Michael D. Freed, M.D.
Associate Professor of Pediatrics, Harvard
Medical School
Senior Associate in Cardiology and Chief,
Inpatient and Outpatient Cardiovascular
Services, Children's Hospital
Boston, Massachusetts

Peter Libby, M.D.
Mallinckrodt Professor of Medicine, Harvard
Medical School
Chief, Cardiovascular Division, Brigham and
Women's Hospital
Boston, Massachusetts

Richard R. Liberthson, M.D.
Associate Professor of Pediatrics, Harvard
Medical School
Director, Congenital Heart Program and
Physician in Medicine, Massachusetts General
Hospital
Boston, Massachusetts

Leonard S. Lilly, M.D.
Associate Professor of Medicine, Harvard
Medical School
Chief, Brigham and Women's/Faulkner
Cardiology
Cardiovascular Division, Brigham and
Women's Hospital
Boston, Massachusetts

Patrick T. O'Gara, M.D.
Associate Professor of Medicine, Harvard
Medical School
Director of Clinical Cardiology, and Vice
Chairman, Clinical Affairs, Department of
Medicine, Brigham and Women's Hospital
Boston, Massachusetts

Marc S. Sabatine, M.D.
Chief Resident in Medicine, Massachusetts
General Hospital
Richard A. Gorlin Fellow in Cardiovascular
Medicine, Brigham and Women's Hospital
Instructor in Medicine, Harvard Medical School
Boston, Massachusetts

William G. Stevenson, M.D.
Associate Professor of Medicine, Harvard
Medical School
Director, Clinical Cardiac Electrophysiology
Program, Brigham and Women's Hospital
Boston, Massachusetts

Gary R. Strichartz, Ph.D.
Professor of Anaesthesia (Pharmacology),
Harvard Medical School
Director, Pain Research Center, and Vice
Chairman of Research, Department of
Anesthesia, Brigham and Women's Hospital
Boston, Massachusetts

Gordon H. Williams, M.D.
Professor of Medicine, Harvard Medical School
Director, Specialized Center of Research in
Hypertension
Director, Center for Clinical Investigation,
Brigham and Women's Hospital
Boston, Massachusetts

Contents

Foreword vii
Preface ix
Contributors xi

Chapter 1
Basic Cardiac Structure and Function 1
Rajeev Malhotra, Elazer R. Edelman,
*   and Leonard S. Lilly*

Chapter 2
Heart Sounds and Murmurs 29
Leonard S. Lilly

Chapter 3
Diagnostic Imaging and Cardiac
**   Catheterization** 45
Patrick Yachimski and Patricia Challender
*   Come*

Chapter 4
The Electrocardiogram 75
Leonard S. Lilly

Chapter 5
Atherosclerosis 111
Mary Beth Gordon and Peter Libby

Chapter 6
Ischemic Heart Disease 131
Anurag Gupta, Marc S. Sabatine, and Leonard
*   S. Lilly*

Chapter 7
Acute Coronary Syndromes 157
Anurag Gupta, Marc S. Sabatine, Patrick T.
*   O'Gara, and Leonard S. Lilly*

Chapter 8
Valvular Heart Disease 185
Patrick Yachimski and Leonard S. Lilly

Chapter 9
Heart Failure 211
George S.M. Dyer and Michael A. Fifer

Chapter 10
The Cardiomyopathies 237
Yi-Bin Chen, G. William Dec, and Leonard S.
*   Lilly*

Chapter 11
Mechanisms of Cardiac Arrhythmias 253
Jennifer E. Ho, William G. Stevenson, Gary R.
*   Strichartz, and Leonard S. Lilly*

Chapter 12
Clinical Aspects of Cardiac
**   Arrhythmias** 269
Jennifer E. Ho, William G. Stevenson, and
*   Leonard S. Lilly*

Chapter 13
Hypertension 289
Rajeev Malhotra, Gordon H. Williams, and
*   Leonard S. Lilly*

Chapter 14
Diseases of the Pericardium 311
Leonard S. Lilly

Chapter 15
Diseases of the Peripheral
**   Vasculature** 325
Mary Beth Gordon and Mark A. Creager

Chapter 16
Congenital Heart Disease 347
Yi-Bin Chen, Richard R. Liberthson, and
*   Michael D. Freed*

Chapter 17
Cardiovascular Drugs 371
Chiadi E. Ndumele, Mark Friedberg, Elliott M.
*   Antman, Gary R. Strichartz, and Leonard*
*   S. Lilly*

Index 423

Basic Cardiac Structure and Function

Rajeev Malhotra, Elazer R. Edelman, and Leonard S. Lilly

Cardiac Anatomy and Histology
  Pericardium
  Surface Anatomy of the Heart
  Internal Structure of the Heart
  Impulse Conducting System
  Cardiac Innervation
  Cardiac Vessels
  Histology of Ventricular Myocardial Cells

Basic Electrophysiology
  Ion Movement and Channels
  Resting Potential
  Action Potential
  Refractory Periods
  Impulse Conduction
  Normal Sequence of Cardiac Depolarization
Excitation-Contraction Coupling
  Beta-Adrenergic and Cholinergic Signaling

A knowledge of normal cardiac structure and function is crucial to understanding diseases that afflict the heart. This chapter reviews basic cardiac anatomy, electrophysiology, and the events that lead to cardiac contraction.

CARDIAC ANATOMY AND HISTOLOGY

Although the study of cardiac anatomy dates back to ancient times, interest in this field has recently gained momentum. The development of sophisticated cardiac imaging procedures such as coronary angiography, echocardiography, computed tomography, and magnetic resonance imaging has made essential an intimate knowledge of the spatial relationships of cardiac structures. Such information also proves helpful in understanding the pathophysiology of heart disease. This section emphasizes the aspects of cardiac anatomy that are important to the clinician; that is, the "functional" anatomy.

Pericardium

The heart and roots of the great vessels are enclosed by a fibroserous sac called the pericardium (Fig. 1.1). This structure consists of two layers: a strong outer fibrous layer and an inner serosal layer. The inner serosal layer adheres to the external wall of the heart and is called the **visceral pericardium.** The visceral pericardium reflects back on itself and lines the outer fibrous layer, forming the **parietal pericardium.** The space between the visceral and parietal layers contains a thin film of pericardial fluid that allows the heart to beat in a minimal-friction environment.

The pericardium is attached to the sternum and the mediastinal portions of the right and left pleurae. Its many connections to surrounding structures keep the pericardial sac firmly anchored within the thorax and therefore help to maintain the heart in its normal position.

Emanating from the pericardium in a superior direction are the aorta, the pulmonary artery, and the superior vena cava (see Fig. 1.1). The inferior vena cava projects through the pericardium inferiorly.

Surface Anatomy of the Heart

The heart is shaped roughly like a cone and consists of four muscular chambers. The right and left ventricles are the main

CHAPTER ONE

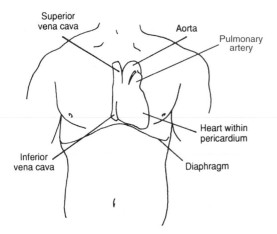

Figure 1.1. The position of the heart in the chest.
The superior vena cava, aorta, and pulmonary artery exit superiorly, whereas the inferior vena cava projects inferiorly.

pumping chambers. The less muscular right and left atria deliver blood to their respective ventricles.

Several terms are used to describe the heart's surfaces and borders (Fig. 1.2). The **apex** is formed by the tip of the left ventricle, which points inferiorly, anteriorly, and to the left. The **base** or posterior surface of the heart is formed by the atria, mainly the left, and lies between the lung hila. The **anterior** surface of the heart is shaped by the right atrium and ventricle. Since the left atrium and ventricle lie more posteriorly, they form only a small strip of this anterior surface. The **inferior** surface of the heart is formed by both ventricles, primarily the left. This surface of the heart lies along the diaphragm; hence, it is also referred to as the "diaphragmatic" surface.

Observing the chest from an anteroposterior view (such as on a chest radiograph, as described in Chapter 3), four recognized borders of the heart are apparent. The right border is established by the right atrium and is almost in line with the superior and inferior vena cavae. The inferior border is nearly horizontal and is formed mainly by the right ventricle, with a slight contribution from the left ventricle near the apex. The left ventricle and a portion of the left atrium make up the left border of the heart, whereas the superior border is shaped by

both atria. From this description of the surface of the heart emerge two basic "rules" of normal cardiac anatomy: 1) right-sided structures lie mostly anterior to their left-sided counterparts, and 2) atrial chambers are located mostly to the right of their corresponding ventricles.

Internal Structure of the Heart

Four major valves are present in the normal heart which direct blood flow in a forward direction and prevent backward leakage. The atrioventricular valves (tricuspid and mitral) separate the atria and ventricles, whereas the semilunar valves (pulmonic and aortic) separate the ventricles from the great arteries. All four heart valves are attached to the fibrous **cardiac skeleton** (Fig. 1.3). The cardiac skeleton is composed of dense connective tissue and serves as a site of attachment for the valves, and for the ventricular and atrial muscles.

The surface of the heart valves and the interior surface of the heart chambers are lined by a single layer of endothelial cells called the **endocardium.** The subendocardial tissue contains fibroblasts, elastic and collagenous fibers, veins, nerves, and branches of the conducting system and is continuous with the connective tissue of the heart muscle layer, the myocardium. The **myocardium** is the thickest layer of the heart and consists of bundles of cardiac muscle cells, the histology of which is described below. External to the myocardium is a layer of connective tissue and adipose tissue through which pass the larger blood vessels and nerves that supply the heart muscle. The **epicardium** is the outermost layer of the heart and is identical to, and just another term for, the visceral pericardium described above.

Right Atrium and Ventricle

Opening into the **right atrium** are the superior and inferior vena cavae and the coronary sinus (Fig. 1.4). The vena cavae return deoxygenated blood from the systemic veins into the right atrium, whereas the coronary

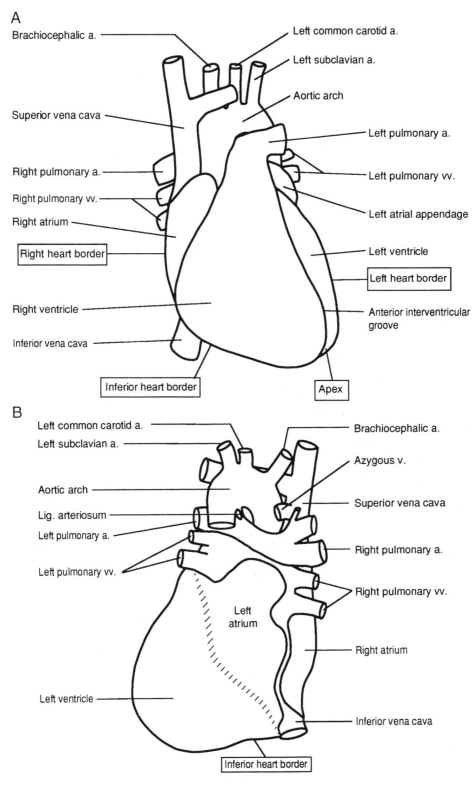

Figure 1.2. **A.** The anterior view of the heart and great vessels. **B.** The posterior aspect (or base) of the heart and great vessels, as viewed from the back. a, artery; vv, veins.

Anterior

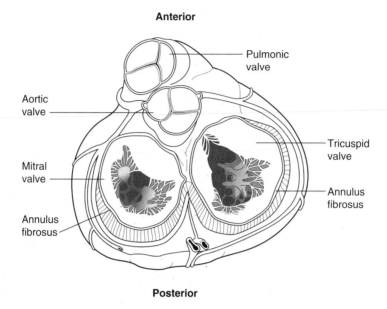

Figure 1.3. **The four heart valves viewed from above with atria removed.** The figure depicts the period of ventricular filling (diastole) during which the tricuspid and mitral valves are open and the semilunar valves (pulmonic and aortic) are closed. Each annulus fibrosus surrounding the mitral and tricuspid valves is thicker than those surrounding the pulmonic and aortic valves.

sinus carries venous return from the coronary arteries. The interatrial septum forms the posteromedial wall of the right atrium and separates it from the left atrium. The **tricuspid valve** is located in the floor of the atrium and opens into the right ventricle.

The **right ventricle** (see Fig. 1.4) is roughly triangular in shape, and its superior aspect forms a cone-shaped outflow tract, which leads to the pulmonary artery. Although the inner wall of the outflow tract is smooth, the rest of the ventricle is covered by a number of irregular bridges (termed **trabeculae carneae**) that give the right ventricular wall a spongelike appearance. A large trabecula that crosses the ven-

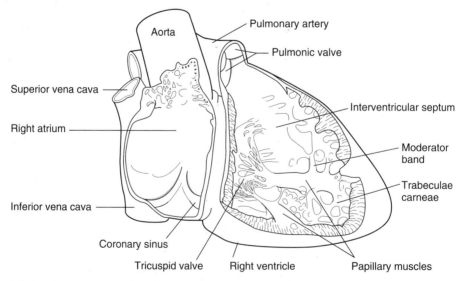

Figure 1.4. **Interior structures of the right atrium and right ventricle.** (Modified from Goss CM. Gray's Anatomy. 29th Ed. Philadelphia: Lea & Febiger, 1973:547.)

tricular cavity is called the **moderator band.** It carries a component of the right bundle branch of the conducting system to the ventricular muscle.

The right ventricle contains three **papillary muscles,** which project into the chamber and via their thin, string-like **chordae tendineae** attach to the edges of the tricuspid valve leaflets. The leaflets, in turn, are attached to the fibrous ring that supports the valve between the right atrium and ventricle. Contraction of the papillary muscles prior to other regions of the ventricle tightens the chordae tendineae, helping to align and restrain the leaflets of the tricuspid valve as they are forced closed. This action prevents blood from regurgitating into the right atrium during ventricular contraction.

At the apex of the right ventricular outflow tract is the **pulmonic valve,** which leads to the pulmonary artery. This valve consists of three cusps attached to a fibrous ring. During relaxation of the ventricle, elastic recoil of the pulmonary arteries forces blood back toward the heart, distending the valve cusps toward one another. This action closes the pulmonic valve and prevents regurgitation of blood back into the right ventricle.

Left Atrium and Ventricle

Entering the posterior half of the **left atrium** are the four pulmonary veins (Fig. 1.5A). The wall of the left atrium is about 2 mm thick, being slightly greater than that of the right atrium. The mitral valve opens into the left ventricle through the inferior wall of the left atrium.

The cavity of the **left ventricle** is approximately cone-shaped and longer than that of the right ventricle. In healthy adult hearts, the wall thickness is 9–11 mm, roughly 3 times that of right. The aortic vestibule is a smooth-walled part of the left ventricular cavity located just inferior to the aortic valve. Inferior to this region, most of the ventricle is covered by trabeculae carneae, which are finer and more numerous than in the right ventricle.

The left ventricular chamber (Fig. 1.5B) contains two large papillary muscles. These are larger than their counterparts in the right ventricle, and their chordae tendineae are thicker but less numerous. The chordae tendineae of each papillary muscle distribute to both leaflets of the **mitral valve.** Similar to the case in the right ventricle, tensing of the chordae tendineae during left ventricular contraction helps restrain and align the mitral leaflets so that they close properly and prevent the backward leakage of blood.

The **aortic valve** separates the left ventricle from the aorta. Surrounding the aortic valve opening is a fibrous ring to which is attached the three cusps of the valve. Just above the right and left aortic valve cusps in the aortic wall are the origins of the right and left coronary arteries (see Fig. 1.5B).

Interventricular Septum

The interventricular septum is the thick wall between the left and right ventricles. It is composed of a muscular and a membranous part (see Fig. 1.5B). The margins of this septum can be traced on the surface of the heart by following the anterior and posterior interventricular grooves. Owing to the greater hydrostatic pressure within the left ventricle, the large muscular portion of the septum bulges toward the right ventricle. The small, oval-shaped membranous part of the septum is thin and located just inferior to the cusps of the aortic valve.

To summarize the functional anatomic points presented in this section, the path of blood flow through the heart will now be reviewed. Deoxygenated blood is delivered to the heart through the inferior and superior vena cavae, which enter into the right atrium. Flow continues through the tricuspid valve orifice into the right ventricle. Contraction of the right ventricle propels the blood across the pulmonic valve to the pulmonary artery and lungs, where carbon dioxide is released and oxygen is absorbed. The oxygen-rich blood returns to the heart through the pulmonary veins to the left atrium and then passes across the mitral valve into the left ventricle. Contraction of the left ventricle pumps the oxygenated blood across the aortic valve into the aorta,

A

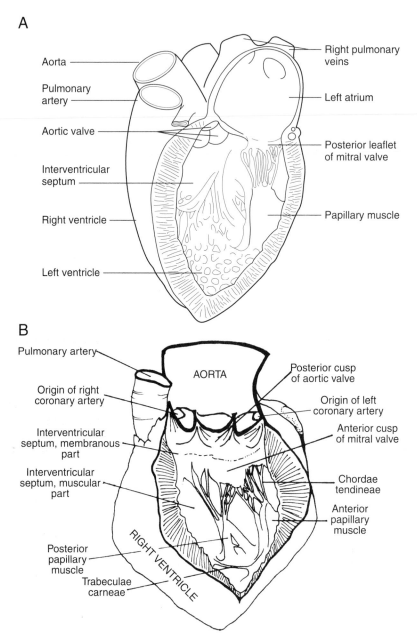

Aorta

Pulmonary
artery

Aortic valve

Interventricular
septum

Right ventricle

Left ventricle

Right pulmonary
veins

Left atrium

Posterior leaflet
of mitral valve

Papillary muscle

B

Pulmonary artery

Origin of right
coronary artery

Interventricular
septum, membranous
part

Interventricular
septum, muscular
part

Posterior
papillary
muscle

Trabeculae
carneae

AORTA

RIGHT VENTRICLE

Posterior cusp
of aortic valve

Origin of left
coronary artery

Anterior cusp
of mitral valve

Chordae
tendineae

Anterior
papillary
muscle

Figure 1.5. **A.** The left atrium and left ventricular (LV) inflow and outflow regions. **B.** Interior structures of the LV cavity. (Modified from Agur AMR, Lee MJ. Grant's Atlas of Anatomy. 9th Ed. Baltimore: Williams & Wilkins, 1991:59.)

whereupon it is distributed to all other tissues of the body.

Impulse Conducting System

The impulse conducting system (Fig. 1.6) consists of specialized cells that initiate the heart beat and electrically coordinate contractions of the heart chambers.

The **sinoatrial (SA) node** is a small mass of specialized cardiac muscle fibers in the wall of the right atrium. It is located to the right of the superior vena cava entrance and normally initiates the electrical impulse for contraction. The **atrioventricular (AV) node** lies beneath the endocardium in the inferoposterior part of the interatrial septum.

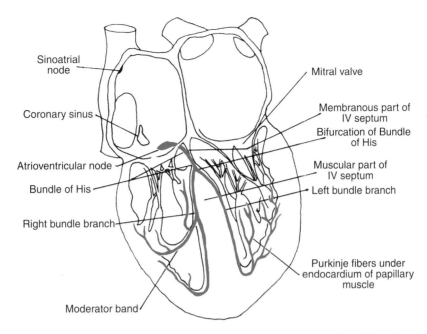

Figure 1.6. **Main components of the cardiac conduction system include the sinoatrial node, atrioventricular node, bundle of His, right and left bundle branches, and the Purkinje fibers.** The moderator band carries a large portion of the right bundle.

Distal to the AV node is the **bundle of His,** which perforates the interventricular septum posteriorly. Within the septum, the bundle of His bifurcates into a broad sheet of fibers that continues over the left side of the septum, known as the **left bundle branch,** and a compact, cablelike structure on the right side, the **right bundle branch.**

The right bundle branch is thick and deeply buried in the muscle of the interventricular septum and continues toward the apex. Near the junction of the interventricular septum and the anterior wall of the right ventricle, the right bundle branch becomes subendocardial and bifurcates. One branch travels across the right ventricular cavity in the moderator band, whereas the other continues toward the tip of the ventricle. These branches eventually arborize into a finely divided anastomosing plexus that travels throughout the right ventricle.

Functionally, the left bundle branch is divided into an anterior and a posterior fascicle and a small branch to the septum. The anterior fascicle runs anteriorly toward the apex, forming a subendocardial plexus in the area of the anterior papillary muscle.

The posterior fascicle travels to the area of the posterior papillary muscle; it then divides into a subendocardial plexus and spreads to the rest of the left ventricle.

The subendocardial plexuses of both ventricles send distributing **Purkinje fibers** to the ventricular muscle. Impulses within the His-Purkinje system are transmitted first to the papillary muscles and then throughout the walls of the ventricles, allowing papillary muscle contraction to precede that of the ventricles. This coordination prevents regurgitation of blood flow through the AV valves, as discussed above.

Cardiac Innervation

The heart is innervated by both parasympathetic and sympathetic afferent and efferent nerves. Preganglionic *sympathetic* neurons located within the upper five to six thoracic levels of the spinal cord synapse with second-order neurons in the cervical sympathetic ganglia. Traveling within the cardiac nerves, these fibers terminate in the heart and great vessels. Preganglionic *parasympathetic* fibers originate in the dorsal motor nucleus of the medulla and pass as branches of the vagus nerve to the heart and great vessels. Here the fibers synapse with second-order neurons located in ganglia within these structures. A rich supply of vagal afferents from the inferior and posterior aspects of the ventricles mediates important cardiac reflexes, whereas the abundant vagal efferent fibers to the SA and AV nodes are active in modulating electrical impulse initiation and conduction.

Cardiac Vessels

The cardiac vessels consist of the coronary arteries and veins and the lymphatic vessels. The largest components of these systems lie within the loose connective tissue in the epicardial fat.

Coronary Arteries

The heart muscle is supplied with oxygen and nutrients by the right and left coronary arteries, which arise from the root of the aorta just above the aortic valve cusps (Figs. 1.5B and 1.7). After their origin, these vessels pass anteriorly, one on each side of the pulmonary artery (see Fig. 1.7).

The large **left main coronary artery** passes between the left atrium and the pulmonary trunk to reach the AV groove. Here, it divides into the **left anterior descending (LAD) coronary artery** and the circumflex artery. The LAD travels within the anterior interventricular groove toward the cardiac apex. During its descent on the anterior surface, the LAD gives off septal branches that supply the anterior two-thirds of the interventricular septum and the apical portion of the anterior papillary muscle. The LAD also gives off diagonal branches that supply the anterior surface of the left ventricle. The **circumflex artery** continues within the left AV groove and passes around the left border of the heart to reach the posterior surface. It gives off large obtuse marginal branches that supply the lateral and posterior wall of the left ventricle.

The **right coronary artery (RCA)** travels in the right AV groove, passing posteriorly between the right atrium and ventricle. It

supplies blood to the right ventricle via acute marginal branches. In most individuals, the distal RCA gives rise to a large branch, the **posterior descending artery** (Fig. 1.7C). This vessel travels from the inferoposterior aspect of the heart to the apex and supplies blood to the inferior and posterior walls of the ventricles and the posterior one-third of the interventricular septum. Just prior to giving off the posterior descending branch, the RCA usually gives off the **AV nodal artery.**

The posterior descending and AV nodal arteries arise from the RCA in 85% of the population. In approximately 8% of individuals, the posterior descending artery arises from the circumflex artery instead. In the remaining population, the heart's posterior blood supply is contributed to from branches of both the RCA and the circumflex.

The blood supply to the SA node is also most often (70% of the time) derived from the RCA. However, in 25% of normal hearts, the **SA nodal artery** arises from the circumflex artery, and in 5% of cases, both the RCA and the circumflex contribute to this vessel.

From their epicardial locations, the coronary arteries send perforating branches into the ventricular muscle which form a richly branching and anastomosing vasculature in the walls of all the cardiac chambers. From this plexus arise a massive number of capillaries that form an elaborate network surrounding each cardiac muscle fiber. The muscle fibers located just beneath the endocardium, particularly those of the papillary muscles and the thick left ventricle, are supplied either by the terminal branches of the coronary arteries or directly from the ventricular cavity through tiny vascular channels, known as **thebesian veins.**

Collateral connections, usually <200 μm in diameter, exist at the subarteriolar level between the coronary arteries. In the normal heart, few of these collateral vessels are visible. However, they may become larger and functional when atherosclerotic disease obstructs a coronary artery, thereby providing flow to distal portions of the vessel from a nonobstructed neighbor.

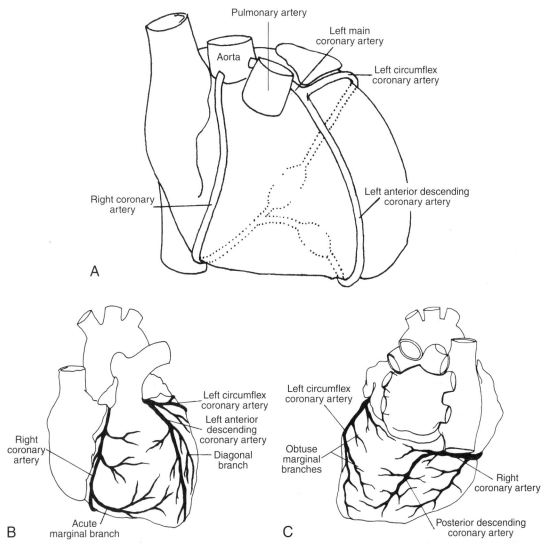

Figure 1.7. Coronary artery anatomy. A. Schematic representation of the right and left coronary arteries demonstrates their orientation to one another; the left main artery bifurcates into the circumflex artery, which perfuses the lateral and posterior regions of the left ventricle (LV), and the anterior descending artery, which perfuses the LV anterior wall, anterior portion of the intraventricular septum, and a portion of the anterior right ventricular (RV) wall. The right coronary artery (RCA) perfuses the right ventricle and variable portions of the posterior left ventricle through its terminal branches. The posterior descending artery most often arises from the RCA. **B.** Anterior view of the heart demonstrating the coronary arteries and their major branches. **C.** Posterior view of the heart demonstrating the terminal portions of the right and circumflex coronary arteries and their branches.

Coronary Veins

The coronary veins follow a distribution similar to that of the major coronary arteries. These vessels return blood from the myocardial capillaries to the right atrium predominantly via the coronary sinus. The major veins lie in the epicardial fat, usually superficial to the coronary arteries. The thebesian veins, mentioned above, provide an addi-

tional potential route for a small amount of direct blood return to the cardiac chambers.

Lymphatic Vessels

The heart lymph is drained by an extensive plexus of valved vessels located in the subendocardial connective tissue of all four chambers. This lymph drains to the epicardial plexus of lymphatic vessels in the interstitial connective tissue. These smaller vessels anastomose to form several large lymphatic vessels that follow the distribution of the coronary arteries and veins. Each of these large vessels then combines in the AV groove to form a single large lymphatic vessel, which eventually exits the heart to reach the mediastinal lymphatic plexus and ultimately the thoracic duct.

Histology of Ventricular Myocardial Cells

The mature myocardial cell (also termed **myocyte**) measures up to 25 μm in diameter and 100 μm in length. The cell shows a cross-striated banding pattern similar to that of skeletal muscle. However, unlike the multinucleated skeletal myofibers, myocardial cells contain only one or two centrally located nuclei. Surrounding each myocardial cell is connective tissue with a rich capillary network.

Each myocardial cell contains numerous **myofibrils,** which are long chains of individual **sarcomeres,** the fundamental contractile units of the cell (Fig. 1.8). Each sarcomere is made up of two groups of overlapping filaments of contractile proteins. Biochemical and biophysical interactions occurring between these myofilaments produce muscle contraction. Their structure and function are described later in this chapter.

Within each myocardial cell the neighboring sarcomeres are all in register, producing the characteristic cross-striated banding pattern seen by light microscopy. The relative densities of the cross bands identify the location of the contractile proteins within the sarcomere. Under physiologic conditions, the overall sarcomere length (Z to Z distance) varies between 2.2 and 1.5 μm during the cardiac cycle. The larger dimension reflects the degree of fiber stretch during ventricular filling, whereas

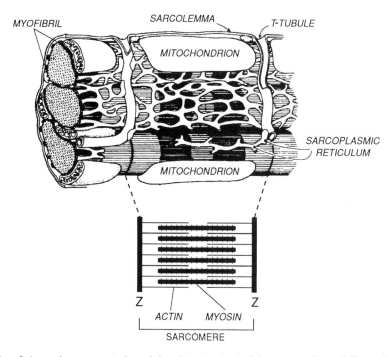

Figure 1.8. Top. Schematic representation of the ultrastructure of the myocardial cell. The cell consists of multiple parallel myofibrils surrounded by mitochondria. The T tubules are invaginations of the cell membrane (the sarcolemma) that increase the surface area for ion transport and transmission of electrical impulses. The intracellular sarcoplasmic reticulum houses the majority of intracellular calcium and abuts the T tubules. (Modified from Katz AM. Physiology of the Heart. 2nd Ed. New York: Raven Press, 1992:21.) **Bottom. Expanded view of a sarcomere, the basic unit of contraction.** Each myofibril consists of serially connected sarcomeres that extend from one Z line to the next. The sarcomere is composed of alternating thin (actin) and thick (myosin) myofilaments.

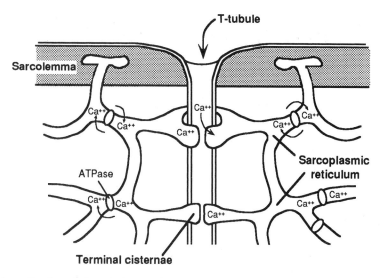

Figure 1.9. Schematic view of the tubular systems of the myocardial cell. The T tubules, invaginations of the sarcolemma, abut the sarcoplasmic reticulum at right angles at the terminal cisternae sacs. This relationship is important in linking membrane excitation with intracellular release of calcium from the sarcoplasmic reticulum.

the smaller one represents the extent of fiber shortening during contraction.

The myocardial cell membrane is termed the **sarcolemma.** A specialized region of the membrane is the **intercalated disk,** a distinct characteristic of cardiac muscle tissue. Intercalated disks are seen on light microscopic study as darkly staining transverse lines that cross chains of cardiac cells at irregular intervals. They represent the gap junction complexes at the interface of adjacent cardiac fibers and establish structural and electrical continuity between the myocardial cells.

Another functional feature of the cell membrane is the **transverse tubular system (or T tubules).** This complex system is characterized by deep, fingerlike invaginations of the sarcolemma (Figs. 1.8 and 1.9). Similar to the intercalated disks, transverse tubular membranes establish pathways for rapid transmission of the excitatory electrical impulses that initiate contraction. The T tubule system increases the surface area of the sarcolemma in contact with the extracellular environment, allowing the transmembrane ion transport accompanying excitation and relaxation to occur quickly and synchronously.

The **sarcoplasmic reticulum** is an extensive intracellular tubular membrane network that complements the T tubule system both structurally and functionally. The sarcoplasmic reticulum abuts the T tubules at right angles in lateral sacs, called the terminal cisternae (see Fig. 1.9). These sacs house the majority of intracellular calcium stores (the release of these stores is important in linking membrane excitation with activation of the contractile apparatus). Lateral sacs also abut the intercalated disks and the sarcolemma, providing each with a complete system for excitation-contraction coupling.

To serve the tremendous metabolic demand placed on the heart and the need for a constant supply of high-energy phosphates, the myocardial cell has an abundant concentration of mitochondria. These organelles are located between the individual myofibrils and constitute approximately 35% of cell volume (see Fig. 1.8).

BASIC ELECTROPHYSIOLOGY

Rhythmic contraction of the heart relies on the organized propagation of electrical impulses along its conduction pathway. The marker of electrical stimulation, the **action potential,** is created by a sequence of ion fluxes through specific channels in the sarcolemma. To provide a basis for understanding how electrical impulses lead to cardiac contraction, the process of cellular depolarization and repolarization is reviewed here. This material serves as an important foundation for topics addressed later in this book, including electrocardiography (Chapter 4) and cardiac arrhythmias (Chapters 11 and 12).

Cardiac cells capable of electrical excitation are of three electrophysiologic types, the properties of which have been studied by intracellular microelectrode and patch-clamp recordings:

1. Pacemaker cells (e.g., SA node, AV node)
2. Specialized rapidly conducting tissues (e.g., Purkinje fibers)
3. Ventricular and atrial muscle cells

The sarcolemma of each of these cardiac cell types is a phospholipid bilayer that is largely impermeable to ions. There are specialized proteins interspersed throughout the membrane that serve as ion channels,

cotransporters, and active transporters (Fig. 1.10). These transporters help maintain ionic concentration gradients and charge differentials between the inside and the outside of the cardiac cells. Normally, Na^+ and Ca^{++} concentrations are much higher outside the cell and K^+ concentration is much higher inside.

Ion Movement and Channels

The movement of specific ions across the cell membrane serves as the basis for action potentials. Ion transport depends on two major factors: 1) the energetic favorability and 2) the permeability of the membrane for the ion.

Energetics (Box 1.1)

The two major forces that drive the energetics of ion transport are the *concentration gradient* and the *transmembrane potential*

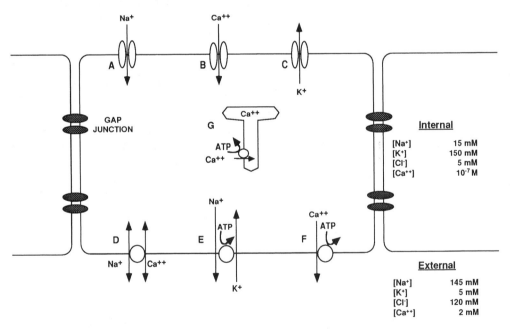

Figure 1.10. **Ion channels, cotransporters, and active transporters of the myocyte. A.** Sodium entry through the "fast" sodium channel is responsible for the rapid upstroke (phase 0) of the action potential (AP) in non-pacemaker cells. **B.** Calcium enters the cell through the "slow" calcium channel during phase 2 of the Purkinje and muscle cell AP, and is the main channel responsible for depolarization of pacemaker cells. **C.** Potassium exits through the potassium channel to repolarize the cell during phase 3 of the AP, and open potassium channels help maintain the resting potential (phase 4) of non-pacemaker cells. **D.** Sodium/calcium exchanger helps maintain the low intracellular calcium concentration. **E.** Sodium/potassium ATPase pump maintains concentration gradients for these ions. **F, G.** Active calcium pumps aid removal of calcium to the external environment and sarcoplasmic reticulum, respectively.

Box 1.1 Energetics of Ion Movement and the Nernst Potential

The energetics of ion transport can be expressed quantitatively by considering the movement of any ion (M^+) across the membrane as a chemical reaction: M^+(outside) $\rightarrow$ M^+(inside).

Calculation of the free energy (ΔG) determines the favorability, or spontaneity, of this reaction. When ΔG is a negative number, the reaction is spontaneous; when a positive number, the *reverse* reaction is spontaneous. ΔG (expressed in J/mol) is dependent on two terms, the **concentration gradient (ΔG_{cg})** and the **membrane potential (ΔG_{mp}).** These terms are defined as follows:

$$\Delta G_{cg} = R \cdot T \cdot \ln Q$$

R = Boltzmann's constant = 8.31 J/mol·°K
T = temperature in °Kelvin
Q = [products]/[reactants] = $[M^+]_{in}/[M^+]_{out}$

$$\Delta G_{mp} = \textbf{charge x voltage} = z \cdot F \cdot V$$

V = membrane potential in volts
F = Faraday's constant = 96,500 J/mol·volt
z = ionic charge

Combining these two terms:

$$\Delta G = R \cdot T \cdot \ln([M^+]_{in}/[M^+]_{out}) + z \cdot F \cdot V$$

For example, if the resting membrane potential of a normal cardiac myocyte at 37°C (310°K) is –90 mV, $[Na^+]_{in}$=15mM and $[Na^+]_{out}$=145 mM, then:

$$\Delta G = (8.31)(310) \cdot \ln(15/145) + (+1)(96,500)(-0.090)$$
$$= -14,529 \text{ J/mol}$$

Since ΔG is negative, this reaction occurs spontaneously (i.e., it is energetically favorable for sodium to enter the cell under these conditions) and 14.5 kJ of energy is released per mole in the process.

Now consider a theoretical situation in which a cell membrane is permeable for Na^+ ions and there are no other types of ions in the vicinity. The Na^+ ions will move into the cell until an equilibrium is reached in which the net flux of sodium into the cell equals the net flux out of the cell. This equilibrium occurs when $\Delta G = 0$. If the concentrations of $[Na^+]_{in}$ = 15mM and $[Na^+]_{out}$ = 145 mM, at what membrane potential is equilibrium achieved? At equilibrium,

$$\Delta G = 0 = R \cdot T \cdot \ln([M^+]_{in}/[M^+]_{out}) + z \cdot F \cdot V$$

and rearranging the terms:

$$V_{NERNST} = (-RT/zF) \cdot \ln([M^+]_{in}/[M^+]_{out})$$
$$= (-26.7 \text{ mV}) \cdot \ln(15/145) = +60.6 \text{ mV}$$

Thus, the equilibrium potential (or Nernst potential) of sodium is +60.6 mV. At this membrane potential, there would be no net current of sodium across the permeable membrane.

(voltage). Molecules diffuse from areas of high concentration to areas of lower concentration—the gradient between these values determines the rate of ion flow. For example, the extracellular Na^+ concentration is normally 145 mM, while the concentration inside the myocyte is 15 mM. Thus, there is a strong force tending to drive Na^+ into the cell, down its concentration gradient. In addition, the transmembrane potential of cardiac cells exerts an electrical force on ions (i.e., like charges repel one another, and opposite charges attract each other). The transmembrane potential of a myocyte at rest is about $-90\,mV$ (negative on the inside of the cell relative to the outside, since there are more positive charges on the outside). Extracellular Na^+, a positively charged ion, is therefore attracted to the relatively negatively charged interior of the cell. Thus, there is a strong tendency for Na^+ to enter the cell because of both the steep concentration gradient and the electrical attraction.

Permeability

If there is such a strong force driving Na^+ into the cell, what keeps this ion from actually moving inside? The membrane of the cell at its resting potential is not permeable to sodium. Cell membranes are made of a phospholipid bilayer with a hydrophobic core that does not allow simple passage of charged, hydrophilic particles. Instead, permeability of the membrane to ions is dependent on **ion channels,** specialized proteins that span the cell membrane and contain hydrophilic pores through which certain charged atoms can pass under specific circumstances.

Most types of ion channels share similar protein sequences and structures, consisting of repeating transmembrane domains (Fig. 1.11). Each of these domains contains six membrane-spanning segments. The fourth segment (see S_4 in Fig. 1.11) contains a sequence of positively charged amino acids (lysine and arginine) that responds to the membrane potential, and that segment is thought to be responsible for voltage-sensitivity of the channel, as described below.

There are several types of cardiac ion channels which vary by two functional properties: selectivity and gating. Each type of channel is normally **selective** for a specific ion, which is a manifestation of the size and structure of its pore. For example, in cardiac cells, some channels permit the passage of sodium ions, some are specific for potassium, and others allow only calcium to pass through.

An ion can pass through its specific channel only at certain times. That is, the ion channel is **gated**—at any given moment, the channel is either open or closed. The more time that a channel is in its open state, the larger the number of ions that pass through it and therefore, the greater the transmembrane current. Each cell contains numerous individual specific ion channels, each of which may be in the open or closed state. It is the voltage across the membrane that determines what fraction of the channels are open at any point. Therefore, the gating of such channels is **voltage-sensitive.** As the membrane voltage changes during depolarization and repolarization of the cell, specific channels open and close, with corresponding alterations in the ion fluxes across the sarcolemma.

As an example of voltage-sensitive gating, the cardiac channel known as the **fast sodium channel** is considered here. The transmembrane protein that forms this channel assumes different conformations depending on the cell's membrane potential (Fig. 1.12). At a potential of $-90\,mV$ (the typical resting voltage of a ventricular muscle cell), the channels are primarily in a closed, *resting state,* such that Na^+ ions cannot pass through. In this resting state, the channels are available for conversion to the open configuration.

A rapid wave of depolarization (which causes the membrane potential to become less negative) "activates" the resting channels to the *open state,* through which Na^+ ions readily permeate; thus, an inward Na^+ current ensues. However, the activated channels remain open for only a brief time, a few thousandths of a second, and then spontaneously close, to an *inactive state* (see Fig. 1.12C). Channels in this

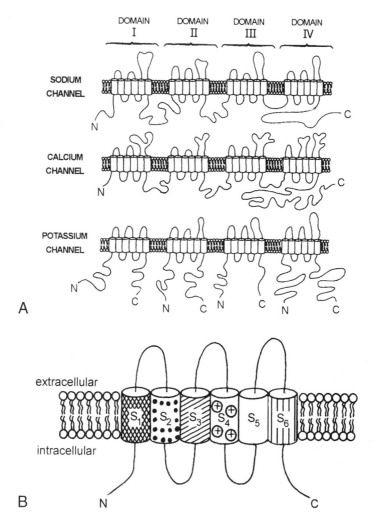

Figure 1.11. Structure of ion channels. A. Ion channels consist of glycosylated proteins arranged as repeating transmembrane domains. Each domain consists of six membrane-spanning segments. The potassium channel has four separate domains in a tetrameric structure, while the sodium and calcium channels contain four domains covalently linked together as a single unit. **B.** Enlarged view of a single domain showing the six membrane-spanning segments. The S_4 segment of each domain contains a sequence of positively charged amino acids that is thought to confer voltage-sensitivity to the channel. (Reproduced with permission from Katz AM. Physiology of the Heart. 2nd Ed. New York: Raven Press, 1992:427, 429.)

closed, inactivated conformation cannot be directly converted back to the open state; the "gating" portions of the channel protein are largely immobilized by the inactivation process.

The inactivated state persists until the membrane voltage has repolarized nearly back to its original resting level. Until it does so, the closed, inactivated channel prevents any flow of sodium ions. Therefore, during normal cellular depolarization, the voltage-dependent fast sodium channels

conduct for a short period and then close and are unable to reopen until the cell membrane has nearly fully repolarized.

Another important attribute of cardiac fast sodium channels should be noted. If the transmembrane voltage of a cardiac cell is *slowly* depolarized and maintained *chronically* at levels less negative than the usual resting potential, inactivation of channels occurs *without* initial opening and current flow (see Fig. 1.12). Furthermore, as long as the less negative potential exists, the closed,

A key characteristic of fast sodium channels is their ability to activate and then inactivate rapidly when the cell is depolarized. The mechanism by which this occurs has been investigated for many decades. In the mid 1900s, Hodgkin and Huxley studied the action potential in giant squid axons (*J. Physiol* (Lond) 1952; 117:500-544). They found that ion channels act as if they contain a series of "gates" that open and close in a specific pattern when the membrane potential is altered. In the case of the sodium channel, they postulated the presence of "m gates" that are closed in the resting state and an "h gate" that is open in the resting state. Depolarization of the membrane causes the m gates to open quickly, which allows Na⁺ ions to pass through the channel (equivalent to the open channel in Figure 1.12B). However, that same depolarization of the cell also causes the h gate to close, which blocks the passage of sodium ions (the closed inactive state in Fig. 1.12C). Na⁺ can flow through the channel only when both sets of gates are open. Since the m gates open faster than the h gate closes, there is a brief period (about 1 millisecond!) during which Na⁺ can pass through. After the membrane repolarizes to voltages more negative than about −60 mV, the m gates shut, the h gate reopens, and the channel returns to the closed, resting state (see Fig. 1.12A), available for activation once again.

More recent research has demonstrated that ion channel activity is actually more complex than suggested by this model, but there are important correlates with current molecular concepts. For example, the cluster of positively charged amino acids on segment 4 of the ion channel domain (see Fig. 1.11) has been suggested as the "m gate" that opens the channel during depolarization (equivalent to the charged portion of the channel in Figure 1.12). Inactivation (the "h gate") is thought to be achieved by a peptide loop that connects domains III and IV of the sodium channel (see Fig. 1.11), that swings into and occludes the channel during depolarization.

inactive state *does not* transition to the resting state. Thus, the fast sodium channels in such a cell are continuously unable to conduct Na⁺ ions. This is the typical case in cardiac pacemaker cells (e.g., SA and AV node) in which the membrane voltage is generally less negative than −70 mV throughout the cardiac cycle. As a result, the fast sodium channels in pacemaker cells are persistently inactivated and do not play a role in the generation of the action potential in these cells.

Calcium and potassium channels in cardiac cells also act in voltage-dependent fashions, but they behave differently than the sodium channels, as will be described in the following sections.

Resting Potential

In cardiac cells at rest, before excitation, the electrical charge differential between the inside and outside of a cell is known as the **resting potential.** The magnitude of the resting potential of a cell depends on two main properties: 1) the concentration gradients for all the different ions between the inside and outside of the cell, and 2) which ion channels are open at rest.

Similar to other tissues such as nerve cells and skeletal muscle, the potassium concentration is much greater inside cardiac cells compared with outside the cells. This is attributed to cell membrane transporters, the most important of which is the ATP-dependent Na⁺/K⁺ "pump" (Na⁺,K⁺-ATPase), which exchanges Na⁺ ions in an outward direction for K⁺ movement inward.

Cardiac myocytes contain potassium channels that are open in the resting state, at a time when other ionic channels (i.e., sodium and calcium) are closed. Therefore, *the resting cell membrane is much more permeable to potassium than to other ions.* As a result of its open channels at rest, K⁺ fluxes in an outward direction down its concentration gradient, removing positive charges from the cell. The predominant counter ions for potassium within the cell are large negatively charged proteins that are unable to diffuse out of the cell along with K⁺. Thus as potassium ions exit the cell, the anions that are left behind cause the interior of the cell to become electrically negative with respect to the outside.

However, as the interior of the cell becomes more and more *negatively* charged by the outward flux of potassium, the *positively* charged K⁺ ions are attracted back toward the cellular interior, an effect that slows their net exit from the cell. Thus, the two opposing forces directing the flux of potassium ions across their open channels in the resting state are (Fig. 1.13): 1) the concentration gradient, which favors outward passage of potassium, and 2) the electrostatic force which attracts potassium back into the cell. At steady state, the balance between these chemical and electrical forces determines the resting potential, which is

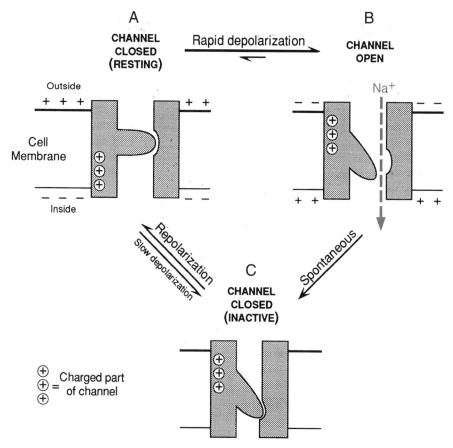

Figure 1.12. **Schematic representation of gating of "fast" sodium channels. A.** In the resting membrane, most channels are in the closed, resting state. **B.** Rapid, large depolarizations force the charged parts of the channel to translocate, activating the channel to the open conformation, and Na^+ ions permeate into the cell. **C.** From the open state, the channels spontaneously close to the inactivated state, from which reopening cannot directly occur. This closed, inactive state persists until repolarization returns the channel to the resting state. Note that when cells are *slowly* depolarized, they may enter the closed, inactive state directly from the resting state, without channel opening.

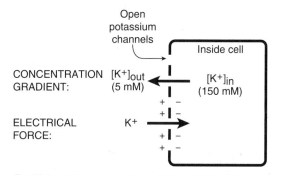

Equilibrium Nernst potential = $-26.7 \ln ([K^+]_{in}/[K^+]_{out})$ = -91 mV

Figure 1.13. **The resting potential of a cardiac muscle cell is determined by the balance between the concentration gradient and electrostatic forces for potassium, because only potassium channels are open at rest.** The concentration gradient favors outward movement of K^+, whereas the electrical force attracts the positively charged K^+ ions inward. The equilibrium (resting) potential can be approximated by the Nernst equation for potassium, as shown in the figure.

approximately −90 mV in ventricular muscle cells, as predicted by the Nernst equation for potassium, as shown in Figure 1.13.

In the resting state, the permeability of the cardiac muscle cellular membrane for sodium is minimal because the channels that conduct that ion are essentially closed. Nonetheless, there is a slight leak of sodium ions through their channels into the cell. This tiny inward current of positively charged sodium ions explains why the actual resting potential is slightly less negative than would be predicted if the cell

membrane were truly only permeable to potassium. The sodium ions that slowly leak into the myocyte at rest (and the much larger amount that enters during the action potential as described below) are continuously removed from the cell and returned to the extracellular environment. This is accomplished by Na$^+$,K$^+$-ATPase, the transmembrane protein that converts chemical energy from hydrolysis of ATP into mechanical energy and transports 3 Na$^+$ ions out of the cell while moving 2 K$^+$ ions into the cell. This net outward flow of cations also contributes to maintaining the cell interior as more negatively charged than the outside.

Action Potential

When the cell membrane voltage is altered, its permeability to specific ions changes. The changes in ion permeability are a reflection of the voltage-gating of the ion channels, and each type of channel has a characteristic pattern of activation and inactivation that determines the progression of the electrical signal. This discussion begins by following the development of the action potential in a typical cardiac muscle cell (Fig. 1.14). The unique characteristics of action potentials in cardiac pacemaker cells will be described below.

Cardiac Muscle Cell

Until otherwise provoked, the resting potential of the cardiac muscle cell remains stable, at approximately −90 mV. This resting state before depolarization is known as **phase 4** of the action potential. Following phase 4, four additional phases characterize depolarization and repolarization of the cell (see Fig. 1.14).

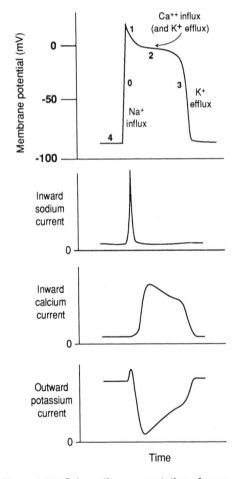

Figure 1.14. **Schematic representation of a myocyte action potential (AP) and relative net ion currents for Na$^+$, Ca^{++}, and K$^+$.** The resting potential is represented by phase 4 of the AP. Following depolarization, Na$^+$ influx results in the rapid upstroke of phase 0; a transient outward potassium current is responsible for partial repolarization during phase 1; slow Ca^{++} influx (and relatively low K$^+$ efflux) results in the plateau of phase 2; and final rapid repolarization is largely due to K$^+$ efflux during phase 3.

Phase 0

At the resting membrane voltage, sodium and calcium channels are closed. Any process that makes the membrane potential less negative than the resting value causes some sodium channels to open. As Na$^+$ channels open, sodium ions rapidly enter the cell, flowing down their concentration gradient, and towards the negatively charged cellular interior. The entry of Na^+ ions into the cell causes the transmembrane potential to become progressively less negative, which in turn causes more sodium channels to open and promotes further sodium entry into the cell. When the membrane voltage approaches the **threshold potential** (approximately -70 mV in cardiac muscle cells), enough of these "fast" Na^+ channels have opened to generate a self-sustaining inward Na^+ current. The magnitude of entry of positively charged Na^+ ions neutralizes the membrane potential to zero, and transiently into the positive range.

This prominent influx of sodium ions is responsible for the rapid upstroke, or phase 0, of the action potential. However, the Na^+ channels remain open for only a few thousandths of a second and are then quickly inactivated, preventing further influx (see Fig. 1.14). Thus, while activation of these fast Na^+ channels causes the rapid early depolarization of the cell, the rapid inactivation makes their major contribution to the action potential short-lived.

Phase 1

Following rapid phase 0 depolarization, a transient current of repolarization returns the membrane potential to approximately 0 mV. The responsible current appears to be due primarily to an outward flow of K^+ ions through a type of transiently activated potassium channel.

Phase 2

This relatively long phase of the action potential is mediated by a balance of persistent outward K^+ current opposed by an inward Ca^{++} current through calcium channels (termed "L-type" calcium channels), which begin to open during phase 0, when the membrane voltage reaches approximately -40 mV. When these channels open, Ca^{++} flows down its concentration gradient into the cell. Ca^{++} entry proceeds in a more gradual fashion than the initial influx of sodium, because the activation of calcium channels is slower and the channel remains open much longer than the fast Na^+ channel (see Fig. 1.14). During this phase, the Ca^{++} influx, and the relatively low permeability to K^+ efflux, maintains a voltage of approximately 0 mV for a prolonged period, known as the **plateau.** Calcium ions that enter the cell during this phase play a critical role in triggering additional internal calcium release from the sarcoplasmic reticulum ("calcium-induced calcium release"), which is important in initiating myocyte contraction, as discussed below.

Phase 3 begins as the Ca^{++} channels gradually inactivate and the efflux of K^+ begins to exceed the influx of calcium.

Phase 3

This is the final period of repolarization that returns the transmembrane voltage back to the resting potential of approximately -90 mV. An outward potassium current and low membrane permeability for other cations are responsible for this rapid repolarization. This phase completes the action potential cycle, with a return to resting phase 4, preparing the cell for the next stimulus for depolarization.

To preserve normal transmembrane ionic concentration gradients, the sodium and calcium that enter the cell during depolarization must be returned to the extracellular environment. Similarly, potassium ions must return to the cell interior. The exchange of Na^+ and K^+ across the cell membrane is mediated via Na^+,K^+-ATPase, as described above. Excess Ca^{++} in the cell is eliminated primarily by Na^+/Ca^{++} exchange and to a lesser extent by the ATP-consuming calcium "pump" (Ca^{++}-ATPase).

Specialized Conduction System

The previous section applies to the action potential of cardiac muscle cells. The cells of the specialized conduction system (e.g., Purkinje fibers) behave similarly, although the resting potential is slightly more negative, and the upstroke of phase 0 is even more rapid.

Pacemaker Cells

The upstroke of the action potential of cardiac muscle cells described in the previous sections does not normally occur spontaneously. Rather, when a wave of depolarization reaches the myocyte from neighboring cells, its membrane potential becomes less negative and an action potential is triggered.

Certain heart cells do not require external provocation to initiate their action potential. Rather, they are capable of self-initiated depolarization in a rhythmic fashion and are known as **pacemaker cells.** They are endowed with the property of **automaticity,** by which the cells undergo *spontaneous* depolarization during phase 4. When the threshold voltage is reached in such cells, the upstroke of an action potential is triggered (Fig. 1.15).

Cells that display pacemaker behavior include the SA node (the "natural pacemaker" of the heart) and the AV node. Although atrial and ventricular muscle cells do not normally display automaticity, they may do so under disease conditions such as ischemia.

The shape of the action potential of a pacemaker cell is different from that of a ventricular muscle cell in three ways.

1. The maximum negative voltage of pacemaker cells is approximately −60 mV, substantially less negative than the resting potential of ventricular muscle cells (−90 mV). *The persistently less negative membrane voltage of pacemaker cells causes the fast sodium channels within these cells to remain inactivated.*
2. Unlike cardiac muscle cells, phase 4 of the pacemaker cell action potential is not flat, but has an upward slope, representing spontaneous gradual depolarization. This spontaneous depolarization is due to an ionic flux known as the **pacemaker current** (termed I_f). Current evidence indicates that the pacemaker current is carried predominantly by Na^+ ions. The ion channel through which the pacemaker current passes is different from the fast sodium channel responsible for phase 0 of cardiac muscle cell depolarization. Rather, this pacemaker channel opens during *repolarization* of the cell, as the membrane potential approaches its most negative values. The inward flow of positively charged Na^+ ions through the pacemaker channel causes the membrane potential to become progressively less negative during phase 4, ultimately depolarizing the cell to its threshold voltage (see Fig 1.15) and gradually deactivating the pacemaker channel.
3. The phase 0 upstroke of the pacemaker cell action potential is less rapid and reaches a lower amplitude than that of a cardiac muscle cell. This is so because the fast sodium channels of the pacemaker cells are inactivated, and the upstroke of the action potential relies solely on Ca^{++} influx through the relatively slow calcium channels.

Repolarization of pacemaker cells occurs in a fashion similar to that of ventricular muscle cells and is due to 1) inactivation of the calcium channels and 2) increased activation of potassium channels with enhanced K^+ efflux from the cell.

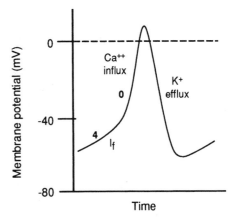

Figure 1.15. **Action potential of a pacemaker cell.** Phase 4 is characterized by gradual, spontaneous depolarization owing to the pacemaker current (I_f). When the threshold potential is reached, at about −40 mV, the upstroke of the action potential follows. The upstroke of phase 0 is less rapid than in non-pacemaker cells, because the current represents Ca^{++} influx through the relatively slow calcium channels.

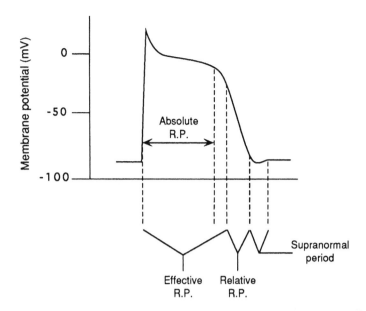

Figure 1.16. Refractory periods (RP) of the myocyte. During the absolute refractory period (ARP), the cell is unexcitable to stimulation. The effective refractory period includes a brief period beyond the ARP during which stimulation produces a localized depolarization that does not propagate. During the relative refractory period, stimulation produces a weak action potential (AP) that propagates, but more slowly than usual. During the supranormal period, a weaker-than-normal stimulus can trigger an AP.

Refractory Periods

Compared with electrical impulses in nerves and skeletal muscle, the cardiac action potential is much longer in duration. This results in a prolonged refractory period during which the muscle cannot be restimulated. These long periods are physiologically necessary, because they allow the ventricles sufficient time to empty their contents and refill before the next cardiac contraction.

There are different levels of refractoriness during the action potential, as illustrated in Figure 1.16. The degree of refractoriness primarily reflects the number of fast Na^+ channels that have recovered from their inactive state and are capable of reopening. As phase 3 of the action potential progresses, an increasing number of Na^+ channels recover and can respond to the next depolarization. This, in turn, corresponds to an increasing probability that a stimulus will trigger an action potential and result in a propagated impulse.

The *absolute* refractory period refers to the time during which the cell is completely unexcitable to a new stimulation. The *effec-* *tive* refractory period includes the absolute refractory period but extends beyond it to include a short interval of phase 3, during which stimulation produces a localized action potential that is not strong enough to propagate further. The *relative* refractory period is the interval during which stimulation triggers an action potential that is conducted, but because the cell is stimulated from a voltage less negative than the resting potential, its upstroke is less steep and of lower amplitude and its conduction velocity slower than normal (see the section on Impulse Conduction below). Following the relative refractory period, a short "supranormal" period is present in which a less-than-normal stimulus can trigger an action potential.

The refractory period of atrial cells is shorter than that of ventricular muscle cells, so that atrial rates can generally exceed ventricular rates during rapid arrhythmias, as is explored in Chapter 11.

Impulse Conduction

During depolarization, the electrical impulse spreads along each cardiac cell, and rapidly from cell to cell, because each myocyte is connected to its neighbors through low-resistance gap junctions. The speed of tissue depolarization (phase 0) and the conduction velocity along the cell depend on the number of sodium channels and on the magnitude of the resting potential. Tissues with a high concentration of Na^+ channels, such as Purkinje fibers, have a large fast inward current, which spreads rapidly within and between cells to support rapid conduction. In contrast, the less negative the resting potential, the greater the number of inactivated fast sodium channels, and therefore the less rapid the upstroke velocity (Fig. 1.17). Thus, alterations in the resting potential greatly affect the upstroke and conduction velocity of the action potential.

Normal Sequence of Cardiac Depolarization

Electrical activation of the heart beat is normally initiated at the SA node (see Fig. 1.6). The impulse spreads to the surrounding atrial muscle through intercellular gap junctions that provide electrical continuity between the cells. Ordinary atrial muscle fibers participate in the propagation of the impulse from the SA to the AV node, although in certain regions the fibers are more densely arranged, facilitating conduction.

Fibrous tissue surrounds the AV valves, such that there is no direct electrical connection between the atrial and ventricular chambers other than through the AV node.

As the electrical impulse reaches the AV node, a delay in conduction (approximately 0.1 sec) is encountered. This delay occurs because the small-diameter fibers in this region conduct slowly, and the action potential is of the "slow" pacemaker type (recall that in pacemaker tissue, the fast sodium channels are permanently inactivated, and the upstroke velocity relies on the slower calcium channels). The pause in conduction at the AV node is beneficial because it allows the atria time to contract and fully empty their contents before ventricular stimulation. In addition, the delay allows the AV node to serve as a "gatekeeper" of conduction from atria to ventricles, which is critical for limiting the rate of ventricular stimulation during abnormally rapid atrial rhythms.

After traversing the AV node, the cardiac action potential spreads into the rapidly conducting bundle of His and Purkinje fibers, which distribute the electrical impulses to the bulk of the ventricular muscle cells. This allows for precisely timed stimulation and smooth contraction of the ventricular myocytes.

EXCITATION-CONTRACTION COUPLING

This section reviews how the action potential leads to physical contraction of cardiac muscle cells, a process known as excitation-contraction coupling. During this process, chemical energy in the form of

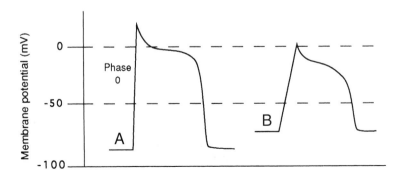

Figure 1.17. **Dependence of speed of depolarization on resting potential. A.** Normal resting potential (RP) and normal rapid rise of phase 0. **B.** Less negative RP results in slower rise of phase 0 and lower maximum amplitude of the action potential.

high-energy phosphate compounds is translated into the mechanical energy of myocyte contraction.

There are several distinct proteins responsible for cardiac muscle cell contraction (Fig. 1.18). Two of the proteins, actin and myosin, are the chief contractile elements. Two other proteins, tropomyosin and troponin, serve regulatory functions.

Myosin is arranged in thick filaments, each composed of lengthwise stacks of approximately 300 molecules. The myosin filament exhibits globular heads that are evenly spaced along its length and contain myosin ATPase, an enzyme that is necessary for contraction to occur. **Actin,** a smaller molecule, is arranged in thin filaments as an alpha-helix consisting of two strands that interdigitate between the thick myosin filaments (see Fig. 1.8). **Titin** (also termed connectin) is a protein that helps tether myosin to the Z-line of the sarcomere and also provides elasticity to the contractile process.

Tropomyosin is a double helix that lies in the grooves between the actin filaments and, in the resting state, inhibits the interaction between myosin heads and actin, thus preventing contraction. **Troponin** sits at regular intervals along the actin strands and is composed of three subunits. The troponin C (TN-C) subunit is responsible for binding calcium ions that regulate the contractile process. The troponin I (TN-I) subunit inhibits the ATPase activity of the actin-myosin interaction. The troponin T (TN-T) subunit links the troponin complex to the actin and tropomyosin molecules.

During phase 2 of the action potential, Ca^{++} enters the myocyte through L-type calcium channels in the sarcolemma and T tubules. The relatively small amount of calcium that enters the cell in this fashion is not sufficient to cause contraction of the myofibrils, but it triggers a much greater Ca^{++} release from the sarcoplasmic reticulum (SR) acting via **ryanodine receptors** (Fig. 1.19). Portions of these receptors extend from the membrane of the SR toward the T tubules. When calcium enters the cell via the T tubules and reaches the ryanodine receptor, the molecular configuration of the receptor changes, causing Ca^{++} to be released from the sarcoplasmic reticulum into the cytosol. As a result of this action, the calcium concentration in the cytosol increases dramatically.

As calcium ions bind to TN-C, the activity of TN-I is inhibited, which induces a conformational change in tropomyosin. The latter event unblocks the active site between actin and myosin, enabling contraction to proceed.

Contraction ensues as myosin heads bind to actin filaments and "flex," thus causing the interdigitating thick and thin filaments to move past each other in an ATP-dependent reaction (Fig. 1.20). The first step in this process is activation of the myosin head by hydrolysis of ATP, following which the myosin head binds to actin and forms a cross bridge. The interaction between the myosin head and actin results in a conformational change in the head, causing it to pull the actin filament inward.

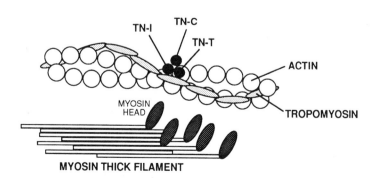

Figure 1.18. Schematic diagram of the main contractile proteins of the myocyte, actin and myosin. Tropomyosin and troponin (components TN-I, TN-C, and TN-T) are regulatory proteins.

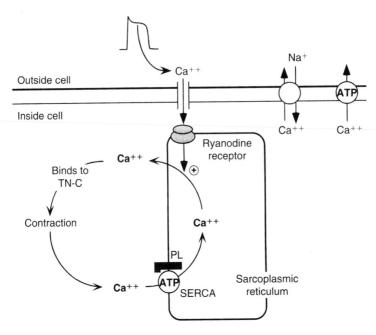

Figure 1.19. Calcium ion movements during excitation and contraction in cardiac muscle cells. Ca^{++} enters the cell through calcium channels during phase 2 of the action potential, triggering a much larger calcium release from the sarcoplasmic reticulum (SR) via the ryanodine receptor complex. The binding of cytosolic Ca^{++} to troponin-C (TN-C) results in contraction. Relaxation occurs as Ca^{++} returns to the SR by sarco(endo)plasmic reticulum calcium ATPase (SERCA). Phospholamban (PL) is a major regulator of this pump, inhibiting Ca^{++} uptake in its dephosphorylated state. Excess intracellular calcium is returned to the extracellular environment by sodium-calcium exchange and to a smaller degree by the sarcolemmal Ca^{++}-ATPase.

Next, while the myosin head and actin are still attached, ADP is released and a new molecule of ATP then binds to the myosin head, causing it to release the actin filament, and the cycle can then repeat. Progressive coupling and uncoupling of actin and myosin causes the muscle fiber to shorten by increasing the overlap between the myofilaments within each sarcomere. In the presence of ATP, this process continues for as long as the cytosolic calcium concentration remains sufficiently high to inhibit the troponin-tropomyosin blocking action.

At the conclusion of phase 2 of the action potential, the Ca^{++} channels close so that there is no further influx into the sarcoplasm. Meanwhile, calcium is continuously pumped back into the sarcoplasmic reticulum and out of the cell (see Fig. 1.19). This restoration of calcium concentration occurs primarily via the sarco(endo)plasmic reticulum Ca^{++}-ATPase (SERCA), which pumps Ca^{++} back into the SR. The small amount of Ca^{++} that entered the cell from extracellular sources is removed from the cell by Na^{+}-Ca^{++} exchange and to a lesser extent by the sarcolemmal ATP-dependent calcium "pump" (Ca^{++}-ATPase).

As calcium ions dissociate from troponin C, tropomyosin once again inhibits the actin-myosin interaction, leading to relaxation of the contracted cell. The contraction-relaxation cycle can then repeat with the next action potential.

There is substantial evidence that the concentration of Ca^{++} within the cytosol is the major determinant of the force of cardiac contraction with each heart beat. Mechanisms that raise intracellular Ca^{++} concentration enhance force development, whereas factors that lower Ca^{++} concentration reduce the contractile force.

β-Adrenergic and Cholinergic Signaling

β-Adrenergic stimulation is one mechanism that enhances calcium fluxes in the myocyte and thereby strengthens the force of ventricular contraction (Fig. 1.21). Catecholamines

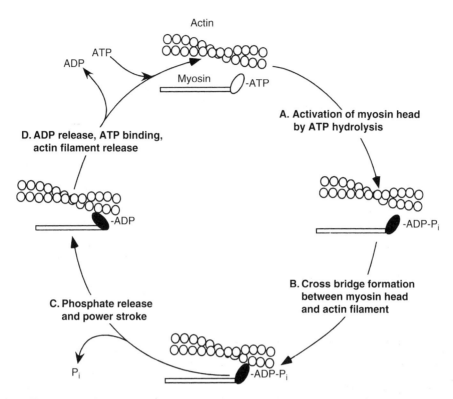

Figure 1.20. **The contractile process. A.** Myosin head is activated by hydrolysis of ATP. **B.** During cellular depolarization, cytoplasmic calcium concentration increases and removes the troponin-tropomyosin inhibition, such that a crossbridge is formed between actin and myosin. **C.** Inorganic phosphate (Pi) is released and a conformational change in the myosin head draws the actin filament inward. **D.** ADP is released and replaced by ATP, causing the myosin head to dissociate from the actin filament. As the process repeats, the muscle fiber shortens. The cycle continues until cytosolic calcium concentration decreases at the end of phase 2 of the action potential.

(e.g., norepinephrine) bind to the myocyte β_1-adrenergic receptor, which is coupled to, and activates, the G protein system (G_s) attached to the inner surface of the cell membrane. G_s in turn stimulates membrane-bound adenylate cyclase to produce cyclic AMP (cAMP) from ATP. cAMP then activates intracellular protein kinases, which phosphorylate cellular proteins, including the L-type calcium channels within the cell membrane. Phosphorylation of the calcium channel augments Ca^{++} influx, which triggers a corresponding increase in Ca^{++} release from the sarcoplasmic reticulum, thereby enhancing the force of contraction.

β-Adrenergic stimulation of the myocyte also enhances myocyte *relaxation*. The return of Ca^{++} from the cytosol to the sarcoplasmic reticulum (SR) is regulated by **phospholamban** (PL), a low molecular weight protein in the SR membrane. In its

dephosphorylated state, PL inhibits Ca^{++} uptake by SERCA (see Fig. 1.19). However, β-adrenergic activation of protein kinases (see Fig. 1.21) causes PL to become phosphorylated, an action that blunts PL's inhibitory effect. The subsequently greater uptake of calcium ions by the SR hastens Ca^{++} removal from the cytosol and therefore promotes myocyte relaxation. The increased cAMP activity also results in phosphorylation of TN-I, an action that inhibits actin-myosin interactions and therefore further enhances relaxation of the cell.

Cholinergic signaling via parasympathetic inputs (mainly from the vagus nerve) opposes the effects of β-adrenergic stimulation (see Fig. 1.21). Acetylcholine released from parasympathetic nerve terminals binds to the muscarinic M_2 receptor on cardiac cells. This receptor also activates G-proteins, but in distinction to the β-adrenergic receptor, it

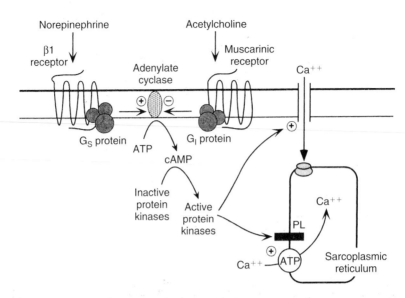

Figure 1.21. Effects of β-adrenergic and cholinergic stimulation on cardiac cellular signaling and calcium ion movement. The binding of a ligand (e.g., norepinephrine) to the β_1-receptor induces G-protein–mediated stimulation of adenylate cyclase and formation of cyclic AMP (cAMP). The latter activates protein kinases, which phosphorylate cellular proteins, including ion channels. Phosphorylation of the slow Ca^{++} channel enhances calcium movement into the cell and therefore strengthens the force of contraction. Protein kinases also phosphorylate phospholamban (PL), reducing the latter's inhibition of Ca^{++} uptake by the sarcoplasmic reticulum. The enhanced removal of Ca^{++} from the cytosol facilitates relaxation of the myocyte. Cholinergic signaling, triggered by acetylcholine binding to the muscarinic receptor, activates inhibitory G proteins that reduce adenylate cyclase activity and cAMP production, thus antagonizing the effects of β-adrenergic stimulation.

is coupled to G_i, an *inhibitory* G protein system. G_i associated with cholinergic stimulation inhibits adenylate cyclase activity and reduces cAMP formation. G_i also activates specific K^+ channels in the plasma membrane which hyperpolarizes the cell. At the sinus node, these actions of cholinergic stimulation serve to reduce heart rate. In the myocardium, the effect is to counteract the force of contraction induced by β-adrenergic stimulation. It should be noted that ventricular cells are much less sensitive to this cholinergic effect than atrial cells, likely reflecting different degrees of G-protein coupling.

Thus, physiologic or pharmacologic catecholamine stimulation of the myocyte β_1-adrenergic receptor enhances contraction of the cell, while cholinergic stimulation opposes that enhancement. These important properties will be referred to in later chapters.

SUMMARY

The anatomic structure, cellular composition, and conduction pathways of the heart form an efficient system for repetitive, organized contractions. As a result, the heart is capable of purposeful stimulation billions of times during the lifespan of a normal individual. With each contraction cycle, the heart receives and propagates blood through the circulation to provide nutrients to and remove waste products from the body's tissues.

The following chapters explore what can go wrong with this extraordinary system.

Acknowledgments   Contributors to the previous editions of this chapter were Stephanie Harper, MD; Scott Hyver, MD; Paul Kim, MD; Laurence Rhines, MD; James D. Marsh, MD; Kirsten Greineder, MD; Gary R. Strichartz, MD; and Leonard S. Lilly, MD.

ADDITIONAL READING

Braunwald E, Ross J, Jr., Sonnenblick EM. Mechanisms of Contraction of the Normal and Failing Heart. Boston: Little, Brown & Co., 1976.

Hille B. Ionic Channels of Excitable Membranes. 2nd Ed. Sunderland, MA: Sinauer Assoc., 1992.

Hodgkin AL, Huxley AF. A quantitative description of membrane current and its application to conduction and excitation in nerve. J Physiol (Lond) 1952;117:500–544.

Katz AM. Physiology of the Heart. 3rd Ed. Philadelphia: Lippincott Williams & Wilkins, 2000.

Katz AM. Cardiac ion channels. N Engl J Med 1993;328:1244–1251.

Linder ME, Gilman AG. G proteins. Sci Am 1992;267(1):36–43.

Opie LH. The Heart: Physiology, From Cell to Circulation. 3rd Ed. Philadelphia: Lippincott Williams & Wilkins, 1998.

Roberts R. Molecular Basis of Cardiology. Boston: Blackwell Scientific Publications, 1993.

Sperelakis N, Kurachi Y, Terzic A, et al. Heart Physiology and Pathophysiology. 4th Ed. San Diego: Academic Press, 2001.

Trautwein W, Hescheler J. Regulation of cardiac L-type calcium current by phosphorylation and G proteins. Ann Rev Physiol 1990;52:257–274.

Heart Sounds and Murmurs

Leonard S. Lilly

Cardiac Cycle
Heart Sounds
  First Heart Sound (S$_1$)
  Second Heart Sound (S$_2$)
  Extra Systolic Heart Sounds
  Extra Diastolic Heart Sounds

Chapter 2

Murmurs
  Systolic Murmurs
  Diastolic Murmurs
  Continuous Murmurs

Diseases of the heart often cause abnormal findings on physical examination, including pathologic heart sounds and murmurs. These findings are clues to the underlying disease pathophysiology, and proper interpretation is essential for successful diagnosis and disease management. This chapter describes heart sounds of the normal cardiac cycle and then focuses on the origins of pathologic heart sounds and murmurs.

In this chapter, many cardiac diseases are mentioned briefly as examples of abnormal heart sounds and murmurs. Each of these conditions is described in greater detail later in this book, so it is not necessary to memorize the examples presented here. Rather, it is preferable to understand the mechanisms by which the abnormal sounds are produced, so that their descriptions will make sense in later chapters.

CARDIAC CYCLE

The cardiac cycle consists of precisely timed electrical and mechanical events that result in the rhythmic atrial and ventricular contractions that propel blood into the pulmonary and systemic circulations. Mechanical **systole** refers to ventricular contraction, and **diastole** to ventricular relaxation and filling (Fig. 2.1). Throughout the cycle, the right and left atria continuously accept blood returning to the heart from the systemic veins and from the pulmonary veins, respectively. During diastole, blood passes from the atria into the ventricles across the open tricuspid and mitral valves. In late diastole, atrial contraction propels a final bolus of blood into the ventricles, which produces a slight pressure rise, termed the *a* wave.

Contraction of the ventricles follows, signaling the onset of mechanical systole. As the ventricles start to contract, the pressures within them rapidly exceed atrial pressures, resulting in the forced closure of the tricuspid and mitral valves. This event produces the first heart sound, termed **S$_1$** (see Fig. 2.1). S$_1$ has two nearly superimposed components: the mitral component slightly precedes the tricuspid component because of the earlier electrical stimulation of left ventricular contraction.

As the ventricular pressures rapidly rise further, they soon exceed the diastolic pressures within the pulmonary artery and aorta, forcing the pulmonic and aortic valves to open, and blood is ejected into the pulmonary and systemic circulations. At the conclusion of the ventricular ejection phase, the ventricular pressures fall below those of the pulmonary artery and aorta, such that the pulmonic and aortic valves are forced to close, producing the second heart sound, termed **S$_2$**. S$_2$ also consists of two components: the aortic component (A$_2$) normally precedes the pulmonic compo-

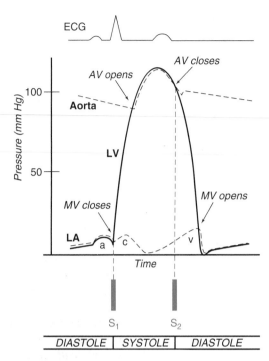

Figure 2.1. The normal cardiac cycle, showing pressure relationships between the left-sided heart chambers. During diastole, the mitral valve (MV) is open, so that the left atrial (LA) and left ventricular (LV) pressures are equal. In late diastole, LA contraction causes a small rise in pressure in both the LA and LV (the *a* wave). During systolic contraction, the LV pressure rises; when it exceeds the LA pressure, the MV closes, contributing to the first heart sound (S₁). As LV pressure rises above the aortic pressure, the aortic valve (AV) opens, which is a silent event. As the ventricle begins to relax and its pressure falls below that of the aorta, the AV closes, contributing to the second heart sound (S₂). As LV pressure falls further, below that of the LA, the MV opens, which is silent in the normal heart. In addition to the *a* wave, the LA pressure curve displays two additional positive deflections: the *c* wave represents a small rise in LA pressure as the MV closes and bulges toward the atrium, and the *v* wave is due to passive filling of the LA from the pulmonary veins during systole, when the MV is closed.

At the bedside, systole can be approximated by the period from S_1 to S_2, and diastole from S_2 to the next S_1. Although the duration of systole remains constant from beat to beat, the length of diastole varies with the heart rate: the faster the heart rate, the shorter the diastolic phase. The main heart sounds, S_1 and S_2, provide a framework from which all other heart sounds and murmurs can be timed.

Typical stethoscopes have two chest pieces for auscultation of the heart. The concave "bell" chest piece is meant to be applied lightly to the skin, whereby it accentuates low-frequency sounds. Conversely, the flat "diaphragm" chest piece should be pressed firmly against the skin to eliminate low frequencies and therefore accentuate high-frequency sounds and murmurs.

HEART SOUNDS

First Heart Sound (S₁)

S_1 is produced by closure of the mitral and tricuspid valves in early systole and is loudest near the apex of the heart (Fig. 2.2). It is a high-frequency sound, best heard with the diaphragm of the stethoscope. Although mitral closure usually precedes tricuspid closure, they are separated by only approximately 0.01 sec, such that the human ear appreciates only a single sound through the stethoscope. An exception oc-

nent (P₂) because the diastolic pressure gradient between the aorta and left ventricle is higher than that between the pulmonary artery and right ventricle. The ventricular pressures continue to fall during the relaxation phase. As they drop below the pressures in the right and left atria, the tricuspid and mitral valves open, followed by diastolic ventricular filling and then repetition of the cycle.

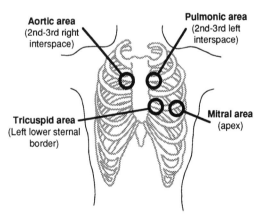

Figure 2.2. Standard positions of stethoscope placement for cardiac auscultation.

curs in patients with right bundle branch block (see Chapter 4), in whom these components *may* be audibly split, because of delayed closure of the tricuspid valve.

Three factors determine the intensity of S_1: 1) the distance separating the individual leaflets of the open valves at the onset of ventricular contraction, 2) the mobility of the leaflets (normal or rigid because of stenosis), and 3) the rate of rise of ventricular pressure (Table 2.1).

The distance between the open valve leaflets at the onset of ventricular contraction is affected by the PR interval on the electrocardiogram, the period between the onset of atrial and ventricular activation. Normal atrial contraction initiated by the P wave forces the tricuspid and mitral valve leaflets apart. As they start to drift back together, ventricular contraction forces them shut, from whatever position they are at, as soon as ventricular pressure exceeds that in the atrium. An *accentuated* S_1 results when the PR interval is shorter than normal because the valve leaflets have not had sufficient time to drift back together, and are forced shut from a relatively wide distance at the onset of ventricular contraction.

Similarly, in *mild* mitral stenosis (see Chapter 8) a prolonged diastolic pressure gradient exists between the left atrium and ventricle, which keeps the mobile portions of the mitral leaflets farther apart than normal during diastole. Since the leaflets are relatively wide apart at the onset of systole, they are forced shut loudly when the left ventricle contracts.

S_1 also may be accentuated when the heart rate is more rapid than normal (i.e., tachycardia), because diastole is shortened and therefore ventricular contraction forces together the tricuspid and mitral leaflets from relatively wide apart positions, because they have had insufficient time to drift together.

Conditions that *reduce* the intensity of S_1 are also listed in Table 2.1. In first-degree atrioventricular (AV) nodal block (discussed in Chapter 12), a diminished S_1 results from an abnormally prolonged PR interval, which delays the onset of ventricular contraction: following atrial contraction, the mitral and tricuspid valves have *additional* time to float back together so that the leaflets are forced closed from only a small distance apart.

In patients with mitral regurgitation (see Chapter 8), S_1 is often diminished in intensity, because the mitral leaflets may not come into full contact with one another as they close. In *severe* mitral stenosis, the leaflets are nearly fixed in position throughout the cardiac cycle, and that reduced movement can also lessen the intensity of S_1.

In patients with a "stiffened" left ventricle (e.g., a hypertrophied or scarred chamber), atrial contraction results in a higher than normal pressure at the end of diastole. This higher pressure accelerates the drifting together of the mitral leaflets, so that when ventricular contraction commences, they are forced closed from a less than normal distance apart, and therefore S_1 may be reduced in intensity.

Second Heart Sound (S_2)

The second heart sound results from the closure of the aortic and pulmonic valves and therefore has aortic (A_2) and pulmonic (P_2) components. Unlike S_1, which is usually auscultated as a single sound, the components of S_2 vary with the respiratory cycle: they are normally fused as one sound during expiration, but become audibly separated during inspiration, a situation termed "normal" or **physiologic splitting** of S_2 (Fig. 2.3).

TABLE 2.1. Causes of Altered Intensity of S_1

Accentuated S_1
1. Shortened PR interval
2. Mild mitral stenosis
3. High cardiac output states or tachycardia (e.g., exercise or anemia)

Diminished S_1
1. Lengthened PR interval: first-degree AV nodal block
2. Mitral regurgitation
3. Severe mitral stenosis
4. "Stiff" left ventricle (e.g., systemic hypertension)

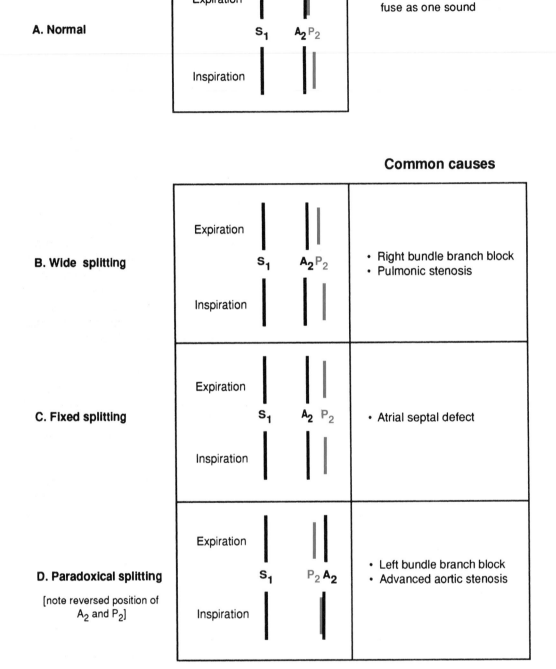

A. Normal

Expiration

S_1 $A_2 P_2$

Inspiration

In expiration, A_2 and P_2
fuse as one sound

Common causes

B. Wide splitting

Expiration

S_1 $A_2 P_2$

Inspiration

• Right bundle branch block
• Pulmonic stenosis

C. Fixed splitting

Expiration

S_1 A_2 P_2

Inspiration

• Atrial septal defect

D. Paradoxical splitting

[note reversed position of
A_2 and P_2]

Expiration

S_1 $P_2 A_2$

Inspiration

• Left bundle branch block
• Advanced aortic stenosis

Figure 2.3. Splitting patterns of the second heart sound (S_2). A_2, aortic component; P_2, pulmonic component of S_2; S_1, first heart sound.

One explanation for normal splitting of S_2 is as follows. Expansion of the chest during inspiration causes the intrathoracic pressure to become more negative. The negative pressure transiently increases the capacitance (and reduces the impedance) of the intrathoracic pulmonary vessels. As a result, there is a temporary delay in the diastolic "back pressure" of the pulmonary artery responsible for closure of the pulmonic valve. Thus, P_2 is delayed; that is, it occurs *later* during inspiration than during expiration.

Inspiration has the *opposite* effect on A_2. Since the capacity of the intrathoracic pulmonary veins is increased by the negative pressure during inspiration, the venous return to the left atrium and ventricle temporarily decreases. Reduced filling of the LV causes a reduced stroke volume during the next systolic contraction and therefore shortens the time required for LV emptying. Therefore, aortic valve closure (A_2) occurs slightly earlier in inspiration than during expiration. The combination of an earlier A_2 and delayed P_2 during inspiration causes audible separation of these two components of the second heart sound. Since the components of S_2 are high-frequency sounds, they are best heard with the diaphragm of the stethoscope, and splitting of the sounds is usually most easily appreciated near the second left intercostal space next to the sternum (the "pulmonic" area).

Abnormalities of S_2 include alterations in its intensity and changes in the pattern of splitting. The intensity of S_2 depends on the velocity of blood coursing back toward the valves from the aorta and pulmonary artery after the completion of ventricular contraction, and the suddenness with which that motion is arrested by the closing valves. In systemic hypertension or pulmonary arterial hypertension, the diastolic pressure in the respective great artery is higher than normal, such that the velocity of the blood surging toward the valve is elevated, and S_2 is accentuated. Conversely, in severe aortic or pulmonic valve stenosis, the valve commissures are nearly fixed in position, such

that the contribution of the stenotic valve to S_2 is diminished.

Widened splitting of S_2 refers to an increase in the time interval between A_2 and P_2, such that the two components are audibly separated *even during expiration* and become more widely separated in inspiration (see Fig. 2.3). This pattern is usually the result of delayed closure of the pulmonic valve, which occurs in right bundle branch block (RBBB) and pulmonic valve stenosis.

Fixed splitting of S_2 is an abnormally widened interval between A_2 and P_2 that persists unchanged through the respiratory cycle (see Fig. 2.3). The most common abnormality that causes fixed splitting of S_2 is an atrial septal defect (see Chapter 16). In that condition, chronic volume overload of the right-sided circulation results in a high-capacitance, low-resistance pulmonary vascular system. This alteration in pulmonary artery hemodynamics delays the "back pressure" responsible for closure of the pulmonic valve. Thus, P_2 occurs later than normal, even during expiration, such that there is wider than normal separation of A_2 and P_2. The pattern of splitting does not change (i.e., it is fixed) during the respiratory cycle because (1) inspiration does not substantially increase further the already elevated pulmonary vascular capacitance, and (2) augmented filling of the right atrium from the systemic veins during inspiration is counterbalanced by a reciprocal decrease in the left-to-right transatrial shunt, eliminating respiratory variations in right ventricular filling.

Paradoxical splitting (or "reversed" splitting) refers to audible separation of A_2 and P_2 during *expiration* that disappears on *inspiration*, the opposite of the normal situation. It reflects an abnormal delay in the closure of the aortic valve such that P_2 *precedes* A_2. In adults, the most common cause is left bundle branch block (LBBB). In LBBB, the spread of electrical activity through the left ventricle is impaired, resulting in delayed ventricular contraction and late closure of the aortic valve such that it *follows* P_2. During inspiration, as in the normal case, the pulmonic valve closure sound is delayed and the aortic valve closure sound moves earlier. This results in *narrowing* and often superimposition of the two sounds; therefore, there is no apparent split at the height of inspiration (see Fig. 2.3). In addition to LBBB, paradoxical splitting may be observed under circumstances in which left ventricular ejection is prolonged, such as aortic stenosis.

Extra Systolic Heart Sounds

Extra systolic heart sounds may occur in early, mid, or late systole.

Early Extra Systolic Heart Sounds

Abnormal early systolic sounds, or "ejection clicks," occur shortly after S_1 and coincide with the opening of the aortic or pulmonic valves (Fig. 2.4). These sounds have

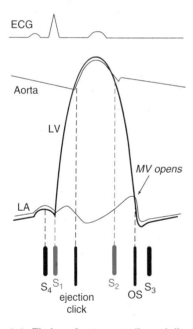

Figure 2.4. Timing of extra systolic and diastolic heart sounds. S_4 is produced by atrial contraction into a "stiff" left ventricle (LV). An ejection click follows the opening of the aortic or pulmonic valve in cases of valve stenosis or dilatation of the corresponding great artery. An S_3 occurs during the period of rapid ventricular filling; it is normal in young individuals, but its presence in adults implies LV contractile dysfunction. The timing of an opening snap (OS) is placed for comparison, but it is not likely that all of these sounds would appear in the same individual. LA, left atrium; MV, mitral valve.

a sharp, high-pitched quality, so they are heard best with the diaphragm of the stethoscope placed over the aortic and pulmonic areas. Ejection clicks indicate the presence of aortic or pulmonic valve stenosis or dilatation of the pulmonary artery or aorta. In stenosis of the aortic or pulmonic valve, the sound occurs as the valve leaflets reach their maximal level of ascent into the great artery, just prior to blood ejection. At that moment, the rapidly ascending valve reaches its elastic limit and decelerates abruptly, an action thought to result in the sound generation. In dilatation of the root of the aorta or pulmonary artery, the sound is associated with sudden tensing of the aortic or pulmonic root with the onset of blood flow into the vessel. The aortic ejection click is heard at both the base and the apex of the heart and does not vary with respiration. In distinction, a pulmonic ejection click is heard only at the base and its intensity *diminishes* during inspiration (see Chapter 16).

Mid or Late Extra Systolic Heart Sounds

Clicks occurring in mid or late systole are usually the result of systolic prolapse of the mitral or tricuspid valves, in which the leaflets bulge abnormally from the ventricular side of the atrioventricular junction to the atrial side during ventricular contraction, often accompanied by valvular regurgitation. They are loudest over the mitral or tricuspid auscultatory regions, respectively (see Fig. 2.2).

Extra Diastolic Heart Sounds

Extra heart sounds in diastole include the opening snap (OS), the third heart sound (S_3), the fourth heart sound (S_4), and the pericardial knock.

Opening Snap

Opening of the mitral and tricuspid valves is normally silent, but mitral or tricuspid valvular stenosis (usually the result of rheumatic heart disease) produces an opening sound, termed a "snap," shortly after S_2. It is a sharp, high-pitched sound, and its timing does not vary significantly with respiration. In mitral stenosis (which is much more common than tricuspid valve stenosis), the OS is heard best between the apex and the left sternal border, just after the aortic closure sound (A_2), when the left ventricular pressure falls below that of the left atrium (see Fig. 2.4). Because of its proximity to A_2, the A_2-OS sequence can be confused with a widely split second heart sound, but careful auscultation at the pulmonic area during inspiration reveals *three* sounds occurring in rapid succession (Fig. 2.5), which correspond to aortic closure (A_2), pulmonic closure (P_2), then the opening snap (OS). The three sounds become two on expiration, as A_2 and P_2 normally fuse.

The severity of stenosis can be approximated by the time interval between A_2 and the opening snap: the more severe the stenosis, the shorter the interval. This occurs because the degree of left atrial pressure elevation corresponds to the severity of mitral stenosis. When the ventricle relaxes in diastole, the greater the left atrial pressure, the earlier the mitral valve opens. Compared with severe stenosis, in mild disease, left atrial pressure is less elevated, so that it takes longer for the left ventricular pressure to fall below that of the atrium. Therefore, in mild mitral stenosis, the opening snap is widely separated from A_2, whereas in more severe stenosis, the A_2-OS interval is narrower.

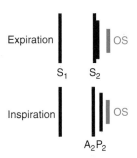

Figure 2.5. Timing of the opening snap (OS) in mitral stenosis does not change with respiration. Upon inspiration, normal splitting of the second heart sound (S_2) is observed so that three sounds are heard. A_2, aortic component; P_2, pulmonic component of S_2; S_1, first heart sound.

Third Heart Sound (S_3)

When present, an S_3 occurs in early diastole, following the opening of the atrioventricular valves, during the ventricular rapid filling phase (see Fig. 2.4). It is a dull, low-pitched sound best heard with the bell of the stethoscope placed over the cardiac apex while the patient lies in the left lateral decubitus position. Production of the S_3 sound appears to result from tensing of the chordae tendinae during rapid filling and expansion of the ventricle.

The third heart sound is a normal finding in children and young adults. In these groups, an S_3 implies the presence of a supple ventricle that is capable of normal rapid expansion in early diastole. Conversely, when heard in middle-aged or older adults, an S_3 is often a sign of disease, indicating volume overload owing to congestive heart failure, or the increased transvalvular flow that accompanies advanced mitral or tricuspid regurgitation. A pathologic S_3 is sometimes referred to as a **ventricular "gallop."**

Fourth Heart Sound (S_4)

When an S_4 is present, it occurs in late diastole and coincides with contraction of the atria (see Fig. 2.4). This sound is generated by the left (or right) atrium vigorously contracting against a *stiffened* ventricle. Thus, an S_4 usually indicates the presence of cardiac disease, specifically a decrease in ventricular compliance, usually due to ventricular hypertrophy or myocardial ischemia. Like an S_3, the S_4 is a dull, low-pitched sound, and is heard best with the bell of the stethoscope. In the case of the left-sided S_4, the sound is loudest at the apex, with the patient lying in the left lateral decubitus position. An S_4 is sometimes referred to as an **atrial "gallop."**

Quadruple Rhythm or Summation Gallop

In a patient with both an S_3 and S_4, those sounds, in conjunction with S_1 and S_2, produce a quadruple beat. If a patient with such a quadruple rhythm develops tachycardia, diastole becomes shorter in duration, the S_3 and S_4 sounds coalesce, and a **"summation gallop"** results. The summation of S_3 and S_4 is heard as a long mid-diastolic, low-pitched sound, often louder than S_1 and S_2.

Pericardial Knock

A pericardial knock is an uncommon, high-pitched sound that occurs in patients with severe constrictive pericarditis (see Chapter 14). It appears early in diastole soon after S_2, and can be confused with an opening snap or an S_3. However, the knock appears slightly later in diastole than the timing of an opening snap and is louder and occurs earlier than the ventricular gallop. It results from the abrupt cessation of ventricular filling in early diastole, which is the hallmark of constrictive pericarditis.

MURMURS

A murmur is the sound generated by turbulent blood flow. Under normal conditions, the flow of blood is laminar (i.e., has a continuous, smooth movement) through the vascular bed and is therefore silent. However, as a result of hemodynamic and/or structural changes in the heart or vasculature, laminar flow can become disturbed and produce an audible noise. Murmurs result from any of the following mechanisms:

1. Flow across a partial obstruction (e.g., aortic stenosis)
2. Increased flow through normal structures (e.g., aortic systolic murmur associated with a high output state, such as anemia)
3. Ejection into a dilated chamber (e.g., aortic systolic murmur associated with aneurysmal dilatation of the aorta)
4. Regurgitant flow across an incompetent valve (e.g., mitral regurgitation)
5. Abnormal shunting of blood from one vascular chamber to a lower-pressure chamber (e.g., ventricular septal defect)

Murmurs are described by their timing, intensity, pitch, shape, location, radiation,

and response to maneuvers. *Timing* refers to whether the murmur occurs during systole, diastole, or is continuous (i.e., begins in systole and continues into diastole). The *intensity* of the murmur is typically quantified by a grading system. In the case of *systolic murmurs:*

Grade 1/6 (or I/VI):	Barely audible (i.e., medical students may not hear it!)
Grade 2/6 (or II/VI):	Faint but immediately audible
Grade 3/6 (or III/VI):	Easily heard
Grade 4/6 (or IV/VI):	Easily heard and associated with a palpable thrill
Grade 5/6 (or V/VI):	Very loud; heard with stethoscope lightly on chest
Grade 6/6 (or VI/VI):	Audible without the stethoscope directly on the chest wall

In the case of *diastolic murmurs:*

Grade 1/4 (or I/IV):	Barely audible
Grade 2/4 (or II/IV):	Faint but immediately audible
Grade 3/4 (or III/IV):	Easily heard
Grade 4/4 (or IV/IV):	Very loud

Pitch refers to the frequency of the murmur, ranging from high to low. High-frequency murmurs are caused by large pressure gradients between chambers (e.g., aortic stenosis) and are best appreciated using the diaphragm chest piece of the stethoscope. Low-frequency murmurs imply less of a pressure gradient between chambers (e.g., mitral stenosis) and are best heard using the stethoscope's bell piece.

Shape describes how the murmur changes in intensity from its onset to its completion. For example, a "crescendo-decrescendo" (or "diamond-shaped") murmur first rises and then falls off in intensity. Other shapes include "decrescendo" (i.e., the murmur begins at its maximum intensity and grows softer) and "uniform" (the intensity of the murmur does not change).

Location refers to the murmur's region of maximum intensity and is usually described in terms of specific auscultatory areas (see Fig. 2.2):

Aortic area:	2nd–3rd right intercostal space, next to sternum
Pulmonic area:	2nd–3rd left intercostal space, next to sternum
Tricuspid area:	Lower left sternal border
Mitral area:	Cardiac apex

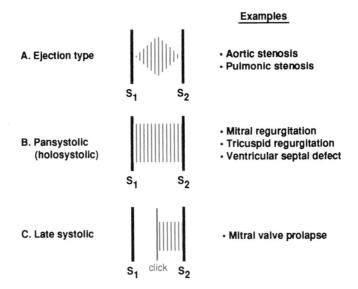

Figure 2.6. **Classification of systolic murmurs.** Ejection murmurs are crescendo–decrescendo in configuration, whereas pansystolic murmurs are uniform throughout systole. A late systolic murmur often follows a midsystolic click and suggests mitral (or tricuspid) valve prolapse.

From their primary locations, murmurs are often heard to *radiate* to other areas of the chest, and such patterns of transmission relate to the direction of the turbulent flow. Finally, similar types of murmurs can be distinguished from one another by simple bedside *maneuvers,* such as standing upright, Valsalva (forceful expiration against a closed airway), or clenching of the fists, each of which alters the heart's loading conditions and can affect the intensity of many murmurs. Examples of the effects of maneuvers on specific murmurs are presented in Chapter 8.

When describing a murmur, some or all of these descriptors are listed. For example, a physician might describe a patient's murmur of aortic stenosis as follows: "A grade III/VI high-pitched, crescendo-decrescendo systolic murmur, heard best at the upper right sternal border, radiating toward the neck."

Systolic Murmurs

Systolic murmurs are subdivided into systolic ejection murmurs, pansystolic murmurs, and late systolic murmurs (Fig. 2.6).

A **systolic ejection murmur** is typical of aortic or pulmonic valve stenosis. It begins after the first heart sound and terminates before or during S2, depending on its severity and whether the obstruction is of the aortic or pulmonic valve. The murmur is of the crescendo-decrescendo type (i.e., its intensity rises and then falls).

The ejection murmur of *aortic stenosis* begins in systole after S_1, from which it is separated by a short audible gap (Fig. 2.7). This gap corresponds to the period of isovolumetric contraction of the left ventricle (the period after the mitral valve has closed, but before the aortic valve has opened). The murmur becomes more intense as flow increases across the aortic valve during the rise in left ventricular pressure (crescendo). Then, as the ventricle relaxes, forward flow decreases, and the murmur lessens in intensity (decrescendo) and finally ends prior to the aortic component of S_2. The murmur may be immediately preceded by an ejection click, especially in mild forms of aortic stenosis.

Although the intensity of the murmur does not correlate well with the severity of aortic stenosis, other features do. For exam-

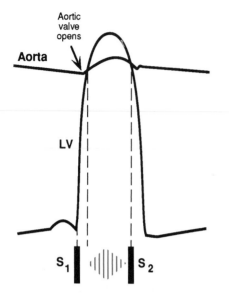

Figure 2.7. **Systolic ejection murmur of aortic stenosis.** There is a short delay between the first heart sound (S_1) and the onset of the murmur. LV, left ventricle; S_2, second heart sound.

ple, the more severe the stenosis, the longer it takes to force blood across the valve, and the later the murmur peaks in systole (Fig. 2.8). As also shown in Figure 2.8, as the severity of stenosis increases, the aortic component of S_2 softens, as the leaflets become more rigidly fixed in place.

Aortic stenosis causes a high-frequency murmur, reflecting the sizable pressure gradient across the valve. It is best heard in the "aortic area" in the second and third right interspaces close to the sternum. The murmur typically radiates toward the neck (the direction of turbulent blood flow) but often can be heard in a wide distribution, including the cardiac apex.

When a systolic ejection murmur is due to *pulmonic stenosis,* it also begins after S_1, may be preceded by an ejection click, but may extend beyond A_2. That is, if the stenosis is severe, it will result in a very prolonged right ventricular ejection time, elongating the murmur, which will continue beyond A_2 and end just prior to closure of the pulmonic valve (P_2). Pulmonic stenosis is usually loudest at the second to third left interspaces close to the sternum. It does not radiate as widely as aortic stenosis, but

sometimes it is transmitted toward the neck or left shoulder.

Young adults often have *benign systolic ejection murmurs* owing to increased systolic flow across normal aortic and pulmonic valves. This type of murmur often becomes softer or disappears when the patient sits upright.

Pansystolic (also termed **holosystolic**) murmurs are caused by regurgitation of blood across an incompetent mitral or tricuspid valve or through a ventricular septal defect (VSD) (see Fig. 2.6). These murmurs are characterized by a uniform intensity throughout systole. In mitral and tricuspid valve regurgitation, as soon as ventricular pressure exceeds atrial pressure (i.e., when

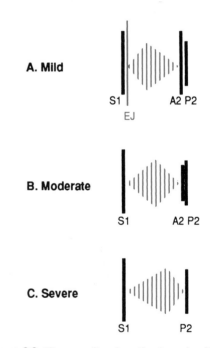

Figure 2.8. **The severity of aortic stenosis affects the shape of the systolic murmur and the heart sounds. A.** In mild stenosis, an ejection click (EJ) is often present, followed by an early peaking crescendo–decrescendo murmur and a normal aortic component of S_2 (A_2). **B.** As stenosis becomes more severe, the peak of the murmur becomes more delayed in systole and the intensity of A_2 lessens. The prolonged ventricular ejection time delays A_2 so that it merges with or occurs after the pulmonic component of S_2 (P_2); the ejection click may not be heard. **C.** In severe stenosis, the murmur peaks very late in systole, and A_2 is usually absent, because of immobility of the valve leaflets. S_1, first heart sound; S_2, second heart sound.

S_1 occurs), there is immediate retrograde flow across the regurgitant valve. Thus, there is no gap between S_1 and the onset of these pansystolic murmurs, in distinction to the systolic ejection murmurs discussed above. Similarly, there is no significant gap between S_1 and the onset of the systolic murmur of a VSD, since left ventricular systolic pressure exceeds right ventricular systolic pressure (and flow occurs) quickly after the onset of contraction.

The pansystolic murmur of advanced *mitral regurgitation* continues through the aortic closure sound because left ventricular pressure remains greater than that in the left atrium at the time of aortic closure. The murmur is heard best at the apex, is high-pitched and "blowing" in quality, and often radiates toward the left axilla; its intensity does not change with respiration.

Tricuspid valve regurgitation is best heard along the left lower sternal border. It generally radiates to the right of the sternum and is high-pitched and "blowing" in quality. The intensity of the murmur *increases* with inspiration, because the negative intrathoracic pressure induced during inspiration enhances venous return to the heart. The latter augments right ventricular stroke volume, thereby increasing the amount of regurgitated blood.

The murmur of a *ventricular septal defect* is heard best at the fourth to sixth left intercostal spaces, is high-pitched, and may be associated with a palpable thrill. The intensity of the murmur does not increase with inspiration and does not radiate to the axilla, which helps distinguish it from tricuspid and mitral regurgitation, respectively. Of note, the *smaller* the VSD, the greater the turbulence of blood flow between the left and right ventricles, and the *louder* the murmur. Some of the loudest murmurs physicians ever hear are those of small VSDs.

Late systolic murmurs begin in mid to late systole and continue to A_2. The most common example is mitral regurgitation due to *mitral valve prolapse*—bowing of abnormally redundant and elongated valve leaflets into the left atrium during ventricular contraction (see Fig. 2.6). This murmur is usually preceded by a midsystolic click and is described further in Chapter 8.

Diastolic Murmurs

Diastolic murmurs are divided into early decrescendo murmurs and mid to late rumbling murmurs (Fig. 2.9). **Early diastolic murmurs** result from regurgitant flow through either the aortic or pulmonic valve, with the former being much more common in adults. If produced by *aortic valve regurgitation,* the murmur begins at A_2, has a decrescendo shape, and terminates prior to the next S_1. Because diastolic relaxation of the left ventricle is rapid, a pressure gradient develops immediately between the aorta and lower-pressured left ventricle in aortic regurgitation, and the murmur therefore displays its maximum intensity at its onset. Thereafter in diastole, as the aortic pressure falls and the LV pressure increases (as blood fills the ventricle), the gradient between the two chambers diminishes and the murmur decreases in intensity. Aortic regurgitation is a high-pitched murmur, best heard using the diaphragm of the stethoscope along the left sternal border with the patient sitting, leaning forward, and exhaling.

Pulmonic regurgitation in adults is usually due to the presence of pulmonary arterial hypertension. It has a similar early diastolic decrescendo murmur profile as aortic regurgitation, but it is best heard in the "pulmonic" area and its intensity may increase with inspiration.

Mid to late diastolic murmurs result from either turbulent flow across a *stenotic mitral or tricuspid valve* or less commonly from abnormally increased flow across a normal mitral or tricuspid valve (see Fig. 2.9). If due to stenosis, the murmur begins after S_2 and is preceded by an opening snap. The shape of this murmur is unique. Following the opening snap, the murmur is at its loudest because the pressure gradient between the atrium and ventricle is at its maximum. The murmur then decrescendos or disappears totally during diastole as the transvalvular gradient decreases. The de-

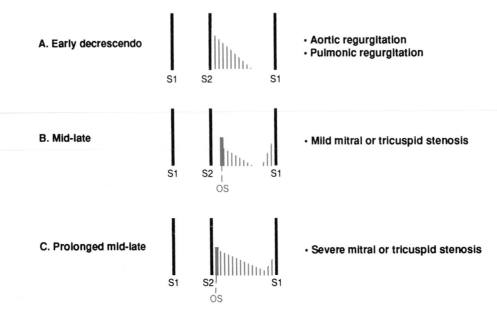

A. Early decrescendo

S1   S2   S1

• **Aortic regurgitation**
• **Pulmonic regurgitation**

B. Mid-late

S1   S2   S1
        OS

• **Mild mitral or tricuspid stenosis**

C. Prolonged mid-late

S1   S2   S1
        OS

• **Severe mitral or tricuspid stenosis**

Figure 2.9. Classification of diastolic murmurs. A. An early diastolic decrescendo murmur is typical of aortic or pulmonic valve regurgitation. **B.** Mid to late low-frequency rumbling murmurs are usually the result of mitral or tricuspid valve stenosis, which follows a sharp opening snap (OS). Presystolic accentuation of the murmur occurs in patients in normal sinus rhythm because of the transient rise in atrial pressure during atrial contraction. **C.** In more severe mitral or tricuspid valve stenosis, the opening snap and diastolic murmur occur earlier and the murmur is prolonged. S_1, first heart sound; S_2, second heart sound.

gree to which the murmur fades depends on the severity of the stenosis. If the stenosis is severe, the murmur is prolonged; if the stenosis is mild, the murmur disappears in mid to late diastole. Regardless of whether the stenosis is mild or severe, the murmur intensifies at the end of diastole in patients in normal sinus rhythm, when atrial contraction accelerates flow across the valve (see Fig. 2.9). The murmur of mitral stenosis is low-pitched and is heard best with the bell of the stethoscope at the apex, while the patient lies in the left lateral decubitus position. The much less common murmur of tricuspid stenosis is better auscultated at the lower sternum, near the xiphoid process.

Hyperdynamic states such as fever, anemia, hyperthyroidism, and exercise cause increased flow across the normal tricuspid and mitral valves and can therefore result in a diastolic murmur. In patients with advanced mitral regurgitation, the expected systolic murmur can be accompanied by an additional diastolic murmur due to the increased volume of blood that must return back across the valve to the left ventricle in diastole. Similarly, patients with either tricuspid regurgitation or an atrial septal defect (see Chapter 16) may display a diastolic flow murmur across the tricuspid valve.

Continuous Murmurs

Continuous murmurs are heard throughout the cardiac cycle without an audible hiatus between systole and diastole. Such murmurs result from conditions in which there is a persistent pressure gradient between two structures during systole and diastole. An example is the murmur of patent ductus arteriosus, in which there is an abnormal communication between the aorta and pulmonary artery (see Chapter 16). During systole, blood flows from the high-pressure ascending aorta through the ductus into the lower-pressure pulmonary artery. During diastole, the aortic pressure remains greater

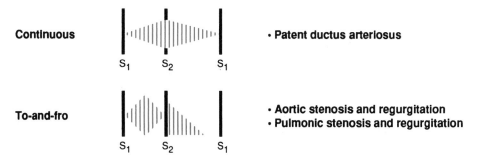

Figure 2.10. **A continuous murmur peaks at, and extends through, the second heart sound (S$_2$).** A "to-and-fro" murmur is not continuous; rather, there is a systolic component and a distinct diastolic component, separated by S$_2$. S$_1$, first heart sound.

than that in the pulmonary artery and flow continues across the ductus. This murmur begins in early systole, crescendos to its maximum at S$_2$, then decrescendos until the next S$_1$ (Fig. 2.10).

The "to-and-fro" combined murmur in a patient with *both* aortic stenosis and aortic regurgitation could be mistaken for a continuous murmur (see Fig. 2.10): During systole there is a diamond-shaped ejection murmur, and during diastole a decrescendo murmur. However, in the case of such a to-and-fro murmur, the sound does not extend through S$_2$, as it has discrete systolic and diastolic components.

SUMMARY

Abnormal heart sounds and murmurs are common in acquired and congenital heart disease. Although it may seem difficult to remember even the basic features presented here, it will become easier as you learn more about the pathophysiology of these conditions, and as your physical diagnosis experience grows. For now, just remember that the information is here and refer to it as needed. Tables 2.2 and 2.3 and Figure 2.11 summarize features of the most common heart sounds and murmurs described in this chapter.

TABLE 2.2 Common Heart Sounds

Sound	Location (& Pitch)	Significance
S$_1$	Apex (high-pitched)	Normal closure of mitral and tricuspid valves
S$_2$	Base (high-pitched)	Normal closure of aortic (A$_2$) and pulmonic (P$_2$) valves
Extra Systolic Sounds		
Ejection clicks	*Aortic:* apex & base	Aortic or pulmonic stenosis, or dilatation of aortic root
	Pulmonic: base	or pulmonary artery
	(both are high-pitched)	
Mid/late click	*Mitral:* apex	Mitral or tricupid valve prolapse
	Tricuspid: left lower	
	sternal border	
	(both are high-pitched)	
Extra Diastolic Sounds		
Opening snap	Apex (high-pitched)	Mitral stenosis
S$_3$	(*left-sided*): Apex	Normal in children
	(low-pitched)	Abnormal in adults: indicates heart failure or volume
		overload state
S$_4$	(*left-sided*): Apex	Reduced ventricular compliance
	(low-pitched)	

TABLE 2.3 Common Murmurs

Murmur Type		Examples	Location & Radiation
Systolic ejection		Aortic stenosis	2nd right interspace → neck (but may radiate widely)
		Pulmonic stenosis	2nd-3rd left interspace
Pansystolic		Mitral regurgitation Tricuspid regurgitation	Apex → axilla Left lower sternal border → right lower sternal border
Late systolic		Mitral valve prolapse	Apex → axilla
Early diastolic		Aortic regurgitation Pulmonic regurgitation	Along left side of sternum Upper left side of sternum
Mid/late diastolic		Mitral stenosis	Apex

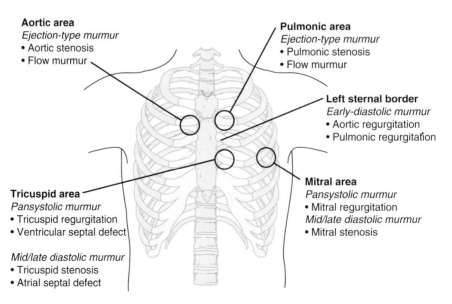

Figure 2.11. Locations of maximum intensity of the murmurs presented in this chapter.

Acknowledgments   Contributors to the previous editions of this chapter were Oscar Benavidez, MD; Bradley S. Marino, MD; Allan Goldblatt, MD; and Leonard S. Lilly, MD.

ADDITIONAL READING

Bickley LS. Bates' Guide to Physical Examination and History Taking. 7th Ed. Philadelphia: Lippincott Williams & Wilkins, 1999.

Constant J. Bedside Cardiology. 5th Ed. Philadelphia: Lippincott Williams & Wilkins, 1999.

DeGowin RL, DeGowin EL. Bedside Diagnostic Examination. New York: Macmillan, 1994.

Marriott HJL. Bedside Cardiac Diagnosis. Philadelphia: JB Lippincott, 1993.

Orient JM, Sapira JD. Sapira's Art and Science of Bedside Diagnosis. 2nd Ed. Philadelphia: Lippincott Williams & Wilkins, 2000.

Diagnostic Imaging and Cardiac Catheterization

Patrick Yachimski and Patricia Challender Come

Chapter
3

Cardiac Radiography
  Cardiac Silhouette
  Pulmonary Manifestations
Echocardiography
  Ventricular Assessment
  Valvular Lesions
  Coronary Artery Disease
  Cardiomyopathy
  Pericardial Disease

Cardiac Catheterization
  Measurement of Pressure
  Measurement of Blood Flow
  Calculation of Vascular Resistance
  Contrast Angiography
Nuclear Imaging
  Assessment of Myocardial Perfusion
  Radionuclide Ventriculography
  Assessment of Myocardial Metabolism
Computed Tomography
Magnetic Resonance Imaging

Imaging plays a central role in the assessment of cardiac function and pathology. Traditional imaging modalities such as chest radiography, echocardiography, cardiac catheterization with cineangiography, and nuclear imaging are fundamental in the diagnosis and management of cardiovascular diseases. However, they are being increasingly supplemented by newer modalities, including computed tomography (CT) and magnetic resonance imaging (MRI).

This chapter presents an overview of these techniques as they are used to assess the cardiovascular disorders described in this book. It would be beneficial to familiarize yourself with the information now, but not to memorize the details. This chapter is meant as a reference, to be looked back to as needed while reading subsequent material.

CARDIAC RADIOGRAPHY

Penetration of x-rays through the body is inversely proportional to tissue density. Air-filled tissues, such as the lung, absorb few x-rays and expose the underlying film, causing it to appear black. In contrast, dense materials, such as bone, absorb more radiation and appear white, or radiopaque. For a boundary to show between two structures, they must differ in density. Myocardium, valves, and other intracardiac structures have densities similar to that of adjacent blood; consequently, radiography cannot delineate these structures unless they happen to be calcified. Conversely, heart borders adjacent to lung are depicted clearly because the heart and an air-filled lung have different densities. If the lung adjacent to the heart is diseased, however (as in pulmonary edema, consolidation, or collapse), the lung density will match that of the heart. In such a case, the cardiac border will be ill-defined.

Frontal and lateral radiographs are routinely used to assess the heart and lungs (Fig. 3.1). The *frontal* view is usually a posterior-anterior (PA) image in which the x-rays are transmitted from behind (i.e., posterior to) the patient, travel through the body, and then expose a sheet of film placed against the anterior chest. In the standard *lateral* view, the patient's left side is placed against the film plate and the x-rays pass through the body from right to left. The

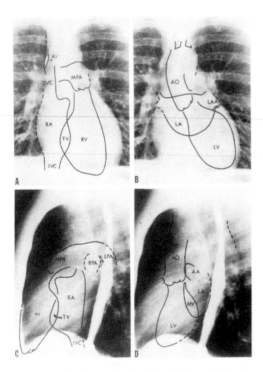

Figure 3.1. Posteroanterior (A and B) and lateral (C and D) chest radiographs from an individual without cardiopulmonary disease illustrating cardiac chambers and valves. AV, azygos vein; SVC, superior vena cava; RA, right atrium; IVC, inferior vena cava; TV, tricuspid valve; RV, right ventricle; MPA, main pulmonary artery; AO, aorta; LA, left atrium; LAA, left atrial appendage; LV, left ventricle; RPA, right pulmonary artery; LPA, left pulmonary artery; MV, mitral valve. (Reprinted with permission from Come PC, ed. Diagnostic Cardiology: Noninvasive Imaging Techniques. Philadelphia: JB Lippincott, 1985.)

frontal radiograph is particularly good for assessing the size of the left ventricle, left atrial appendage, pulmonary artery, aorta, and superior vena cava; the lateral view evaluates right ventricular size, posterior borders of the left atrium and ventricle, and PA diameter of the thorax. In some cases, optimal evaluation of the heart requires right and left anterior oblique views as well.

Cardiac Silhouette

Chest radiographs are used to evaluate the size of heart chambers and the pulmonary consequences of heart disease. Alterations in chamber size are reflected by changes in the cardiac silhouette. In the

frontal view of adults, the heart shadow should occupy 50% or less of the maximal width of the thorax, measured between the inner margins of the ribs (although in children, normal cardiac diameter may be up to 60% of the thoracic width). Thus, the *cardio/thoracic ratio* is used instead of absolute measurements to account for differences in body habitus.

There are several situations in which the cardiac silhouette inaccurately reflects heart size. An elevated diaphragm or narrow chest PA diameter, for example, may cause the heart to appear to spread out transversely. Consequently, the silhouette on a PA chest film may be greater than 50% of the thorax even though the *actual* heart size is normal. Therefore, the chest PA diameter should be assessed on the lateral view before one concludes that a frontal image truly represents an enlarged heart. The presence of a pericardial effusion around the heart can also enlarge the cardiac silhouette, because fluid and myocardium affect x-ray penetration similarly.

Radiographs can depict dilatation of the cardiac chambers and great vessels. Hypertrophy alone *may not* result in radiographic abnormalities, because it generally occurs at the expense of the cavity's internal volume and produces little or no change in overall cardiac size. Hypertrophy is more readily suspected from abnormalities on the electrocardiogram or by directly measuring wall thickness by echocardiography (see below). Major causes of chamber and great vessel dilatation include heart failure, valvular lesions, abnormal intracardiac and extracardiac communications (shunts), and certain pulmonary disorders. Because dilatation takes time to develop, recent lesions, such as *acute* mitral insufficiency, may present without apparent cardiac enlargement.

The pattern of chamber enlargement may suggest specific disease entities. For example, dilatation of the left atrium and right ventricle, accompanied by signs of pulmonary hypertension, suggests mitral stenosis (Fig. 3.2). In contrast, dilatation of the pulmonary artery and right heart chambers, but without enlargement of the left-

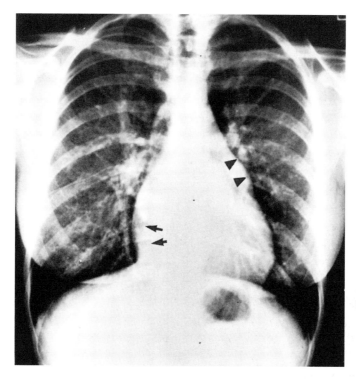

Figure 3.2. Posteroanterior chest radiograph from a patient with severe mitral stenosis and secondary pulmonary vascular congestion. The radiograph shows a prominent left atrial appendage (arrowheads) with consequent straightening of the left heart border and suggestion of a double density right cardiac border (arrows) produced by the enlarged left atrium. The aortic silhouette is small, which suggests chronic low cardiac output. Radiographic signs of pulmonary vascular congestion include increased caliber of upper zone pulmonary vessel markings and decreased caliber of lower zone vessels.

sided heart dimensions, suggests pulmonary vascular obstruction or increased pulmonary artery blood flow (e.g., due to an atrial septal defect; see Fig. 3.3).

The shape of the dilated chamber may also provide etiologic clues. For instance, in left ventricular volume overload due to valvular insufficiency, the ventricle tends to enlarge primarily in its long axis, displacing the apex downward and to the left. In contrast, when left ventricular dilation results from primary myocardial dysfunction, left ventricular length and width are generally both increased, causing the heart to appear globular.

Dilatation of the aorta and pulmonary artery can also be detected by chest radiographs. Causes of aortic dilatation include aneurysm, dissection, and aortic valve disease (Fig. 3.4). The pulmonary artery may be enlarged in patients with left-to-right shunts, which cause increased pulmonary

blood flow (see Fig. 3.3), and in those with pulmonary hypertension of diverse causes. Isolated enlargement of the proximal left pulmonary artery is seen in some patients with pulmonic stenosis.

Pulmonary Manifestations

The appearance of the pulmonary vasculature reflects abnormalities of pulmonary arterial and venous pressures and pulmonary blood flow. Increased pulmonary venous pressure, as occurs in left heart failure, causes increased vascular markings, redistribution of blood flow from the bases to the apices of the lungs (termed "cephalization" of vessels), pulmonary edema, the presence of abnormal septal lines (Kerley lines), and pleural effusions (Fig. 3.5). Blood flow redistribution appears as an increase in the number or width of vascular markings at the apex. Interstitial and alveolar

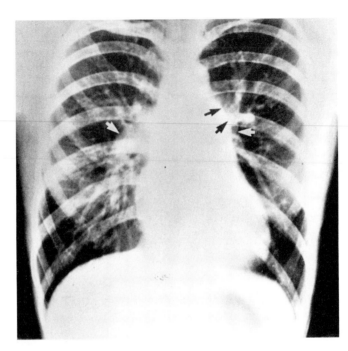

Figure 3.3. Posteroanterior chest radiograph of a patient with pulmonary hypertension secondary to an atrial septal defect. Radiographic signs of pulmonary hypertension include pulmonary artery dilatation (black arrows) (compare with the appearance of left atrial appendage dilatation in Fig. 3.2) and large central pulmonary arteries (white arrows) associated with small peripheral vessels (a pattern known as "peripheral pruning").

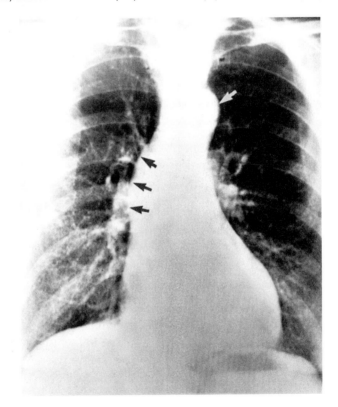

Figure 3.4. Posteroanterior chest radiograph from a patient with aortic stenosis and insufficiency secondary to a bicuspid aortic valve. In addition to poststenotic dilatation of the ascending aorta (black arrows), the transverse aorta (white arrow) is prominent, which suggests aortic insufficiency in addition to stenosis.

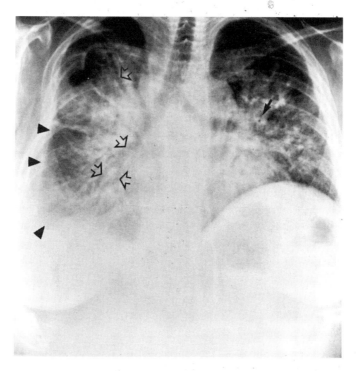

Figure 3.5. **Posteroanterior radiograph of a patient with severe congestive heart failure.** Pulmonary vascular congestion is indicated by vascular redistribution from the bases to the apices of the lungs (although in severe CHF there is increased pulmonary vascular markings throughout the lung fields), peribronchiolar cuffing (black arrow), and pleural effusion, which is indicated by blunting of the costodiaphragmatic angle and tracking up the right lateral hemithorax (black arrowheads). The presence of interstitial and alveolar edema produces perihilar haziness and air bronchograms (open arrows), which occur when the radiolucent bronchial tree is contrasted with opaque edematous lung tissue. (Courtesy of Robert Pugatch, MD, Brigham and Women's Hospital, Boston, MA.)

pulmonary edema produce opacity radiating from the hilar region bilaterally (known as a "butterfly pattern") and air bronchograms, respectively. Septal lines, which depict fluid in interlobular spaces, result from interstitial edema. Pleural effusions cause blunting of the costodiaphragmatic angles.

Changes in pulmonary blood flow may also alter the appearance of the pulmonary vessels. Focal oligemia (decreased flow) may result from pulmonary embolism or replacement of functioning lung tissue by emphysematous bullae. The finding of enlarged central pulmonary arteries, but small peripheral vessels (termed "peripheral pruning"), suggests pulmonary hypertension (see Fig. 3.3).

Table 3.1 summarizes the major radiographic findings in common forms of cardiac disease.

ECHOCARDIOGRAPHY

Echocardiography plays an essential role in the diagnosis and serial evaluation of many cardiac disorders. It is safe, noninvasive, relatively inexpensive, and capable of accurately depicting a wide array of heart diseases. High-frequency (ultrasonic) waves, generated by a piezoelectric transducer, travel through body tissue and are reflected at interfaces where there are differences in the acoustic impedance of adjacent tissues. The reflected waves return to the transducer and cause mechanical deformation of the piezoelectric ceramic. The machine measures the time elapsed between the initiation and reception of the sound waves, and calculates the distance between the transducer and each anatomic reflecting surface. Images are then constructed from these calculations.

TABLE 3.1 Chest Radiography of Common Cardiac Disorders

Congestive heart failure	• Vascular redistribution from bases to apices of the lungs • Perivascular haziness • Peribronchiolar cuffing • Air bronchograms • Pleural effusions
Pulmonic valve stenosis	• Poststenotic dilatation of pulmonary artery • Normal cardiac chamber sizes • Clear lung fields
Aortic valve stenosis	• Poststenotic dilatation of ascending aorta • Normal cardiac chamber sizes (until heart fails) • Normal pulmonary vasculature
Aortic regurgitation	• Left ventricular enlargement • Dilated aorta
Mitral stenosis	• Enlarged left atrium • Small aorta (if chronic low cardiac output) • Signs of pulmonary venous congestion

Mitral regurgitation	• Left atrial dilatation
	• Left ventricular dilatation
	• If severe:
	  • Right ventricular dilatation
	  • Signs of congestive heart failure

Three types of echocardiographic modalities are generally performed: 1) M-mode, 2) two-dimensional (2-D), and 3) Doppler imaging. Each type of imaging can be performed from a variety of locations. Most commonly, *transthoracic* studies are performed, in which images are obtained by placing the transducer on the surface of the chest. When greater structural detail is required, *transesophageal* imaging is performed, as described below.

M-mode echocardiography was the first cardiac application of ultrasonography. It is now used rarely by itself because it provides limited data from one narrow ultrasonic beam, and only images along that single line are displayed. M-mode techniques continue to be valuable for measurement of wall thicknesses and chamber diameters and for accurate timing of valve movements (Fig. 3.6).

In **2-D echocardiography,** multiple ultrasonic beams are transmitted through a wide arc. The returning signals are integrated to produce two-dimensional images of the heart on a video monitor. As a result, this technique depicts anatomic relationships and defines the movement of cardiac structures relative to one another. The wide fields of view enhance the ability of 2-D echocardiograms to detect and display wall and valve motion, abnormal shunts, and intracardiac masses such as vegetations, thrombi, and tumors.

Each two-dimensional plane (Fig. 3.7) delineates only part of a given cardiac structure. Optimal evaluation of the entire heart is achieved by using combinations of views. In transthoracic echocardiography (TTE), in which the transducer is placed against the patient's skin, these include the standard parasternal long axis, parasternal short axis, apical four-chamber, apical two-chamber, and subcostal views. The *parasternal long axis* view is recorded with the transducer in the third or fourth intercostal space to the left of the sternum. This view is particularly useful for evaluation of the left atrium, mitral valve, left ventricle, and left ventricular outflow tract, which includes the aortic valve and adjacent interventricular septum. To obtain the *parasternal short axis* views, the transducer is rotated 90° from its position for the parasternal long axis view. The short axis images depict transverse planes of the heart. Several different levels are imaged to assess the aortic valve, mitral valve, and left ventricular wall

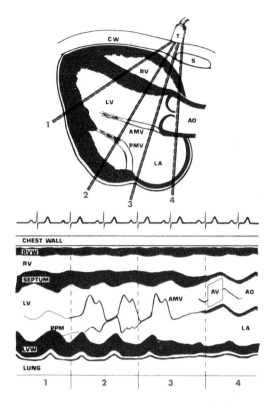

Figure 3.6. A schematic diagram of the heart in a parasternal long axis view is illustrated in the upper drawing. Below it is an electrocardiogram and an M-mode echocardiogram generated by changes in the direction of the transducer from position 1 to position 4. Chamber sizes and wall thicknesses can be measured along the vertical axis. Wall thickening and wall thinning with ventricular contraction and relaxation are evident, as is movement of the aortic and mitral valves. CW, chest wall; T, echocardiographic transducer; S, sternum; RV, right ventricle; LV, left ventricle; AO, aortic root; AMV, anterior mitral valve leaflet; LA, left atrium; RVW, right ventricular wall; AV, aortic valve; PPM, posterior papillary muscle region; LVW, left ventricular wall. (Reprinted with permission from Come PC. Echocardiography in diagnosis and management of cardiovascular disease. Compr Ther 1980;6:7–17. By permission of International Publishing Group, Cleveland, OH.)

motion. *Apical views* are produced when the transducer is placed at the point of maximal cardiac impulse. The apical four-chamber view evaluates the mitral and tricuspid valves as well as the atrial and ventricular chambers, including the motion of the lateral, septal, and apical left ventricular walls. The apical two-chamber view shows only the left side of the heart, and it depicts movement of the anterior, inferior, and api-

cal walls. In some patients, such as those with obstructive airways disease or obesity, the above views do not provide adequate depiction of cardiac structures because of signal attenuation caused by the increased air or adipose tissue. In such patients the *subcostal view*, in which the transducer is placed inferior to the rib cage, may provide a better ultrasonic window, allowing visualization of all four cardiac chambers.

Doppler ultrasonography evaluates blood flow direction, turbulence, and velocity, and it permits estimation of pressure gradients within the heart and great vessels. Doppler studies are based on the physical principle that waves reflected from a moving object undergo a frequency shift according to the moving object's velocity relative to the source of the waves. Color flow mapping converts the Doppler signals to an arbitrarily chosen scale of colors that represent direction, velocity, and turbulence of blood flow in a semiquantitative way. The colors are superimposed on 2-D images and show the location of stenotic and regurgitant valvular lesions and of abnormal communications within the heart and great vessels. For example, Doppler echocardiography in a patient with mitral regurgitation shows a jet of retrograde flow into the left atrium during systole (Fig. 3.8).

Sound frequency shifts are converted into blood flow velocity measurements (automatically calculated by the echo machine), by the relationship:

$$v = \frac{fs \cdot c}{2f_o(\cos \theta)}$$

in which v equals blood flow velocity (m/sec); fs, Doppler frequency shift (kHz); c, velocity of sound in body tissue (m/sec); f_o, frequency of the sound pulse emitted from the transducer (MHz); and θ, angle between the transmitted sound pulse and the mean axis of blood flow.

Transesophageal echocardiography (TEE) uses a miniaturized transducer mounted at the end of a modified endoscope to transmit and receive ultrasound waves from within the esophagus, thus producing very clear images of the neigh-

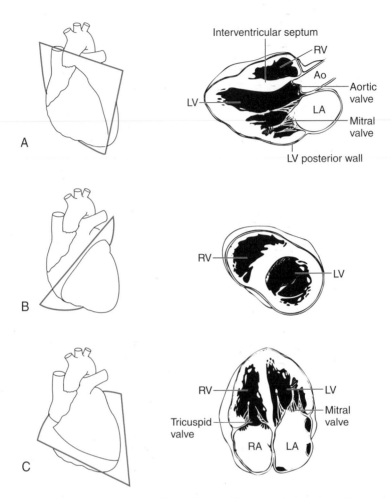

Figure 3.7. Transthoracic two-dimensional echocardiographic views. A. Parasternal long axis view.
B. Parasternal short axis view. **C.** Apical four-chamber view. LA, left atrium; RA, right atrium; LV, left ventricle; RV, right ventricle; Ao, aorta. (Modified from Sahn DJ, Anderson F. Two-Dimensional Anatomy of the Heart. New York: John Wiley & Sons, 1982.)

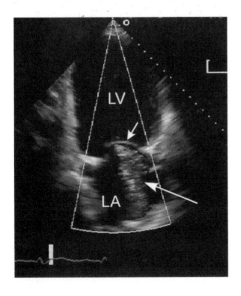

Figure 3.8. Doppler color-flow mapping (reproduced in gray tones) of mitral regurgitation (MR). The Doppler image, recorded in systole, is superimposed on an apical view of the left ventricle (LV), left atrium (LA), and mitral valve (short arrow). The retrograde flow of MR into the LA is indicated by the long arrow.

boring cardiac structures (Fig. 3.9) and much of the thoracic aorta. Modern probes permit multiplanar imaging and Doppler interrogation. TEE is particularly helpful in the assessment of aortic and atrial abnormalities, conditions that are less well-visualized by conventional transthoracic echo imaging. For example, TEE is more sensitive than transthoracic echo for the detection of thrombus within the left atrial appendage (Fig. 3.10), which is of great importance in patients with atrial fibrillation (see Chapter 12). The proximity of the esophagus to the heart makes TEE imaging particularly advantageous in patients in whom transthoracic echo images are unsatisfactory (e.g., patients with chronic obstructive lung disease).

TEE is also advantageous in the evaluation of patients with prosthetic heart valves. During standard transthoracic imaging, artificial mechanical valves reflect a large portion of ultrasound waves, thus masking visualization of more posterior structures. TEE aids visualization of the posterior chambers in such patients and is therefore the most sensitive noninvasive technique for evaluating perivalvular leaks.

TEE is commonly used to evaluate patients with cerebral ischemia of unexplained etiology, because it can identify cardiovascular causes of emboli with a high sensitivity. These etiologies include intracardiac thrombi or tumors, atherosclerotic debris within the aorta, and valvular vegetations. It is also highly sensitive and specific for the detection of aortic dissection.

In the operating room, TEE permits evaluation of surgical repair of congenital and valvular lesions. In addition, imaging of ventricular wall motion can identify periods of myocardial ischemia during high-risk surgery.

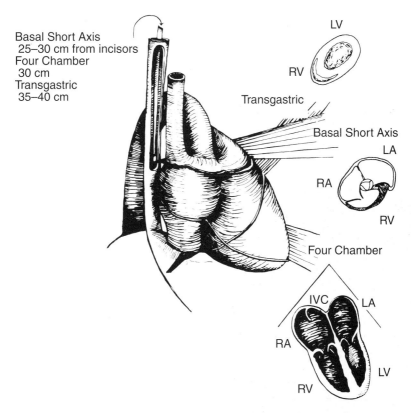

Figure 3.9. Transesophageal echocardiographic views. LA, left atrium; RA, right atrium; LV, left ventricle; RV, right ventricle; IVC, inferior vena cava. (Courtesy of Jane Freedman, MD, Boston University Medical Center, Boston, MA.)

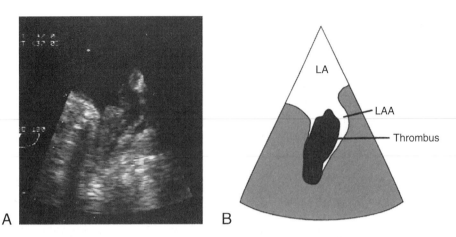

Figure 3.10. Echocardiographic assessment of intracardiac thrombus. A. Transesophageal echocardiographic image illustrating thrombus within the left atrial appendage. **B.** Schematic drawing of same image. LA, left atrium; LAA, left atrial appendage. (Courtesy of Scott Streckenbach, MD, Massachusetts General Hospital, Boston, MA.)

Contrast echocardiography is frequently used in the evaluation of congenital heart disease, as it is highly sensitive for the detection of abnormal intracardiac shunts. In this technique, an echocardiographic contrast agent (e.g., agitated saline) is rapidly injected into a peripheral (usually a brachial) vein. Using standard echocardiographic imaging, the "contrast" can be visualized passing through the cardiac chambers. Normally, there is rapid opacification of the right-sided chambers, but because the contrast is filtered out (harmlessly) in the lungs, it does not reach the left-sided chambers. However, in the presence of an intracardiac shunt with abnormal right-to-left heart blood flow, or the presence of an intrapulmonary shunt, contrast will appear in the left-sided chambers as well. Newer contrast agents have been developed with sufficiently small particle size to actually pass through the pulmonary circulation. Such agents are sometimes used to opacify the left ventricle and, via the coronary arteries, the myocardium, enabling superior assessment of LV contraction and myocardial perfusion.

Echocardiographic techniques can identify valvular lesions, complications of coronary artery disease, septal defects, intracardiac masses, cardiomyopathy, ventricular hypertrophy, pericardial disease, aortic disease, and congenital heart disease. Evalua-

tion includes assessment of cardiac chamber sizes, wall thicknesses, wall motion, valvular function, blood flow, and intracardiac hemodynamics. A few of these topics are highlighted below.

Ventricular Assessment

Two-dimensional echocardiography measures left ventricular systolic function by computing fractional changes between end-diastolic and end-systolic measurements. Left ventricular width, area, and volume in diastole and systole can be measured to assess contractile function and generate estimates of the ventricular ejection fraction. Two-dimensional echocardiography also depicts regional ventricular wall motion abnormalities, a common sign of coronary artery disease. Right ventricular (RV) function is generally assessed qualitatively, because the RV does not lend itself as easily to geometric modeling as does the left ventricle. Two-dimensional echocardiography is also useful in evaluating ventricular wall thickness and mass, important in patients with hypertension, aortic stenosis, or hypertrophic cardiomyopathy (Fig. 3.11).

Valvular Lesions

Echocardiography can assess underlying causes of valvular abnormalities. It also

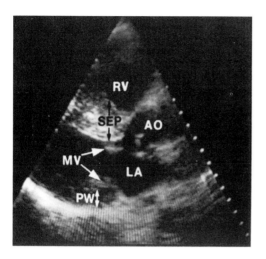

Figure 3.11. Diastolic parasternal long axis two-dimensional echocardiographic image of a patient with hypertrophic cardiomyopathy. A thickened septum (SEP), slight hypertrophy of the posterior ventricular wall (PW), and increased echogenicity of the septum are characteristic of hypertrophic cardiomyopathy. RV, right ventricle; AO aorta; MV mitral valve; LA, left atrium. (Reprinted with permission from Come PC, ed. Diagnostic Cardiology: Noninvasive Imaging Techniques. Philadelphia: JB Lippincott, 1985.)

helps to quantitate the severity of certain lesions, such as mitral stenosis and aortic stenosis. The pressure gradient across a stenotic valve can be easily calculated from the maximum blood flow velocity (v) measured distal to the valve, using the simplified Bernoulli equation:

$$\text{Pressure gradient} = 4 \times v^2$$

For example, if the peak velocity recorded distal to a stenotic aortic valve is 4 m/sec, then the calculated peak pressure gradient across the valve = $4 \times 4^2 = 64$ mm Hg. Other calculations (beyond the scope of this book) yield fairly accurate noninvasive measurements of aortic, mitral, and tricuspid valve areas. In addition, color Doppler analysis provides a qualitative assessment of the severity of regurgitant valve lesions.

Coronary Artery Disease

Echocardiography demonstrates ventricular wall motion abnormalities associated with infarcted or transiently ischemic myocardium. The location and degree of abnormal systolic contraction and de-

creased systolic wall thickening can estimate the extent of an infarction and implicate the responsible coronary artery. Infarct size measured by 2-D echocardiography correlates well with other methods of quantification.

Echocardiography is also used to detect complications of acute myocardial infarction, including intraventricular thrombus formation, papillary muscle rupture, valvular dysfunction, ventricular septal rupture, aneurysm formation, and pericardial effusion.

Although echocardiography can depict these *consequences* of coronary artery disease, transthoracic echo resolution is usually insufficient to directly image the coronary arteries themselves. In occasional patients, the most proximal portions of the coronaries can be delineated by this technique.

Stress echocardiography can be used to indirectly evaluate coronary artery disease. This technique assesses the development of left ventricular regional wall motion abnormalities induced by exercise or by the infusion of specific pharmacologic agents, such as dobutamine, dipyridamole, or adenosine (see Chapter 6). Reversible myocardial ischemia is recognized by a stress-induced wall motion abnormality.

Cardiomyopathy

Cardiomyopathies are heart muscle disorders that occur in three forms: dilated, hypertrophic, and restrictive (see Chapter 10). Echocardiography can often distinguish among these and permits assessment of the severity of myocardial dysfunction. For example, Figure 3.11 demonstrates the thickened ventricular walls typical of hypertrophic cardiomyopathy.

Pericardial Disease

Two-dimensional echocardiography can identify abnormal substances in the pericardial cavity (e.g., excessive pericardial fluid, fibrous material, tumor, clot). Tamponade and constrictive pericarditis, the main functional consequences of pericardial disease, are associated with particular echocardiographic abnormalities. In tamponade, the increased intrapericardial pressure compresses the cardiac chambers and results in cyclical "collapse" of the right atrium, right ventricle, and sometimes (in more extreme cases) of the left-sided chambers (Fig. 3.12). Constrictive pericarditis is associated with increased thickness or reflectiveness of the pericardial echo, abnormal patterns of diastolic left ventricular wall motion, and exaggerated changes in mitral and tricuspid valve inflow velocities during respiration.

Table 3.2 summarizes the salient echocardiographic features of common cardiac diseases.

CARDIAC CATHETERIZATION

In the diagnosis of many cardiovascular abnormalities, intravascular catheters are inserted to measure pressures in the heart chambers, to determine cardiac out-

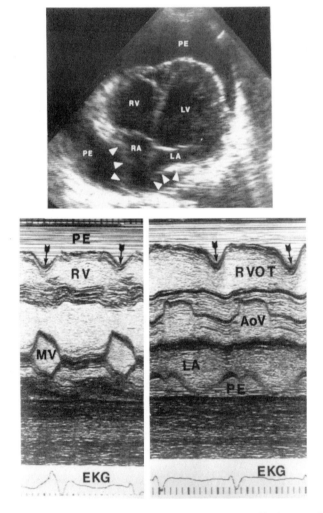

Figure 3.12. **Echocardiographic studies from a patient with pericardial effusion causing cardiac tamponade.** The apical four-chamber two-dimensional image (**upper panel**) shows a large pericardial effusion (PE) and inward collapse (white arrowheads) of the right atrium (RA) and left atrium (LA). M-mode tracings (**lower panels**) indicate early diastolic collapse of the right ventricular wall (black arrows). RV, right ventricle; LV, left ventricle; RVOT, right ventricular outflow tract; MV, mitral valve; AoV, aortic valve; EKG, electrocardiogram. (Reprinted with permission from Cunningham MJ, Safian RD, Come PC, et al. Absence of pulsus paradoxus in a patient with cardiac tamponade and coexisting pulmonary artery obstruction. Am J Med 1987; 83:973–976.)

TABLE 3.2 Echocardiography in Common Cardiac Disorders

	Valvular Lesions
Mitral stenosis	• Enlarged left atrium • Thickened mitral valve leaflets • Decreased movement and separation of mitral valve leaflets • Decreased mitral valve orifice
Mitral regurgitation	• Enlarged left atrium (if chronic) • Enlarged left ventricle (if chronic) • Systolic flow from left ventricle into left atrium (by Doppler)
Aortic stenosis	• Thickened aortic valve cusps • Decreased valve orifice • Increased ventricular wall thickness
Aortic regurgitation	• Enlarged left ventricle • Abnormalities of aortic valve or aortic root
	Left Ventricular Function
Myocardial infarction and complications	• Hypokinetic, dyskinetic, or akinetic ventricular wall motion • Decreased ejection fraction • Thrombus within left ventricle • Aneurysm of ventricular wall • Septal rupture (abnormal Doppler flow) • Papillary muscle rupture • Pericardial effusion
Cardiomyopathies **Dilated**	• Enlarged ventricular chamber sizes • Normal ventricular wall thicknesses • Decreased systolic contraction
Hypertrophic	• Normal or decreased ventricular chamber sizes • Increased ventricular wall thickness • Diastolic dysfunction (assessed by Doppler)
Restrictive	• Normal or decreased ventricular chamber sizes • Enlarged atria • Increased ventricular wall thickness • Ventricular contractile function usually normal

put and vascular resistances, and to inject radiopaque material to examine heart structures and blood flow. In 1929, Werner Forssmann performed the first cardiac catheterization, *on himself*, and humbly ushered in the era of invasive cardiology. Much of what is known about the pathophysiology of valvular heart disease and congestive heart failure comes from decades of subsequent hemodynamic research.

Measurement of Pressure

Before catheterization of an artery or vein, the patient is mildly sedated, and a local anesthetic is used to numb the skin site of catheter entry. The catheter, attached to a pressure transducer outside the body, is then introduced into the appropriate blood vessel. To measure pressures in the right atrium, right ventricle, and pulmonary artery, a catheter is usually inserted into a femoral, brachial, or jugular *vein*. Pressures in the aorta and left ventricle are measured via catheters inserted into a brachial or femoral *artery*. Once in the blood vessel, the catheter is guided by fluoroscopy (x-ray images) to the area of study, where pressure measurements are made. Figure 3.13 depicts normal intracardiac pressures.

The measurement of right heart pressures is performed with a specialized balloon-tipped catheter (e.g., a Swan Ganz catheter) that is advanced through the right side of the heart with the aid of normal blood flow. The catheter is typically inserted percutaneously into a peripheral vein (e.g., femoral, brachial, or internal jugular) and advanced toward the chest. When it reaches a vein of suitable size (e.g., the inferior or superior vena cava), the balloon is manually inflated so that venous re-

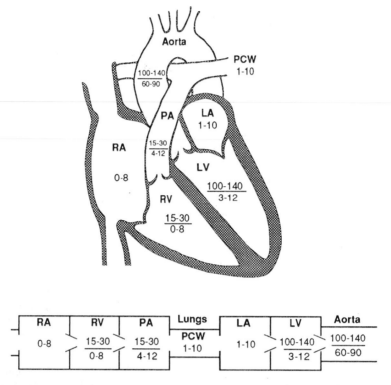

Figure 3.13. Diagrams indicating normal intracardiac chamber pressures. The top figure shows the normal anatomic relationship of the cardiac chambers, whereas the figure on the bottom shows a simplified schematic to clarify the pressure relationships. Numbers indicate pressures in mm Hg. RA, right atrial mean pressure; RV, right ventricular pressure; PA, pulmonary artery pressure; PCW, pulmonary capillary wedge mean pressure; LA, left atrial mean pressure; LV, left ventricular pressure.

turn of blood helps direct the catheter into the right-sided heart chambers and into the pulmonary artery. As it travels through the right side of the heart, recorded pressure measurements identify the catheter tip's position (Box 3.1).

Right Atrial Pressure

Right atrial pressure is equal to the central venous pressure (estimated by the jugular venous pressure on physical examination), because no obstructing valves impede blood return into the right atrium. Similarly, right atrial pressure normally equals right ventricular pressure in diastole, because the right heart functions as a common chamber when the tricuspid valve is open. The mean right atrial pressure is *reduced* when there is intravascular volume depletion. It is *elevated* in right ventricular failure, right-sided valvular dis-

ease, and cardiac tamponade (in which the cardiac chambers are surrounded by high-pressure pericardial fluid, as described in Chapter 14).

Certain abnormalities cause characteristic changes in individual components of the right atrial (and therefore jugular venous) pressure (Table 3.3). For example, a prominent *a* wave is seen in tricuspid stenosis and right ventricular hypertrophy. In these conditions, the right atrium contracts vigorously against the obstructing tricuspid valve or a stiff right ventricle, respectively, generating a prominent pressure wave. Similarly, amplified "cannon" *a* waves may be produced by conditions of atrioventricular dissociation (see Chapter 12), when the right atrium contracts against a closed tricuspid valve. A prominent *v* wave is observed in tricuspid regurgitation because normal right atrial filling is augmented by the regurgitated blood.

Box 3.1 Intracardiac Pressure Tracings

When a catheter is inserted into a systemic vein and advanced into the right side of the heart, each cardiac chamber produces a characteristic pressure tracing. It is important to distinguish these tracings from one another to localize the position of the catheter tip and to derive appropriate physiologic information.

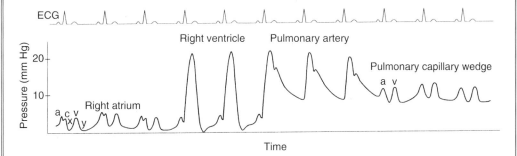

The normal *right atrial* (RA) pressure demonstrates three positive deflections (see Fig. 2.1): the *a* wave reflects right atrial contraction at the end of diastole, the *c* wave results from bulging of the tricuspid valve toward the right atrium as it closes in early systole, and the *v* wave represents passive filling of the right atrium from the systemic veins during systole, when the tricuspid valve is closed. The negative deflection that follows the *c* wave is known as the *x* descent, and the negative deflection after the *v* wave is called the *y* descent. Often, the *a* and *c* waves merge together so that only two major positive deflections are seen. In patients with atrial fibrillation (see Chapter 12), the *a* wave is absent because there is no organized left atrial contraction at the end of diastole.

As the catheter is advanced into the *right ventricle* (RV), a dramatic increase in systolic pressure is seen. The RV systolic waveform is characterized by a rapid upstroke and downstroke. In diastole, there is a gradual continuous increase in RV pressure as the chamber fills with blood.

As the catheter is moved forward into the *pulmonary artery* (PA), the systolic pressure remains the same as that in the RV (as long as there is no obstruction to RV outflow, such as pulmonic valve stenosis). However, three characteristics of the tracing indicate entry into the pulmonary artery: 1) the PA diastolic pressure is higher than that of the RV; 2) the descending systolic portion of the PA tracing inscribes a dicrotic notch—a small transient pressure increase that occurs after the systolic peak and is related to pulmonic valve closure; and 3) the diastolic portion of the PA tracing is downsloping compared with the upsloping RV diastolic pressure.

Further advancement of the catheter into a branch of the pulmonary artery results in the *pulmonary capillary wedge* (PCW) tracing, which reflects the left atrial pressure (see Fig. 3.14). Its characteristic shape is similar to the RA tracing, but the pressure values are usually higher and the tracing is often less clear (with the *c* wave not observed) because of damped transmission through the capillary vessels.

Right Ventricular Pressure

Right ventricular systolic pressure is increased by pulmonic valve stenosis or pulmonary hypertension. Right ventricular diastolic pressure increases when the right ventricle is subjected to pressure or volume overload and may be a sign of right-heart failure.

TABLE 3.3 Causes of Increased Intracardiac Pressures

Chamber and Measurement	Causes
Right atrial pressure	• Right ventricular failure • Cardiac tamponade
a wave	• Tricuspid stenosis • Right ventricular hypertrophy • Atrioventricular dissociation
v wave	• Tricuspid regurgitation • Right ventricular failure
Right ventricular pressure Systolic	• Pulmonic stenosis • Right ventricular failure • Pulmonary hypertension
Diastolic	• Right ventricular failure • Cardiac tamponade • Right ventricular hypertrophy

Pulmonary artery pressure
  Systolic and diastolic
	• Pulmonary hypertension
	  • Left-sided CHF
	  • Chronic lung disease
	  • Pulmonary vascular disease

Systolic only	• Increased flow (L → R shunt)
Pulmonary artery wedge pressure	• Left-sided CHF • Mitral stenosis or regurgitation • Cardiac tamponade
a wave	• Left ventricular hypertrophy
v wave	• Mitral regurgitation • Ventricular septal defect

Pulmonary Artery Pressure

Elevation of systolic and diastolic pulmonary artery pressures occurs in three conditions: 1) *left*-sided heart failure, 2) parenchymal lung disease (e.g., chronic bronchitis or end-stage emphysema), and 3) pulmonary vascular disease (e.g., pulmonary embolism or primary pulmonary hypertension). Normally, the pulmonary artery diastolic pressure is equivalent to the left atrial pressure because of the low resistance of the pulmonary vasculature that separates them. If the left atrial pressure rises because of left-sided heart failure, both systolic and diastolic pulmonary artery pressures increase in an obligatory manner to maintain forward flow through the lungs. This situation leads to "passive" pulmonary hypertension.

In certain conditions, however, pulmonary vascular resistance becomes abnormally high, causing pulmonary artery diastolic pressure to be elevated compared with left atrial pressure. For example, pulmonary vascular obstructive disease may develop as a complication of a chronic left-to-right cardiac shunt, such as an atrial or ventricular septal defect (see Chapter 16).

Pulmonary Artery Wedge Pressure

If a catheter is advanced into the right or left pulmonary artery, its tip will ultimately reach one of the small pulmonary artery branches and temporarily occlude forward blood flow beyond it. During that time, a column of stagnant blood stands between the catheter tip and the portions of the pulmonary capillary and pulmonary venous segments distal to it (Fig. 3.14). That column of blood acts as an "extension" of the catheter, and the pressure recorded through the catheter reflects that of the

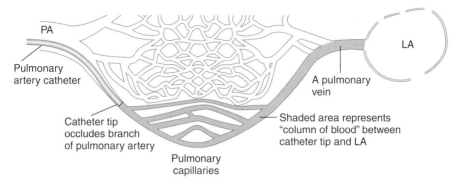

Figure 3.14. Diagram of a pulmonary artery catheter inserted into a branch of the pulmonary artery (PA). Flow is occluded in the arterial, arteriolar, and capillary vessels beyond the catheter; thus, these vessels act as a conduit that transmits the left atrial (LA) pressure to the catheter tip.

downstream chamber, namely the left atrium (LA). Such a pressure measurement is termed the "pulmonary artery wedge pressure" or "pulmonary capillary wedge pressure (PCW)" and closely matches the left atrial pressure in most individuals. Furthermore, while the mitral valve is open during diastole, the pulmonary venous bed, left atrium, and left ventricle normally share equal pressures. Thus, the PCW is also used to estimate the left ventricular diastolic pressure, a measurement of ventricular preload (see Chapter 9). As a result of this important feature, monitoring of PCW pressure is often useful in managing critically ill patients in the intensive care unit.

Elevation of the mean PCW is seen in left-sided heart failure and in mitral stenosis or regurgitation. The individual components of the PCW tracing may also become abnormally high. The *a* wave may be increased in conditions of decreased left ventricular compliance, such as left ventricular hypertrophy or acute myocardial ischemia. The *v* wave is greater than normal when there is increased left atrial filling during ventricular contraction, such as in mitral regurgitation.

Measurement of Blood Flow

Cardiac output is measured by either the thermodilution method or the Fick technique. In the thermodilution method, saline of a known temperature is injected rapidly into the right heart via a catheter side hole located a specific distance proximal to its tip. At the catheter tip, a thermistor registers the surrounding temperature in the pulmonary artery, which is transiently altered by the injected saline. The cardiac output is electronically calculated from the slope of the decay of the temperature change.

The Fick method is derived from the principle that consumption of oxygen by tissues is related to the O_2 content removed from blood as it flows through the capillary bed:

$$O_2 \text{ consumption} = O_2 \text{ content removed} \times \text{Flow}$$

$$\left(\frac{\text{ml } O_2}{\text{min}} \right) \qquad \left(\frac{\text{ml } O_2}{\text{ml blood}} \right) \left(\frac{\text{ml blood}}{\text{min}} \right)$$

Or, in other terms:

$$O_2 \text{ consumption} =$$
$$\text{AV } O_2 \text{ difference} \times \text{Cardiac output}$$

in which arteriovenous O_2 (AVO_2) difference equals the difference in oxygen content between the arterial and venous compartments. Total body oxygen consumption can be determined by analyzing expired air, and arterial and venous O_2 content is measured in blood samples. By rearranging the terms, the cardiac output can then be calculated:

$$\text{Cardiac output} = \frac{O_2 \text{ consumption}}{\text{AV } O_2 \text{ difference}}$$

For example, if the arterial blood in a normal adult contains 190 ml O_2/L and the venous blood contains 150 ml O_2/L, the arteriovenous difference is 40 ml O_2/L. If this patient has a measured O_2 consumption of 200 ml/min, then the cardiac output is 5 L/min.

In many forms of heart disease the cardiac output is lower than normal. In that situation, the total body oxygen consumption does not change significantly; however, a greater percentage of O_2 is extracted per volume of circulating blood by the metabolizing tissues. This leads to a lower than normal venous O_2 content and, therefore, an increased arteriovenous O_2 difference. In our example, if the venous blood contained only 100 ml O_2/L, the arteriovenous O_2 difference would be increased to 90 ml O_2/L, and the calculated cardiac output would be reduced to 2.2 L/min.

Since the normal range of cardiac output varies with a patient's size, it is common to report the *cardiac index*, which is equal to the cardiac output divided by the patient's body surface area (normal range of cardiac index = 2.6–4.2 L/min/M^2).

Calculation of Vascular Resistance

Once pressures and cardiac output have been determined, pulmonary and systemic vascular resistances can be calculated from the following formulas:

$$PVR = \frac{MPAP\text{-}LAP}{CO} \times 80$$

PVR, pulmonary vascular resistance (dynes-sec-cm^{-5})
MPAP, mean pulmonary artery pressure (mm Hg)
LAP, mean left atrial pressure (mm Hg)
CO, cardiac output (L/min)

$$SVR = \frac{MAP\text{-}RAP}{CO} \times 80$$

SVR, systemic vascular resistance (dynes-sec-cm^{-5})
MAP, mean arterial pressure (mm Hg)
RAP, mean right atrial pressure (mm Hg)
CO, cardiac output (L/min)
The normal PVR ranges from 20–130 dynes-sec-cm^{-5}. The normal SVR is 700–1600 dynes-sec-cm^{-5}.

Contrast Angiography

This technique, performed at the time of catheterization, uses radiopaque contrast material to visualize regions of the cardiovascular system. A catheter is introduced into an appropriate vessel and guided under fluoroscopy to the site where the contrast will be injected. Following administration of the contrast agent, x-rays are transmitted through the area of interest. A single exposure produces one film image, whereas a series of x-ray exposures are recorded to produce a "motion picture," termed a cineangiogram.

A specialized type of contrast angiography, termed digital subtraction angiography (DSA), was developed to provide a clear image using less contrast material. In this technique, a computer processes the digitalized x-ray images and subtracts the background of soft tissue and bone, thus enhancing the image of the blood vessel or chamber into which contrast material was injected. DSA has certain advantages over conventional angiography: the techniques used to introduce contrast are often less invasive (e.g., use of smaller catheters), a lower concentration of contrast agent can be used, and greater image resolution may be achieved.

Selective injection of contrast material into the heart chambers is used to recognize valvular insufficiency, abnormal wall thickening, intracardiac shunts, thrombi within the heart, and congenital malformations and to measure ventricular contractile function. To image the right heart chambers, injection is made through a catheter inserted into the inferior or superior vena cava, the right atrium, or the right ventricle. The left side of the heart can be imaged by contrast injection through a catheter advanced into the left ventricle (Fig. 3.15).

A widespread application of contrast angiography is coronary artery angiography. Contrast injection into the coronary arteries is used to examine the location and severity of coronary atherosclerotic lesions (Figs. 3.16 and 3.17).

There is some risk associated with catheterization and contrast angiography. Complications are uncommon but include

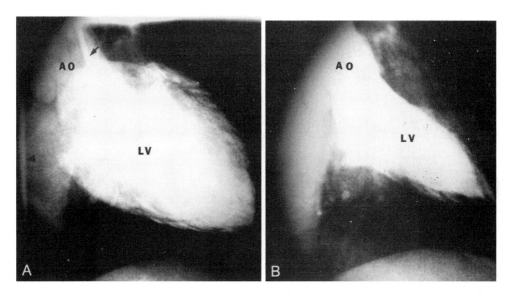

Figure 3.15. **Left ventriculograms in diastole (A) and systole (B) in the right anterior oblique projection from a patient with normal ventricular contractility.** This view depicts movement of the anterior apical and inferior walls. A catheter (arrow) is used to inject contrast into the left ventricle (LV). The catheter can also be seen in the descending aorta (arrowhead). AO, aortic root.

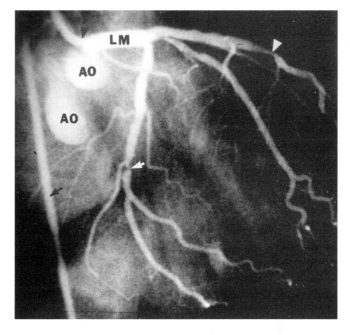

Figure 3.16. **Left coronary artery angiogram in the right anterior oblique projection from a patient with diffuse coronary artery disease.** The tip of the catheter (black arrowhead) is in the ostium of the left main (LM) coronary artery. The more distal catheter (black arrow) is seen within the descending aorta. The most critical stenoses are present in the left anterior descending coronary artery (white arrowhead) and at the origin (white arrow) of the third obtuse marginal branch of the left circumflex coronary artery. Some contrast can also be visualized in two of the aortic sinuses (AO) just above the aortic valve. (Courtesy of John Bittl, MD, Brigham and Women's Hospital, Boston, MA.)

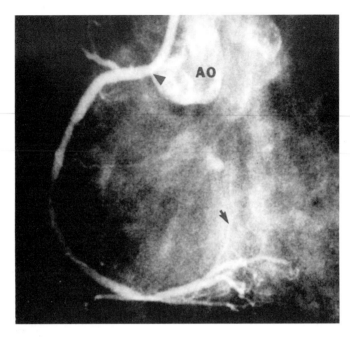

Figure 3.17. Right coronary artery angiogram in the left anterior oblique projection visualized with contrast injected by a catheter (arrowhead) positioned in the ostium of the dominant right coronary artery. Multiple areas of irregularities and stenosis can be seen. The AV nodal artery branches from the right coronary artery (arrow). AO, aorta. (Courtesy of John Bittl, MD, Brigham and Women's Hospital, Boston, MA.)

myocardial perforation by the catheter, precipitation of arrhythmias and conduction blocks, damage to vessel walls, dislodgement of atherosclerotic plaques, and infection. Complications resulting from the contrast medium itself include anaphylaxis and renal toxicity.

Table 3.4 summarizes the catheterization findings in common cardiac abnormalities. Therapeutic interventional catheterization techniques, such as percutaneous transluminal coronary angioplasty, are discussed in Chapter 6.

NUCLEAR IMAGING

Heart function can be evaluated using injected, radioactively labeled tracers and gamma-camera detectors. The resulting images reflect the distribution of the tracers within the cardiovascular system. Nuclear techniques are used to assess myocardial perfusion, to image blood passing through the heart and great vessels, to localize and quantify myocardial ischemia and infarction, and to assess myocardial metabolism.

TABLE 3.4. Cardiac Catheterization and Angiography in Cardiac Disorders

Coronary artery disease	• Identification of atherosclerotic lesions
Mitral regurgitation	• Large systolic v wave in left atrial pressure tracing
Mitral stenosis	• Abnormally high pressure gradient between left atrium and left ventricle in diastole
Tricuspid insufficiency	• Large systolic v wave in the right atrial pressure tracing
Aortic stenosis	• Systolic pressure gradient between left ventricle and aorta
Congestive heart failure	• Estimation of cardiac output • Calculation of systemic and pulmonary vascular resistances

Assessment of Myocardial Perfusion

Ischemia and infarction resulting from coronary artery disease can be detected by myocardial perfusion imaging using various radioisotopes, including thallium-201 (^{201}Tl) and technetium-99m labeled compounds (currently, ^{99m}Tc-sestamibi and ^{99m}Tc-tetrofosmin are widely used). Both ^{201}Tl and ^{99m}Tc-labeled compounds are sensitive for the detection of ischemic or scarred myocardium, but each of these types has certain advantages. For example, the ^{99m}Tc-labeled agents provide better image quality and are superior for detailed single photon emission computed tomography (SPECT) imaging (Fig. 3.18). Conversely, detection of myocardial cellular viability has been best documented by ^{201}Tl imaging.

In the case of ^{201}Tl imaging, the radioisotope is injected intravenously while a patient is exercising on a treadmill or stationary bicycle. Because thallium is a potassium analogue, it enters into normal myocytes, a process thought to be partially governed by the sodium-potassium ATPase pump. The intracellular concentration of thallium, estimated by the density of the image, depends on vascular supply (perfusion) and membrane function (tissue viability). In the normal heart, the radionuclide scan shows a homogenous distribution of thallium in the myocardial tissue. Conversely, myocardial

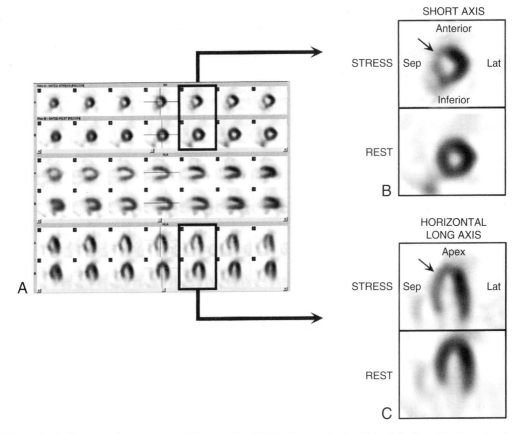

Figure 3.18. Stress and rest myocardial perfusion SPECT images (using ^{99m}Tc-tetrofosmin) of a patient with a high-grade stenosis within the proximal left anterior descending coronary artery. A. Miniaturized reproduction of the complete scan showing tomographic images in each of three views. The first, third, and fifth rows demonstrate images during stress, while the second, fourth, and sixth rows are matching images acquired at rest. **B and C.** Enlarged selected panels from part A showing stress and rest images in the short axis and horizontal long axis views. The arrows indicate regions of decreased perfusion during stress but normal perfusion on the matching resting scans, consistent with inducible ischemia. Sep, septal wall; Lat, lateral wall of the LV. (Courtesy of Marcelo Di Carli, MD, Brigham and Women's Hospital, Boston, MA.)

regions that are scarred (by previous infarction) or have reduced perfusion during exercise (i.e., myocardial ischemia) do not accumulate as much thallium as normal heart muscle. Consequently, these areas will appear on the thallium scan as light, or "cold" spots.

When evaluating for myocardial ischemia, an initial set of images is taken right after exercise and ^{201}Tl injection. Delayed images are acquired several hours later, because ^{201}Tl accumulation does not remain fixed in myocytes. Rather, there is continuous redistribution of the isotope across the cell membrane. After 3–4 hours of redistribution, when additional images are obtained, all viable myocytes should have equal concentrations of [201]Tl. Consequently, any defects due to myocardial *ischemia* on the initial postexercise scan will fill in on the delayed scan (and are therefore termed "reversible" defects), while those representing *infarcted* or scarred myocardium will persist as "cold" spots.

Of note, some myocardial segments that demonstrate persistent ^{201}Tl defects on both stress and redistribution imaging are falsely characterized as nonviable, scarred tissue. Sometimes, these areas represent ischemic, noncontractile but metabolically active areas that have the potential to regain function if an adequate blood supply is restored. For example, such areas may represent *hibernating* myocardium, segments that demonstrate diminished contractile function due to chronic reduction of coronary blood flow. This viable state can be differentiated from irreversibly scarred myocardium by repeat imaging after the injection of additional ^{201}Tl at rest to enhance uptake by viable cells.

[99m]Tc-sestamibi (commonly referred to as MIBI) typifies the use of ^{99m}Tc-labeled compounds. This compound is a large lipophilic molecule that, like thallium, is taken up in the myocardium in proportion to blood flow. The uptake mechanism differs in that the compound crosses the myocyte membrane passively, driven by the negative membrane potential. Once intracellular, it further accumulates in the mitochondria, driven by the even more negative mitochondrial membrane potential. The myocardial distribution of MIBI reflects perfusion at the moment of injection and in distinction to thallium, it remains fixed intracellularly. Consequently, obtaining MIBI images is more flexible: stress injection and imaging can be performed one day, and rest injection and imaging performed the next. Alternatively, MIBI imaging can be undertaken as a one-day protocol in which an injection and imaging are performed at rest, using a small tracer dose, followed a few hours later by injection and imaging after exercise using a larger tracer dose.

Stress nuclear imaging studies with either ^{201}Tl or ^{99m}Tc-labeled compounds have greater sensitivity and specificity (but are more expensive) than standard exercise electrocardiography for detecting ischemia due to coronary artery disease. Nuclear imaging for detection of coronary artery disease is particularly useful for patients with certain baseline ECG abnormalities that preclude accurate interpretation of a standard exercise test. Examples include patients with electronic pacemaker rhythms, those with left bundle branch block, and individuals who take certain medications that alter the ST segment, such as digoxin. In addition, nuclear scans provide more accurate anatomic localization of the ischemic segment(s) and quantification of the extent of ischemia compared with standard exercise testing. False-positive results, however, may still occur, particularly in obese patients or those in whom breast tissue attenuates the radioisotope signal.

Patients with orthopedic or neurologic conditions, as well those with severe physical deconditioning, may be unable to perform an adequate exercise test on a treadmill or bicycle. In such patients, stress images can instead be obtained by administering pharmacologic agents, such as adenosine or dipyridamole. These agents induce diffuse coronary vasodilation, which augments blood flow to myocardium perfused by healthy coronary arteries. Since ischemic regions are already maximally dilated (because of local metabolite accumulation), the drug-induced vasodilation causes a "steal" phenomenon, producing reduced isotope up-take in regions distal to significant coronary stenoses (described further in Chapter 6). Alternatively, dobutamine (see Chapter 17) can be infused intravenously to increase myocardial oxygen demand to test for ischemia.

In addition to its role in diagnosis of myocardial ischemia, nuclear imaging can also be used to assess the effectiveness of thrombolytic therapy after acute myocardial infarction (AMI), to risk-stratify patients after AMI, and to predict which patients would benefit from early mechanical revascularization.

Radionuclide Ventriculography

Radionuclide ventriculography (also known as blood pool imaging) is used to analyze right and left ventricular function (Fig. 3.19). A radioisotope (usually ^{99m}Tc) is bound to red blood cells or to human serum albumin and then injected as a bolus. Nuclear images are obtained at fixed time intervals as the labeled material passes through the heart and great vessels. Multiple images are displayed sequentially to produce a dynamic picture of blood flow. Calculations, such as the determination of ejection fraction, are based on the difference between radioactive counts present in the ventricle at end-diastole and at end-systole. Therefore, measurements are largely independent of any assumptions of ventricular geometry.

Radionuclide ventriculography is useful in assessing baseline cardiac function in patients scheduled to undergo potentially cardiotoxic chemotherapy (e.g., doxorubicin)

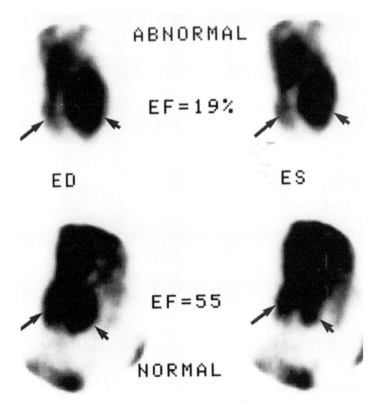

Figure 3.19. Gated blood pool scans in the left anterior oblique projection in diastole (left panels) and systole (right panels) of a patient with ischemic cardiomyopathy (top panels) and of a normal individual (lower panels). The patient with ischemic cardiomyopathy has a dilated left ventricle (short arrows) with globally reduced contraction. The right ventricle (long arrows) is normal in size, but its contraction is also diminished. Normal contraction of the right ventricle (long arrows) and the left ventricle (short arrows) is evident in the normal subject. EF, ejection fraction; ED, end diastole; ES, end systole.

and in following cardiac function over time in such patients. In addition, first-pass imaging and scans gated to the electrocardiogram permit recognition of abnormal cardiac and vascular shunts.

Assessment of Myocardial Metabolism

Positron emission tomography (PET) is a specialized nuclear imaging technique used to assess myocardial perfusion and viability. PET imaging employs positron-emitting isotopes (e.g., oxygen-15, carbon-11, rubidium-82, nitrogen-13, and fluorine-18) attached to a metabolic tracer. Sensitive detectors measure positron emission from the tracer molecules.

Myocardial perfusion is commonly assessed using nitrogen-13 labeled ammonia or rubidium-82. These flow tracers are taken up by myocytes in proportion to blood flow. *Myocardial viability* can be determined by studying glucose utilization in myocardial tissue. In normal myocardial metabolism, glucose is utilized for approximately 20% of energy production, with free fatty acids providing the remaining 80%. In ischemic conditions, however, metabolism shifts toward glucose use, and the more ischemic the myocardial tissue, the stronger the reliance on glucose. Fluoro-18 de-

oxyglucose (^{18}FDG), created by substituting fluorine-18 for hydrogen in 2-deoxyglucose, is used to study glucose uptake. This substance competes with glucose both for transport into myocytes and for subsequent phosphorylation. Unlike glucose, however, ^{18}FDG is not metabolized and becomes trapped within the myocyte.

Combining both perfusion and ^{18}FDG metabolism in a single PET study allows assessment of both regional blood flow and glucose uptake. PET scanning in this manner helps determine whether areas of ventricular contractile dysfunction due to decreased flow represent scar tissue, or whether the region is still viable (e.g., "hibernating" myocardium). In scar tissue, both blood flow to the affected area and ^{18}FDG uptake are decreased. Since the myocytes in this region are permanently scarred, such tissue is not likely to benefit from a revascularization procedure. Hibernating myocardium, in contrast, shows decreased blood flow but normal or elevated ^{18}FDG uptake.

PET imaging is limited by its expense and by the short half-life of the isotopes, which necessitates production by a nearby linear accelerator.

Table 3.5 summarizes the radionuclide imaging abnormalities associated with common cardiac conditions.

TABLE 3.5. Nuclear Imaging in Cardiac Disorders

Myocardial Ischemia:
Stress-delayed-re-injection T1-201
- Low uptake during stress with complete or partial fill-in with delayed or re-injection images
Rest-stress Tc-99m labeled compounds
- Normal uptake at rest with decreased uptake during stress
PET (N-13 ammonia/^{18}FDG)
- Decreased flow with normal or increased ^{18}FDG uptake during stress

Myocardial Infarction:
Stress-delayed-re-injection T1-201
- Low uptake during stress and low uptake after re-injection
Rest-stress Tc-99m labeled compounds
- Low uptake in rest and stress images
PET (N-13 ammonia/^{18}FDG)
- Decreased flow and decreased ^{18}FDG uptake at rest

"Hibernating" Myocardium:
Rest-delayed T1-201
- Complete or partial fill-in of defects after re-injection
PET (N-13 ammonia/^{18}FDG)
- Decreased flow and increased ^{18}FDG uptake at rest

Assessment of Ventricular Function:
Tc-99m RBC gated radionuclide ventriculography
- Assessment of global left and right ventricular function at rest or during exercise
- Regional wall motion

COMPUTED TOMOGRAPHY

Computed tomography (CT) uses thin x-ray beams to obtain axial plane images. An x-ray tube is programmed to rotate around the body, and the generated x-ray beams are partially absorbed by body tissues. The remaining beams emerge and are captured by electronic detectors, which relay information to a computer for image composition. CT scanning typically requires administration of an intravenous contrast agent to distinguish intravascular contents (e.g., LV blood volume) from neighboring soft tissue structures (e.g., LV myocardium).

Applications of standard CT in cardiac imaging include assessment of the great vessels, pericardium, and myocardial structures. CT can accurately diagnose aortic dissections and aneurysms (Fig. 3.20), and it can be used to monitor patients who have undergone surgical repair of these conditions. CT clearly delineates pericardial effusions as well as pericardial thickening and calcification. Myocardial abnormalities, such as regional hypertrophy or ventricular aneurysms, and intracardiac thrombus formation, can be distinctly visualized on CT images.

A limitation of conventional CT techniques is artifact generated by patient motion (i.e., breathing) during image acquisition. *Spiral CT* imaging utilizes newer technology that allows more rapid image acquisition, often during a single breath-hold period, at relatively lower radiation doses than conventional CT. Spiral CT has become increasingly important for its role in the diagnosis of pulmonary embolism. Such emboli create the appearance of "filling defects" in otherwise contrast-enhanced pulmonary vessels (Fig. 3.21).

Electron beam computed tomography (EBCT), or ultrafast CT, refers to an emerging CT technology that uses a direct electron beam to acquire images in a matter of milliseconds. Rapid succession of images depicts cardiac structures at multiple time points during a single cardiac cycle. Displaying these images in a cine "motion picture" format can provide estimates of left

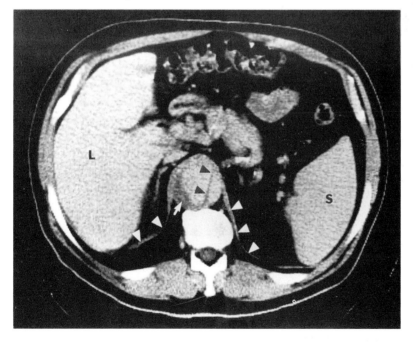

Figure 3.20. Abdominal CT scan of a patient with dissecting aortic aneurysm. Contrast has been injected that delineates the intimal flap (black arrowheads), which separates the opacified true and false lumens of the descending aorta. The nonopacified area in one lumen may represent a thrombus (white arrow). L, liver; S, spleen; white arrowheads, crura of the diaphragm.

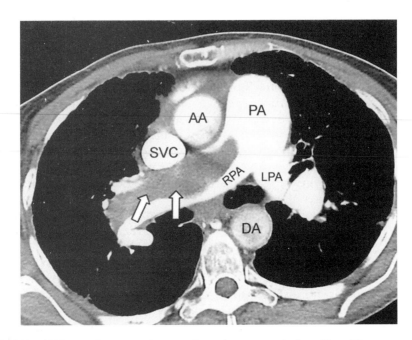

Figure 3.21. **Spiral CT image demonstrating massive pulmonary embolism.** The white arrows point to a large thrombus within the right pulmonary artery. It appears as a filling defect relative to the otherwise contrast-enhanced pulmonary vasculature. SVC, superior vena cava; AA, ascending aorta; PA, main pulmonary artery; RPA, right pulmonary artery; LPA, left pulmonary artery; DA, descending aorta.

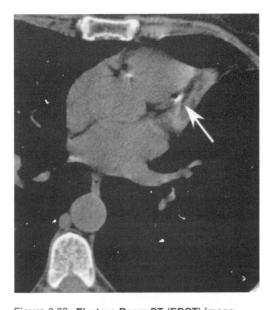

Figure 3.22. **Electron Beam CT (EBCT) image demonstrating coronary artery calcification.** Calcification of the left anterior descending coronary artery is indicated by the white arrow. (Courtesy of Melvin Clouse, MD, Beth Israel Deaconess Medical Center, Boston, MA.)

ventricular volumes, including stroke volume, and ejection fraction, expanding the application of CT to include not only heart structure but also cardiac function.

EBCT is also used to screen for atherosclerotic coronary artery disease by virtue of its ability to detect coronary artery calcification (Fig. 3.22). Calculation of a "calcium score" enables assessment of atherosclerotic plaque burden in the coronary vasculature. EBCT is rapid and relatively inexpensive, and it is significantly less invasive than fluoroscopy and contrast angiography. It is less clear, however, how well coronary artery calcification detected by EBCT correlates with clinically important stenoses. Thus, the use of EBCT as a screening test for coronary artery disease is currently controversial.

MAGNETIC RESONANCE IMAGING

Magnetic resonance imaging (MRI) uses a powerful magnetic field to obtain detailed images of internal structures. This technique is based on the magnetic polarity of hydrogen nuclei, which align themselves with an applied magnetic field. Radiofrequency excitation causes the nuclei to move out of alignment momentarily. As they return to their resting states, the nuclei emit radio waves, which are translated into computer-generated images. Therefore, MR imaging requires no ionized radiation. Furthermore, distinguishing water (i.e., blood) from soft tissue (e.g., myocardium) density does not require exogenous contrast, making standard MRI a completely noninvasive imaging modality.

The detail of soft tissue structures is often exquisitely demonstrated in MR images (Fig. 3.23). Cardiac MRI has an established role in the assessment of congenital anomalies and of diseases of the aorta, including aneurysm and dissection. It is also used to assess left and right ventricular mass and volumes, intravascular thrombus, neoplastic disease, and cardiomyopathies. "ECG-gated" and cine MRI techniques capture images at discrete time points in the cardiac cycle, and therefore permit evaluation of valvular and ventricular function.

Two applications of cardiac MRI deserve special mention. *Coronary magnetic reso-nance angiography* (coronary MRA) is a noninvasive, contrast-free angiographic imaging modality. Laminar blood flow appears as a bright signal intensity in coronary MRA, whereas turbulent blood flow, at the site of stenosis, results in less bright or absent signal intensity. In recent studies, this technique has shown high sensitivity and accuracy for the detection of important coronary artery disease in the left main coronary and of atherosclerotic blockages in the proximal or mid-portions of the three major coronary vessels. Coronary MRA is also useful in delineating coronary artery congenital anomalies.

In *contrast-enhanced MRI*, a gadolinium-based agent is administered intravenously to assess for myocardial viability (an exception to the rule that MRI is completely noninvasive). This technique is based on findings that gadolinium is excluded from viable cells with intact cell membranes, but can permeate and concentrate in nonviable, infarcted (i.e., irreversibly damaged) areas. Nonviable myocardial segments therefore appear "hyperenhanced" relative to viable, reversibly impaired myocardium (Fig. 3.24). Therefore, gadolinium-enhanced MRI can

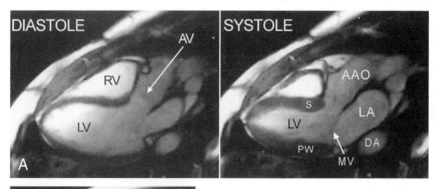

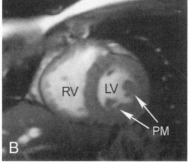

Figure 3.23. **Cardiac magnetic resonance images from a normal individual. A.** Three-chamber long-axis view of the heart in diastole and systole showing the left ventricle (LV), right ventricle (RV), and left atrium (LA). The mitral valve (MV), aortic valve (AV), ascending aorta (AAO), and descending aorta (DA) are also imaged. **B.** Mid-ventricular short-axis view demonstrating the LV, RV, and left ventricular papillary muscles (PM). (Courtesy of Raymond Y. Kwong, MD, Brigham and Women's Hospital, Boston, MA.) S, septum; PW, posterior wall.

TABLE 3.6 Summary of Cardiac Imaging Techniques

Imaging Technique	Cardiac Information Obtained	Examples of Clinical Uses
Chest radiography	• Cardiac and mediastinal contours • Pulmonary vascular markings	• Detect chamber dilatation • Identify consequences of stenotic and regurgitant valve lesions and intracardiac shunts • Visualize pulmonary signs of heart failure
Transthoracic echo-cardiography (TTE)	• Wall thickness, chamber dimensions • Anatomic relationships and motion of cardiac structures • Flow direction, turbulence, and velocity measurements • Echocontrast studies • Stress echocardiography	• Assess global and segmental ventricular contraction • Identify valvular abnormalities and vegetations • Diagnose consequences of myocardial infarction (e.g., ventricular aneurysm, papillary muscle rupture, intraventricular thrombus) • Identify myocardial, pericardial, and congenital abnormalities
Transesophageal echo-cardiography (TEE)	• Similar to TTE but higher resolution	• Visualize intracardiac thrombus • Evaluate prosthetic valves and peri-valvular leaks • Identify valvular vegetations and myo-cardial abscess in endocarditis • Diagnose aortic dissection • Monitor intraoperatively
Cardiac catheterization	• Pressure measurement • Contrast angiography	• Evaluate intracardiac pressures (e.g., in valvular disease, heart failure, pericardial disease) • Perform hemodynamic assessment (calcu-lation of cardiac output, vascular resis-tances) • Visualize ventricular contractile function, regurgitant valve lesions • Identify coronary artery anatomy and severity of stenoses
Nuclear SPECT imaging (using ^{99m}Tc-labeled compounds or ^{201}Thallium)	• Regional myocardial perfusion • Myocardial viability	• Detect, quantify, and localize myocardial ischemia • Perform stress testing in patients with baseline ECG abnormalities • Achieve risk stratification after MI • Distinguish viable myocardium from scar tissue
Radionuclide ven-triculography	• Ventricular contractile function	• Calculate ventricular ejection fraction and quantitate intracardiac shunts
Positron emission tomography (PET)	• Myocardial perfusion and metabolism	• Evaluate contractile function • Distinguish viable myocardium from scar tissue
Computed tomo-graphy (CT)	• Anatomy and structural relationships	• Diagnose disease of the great vessels (aortic dissection, pulmonary embolism) • Assess pericardial disease and myocardial abnormalities (hypertrophy, aneurysm, intraventricular thrombus) • Detect coronary artery calcification (EBCT)
Magnetic resonance imaging (MRI)	• Detailed soft tissue anatomy	• Assess myocardial structure and function (e.g., ventricular mass and volume, neo-plastic disease, intracardiac thrombus, cardiomyopathies) • Diagnose aortic and pericardial disease *Emerging uses:* • Identify coronary artery disease • Determine myocardial viability

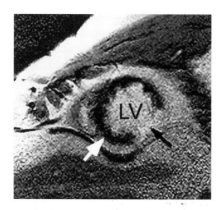

Figure 3.24. Gadolinium-enhanced magnetic resonance image demonstrating region of nonviable myocardium. This delayed-contrast cardiac magnetic resonance image shows the heart in short-axis view. The white arrow points to a nearly concentric ring of normal, viable myocardium. Contrast administration reveals transmural enhancement of the inferolateral ventricular wall (black arrow). Revascularization would not likely result in recovery of function of this myocardial segment. The left ventricular (LV) cavity is contrast-enhanced. (Courtesy of Warren Manning, MD, Beth Israel Deaconess Medical Center, Boston, MA.)

help select patients who will benefit from revascularization procedures.

SUMMARY

This chapter presented an overview of imaging and catheterization techniques currently available to assess cardiac structure and function. Many of these tools are expensive and yield similar information. For example, estimates of ventricular contractile function can be made by echocardiography, nuclear imaging, contrast angiography, gated CT, or MRI. Myocardial viability can be assessed using nuclear imaging studies, gadolinium MRI, or dobutamine echocardiography.

Determining the single best test for any given patient depends on a number of factors. One is the ease by which images may be obtained. In a critically ill patient, bedside echocardiography provides an easily obtained measure of LV systolic function. Obtaining similar information from a nuclear study would require radioisotope administration and a trip to the nuclear scanner. Another factor to consider is the degree of invasiveness of a given imaging tech-

nique. Expense, available equipment, and institutional preference and expertise also play roles in determining the choice of an imaging approach. When used appropriately, each imaging tool can provide important information to guide the diagnosis and management of cardiovascular disorders.

Table 3.6 summarizes the uses of imaging techniques described in this chapter.

Acknowledgments   The authors are grateful to Dr. Warren Manning and Dr. Marcelo Di Carli for their helpful suggestions. Contributors to the previous editions of this chapter were Deborah Bucino, MD; Albert S. Tu, MD; Sharon Horesh, MD; Shona Pendse, MD; and Patricia C. Come, MD.

ADDITIONAL READING

American College of Cardiology/American Heart Association expert consensus document on electron-beam computed tomography for the diagnosis and prognosis of coronary artery disease. Circulation 2000;102:126–140.

Baim D, Grossman W. Grossman's Cardiac Catheterization, Angiography and Intervention. 6th Ed. Philadelphia: Lippincott Williams & Wilkins, 2000.

Daniel WG, Mügge A. Medical progress: transesophageal echocardiography. N Engl J Med 1995;332:1268–1279.

Feigenbaum H. Echocardiography. 5th Ed. Philadelphia: Lippincott Williams & Wilkins, 1995.

Jain D, Zaret BL. Nuclear imaging techniques for the assessment of myocardial viability. Cardiol Clin 1995;13:43–56.

Kim RJ, Wu E, Rafael A, et al. The use of contrast-enhanced magnetic resonance imaging to identify reversible myocardial dysfunction. N Engl J Med 2000;343:1445–1453.

Kim WY, Danias PG, Stuber M, et al. Coronary magnetic resonance angiography for the detection of coronary stenoses. N Engl J Med 2001;345:1863–1869.

Lee TH, Boucher CA. Noninvasive tests in patients with stable coronary artery disease. N Engl J Med 2001;344:1840–1845.

McConnell MV, Ganz P, Selwyn AP, et al. Identification of anomalous coronary arteries and their anatomic course by magnetic resonance coronary angiography. Circulation 1995;92:3158–3162.

Ritchie JL, Bateman TM, Bonow RO, et al. Guidelines for clinical use of cardiac radionuclide imaging. Report of the American College of Cardiology/American Heart Association Task Force on Assessment of Diagnostic and Therapeutic Cardiovascular Procedures (Committee on Radionuclide Imaging). J Am Coll Cardiol 1995;25:521–547.

Weyman AE. Principles and Practice of Echocardiography. 2nd Ed. Philadelphia: Lippincott Williams & Wilkins, 1994.

The Electrocardiogram

Leonard S. Lilly

Electrical Measurement—Single Cell Model
ECG Lead Reference System
Sequence of Normal Cardiac Activation
   Technical Considerations
Interpretation of the Electrocardiogram
   Calibration
   Heart Rhythm

Heart Rate
Intervals (PR, QRS, ST)
Mean QRS Axis
Abnormalities of the P Wave
Abnormalities of the QRS Complex
ST Segment and T Wave Abnormalities

Cardiac contraction relies on the organized flow of electrical impulses through the heart. The electrocardiogram (ECG or EKG) is an easily obtained recording of that activity, and it provides a wealth of information about cardiac structure and function. This chapter presents the electrical basis of the ECG in health and disease and leads the reader through the basics of interpretation. To become fully adept at this technique and to practice the principles described here, the reader may wish to consult one of the complete electrocardiographic textbooks listed at the end of the chapter.

ELECTRICAL MEASUREMENT— SINGLE CELL MODEL

This section begins by observing the propagation of an electrical impulse within a single cardiac muscle cell, illustrated in Figure 4.1. On the right side of the diagram, a voltmeter records the electrical potential across the cell on graph paper. In the resting state, the cell is *polarized,* that is, the entire outside of the cell is electrically positive with respect to the inside, because of the ionic distribution across the cell membrane as described in Chapter 1. In this resting state, the voltmeter electrodes, which are placed on opposite outside surfaces of the cell, do not detect any electrical activity, because there is no electrical potential difference between them (the myocyte surface is homogeneously charged).

This equilibrium is disturbed, however, by stimulation of the cell (see Fig. 4.1B). During the action potential, as cations rush across the sarcolemma into the cell, the polarity at the stimulated region transiently reverses, such that the outside becomes negatively charged with respect to the inside; that is, the region **depolarizes.** At that moment, an electrical potential is created on the cell surface between the depolarized area (negatively charged surface) and the still polarized (positively charged surface) portions of the cell. An electrical current is therefore caused to flow between these two regions.

By convention, the direction of electrical current is said to flow from the negatively charged areas to the positively charged regions. Because the depolarization current in this example proceeds from left to right, that is, toward the (+) electrode of the voltmeter, an upward deflection is recorded. As the wave of depolarization spreads along the cell, additional electrical forces directed toward the (+) electrode record even a greater upward deflection (see Fig. 4.1C). Once the cell has become fully depolarized (see Fig. 4.1D), its outside is completely negatively charged with respect to the inside, the opposite of the initial resting condition. However, since the surface charge is homogeneous once again, the external electrodes measure a potential difference of zero and the voltmeter records a neutral "flat line" during this period.

Note that in Figure 4.1E, if the electrode wires of the voltmeter had been reversed so

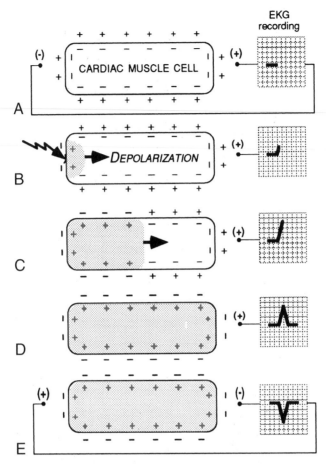

Figure 4.1. Depolarization of a single cardiac muscle cell. A. In the resting state, the surface of the cell is positively charged relative to the inside. Because the surface is homogeneously charged, the voltmeter electrodes outside the cell do not record any electrical potential difference ("flat line" recording). **B.** Stimulation of the cell initiates depolarization (shaded area); the outside of the depolarized region becomes negatively charged relative to the inside. Because the current of depolarization is directed toward the (+) electrode of the voltmeter, an upward deflection is recorded. **C.** Depolarization spreads, creating a greater upward deflection by the recording electrode. **D.** The cell has become fully depolarized. The surface of the cell is now completely negatively charged compared with the inside. Because the surface is again homogeneously charged, a flat line is recorded by the voltmeter. **E.** Note that if the position of the voltmeter electrodes had been reversed, the wave of depolarization would have traveled away from the (+) electrode so that the ECG deflection would be downward.

that the (+) pole was placed to the *left* of the cell, then as the wave of depolarization proceeded toward the right, it would have headed *away* from the (+) electrode and the recorded deflection would have been *downward*. This relationship should be kept in mind when the polarity of ECG leads is discussed below.

Depolarization of the cell initiates cardiac muscle contraction and is then followed by **repolarization,** the process by which the cellular charges return to the resting state (Fig. 4.2). As the left side of the cell begins to repolarize, its surface charge becomes positive once again. A current is therefore generated from the still negatively charged surface toward the positively charged area. Because this current is directed away from the voltmeter's (+) electrode, a downward deflection is recorded, opposite to that which was observed during the process of depolarization. Repolarization is a slower process than depolarization, so that the inscribed deflection of repolarization is wider and of lower magnitude. Once the cell has returned to the resting state, the surface charges are once again homogeneous, and no further electrical potential is detected, resulting in a "flat line" on the voltmeter recording (see Fig. 4.2C).

It is important to note that in the intact human heart, the sequence of repolarization actually proceeds in the direction *opposite* that of depolarization. This is so because myocardial action potential durations are more prolonged in cells near the endocardium (the first cells stimulated by Purkinje fibers) than in myocytes near the outer epicardium (the last cells to depolarize). As a result, the recorded pattern of repolarization is usually the inverse of what

was presented in this example. That is, the current of repolarization (negative to positive flow) in Figure 4.2 would be directed *toward* the (+) electrode and would therefore inscribe an *upright* deflection on the recording. Thus, in a normal individual, the forces of depolarization and repolarization are usually oriented in the *same* direction on the ECG recording (see Fig. 4–2D).

The depolarization and repolarization of a single cardiac muscle cell have been considered here. As the wave of depolarization spreads rapidly through the heart, electrical forces are generated by each cell, and it is the sum of these forces, measured at the skin's surface, that is recorded by the ECG

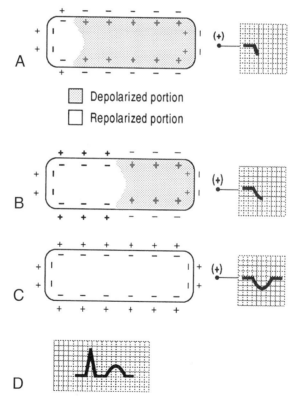

Figure 4.2. **Sequence of repolarization of a single cardiac muscle cell. A.** As repolarization commences, positive charges re-emerge on the surface of the cell, and a current flows from the still negatively charged surface areas to the repolarized region. Because the current is directed away from the (+) electrode of the voltmeter, a downward deflection is recorded. **B.** Repolarization progresses. **C.** Repolarization has been completed and the outside surface of the cell is once again homogeneously charged, so that no further electrical potential is detected ("flat line" once again). **D.** In the human heart, repolarization proceeds in a direction *opposite* that of depolarization (would be from right to left in this example, and the wave of repolarization would be upright). Therefore, the *deflections of depolarization and repolarization of the normal intact heart are in the same direction*, as shown here. Note that the wave of repolarization is of lower amplitude and more prolonged than that of depolarization.

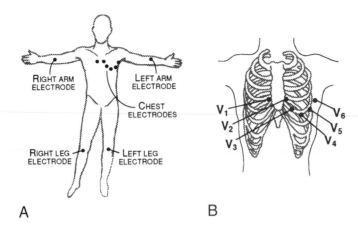

Figure 4.3. **A.** Standard positions of the ECG electrodes. **B.** Close-up view of chest electrode placement.

machine. The direction and magnitude of the deflections on the ECG recording depend on how the electrical forces are aligned to a set of specific reference axes, known as ECG leads.

ECG LEAD REFERENCE SYSTEM

When the ECG was first invented, the recording was made by dunking the patient's arms and legs into large buckets of electrolyte solution that were wired to the machine. As can be imagined, that was fairly messy and fortunately is no longer necessary. Instead, wire electrodes are placed directly on the skin, held in place by adhesive tabs, in the arrangement shown in Figure 4.3. The right leg electrode is not used for measurement but serves as an electrical ground.

The complete ECG tracing is formed by recording the electrical forces between standard positions of the skin electrodes. Figure 4.4 demonstrates the orientation of the six standard reference axes (termed ECG leads), which are electronically constructed by recording between the wire electrodes on the arms and left leg.

The ECG machine records lead **aVR** by selecting the *right* arm electrode as the (+) pole with respect to the other electrodes. This is known as a **unipolar** lead, because there is no single (−) pole; rather, all the other electrodes are averaged together to create a composite (−) reference. When the

instantaneous electrical activity of the heart points in the direction of the right arm, an upward deflection is recorded in lead aVR. However, when the electrical forces are heading away from the right arm, the ECG inscribes a downward deflection in aVR.

Similarly, lead **aVF** is recorded by setting the left leg as the (+) pole, such that a positive deflection is recorded when forces are directed toward the *feet*. **aVL** is selected when the *left* arm electrode is made the (+) pole and records an upward deflection when electrical activity is aimed in that direction.

In addition to these three unipolar limb leads, three **bipolar** leads are also part of the standard ECG recording (see Fig. 4.4). Bipolar indicates that one limb electrode is the (+) pole and another *single* electrode provides the (−) reference. In this case, the ECG machine inscribes an upward deflection if electrical forces are heading toward the (+) electrode and records a downward deflection if the forces are heading toward the (−) electrode. A simple mnemonic to remember the placement of the bipolar leads is that the lead name indicates the number of Ls in the placement sites. For example, lead III connects the *left* arm to the *left leg*, lead II connects the right arm to the *left leg*, and lead I connects the *left* arm to the right arm. Table 4.1 lists how the six limb leads are derived.

By overlaying the six limb leads together, a reference system is established (Fig. 4.5). In

Unipolar Limb Leads

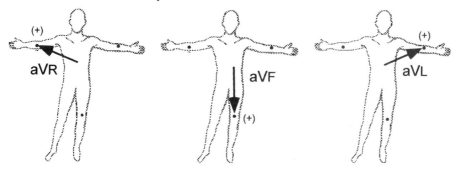

Bipolar Limb Leads

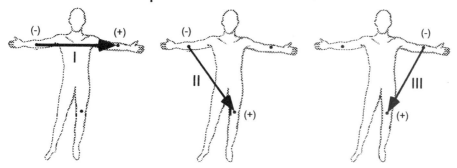

Figure 4.4. The six limb leads are formed from the electrodes placed on the arms and left leg. Each unipolar lead has a (+) designated electrode (for the unipolar leads, the (−) pole is an average of the other electrodes). Each bipolar lead has specific (−) and (+) designated electrodes.

this figure, each lead is presented with its (+) pole designated by an arrowhead, and the (−) aspect by dashed lines. Note that each 30° sector of the circle falls along the (+) or (−) pole of one of the standard six electrocardiographic leads. Also note that

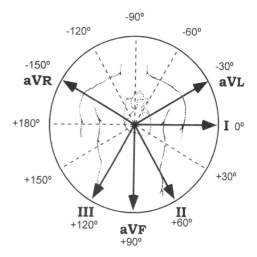

Figure 4.5. The axial reference system is created by combining together the leads shown in Figure 4.4. Each lead has a (+) region indicated by the arrowhead and a (−) region indicated by the dashed line.

TABLE 4.1. The Limb Leads

	(+) electrode	(−) electrode
Bipolar leads		
I	LA	RA
II	LL	RA
III	LL	LA
Unipolar leads		
aVR	RA	*
aVL	LA	*
aVF	LL	*

LA, left arm; *LL*, left leg; *RA*, right arm; *, (−) electrode constructed by combining all other electrodes together.

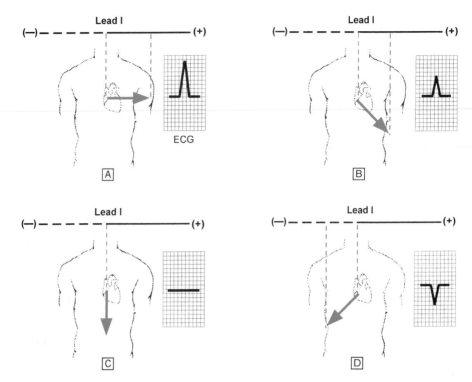

Figure 4.6. Relationship of the magnitude and direction of electrical activity to the ECG lead. A. The electrical vector is oriented parallel to lead I and aimed toward the (+) electrode; therefore, a tall, upward deflection is recorded by the lead. **B.** The vector is still oriented toward the (+) region of lead I but not *parallel* to the lead, so that only a component of the force is recorded. The recorded deflection is still upward but less tall compared with A. **C.** The electrical vector is perpendicular to lead I so that no deflection is generated. **D.** The vector is directed toward the (−) region of lead I so that a downward deflection is recorded by the ECG.

the (+) pole of lead I points to 0° and that, by convention, measurement of the angles proceeds clockwise as +30°, +60°, and so forth. The complete ECG recording provides a simultaneous "snapshot" of the heart's electrical activity, taken from the perspective of each of these lead reference lines.

Figure 4.6 demonstrates how the magnitude and direction of electrical activity are represented by the ECG recording in each lead. Figure 4.6 should be studied until the following four points are clear:

1. An electrical force directed toward the (+) pole of a lead results in an upward deflection on the ECG recording of that lead.
2. Forces that head away from the (+) electrode result in a downward deflection in that lead.
3. The magnitude of the deflection, either upward or downward, reflects how parallel the electrical force is to the axis of the lead being examined. The more parallel the electrical force is to the lead, the greater the magnitude of the deflection.
4. An electrical force directed perpendicular to an electrocardiographic lead does not register any activity by that lead (a "flat line" on the recording).

The six standard limb leads examine the electrical forces in the frontal plane of the body. However, since electrical activity travels in three dimensions, recordings from a perpendicular plane (Fig 4.7A) are also essential. This is accomplished by the use of six electrodes placed on the anterior and left lateral aspect of the chest (see Fig. 4.3B), creating the **chest** (or **precordial**) leads. The orientation of these leads around the heart is shown in Figure 4.7B. These are unipolar leads and, as with the unipolar limb leads, electrical forces that are directed

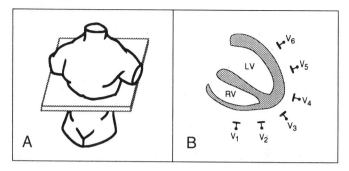

Figure 4.7. The chest (precordial) leads. A. The cross-sectional plane of the chest. **B.** Arrangement of the six chest electrodes shown in the cross-sectional plane.

toward these individual (+) electrodes result in an upward deflection on the recording of that lead; forces heading *away* record a downward deflection.

The standard complete electrocardiogram prints samples from each of the six limb leads and each of the six chest leads, examples of which are presented later in this chapter.

SEQUENCE OF NORMAL CARDIAC ACTIVATION

Conduction of electrical impulses through the heart is an orderly process. The normal beat begins at the sinoatrial node, located at the junction of the right atrium and the superior vena cava (Fig. 4.8). The wave of depolarization rapidly spreads through the right and left atria and then reaches the atrioventricular (AV) node, where it encounters an expected delay. The impulse then travels rapidly through the bundle of His and into the right and left bundle branches. These divide into the Purkinje fibers, which radiate toward the myocardial fibers, stimulating them to contract.

Each heart beat is represented on the ECG by three major deflections that record the sequence of electrical propagation (see Fig. 4.8). The **P wave** represents depolarization of the atria. Following the P wave, the tracing returns to the flat baseline, due to the conduction delay at the AV node. The second deflection of the ECG, the **QRS complex,** represents depolarization of the ventricular muscle cells. After the QRS

complex, the tracing returns to baseline once again, and after a brief delay, repolarization of the ventricular cells is signaled by the **T wave.** Occasionally, an additional small deflection follows the T wave (the **U wave**), which is believed to represent late phases of ventricular repolarization.

The QRS complex may take one of several shapes but can always be subdivided into individual components (Fig. 4.9). If the first deflection of a QRS complex is downward, it is known as a Q wave. However, if the initial deflection is upward, then that particular complex does not have a Q wave. The R wave is defined as the first upward deflection, whether or not a Q wave is present. Any downward deflection following the R wave is known as the S wave. Figure 4.9 demonstrates several variations of the QRS complex. In certain pathologic states, such as bundle branch blocks, additional deflections may be inscribed, as shown in the figure. Figure 4.9 should be studied until the reader can confidently differentiate a Q from an S wave.

The following describes the course of normal ventricular depolarization as it is recorded by two of the ECG leads, aVF and aVL (Fig. 4.10). In the resting state, the surface of the myocardial cells is positively charged compared with the inside, and the ECG leads record zero voltage, as electrical forces in each region are canceled by equal and opposite forces.

The initial portion of ventricular myocardium that is stimulated to depolarize is the mid portion of the interventricular sep-

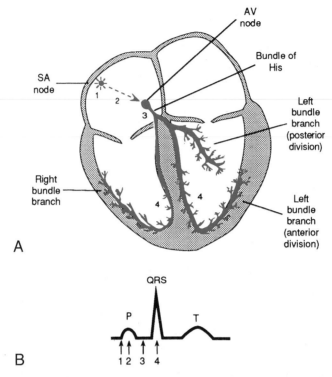

Figure 4.8. **Cardiac conduction pathway. A.** The electrical impulse begins at the sinoatrial (SA) node (1) then traverses the atria (2). After a delay at the AV node (3), conduction continues through the bundle of His and into the right and left bundle branches (4). The latter divide into Purkinje fibers, which stimulate contraction of the myocardial cells. **B.** Corresponding waveforms on the ECG recording: (1) the SA node discharges (too small to generate any deflection on ECG), (2) P wave inscribed by depolarization of the atria, (3) delay at the AV node, and (4) depolarization of the ventricles (QRS complex). The T wave represents ventricular repolarization.

tum, on the left side. Because depolarization reverses the cellular charge, the surface of that region becomes negative with respect to the inside, and an electrical current is generated (Fig. 4.10B, arrow). This initial force heads away from the left ventricle, toward the right ventricle and inferiorly. Because the force is heading *away* from the (+) pole region of lead aVL, an initial *downward* deflection is recorded in

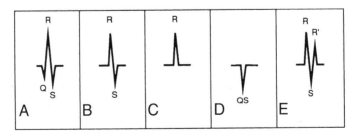

Figure 4.9. **Examples of QRS complexes. A.** The first deflection is downward (Q wave), followed by an upward deflection (R wave), and then another downward wave (S wave). **B.** Because the first deflection is upward, this complex does *not* have a Q wave; rather, the downward deflection *after* the R is an S wave. **C.** A QRS complex without downward deflections lacks Q and S waves. **D.** QRS composed of only a downward deflection; this is a Q wave but is often referred to as a QS complex. **E.** A second upward deflection (seen in bundle branch blocks) is labeled R'.

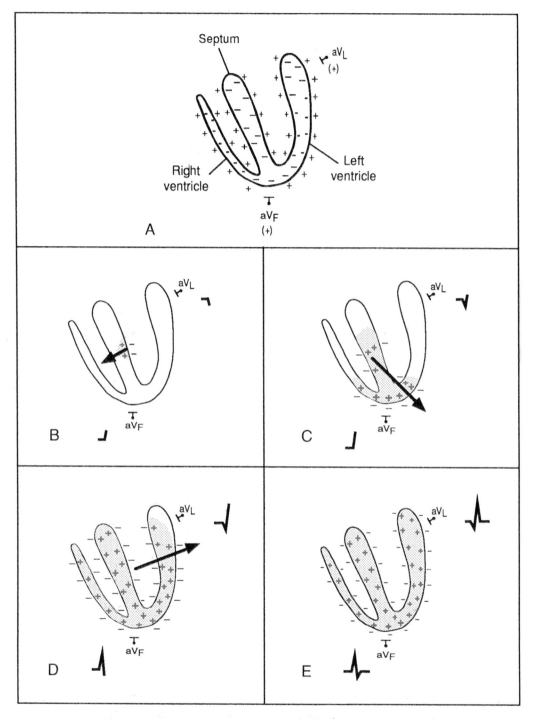

Figure 4.10. Normal ventricular depolarization as recorded by leads aV$_L$ and aV$_F$. A. In the resting state, the surface is homogeneously charged so that the leads do not record any electrical potential. **B.** The first area to depolarize is the left side of the ventricular septum. This results in forces heading away from aV$_L$ (downward deflection on aV$_L$ recording), but toward the (+) region of aV$_F$, such that an upward deflection is recorded by that lead. **C** and **D.** Depolarization continues; the forces from the thicker-walled left ventricle outweigh those of the right, such that the electrical vector swings leftward and posteriorly toward aV$_L$ (upward deflection) and away from aV$_F$. **E.** At the completion of depolarization, the surface is again homogeneously charged, and no further electrical voltage is recorded.

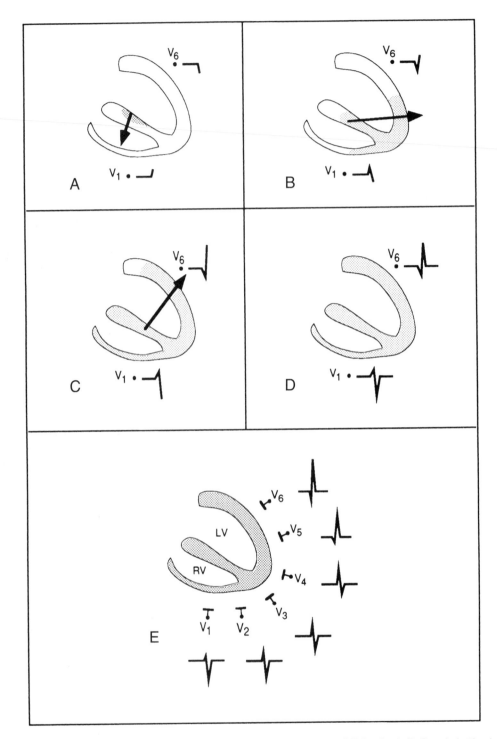

Figure 4.11. **Sequence of depolarization recorded by the chest (precordial) leads. A–D.** Depolarization begins at the left side of the septum, then the forces progress posteriorly toward the left ventricle. Thus, V$_1$, which is an anterior lead, records an initial upward deflection, followed by a downward wave, whereas V$_6$, a posterior lead, inscribes the opposite. **E.** Normal pattern of the QRS from V$_1$ to V$_6$: the R wave becomes progressively taller, and the S wave less deep.

that lead. At the same time, forces are heading *in* the direction of the (+) pole region of lead aVF, so that an initial *upward* deflection is recorded there. As the wave of depolarization spreads through the myocardium, the sequence of net electrical charge is depicted by the series of arrows in Figure 4.10.

As the lateral walls of the ventricles are depolarized, the forces of the thicker left side start outweighing those of the right. Therefore, the arrow swings further and further toward the left ventricle (leftward and posteriorly). At the completion of depolarization, no further net electrical force is generated and the ECG voltage recording returns to baseline in both leads. Thus, in this example of depolarization in a normal heart, lead aVL inscribes an initial small Q wave followed by a tall R wave; in lead aVF, there is an initial upward deflection (R wave) followed by a downward S wave.

One can also record the sequence of depolarization in the cross-sectional plane of the body by studying the six chest leads (Fig. 4.11). Once again, recall that the first region to depolarize is the left ventricular aspect of the interventricular septum. The sequence of depolarization proceeds from the midventricular septum toward the anteriorly placed right ventricle, then toward the cardiac apex, and then around to the lateral walls of both ventricles. Because the initial forces are directed anteriorly, that is, toward the (+) pole of V_1, the initial deflection recorded by lead V_1 is upward. Since these same initial forces are heading *away* from V_6, an initial downward deflection is recorded there. As the wave of depolarization spreads, the forces of the left ventricle outweigh those of the right, and the vector swings posteriorly toward the bulk of the left ventricular muscle. As the forces swing *away* from lead V_1, the deflection there becomes *downward,* whereas it becomes more *upright* in lead V_6. Leads V_2 through V_5 record intermediate steps in this process, such that the R wave becomes progressively taller from lead V_1 through lead V_6 (see Fig.

4.11E). Typically, the height of the R wave becomes greater than the depth of the S wave in lead V_3 or V_4; the lead in which this occurs is termed the "transition" lead.

A normal complete 12-lead ECG is shown at the end of the chapter (see Fig. 4.28).

Technical Considerations

ECG graph paper is divided into lines spaced 1 mm apart in both the horizontal and vertical directions. Each fifth line is made heavier to facilitate measurement. On the vertical axis, voltage is measured in millivolts (mV), and in the standard case, each 1-mm line separation represents 0.1 mV. The horizontal axis represents time. Because the standard paper speed is 25 mm/sec, each 1 mm division represents 0.04 sec and each heavy line (5 mm) represents 0.2 sec (Fig. 4.12).

INTERPRETATION OF THE ELECTROCARDIOGRAM

Many cardiac disorders alter the ECG recording in a diagnostically useful way, and it is important to interpret each tracing in a standard fashion, so as to not miss subtle abnormalities. A commonly followed sequence of analysis is as follows:

1. Check voltage calibration
2. Heart rhythm
3. Heart rate
4. Intervals (PR, QRS, ST)
5. Mean QRS axis
6. Abnormalities of the P wave
7. Abnormalities of the QRS (hypertrophy, bundle branch block, infarction)
8. ST and T wave abnormalities

Calibration

ECG machines routinely inscribe a 1.0 mV vertical signal at the beginning or end of each 12-lead tracing to document the voltage calibration of the machine. In the normal case, each 1-mm vertical box on the ECG paper represents 0.1 mV, so that

Paper Speed: 25 mm/sec ───────────▶

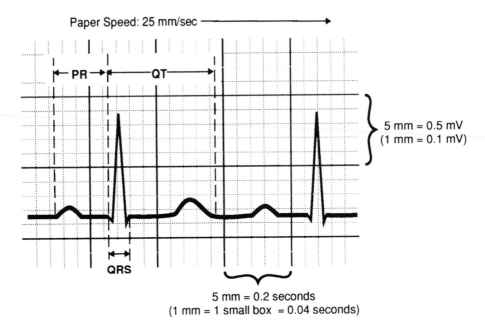

Figure 4.12. Enlarged view of an ECG strip. The paper travels through the machine at 25 mm/sec, so that each 1 mm on the horizontal axis represents 0.04 sec. Each 1 mm on the vertical axis represents 0.1 millivolt (mV). Interval measurements are: PR (from the beginning of the P wave to the beginning of the QRS) = 4 small boxes = 0.16 sec; QRS duration (from the beginning to the end of the QRS complex) = 1.75 small boxes = 0.07 sec; and QT interval (from the beginning of the QRS to the end of the T wave) = 8 small boxes = 0.32 sec. The corrected QT = $\dfrac{QT}{\sqrt{R\text{-}R}}$. Since the R-R = 15 small boxes (0.6 sec), the corrected QT = $\dfrac{0.32}{\sqrt{0.6}}$ = 0.41 sec.

the calibration signal records a 10-mm deflection (e.g., see Fig. 4.28). However, in patients with markedly increased voltage of the QRS complex (e.g., some patients with left ventricular hypertrophy or bundle branch blocks), the very large deflections would not fit on the ECG tracing. To facilitate interpretation in such a case, the recording is purposefully made at half the standard voltage (i.e., each 1-mm box = 0.2 mV), and this is indicated on the ECG tracing by a change in the height of the 1.0 mV calibration signal (at half standard voltage, the signal would be 5 mm tall). It is important to check the height of the calibration signal on each ECG, so that the voltage criteria used to define specific abnormalities will be applicable.

Heart Rhythm

The normal cardiac rhythm, initiated by depolarization of the sinus node, is known as **sinus rhythm** and is present if: 1) every P wave is followed by a QRS; 2) every QRS is preceded by a P wave; 3) the P wave is upright in leads I, II, and III; and 4) the PR interval is greater than 0.12 sec (three small boxes). If the heart rate in sinus rhythm is between 60 and 100 beats per minute (bpm), then **normal sinus rhythm** is present. If less than 60 bpm, the rhythm is **sinus bradycardia;** if greater than 100 bpm, the rhythm is **sinus tachycardia.** Other abnormal rhythms (termed *arrhythmias* or *dysrhythmias*) are described in Chapters 11 and 12.

Heart Rate (Fig. 4.13)

The standard ECG paper speed is 25 mm/sec. Therefore,

Heart rate *(beats per minute)* =

$$\frac{25 \text{ mm/sec} \times 60 \text{ sec/min}}{\text{Number of mm between beats}}$$

Method 1

First, count the number of small boxes (1 mm each) between two adjacent QRS complexes (i.e., between 2 "beats"). Then, since the standard paper speed is 25 mm/sec:

$$\frac{\text{Heart Rate}}{\text{(beats/min)}} = \frac{(25 \text{ mm/sec} \times 60 \text{ sec/min})}{\text{Number of mm between beats}} = \frac{1500}{\text{number of mm between beats}}$$

In this example, there are 23 mm between the first 2 beats:

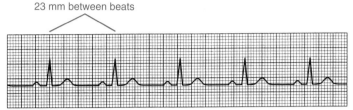

23 mm between beats

Therefore, the heart rate = $\frac{1500}{23}$ = 65 beats/min

Method 1 is particularly helpful for measuring fast heart rates (>100 beats/min)

Method 2

The "count-off" method requires memorizing the sequence:

300 - 150 - 100 - 75 - 60 - 50

Then use this sequence to count the number of large boxes between two consecutive beats:

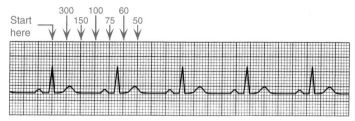

Start here 300 150 100 75 60 50

The second QRS falls between the "75" and "60" beats/min; therefore, the heart rate is approximately mid-way between them ≈ 67 beats/min. Knowing that the heart rate is approximately 60-70 beats/min is certainly close enough.

Method 3

ECG recording paper usually indicates 3-second time markers at the top or bottom of the tracing:

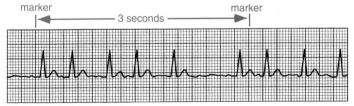

marker ← 3 seconds → marker

To calculate the heart rate, count the number of QRS complexes between the 3 second markers (= 6 beats in this example) and multiply by 20. Thus, the heart rate here is approximately 120 beats/min.

It's even easier (and more accurate) to count the number of complexes between the first and third markers on the strip (representing 6 seconds of the recording) and then multiply by 10 to determine the heart rate.

Method 3 is particularly helpful for measuring irregular heart rates

Figure 4.13. Methods to calculate heart rate.

or more simply:

Heart rate =

$$\frac{1500}{\text{Number of small boxes between 2 consecutive beats}}$$

It is rarely necessary, however, to determine the *exact* heart rate, and a more rapid determination can be made, if one does not mind a bit of memorization. Simply "count off" the number of large boxes between two consecutive QRS complexes, using the sequence:

300 — 150 —100 —75 —60 —50

which corresponds to the heart rate in beats/min and is illustrated in Figure 4.13.

When the rhythm is *irregular,* the heart rate may be approximated by taking advantage of the time markers, spaced 3 seconds apart, printed at the top or bottom of the ECG paper (Fig. 4.13, Method 3).

Intervals (PR, QRS, ST)

The PR interval, QRS interval, and QT interval (see Fig. 4.12) are measured from the *limb* lead recordings. For each of these intervals, the practitioner first glances at all six limb lead recordings and takes the measurement in the lead where the interval is the *longest* in duration. The **PR interval** is measured from the onset of the P wave to the onset of the QRS. The **QRS interval** is measured from the beginning to the end of the QRS complex. The **QT interval** is measured from the beginning of the QRS to the end of the T wave. The normal ranges of the intervals are listed in Table 4.2, along with conditions associated with abnormal values.

Since the QT interval varies with heart rate (the faster the heart rate, the shorter the QT), the **corrected QT interval** is determined by dividing the measured QT by the square root of the R–R interval (see example in Fig. 4.12). When the heart rate is in the normal range (60–100 bpm), a rapid rule can be applied: if the QT interval is visually less than half the interval between two consecutive QRS complexes, then the QT interval is within the normal range.

Mean QRS Axis

The mean QRS electrical axis represents the average of the instantaneous forces generated during the sequence of ventricular depolarization. The normal value is between $-30°$ and $+90°$ (Fig. 4.14). A mean axis that is more negative than $-30°$ implies **left axis deviation,** whereas an axis greater than $+90°$ represents **right axis deviation.** The axis can be accurately determined by plotting the QRS complexes of different leads on the axial reference diagram (see Fig. 4.5), but this is tedious and rarely necessary. It is generally sufficient to note whether the axis is

TABLE 4.2. Electrocardiographic Intervals

Interval	Normal	Decreased in	Increased in
PR	0.12–0.20 sec (3–5 small boxes)	• Pre-excitation syndrome • Junctional rhythm	• First-degree AV block
QRS	≤0.10 sec (≤2.5 small boxes)		• Bundle branch blocks • Ventricular ectopic beat • Toxic drug effect (e.g., quinidine) • Severe hyperkalemia
QT	Corrected QT* ≤0.44 sec	• Hypercalcemia • Tachycardia	• Hypocalcemia • Hypokalemia (↑ QU interval due to ↑ U wave) • Hypomagnesemia • Myocardial ischemia • Congenital prolongation of QT • Toxic drug effect (e.g., quinidine)

*Corrected QT = $\dfrac{QT}{\sqrt{R\text{-}R}}$

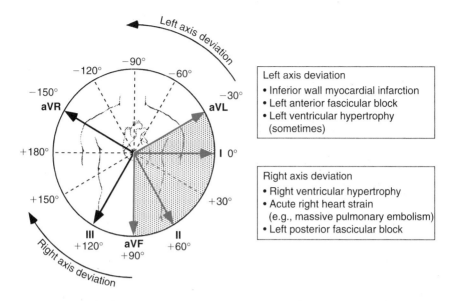

Figure 4.14. **A normal mean QRS axis falls within the shaded area (between −30° and +90°).** A mean axis more negative than −30° is termed *left axis deviation*, whereas an axis > +90° is *right axis deviation*. The figure shows common conditions that result in axis deviation.

normal, deviated to the left, or deviated to the right. If a more precise measurement is needed, the simplified approach described below can be employed.

Recall from Figure 4.5 that each ECG lead has a (+) region and a (−) region. Electrical activity directed toward the (+) half results in an upward deflection, whereas activity toward the (−) half results in a downward deflection on the ECG recording of that lead.

To determine whether the axis is normal or abnormal, examine the QRS complexes in limb leads I and II. If the QRS is primarily positive in both of these leads (upward deflection greater than downward deflection), then the mean vector falls within the normal range (Fig. 4.15). If the QRS in *either* lead I or II is not primarily upward, then the axis is *abnormal*, and the approximate axis should then be determined by the rapid method described here.

First, consider a special example (Fig. 4.16). A sequence of ventricular depolarization is represented in this figure by arrows a–e. The initial deflection (representing left septal depolarization) points to the patient's right side. Because it is directed away from the (+) pole of lead I, a strong

downward deflection is recorded by the lead. As depolarization continues, the arrow swings downward and to the left, resulting in less negative deflections in lead I. After arrow c, the electrical vector swings into the positive region of lead I so that upward deflections are recorded.

In this special example, in which electrical forces begin exactly opposite the (+) electrode and terminate when pointed directly at that electrode, note that the mean electrical vector points straight downward (in the direction of arrow c), *perpendicular* to the lead I axis. Also note the configuration of the inscribed QRS complex. There is a downward deflection, followed by an upward deflection of equal magnitude (when the upward and downward deflections of a QRS are of equal magnitude, it is termed an **isoelectric complex**). Thus, when an ECG lead inscribes an isoelectric QRS complex, it means that the average electrical axis of the ventricles is *perpendicular* to that lead.

Therefore, an easy way to determine the mean QRS axis is to glance at the six limb lead recordings and observe which one has the most isoelectric-appearing complex: the mean axis is simply perpendicular to it. There is then one more step. When the

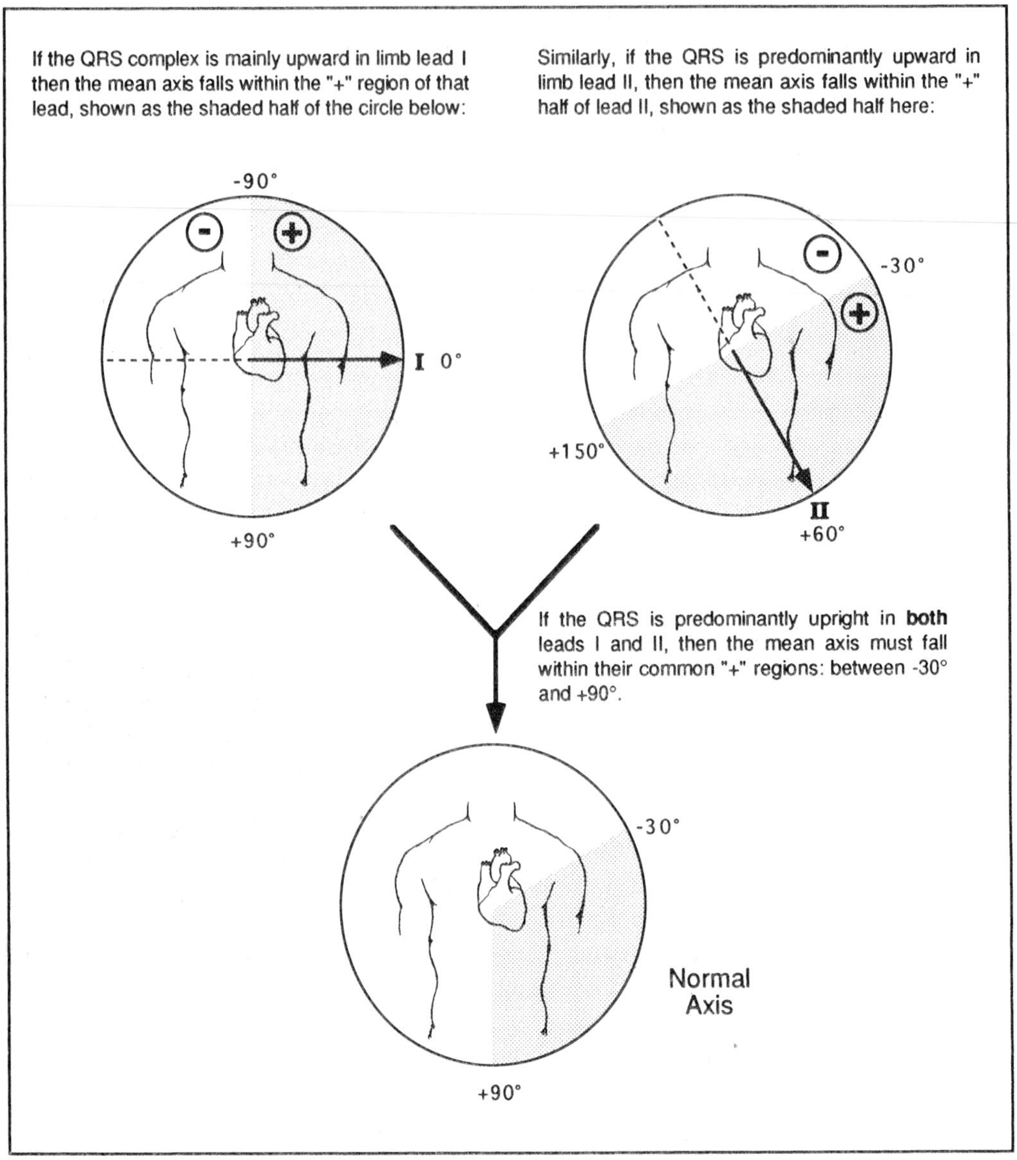

If the QRS complex is mainly upward in limb lead I then the mean axis falls within the "+" region of that lead, shown as the shaded half of the circle below:
Similarly, if the QRS is predominantly upward in limb lead II, then the mean axis falls within the "+" half of lead II, shown as the shaded half here:
-90°
I 0°
+90°
-30°
+150°
II
+60°
If the QRS is predominantly upright in **both** leads I and II, then the mean axis must fall within their common "+" regions: between -30° and +90°.
-30°
Normal Axis
+90°

Figure 4.15. **The mean axis is within the normal range if the QRS complex is predominantly upright in limb leads I and II.**

(-)
a
e
b
c
d
Lead I
(+)
Mean axis
(+)
Lead aVF

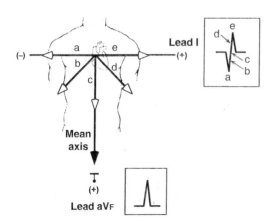

Figure 4.16. **Sequence of ventricular depolarization when the mean axis is +90°.** Because the mean axis is perpendicular to limb lead I, an isoelectric QRS complex (height of upward deflection = height of downward deflection) is recorded by that lead (see text for details).

mean axis is perpendicular to a lead, it could be perpendicular in either a clockwise *or* a counterclockwise direction. In the example, as the isoelectric complex appears in lead I, the mean vector could be at +90° *or* it could be at −90°, since both are perpendicular. To determine which of these it is, the next step is to inspect the recording of the ECG lead that is perpendicular to the one inscribing the isoelectric complex (and is therefore parallel to the mean axis). If the QRS is predominantly upright in that perpendicular lead, then the mean vector points toward the (+) pole of that lead. If it is predominantly negative, then it points away from the lead's (+) pole. In the example, the isoelectric complex appears in lead I; therefore, the next step is to inspect the perpendicular lead, which is aVF (see Fig. 4.5 if this relationship is not clear). Because the QRS complex in aVF is primarily upward, then the mean axis points toward its (+) pole, which is in fact located at +90°.

To summarize, the mean QRS axis is calculated as follows:

1. Inspect limb leads I and II. If the QRS is primarily upward in both, then the axis is normal and you are done. If not, then proceed to the next step.
2. Inspect the six limb leads and determine which one contains the QRS that is most isoelectric. The mean axis is perpendicular to that lead.
3. Inspect the lead that is perpendicular to the lead containing the isoelectric complex. If the QRS in that perpendicular lead is primarily upward, then the mean axis points to the (+) pole of that lead. If primarily negative, then the mean QRS points to the (−) pole of that lead.

Conditions that result in left or right axis deviation are listed in Figure 4.14. In addition, the vertical position of the heart in many normal children and adolescents may result in a rightward mean axis (> +90°).

In some patients, isoelectric complexes are inscribed in *all* of the limb leads. That situation arises when the heart is tilted, so that the mean QRS is pointing straight forward or back from the chest, as it may be in patients with chronic obstructive lung disease; in such a case, the mean axis is said to be *indeterminate.*

Abnormalities of the P Wave

The P wave represents depolarization of the right atrium followed quickly by depolarization of the left atrium—the two components are nearly superimposed on one another (Fig. 4.17). The P wave is usually best visualized in lead II, the lead that runs most parallel to the flow of electrical current through the atria from the sinoatrial to the AV node. When the *right* atrium is enlarged, the initial component of the P wave is larger than normal (taller than 2.5 mm in lead II).

Left atrial enlargement is best observed in lead V_1. Normally, V_1 inscribes a P wave with an initial positive deflection reflecting right atrial depolarization (directed anteriorly), followed by a negative deflection, owing to the left atrial forces oriented posteriorly (see Fig. 1.2 for anatomic relationships). Left atrial enlargement is therefore manifested by a greater than normal negative deflection (at least 1 mm wide and 1 mm deep) in lead V_1 (Fig. 4.17).

Abnormalities of the QRS Complex

Ventricular Hypertrophy

Hypertrophy of the left or right ventricle results in greater than normal electrical forces generated by the hypertrophied chamber. Normally, the forces of the thicker-walled left ventricle are greater than those of the right. However, in **right ventricular hypertrophy** (RVH), the added right-sided forces may outweigh those of the left. Therefore, chest leads V_1 and V_2, which overlie the right ventricle, record greater than normal upward deflections: the R wave becomes taller than the S wave in those leads, the reverse of the normal situation (Fig. 4.18). In addition, the increased right ventricular mass shifts the mean axis of the heart toward the right (greater than +90°).

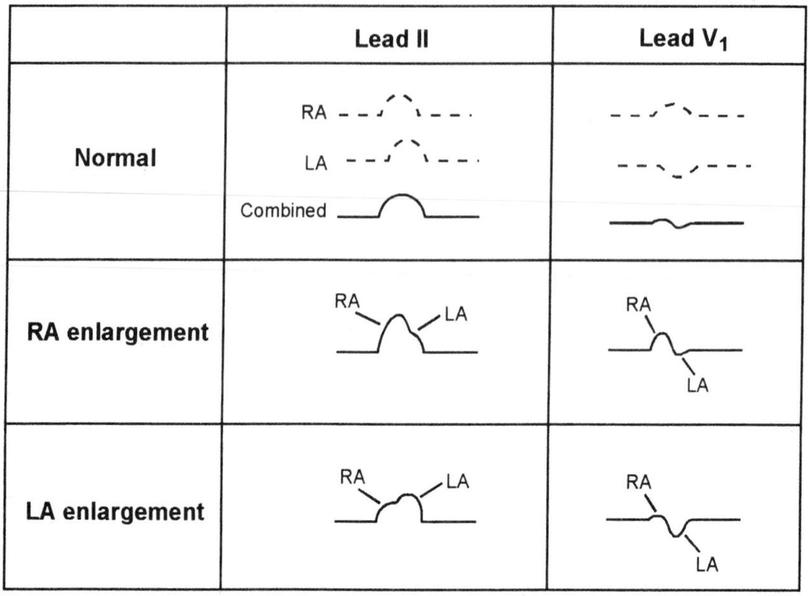

	Lead II	Lead V$_1$
Normal	RA $- -\sim\frown\ \frown -\ -$ LA $- -\sim\frown\ \frown -\ -$ Combined $\underline{\quad\frown\quad}$	$- - \sim\frown\ \frown - - -$ $- - \smile\ \smile - - -$ $\underline{\quad\smile\quad}$
RA enlargement	RA $\frown$ LA	RA LA
LA enlargement	RA $\frown$ LA	RA LA

Figure 4.17. **The P wave represents superimposition of right atrial (RA) and left atrial (LA) depolarization.** RA depolarization occurs slightly earlier than LA depolarization. In RA enlargement, the initial component of the P is prominent (>2.5 mm tall) in lead II. In LA enlargement, there is a large terminal downward deflection in lead V, (>1 mm wide and >1 mm deep).

In **left ventricular hypertrophy,** greater than normal forces are generated by the massive LV, which simply exaggerates the normal situation. Leads that overlie the left ventricle (chest leads V$_5$ and V$_6$ and limb leads I and aVL) show taller R waves than normal. Leads on the other side of the heart (V$_1$ and V$_2$) demonstrate the opposite: deeper than normal S waves. Many criteria exist for the diagnosis of left ventricular hypertrophy, and three of the most helpful are listed in Figure 4.18.

Bundle Branch Blocks

Interruption of conduction through the right or left bundle branches may develop from ischemic or degenerative damage. As a result, the affected ventricle does not depolarize in the normal sequence. Rather than rapid uniform stimulation by the Purkinje fibers, the cells of that ventricle must rely on a more gradual myocyte-to-myocyte spread of electrical activity traveling from the unaffected ventricle. This is a slow process, which prolongs depolar-

ization and widens the QRS complex. When bundle branch block widens the QRS duration to 0.10–0.12 sec (2.5–3 small boxes), *incomplete* bundle branch block is present. If greater than 0.12 sec (3 small boxes), *complete* bundle branch block is identified.

In **right bundle branch block** (Fig. 4.19A; see also Fig. 4.29), initial depolarization of the ventricular septum (which is stimulated by a branch of the left bundle) is unaffected so that the normal small R wave in lead V$_1$ and small Q wave in lead V$_6$ are recorded. Furthermore, as the wave of depolarization spreads down the septum and into the left ventricular free wall, the sequence of depolarization is indistinguishable from normal, because LV forces *normally* outweigh those of the right. However, at the time when the LV has almost fully depolarized, the slow cell-to-cell spread finally reaches the right ventricle and depolarization of that chamber begins, unopposed by LV activity (since that chamber has nearly fully depolarized). Therefore, the QRS complex is widened by this pro-

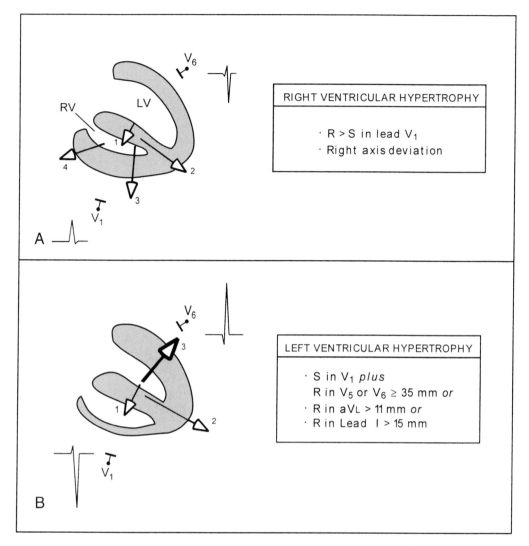

Figure 4.18. Ventricular hypertrophy. The arrows indicate the sequence of average electrical forces during ventricular depolarization. **A.** Right ventricular (RV) hypertrophy. The RV forces outweigh those of the left, resulting in tall R waves in leads V_1 and V_2 and a deep S wave in lead V_6. **B.** Left ventricular (LV) hypertrophy exaggerates the normal pattern of depolarization, with stronger than usual forces directed toward the LV, resulting in a tall R wave in V_6 and deep S in lead V_1.

longed depolarization process. Since the terminal portion of the QRS complex in this case represents right ventricular forces acting alone, there is a terminal *upward* deflection (known as R') over the RV in lead V_1, and a downward deflection (S wave) in V_6 on the opposite side of the heart.

Left bundle branch block produces even greater QRS abnormalities. In this situation, normal initial depolarization of the left septum does *not* occur; rather, the right side of the ventricular septum is first to de-

polarize, through branches of the right bundle. Thus, the initial forces of depolarization are directed toward the left ventricle instead of the right (see Fig. 4.19B; see also Fig. 4.30). Therefore, an initial *downward* deflection is recorded in V_1 and the normal small Q wave in V_6 is absent. Only after depolarization of the right ventricle does slow cell-to-cell spread reach the left ventricular cells. These slowly conducted forces inscribe a widened QRS complex with terminally upward deflections in the leads over-

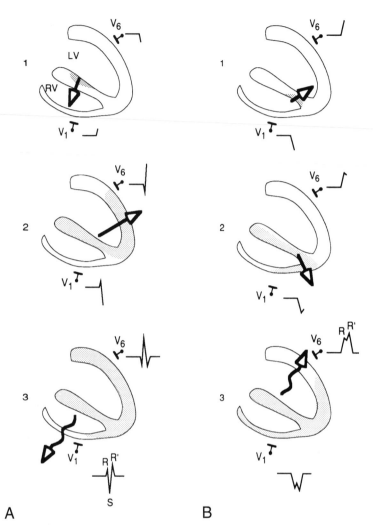

Figure 4.19. Bundle branch blocks. Interruption of conduction through the right (RBBB) or left (LBBB) bundles results in delayed, slowed activation of the respective ventricle and widening of the QRS complex. **A.** In RBBB there is normal initial activation of the septum (1) followed by depolarization of the left ventricle (2). Slow cell-to-cell spread activates the right ventricle (RV) *after* the left ventricle (LV) has nearly fully depolarized, so that the late forces generated by the RV are unopposed. Therefore, V$_1$ records an abnormal terminal upward deflection (R'), and V$_6$ records an abnormal, terminal deep S wave (3). **B.** In LBBB the initial septal depolarization is blocked, such that initial forces are oriented from right to left. Thus, the normal initial R in V$_1$ and Q in V$_6$ are absent (1). After the RV depolarizes, late, slow activation of the LV results in a terminal upward deflection in V$_6$ and downward deflection in V$_1$ (3).

lying the left ventricle (V$_5$ and V$_6$), as shown in Figure 4.19.

A more limited form of conduction block can affect either the anterior or posterior fascicle (division) of the left bundle, resulting in left anterior or left posterior fascicular block (these are also termed *hemiblocks*). Anatomically, the anterior fascicle of the left bundle runs anteriorly toward the anterior

papillary muscle, whereas the posterior fascicle travels to the posterior papillary muscle. As a result, electrical activation of the LV normally spreads simultaneously from the base of the two papillary muscles. If conduction is impaired in one of these divisions, then initial LV depolarization arises exclusively from the unaffected zone. For example, in the case of **left anterior fascic-**

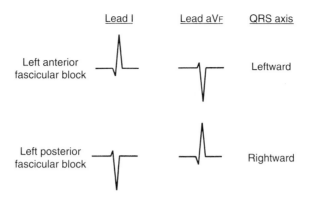

Figure 4.20. **Electrocardiographic patterns in left anterior and left posterior fascicular blocks.**

ular block (LAFB), activation begins at the posterior papillary muscle and then spreads to the rest of the ventricle. Since the posterior papillary muscle is located below and medial to the anterior papillary muscle, the initial depolarization will be downward (i.e., toward the feet) and toward the patient's right side. This results in a positive deflection (initial R wave) in the inferior leads (II, III, aVF) and a small Q wave in leads I and aVL (Fig. 4.20). As the electrical forces then spread upward and to the left, an R wave is inscribed in leads I and aVL while an S wave appears in the inferior leads. The predominance of these leftward forces results in left axis deviation of the QRS mean axis.

In the less common **left posterior fascicular block (LPFB)**, left ventricular activation starts at the base of the anterior papillary muscle, so the initial forces are directed upward and to the patient's left (creating an R in lead I and aVL, and Q waves in the inferior leads). As the impulse spreads downward and to the right, an S wave is inscribed in leads I and aVL, while an R is recorded in leads II, III, and aVF. Since the bulk of these forces head rightward, right axis deviation of the QRS mean axis is expected.

LAFB and LPFB do not result in significant widening of the QRS (in distinction to right or left bundle branch blocks) because rapidly conducting Purkinje fibers bridge the territories served by the anterior and posterior fascicles. Therefore, al-

though the sequence and pathway of conduction are altered, the total time required for depolarization is usually only slightly prolonged.

Myocardial Infarction

The hallmark of transmural myocardial infarction (MI) is the **pathologic Q wave.** Recall that an initial Q wave is normal in some leads. For example, initial septal depolarization routinely inscribes a small Q wave in leads V_6 and aVL. *Normal* Q waves are of *short* duration (≤0.04 sec, or 1 small box) and of *low* magnitude (<25% of the QRS total height). A pathologic Q wave is more prominent (Fig. 4.21), having a width ≥1 small box in duration, and a depth

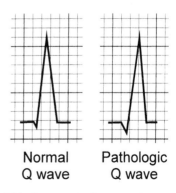

Normal   Pathologic
Q wave   Q wave

Figure 4.21. **Compared with small Q waves generated during normal depolarization, pathologic Q waves are more prominent with a width ≥1 mm (1 small box) and depth >25% of the height of the QRS complex.**

TABLE 4.3. Localization of Myocardial Infarction

Anatomic Site	Leads with Abnormal ECG Complexes[a]	Coronary Artery Most Often Responsible
Inferior	II, III, aV$_F$	RCA
Anteroseptal	V$_1$–V$_2$	LAD
Anteroapical	V$_3$–V$_4$	LAD (distal)
Anterolateral	V$_5$–V$_6$, I, aV$_L$	CFX
Posterior	V$_1$–V$_2$ [tall R, not Q]	RCA

[a]Pathologic Q waves in all of leads V$_1$–V$_6$ implies an "extensive anterior MI" usually associated with a proximal left coronary artery occlusion.
[b]RCA = Right coronary artery, LAD = Left anterior descending coronary artery, CFX = Left circumflex coronary artery

>25% of the total height of the QRS. The ECG leads in which pathologic Q waves appear reflect the anatomic site of an infarction (Table 4.3; see also Fig. 4.23).

Pathologic Q waves develop in the leads overlying infarcted tissue because necrotic muscle does not generate electrical forces. Rather, the ECG electrode over that region detects electrical currents from the healthy tissue on *opposite* regions of the ventricle, which are directed *away* from the infarct and the recording electrode, thus inscribing the downward deflection (Fig. 4.22). Q waves are permanent evidence of a myocardial infarction; only rarely do they disappear over time.

Note in Table 4.3 that in the case of a posterior wall myocardial infarction (Fig. 4.23) it is not pathologic Q waves that are evident on the ECG. Because no standard electrodes are placed on the patient's back overlying the posterior wall, one must rely on other leads to indirectly identify the presence of such an infarction. Since chest leads V$_1$ and V$_2$ are directly opposite the posterior wall, they record the *inverse* of what leads placed on the back would demonstrate. Therefore, *taller than normal R waves in leads V$_1$ and V$_2$* are the equivalent of a pathologic Q wave in the diagnosis of a posterior wall MI. It may be recalled that right ventricular hypertrophy also produces tall R waves in leads V$_1$ and V$_2$, but unlike RVH, right axis devia-

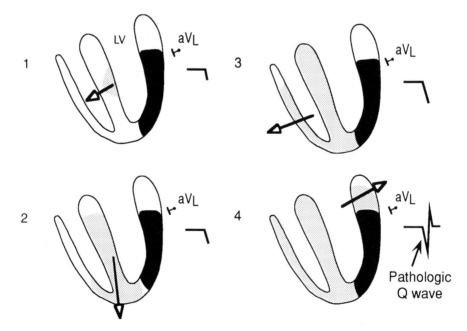

Figure 4.22. Sequence of depolarization recorded by lead aVL, overlying a lateral wall infarction (black region). A pathologic Q wave is recorded because the necrotic muscle does not generate electrical forces; rather, at the time when the lateral wall *should* be depolarizing (**panel 3**), the activation of the healthy muscle on the *opposite* side of the heart is unopposed, such that forces head away from aVL. The terminal R wave recorded by aVL reflects depolarization of the remaining viable myocardium beyond the infarct.

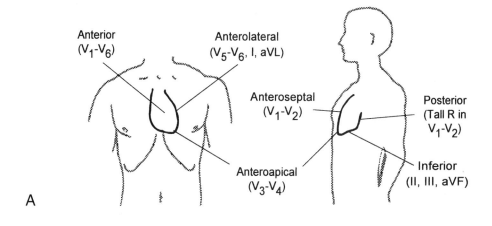

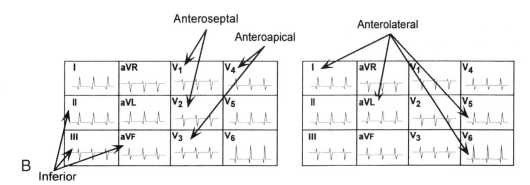

Figure 4.23. **A.** Relationship between ECG leads and cardiac anatomic regions. The leads listed in parentheses are those that reflect infarction of these regions. **B.** Miniaturized schematic drawings of a 12-lead ECG showing the standard orientation of printed samples from each lead. The major anatomic groupings are indicated. Note that while the presence of pathologic Q waves in leads V_1 and V_2 are indicative of anteroseptal infarction, *tall initial R waves* in those leads are seen in posterior wall infarction.

tion is not usually a feature of posterior wall MI.

It is important to note that if a pathologic Q wave appears in only a single ECG lead, it is not diagnostic of an infarction. True pathologic Qs should appear in the groupings listed in Table 4.3 and Figure 4.23. For example, if a pathologic Q wave is present in lead III, but not in II or aVF, it likely does not indicate an infarction. Also, Q waves are *disregarded* in lead aVR, as electrical forces are *normally* directed away from the right arm. Finally, in the presence of left bundle branch block, Q waves are usually not helpful in the diagnosis of MI, because of the markedly abnormal pattern of depolarization in that condition.

The discussion thus far has considered infarctions in which Q waves develop, and these are therefore termed **Q-wave infarctions.** Pathologically, in such infarctions, the entire thickness of a myocardial segment is usually involved, so that this type of MI is often also termed a "transmural" infarct. As described in Chapter 7, infarctions are not always transmural, but may involve only the subendocardial layers of the myocardium. In the latter case, pathologic Q waves do *not* develop, because the remaining viable cells are able to generate some electrical activity; such MIs are therefore called **non–Q-wave infarctions.** In either case, certain ST and T wave abnormalities evolve during Q-wave and non–Q-wave infarctions, as discussed in the next section. The electrocardiographic differences between these types of MI are summarized as follows:

	Q waves	Acute ST deviation
Q-wave MI	Yes	ST elevation
Non–Q-wave MI	No	ST depression (and/or T wave inversion)

ST Segment and T Wave Abnormalities

Among the most common important abnormalities of the ST and T waves are those that represent myocardial ischemia and infarction. Because ventricular repolarization is very sensitive to myocardial perfusion, patients with coronary artery disease often demonstrate reversible deviations of the ST segments and T waves during myocardial ischemia.

As described in the previous section, pathologic Q waves are indicative of an MI but do not differentiate between an acute event and an MI that occurred weeks or years earlier. However, acute MI does result in a sequence of ST and T wave abnormalities that permit this distinction (Fig. 4.24). The initial abnormality during an acute Q-wave MI is elevation of the ST segment, often with a peaked appearance of the T wave. At this early stage, myocardial cells are still viable and Q waves have not yet developed. Within several hours, however, myocyte death leads to loss of the amplitude of the R wave, and pathologic Q waves begin to be inscribed by the ECG

leads positioned over the infarct territory. During the first 1–2 days following infarction, the ST segments remain elevated, the T wave inverts, and the Q wave deepens. Several days later, the ST segment elevation returns to baseline, but the T waves remain inverted. Weeks or months following the infarct, the ST segment and T waves have often returned to normal, but the pathologic Q waves persist, a permanent marker of the MI. If the ST segment *remains* elevated several weeks later, it is likely that a bulging fibrotic scar (ventricular aneurysm) has developed at the site of infarction.

These evolutionary changes of the QRS, ST, and T waves are recorded by the leads overlying the zone of infarction (see Table 4.3). Typically, *reciprocal* changes are seen in leads opposite to that site. For example, in acute anteroseptal MI, ST segment elevation is expected in chest leads V_1 and V_2; simultaneously, however, reciprocal changes (ST *depression*) may be inscribed by the leads overlying the opposite (inferior) region, namely in leads II, III, and aVF.

The mechanism by which ST segment deviations develop during acute MI has not been established with certainty. It is believed, however, that the abnormality results from injured myocardial cells immediately adjacent to the infarct zone producing abnormal systolic or diastolic currents. One explanation, the *diastolic current theory*, contends that these cells are capable of depolarization but are abnormally "leaky" for potassium ions so that they never fully repolarize (Fig. 4.25). Since the surface of such partially depolarized cells in the rest-

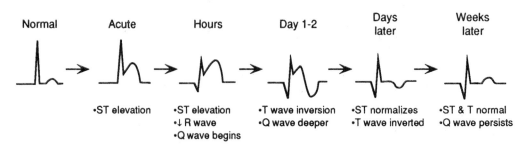

Figure 4.24. **ECG evolution during acute Q-wave myocardial infarction (also termed "acute ST segment elevation MI").**

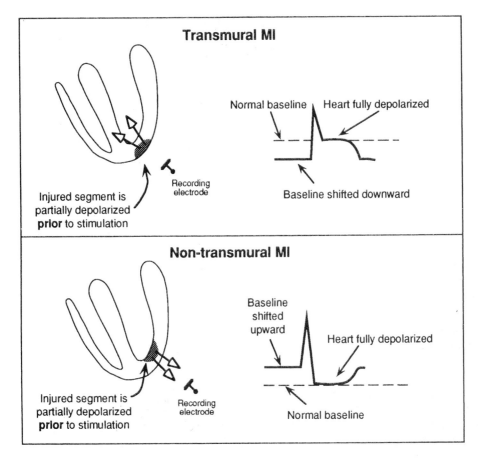

Figure 4.25. ST deviations in acute MI: diastolic injury current. Top. Ionic leak results in partial depolarization of injured myocardium in diastole, prior to electrical stimulation, which produces forces heading away from that site and shifts the ECG baseline downward. This is not noticeable on the ECG because only relative, not absolute, voltages are recorded. Following stimulation, when the entire myocardium has fully depolarized, the voltage is true zero but gives the appearance of ST elevation compared with the abnormally depressed baseline. **Bottom.** In non-transmural MI, the process is similar, but the ionic leak arises from the subendocardial tissue so that the partial depolarization before stimulation is directed *toward* the recording electrode; hence, the baseline is shifted *upward.* When fully depolarized, the voltage is true zero, but the ST segment has the *appearance* that it is depressed compared with the shifted baseline.

ing (diastolic) state would be relatively negatively charged compared with the normal fully repolarized areas, an electrical current is generated between the two regions. This current is directed *away* from the more negatively charged ischemic area, causing the baseline of the ECG leads overlying that region to *shift downward.* Since the ECG machine records only *relative* position, rather than absolute voltages, the downward deviation of the baseline is not noticed. Following ventricular depolarization (indicated by the QRS complex), after *all* the myocardial cells have fully depolarized (including those of the injured zone), the net

electrical potential surrounding the heart is *true* zero. However, compared with the abnormally displaced downward baseline, there is the *appearance* of ST segment elevation (see Fig. 4.25). As the myocytes then repolarize, the injured cells return to the abnormal state of diastolic potassium ion leak, and the ECG again inscribes the abnormally depressed baseline. Thus, ST elevation in acute MI may in part reflect an abnormal shift of the recording baseline.

In *non–Q-wave* myocardial infarctions, it is ST segment *depression*, rather than elevation, that often develops in the leads overlying the infarct (see Fig. 7.7, page 170). In

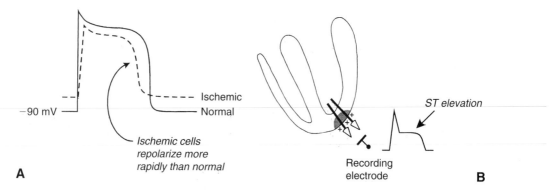

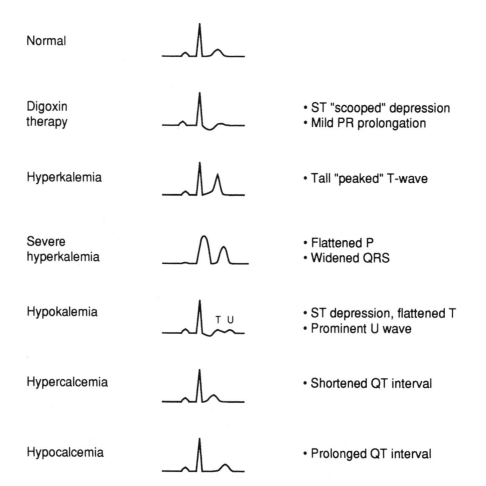

Figure 4.26. ST deviation in acute MI: systolic injury current. A. Compared with normal myocytes (solid line), ischemic myocytes (dashed line) display a reduced resting membrane potential and repolarize more rapidly. **B.** More rapid repolarization causes the surface of the ischemic zone to be relatively positively charged at the time the ST segment is inscribed. The associated electrical current (arrows) is directed *toward* the recording electrode overlying that site, so that the ST segment is abnormally elevated.

Normal		
Digoxin therapy		• ST "scooped" depression • Mild PR prolongation
Hyperkalemia		• Tall "peaked" T-wave
Severe hyperkalemia		• Flattened P • Widened QRS
Hypokalemia		• ST depression, flattened T • Prominent U wave
Hypercalcemia		• Shortened QT interval
Hypocalcemia		• Prolonged QT interval

Figure 4.27. Conditions that alter repolarization of myocytes and therefore result in ST segment and T wave abnormalities.

this situation, the diastolic potassium leak of injured cells adjacent to the infarct generates electrical forces heading from the inner endocardium to the outer epicardium and therefore toward the overlying ECG electrode. Thus, the baseline of the ECG is shifted *upward* (Fig. 4.25). Following full cardiac depolarization, the electrical potential of the heart returns to true zero, but relative to the abnormal baseline, gives the appearance of ST segment *depression.*

The *systolic current theory* of ST segment shifts contends that in addition to reducing the resting membrane potential, ischemic injury also shortens the action potential duration of affected cells. As a result, the ischemic cells repolarize faster than neighboring normal myocytes; therefore, a voltage gradient develops between the two zones, creating an electrical current directed *toward* the ischemic area. This gradient occurs during the ST interval of the ECG, resulting in ST elevation in the leads overlying the ischemic region. (Fig. 4.26)

As discussed in Chapter 7, when evaluating a patient with acute chest pain, it is very important to identify and rapidly distinguish between Q-wave and non–Q-wave myocardial infarctions, because the initial therapeutic approaches are different. Decisions about therapy must be made within minutes of evaluating the patient, usually while acute ST and T wave deviations are present on the ECG but before Q waves would be expected to have formed. Thus, for the purpose of such decision-making, it has become common to refer to an evolving Q-wave MI as an "acute ST segment elevation MI." Similarly, a non–Q-wave MI is now often labeled a "non–ST segment elevation MI."

Other common causes of ST segment and T wave abnormalities due to alterations in myocyte repolarization are illustrated in Figure 4.27.

SUMMARY

The electrocardiogram provides a wealth of important information regarding the structure and integrity of the heart and remains one of the simplest but most important diagnostic tools in cardiology. With the knowl-

---

TABLE 4.4. Summary: Sequence of ECG Interpretation

1. **Calibration**
   - Check 1.0 mV vertical box inscription (normal standard = 10 mm)
2. **Rhythm**
   - Sinus rhythm is present if:
     - each P wave is followed by a QRS complex
     - each QRS is preceded by a P wave
     - the P wave is upright in leads I, II, and III
     - the PR interval is > 0.12 sec (3 small boxes)
   - If these criteria are not met, determine type of arrhythmia (Chapter 12)
3. **Heart rate**
   - Use one of three methods:
     - 1500/(number of mm between beats)
     - Count off method: 300—150—100—75—60—50
     - Number of beats in 6 seconds × 10
   - Normal rate = 60–100 beats/min (bradycardia < 60, tachycardia > 100)
4. **Intervals**
   - Normal PR = 0.12–0.20 sec (3–5 small boxes)
   - Normal QRS ≤ 0.10 sec (≤ 2.5 small boxes)
   - Normal QT ≤ half the R–R interval, if heart rate normal
5. **Mean QRS axis**
   - Normal if QRS is primarily upright in leads I and II (+90° to -30°)
   - Otherwise, determine axis by isoelectric/perpendicular method
6. **P wave abnormalities**
   - Inspect P in leads II and V_1 for left and right atrial enlargement
7. **QRS wave abnormalities**
   - Inspect for left and right ventricular hypertrophy
   - Inspect for bundle branch blocks (BBB)
   - Inspect for pathologic Q waves: What anatomic distribution?
8. **ST segment/T wave abnormalities**
   - Inspect for ST elevations:
     - transmural infarct pattern
     - pericarditis (described in Chapter 14)
   - Inspect for ST depressions/T wave inversions:
     - subendocardial ischemia or infarct
     - commonly accompany ventricular hypertrophy or BBBs
     - metabolic/chemical abnormalities (Fig. 4.27)
9. **Compare** with patient's previous ECGs

---

edge of this chapter in hand, the reader should be well suited to practice analyzing electrocardiograms in any of the excellent texts listed below. Table 4.4 summarizes the suggested sequence of ECG interpretation. Sample ECGs follow, with their interpretations, in Figures 4.28 through 4.35.

Disturbances of the cardiac rhythm (arrhythmias) identified by ECG are discussed in Chapters 11 and 12.

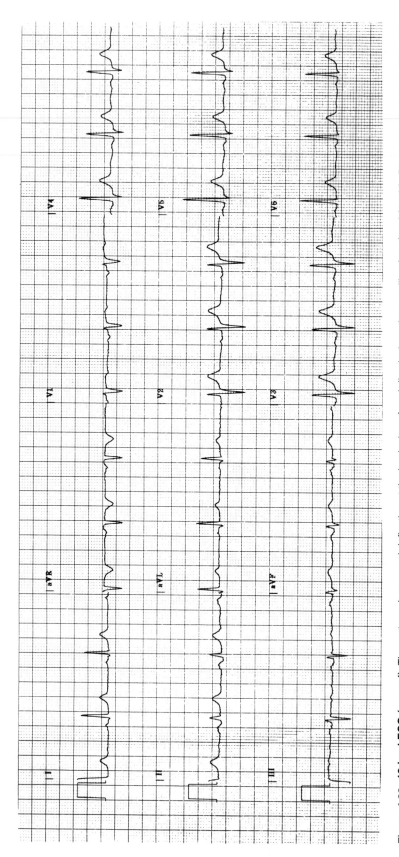

Figure 4.28. 12-lead ECG (normal). The rectangular upward deflection at the beginning of each line is the voltage calibration signal (1 mV). *Rhythm:* normal sinus. *Rate:* 70 bpm. *Intervals:* PR 0.17, QRS 0.06, QT 0.40 sec. *Axis:* 0° (QRS is isoelectric in lead aVF). The P wave, QRS complex, ST segment, and T waves are normal. Note the gradual increase in R wave height between leads V$_1$ through V$_6$.

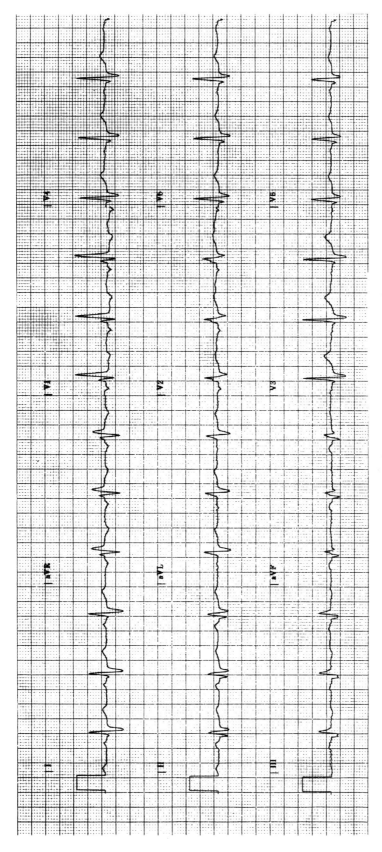

Figure 4.29. **12-lead ECG (abnormal).** *Rhythm:* normal sinus. *Rate:* 75 bpm. *Intervals:* PR 0.16, QRS 0.15, QT 0.42 sec. *Axis:* indeterminate (isoelectric in all limb leads). *P wave:* left atrial enlargement (1 mm wide and 1 mm deep in lead V_1). *QRS:* widened with RSR' in lead V_1 consistent with right bundle branch block (RBBB). Also, pathologic Q waves in leads II, III, and aVF, consistent with inferior wall myocardial infarction (an old one, because the ST segments do not demonstrate an acute injury pattern).

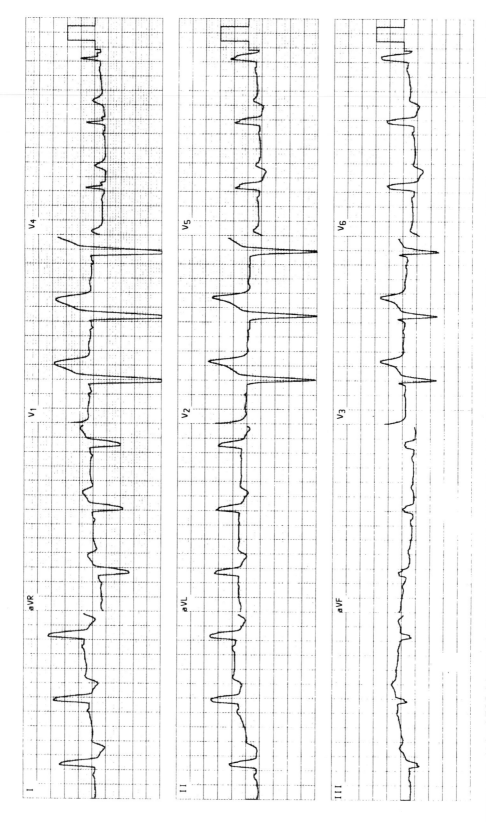

Figure 4.30. **12-lead ECG (abnormal).** *Rhythm:* normal sinus. *Rate:* 68 bpm. *Intervals:* PR 0.16, QRS 0.16, QT 0.40 sec. *Axis:* +15°. *P wave:* normal. *QRS:* widened with RR′ in leads V₄–V₆ consistent with left bundle branch block (LBBB). The *ST segment and T wave* abnormalities are secondary to LBBB.

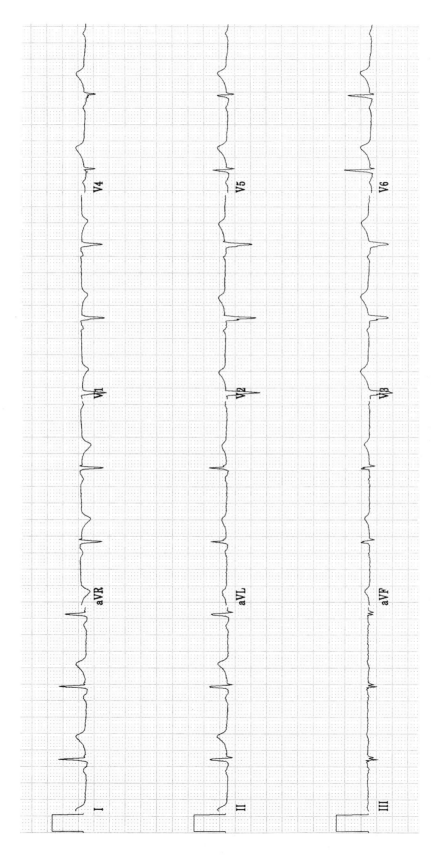

Figure 4.31. **12-lead ECG (abnormal).** *Rhythm:* normal sinus. *Rate:* 66 bpm. *Intervals:* PR 0.16, QRS 0.08, QT 0.40 sec. *Axis:* +10°. *P wave:* normal. *QRS:* pathologic Q waves in leads V₁–V₄, consistent with anteroseptal and anteroapical myocardial infarction (MI). The *ST segment and T waves* do not demonstrate an acute injury pattern, so that the MI is old.

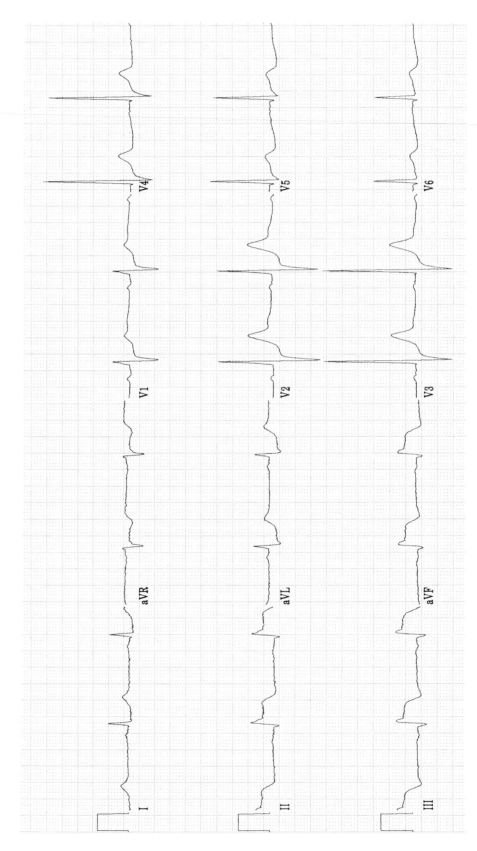

Figure 4.32. 12-lead ECG (abnormal). *Rhythm:* sinus bradycardia. *Rate:* 55 bpm. *Intervals:* PR 0.20 (in aVF), QRS 0.10, QT 0.44 sec. *Axis:* normal (QRS is predominantly upright in leads I and II). *P wave:* normal. *QRS:* prominent voltage in chest leads but does not meet criteria for ventricular hypertrophy; pathologic Q waves are present in II, III, and aVF, indicative of inferior wall MI, and the tall R waves in V_1 and V_2 are consistent with posterior MI involvement as well. There is marked *ST segment elevation* in II, III, and aVF, indicating that this is an *acute* MI.

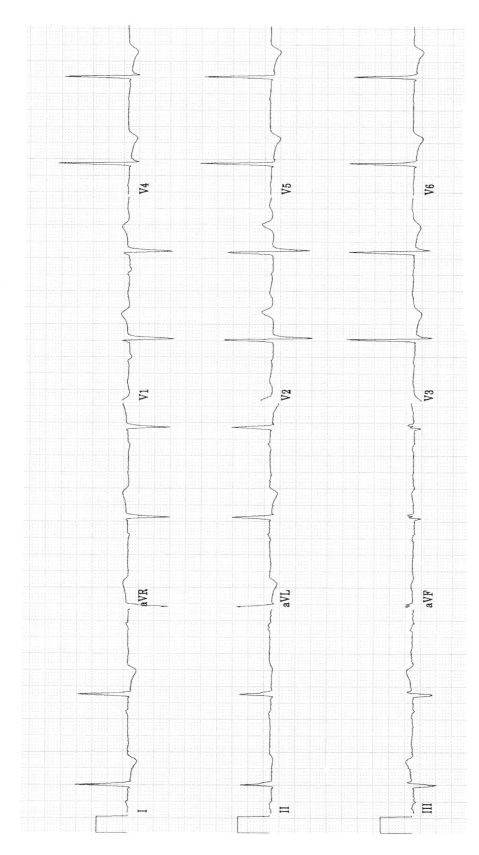

Figure 4.33. **12-lead ECG (abnormal).** *Rhythm:* sinus bradycardia. *Rate:* 55 bpm. *Intervals:* PR 0.24 (first-degree AV block—see Chapter 12), QRS 0.09, QT 0.44 sec. *Axis:* 0°. *P wave:* normal. *QRS:* left ventricular hypertrophy (LVH): S in V_1 (14 mm) + R in V_5 (22 mm) > 35 mm. There are pathologic Q waves in leads III and aVF raising the possibility of an old inferior MI. The *ST segment depression and T wave inversion* are secondary to the abnormal repolarization due to LVH.

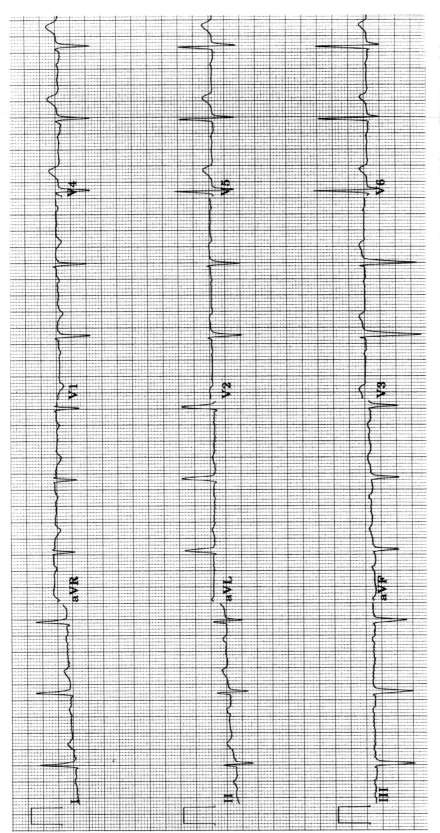

Figure 4.34. **12-lead ECG (abnormal).** *Rhythm:* normal sinus. *Rate:* 68 bpm. *Intervals:* PR 0.24 (first-degree AV block—see Chapter 12), QRS 0.10, QT 0.36 sec. *Axis:* −45° (left axis deviation). *P wave:* left atrial enlargement (terminal deflection of P wave in V₁ is 1 mm wide and 1 mm deep—just barely). *QRS:* pattern of left anterior fascicular block (LAFB; see Fig. 4.20). The abnormally small R waves in leads V₂–V₄ are associated with LAFB, due to the reduction of initial anterior forces. The *ST segment and T waves* are unremarkable.

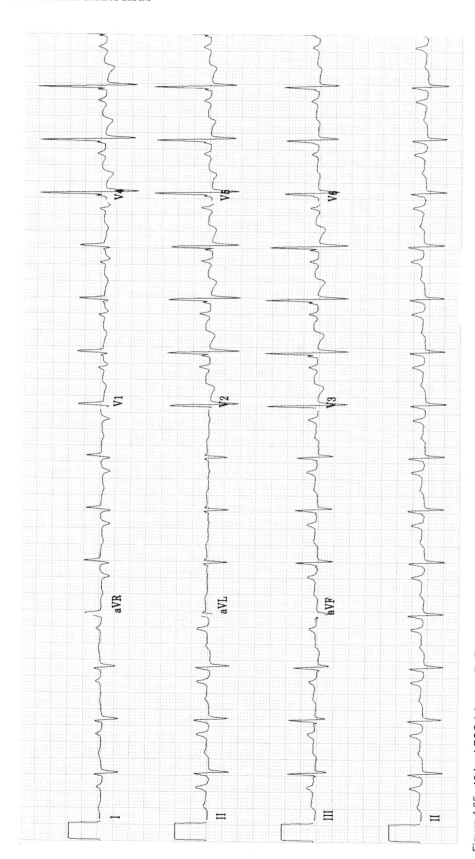

Figure 4.35. 12-lead ECG (abnormal). *Rhythm:* normal sinus. *Rate:* 95 bpm. *Intervals:* PR 0.20, QRS 0.10, QT 0.34 sec. *Axis:* +160° (right axis deviation [RAD]). *P wave:* right atrial enlargement (P in II is > 2.5 mm tall). *QRS:* right ventricular hypertrophy (RVH): R > S in V₁ with RAD. The *T waves* are inverted in the anterior leads, at least in part reflecting abnormal repolarization due to RVH.

Acknowledgments   Contributors to the previous editions of this chapter were Kyle Low, MD; Price Kerfoot, MD; and Leonard S. Lilly, MD.

ADDITIONAL READING

Dubin D. Rapid Interpretation of EKGs. 6th Ed. Tampa: Cover Publishing, 2000.

Goldberger AL, Goldberger E. Clinical Electrocardiography: A Simplified Approach. 6th Ed. St. Louis: Mosby Year Book, 1999.

Mudge GH. Manual of Electrocardiography. 2nd Ed. Boston: Little, Brown & Co., 1991.

Stein E. Rapid Analysis of Electrocardiograms: A Self-Study Course. 3rd Ed. Baltimore: Lippincott Williams & Wilkins, 2000.

Wagner GS. Marriott's Practical Electrocardiography. 10th Ed. Baltimore: Lippincott Williams & Wilkins, 2001.

Atherosclerosis

Mary Beth Gordon and Peter Libby

Chapter 5

The Arterial Wall
Endothelial Cells
Vascular Smooth Muscle Cells
Extracellular Matrix
Pathogenesis of Atherosclerosis
Endothelial Dysfunction
Lipoprotein Entry and Modification
Recruitment of Leukocytes
Recruitment of Smooth Muscle Cells

Complications of Atherosclerosis
Risk Factors for Atherosclerosis and Prevention
Strategies
Dyslipidemia
Tobacco Smoking
Hypertension
Diabetes Mellitus
Physical Activity
Estrogen Status
Emerging Risk Factors

Atherosclerosis, a disease of blood vessels, is known colloquially as "hardening of the arteries." Current models of atherogenesis postulate that various stressors corrupt vascular integrity and allow the abnormal accumulation of lipids, cells, and extracellular matrix within the arterial wall. These unwanted components form lesions known as atherosclerotic plaques. Such plaques may directly cause arterial narrowing, or they may rupture and provoke thrombosis; both mechanisms can limit blood supply to distal tissues. As a result, major complications of atherosclerosis include angina pectoris, myocardial infarction, stroke, and impaired blood flow to the kidneys or lower extremities, making it the leading cause of morbidity and mortality in the developed world.

Despite the prevalence of this disease and the recognition of its pathologic hallmarks for more than a century, the pathophysiology of atherosclerosis remains a topic of active investigation. Many new advances in the field have generated considerable excitement. This chapter describes normal vascular structure and function and then considers the processes associated with atherogenesis, which will help place new advances in context.

THE ARTERIAL WALL

The arterial wall consists of three layers (Fig. 5.1): the **intima,** closest to the arterial lumen and therefore most "intimate" with the blood; the **media,** which is the middle layer; and the outer **adventitia.** The intima is composed of a single layer of endothelial cells that acts as a metabolically active barrier between circulating blood and the vessel. The media is the thickest layer of the normal arterial wall. Boundaries of elastin, known as the internal and external elastic laminae, separate this layer from the intima and adventitia, respectively. These laminae contain openings, termed fenestrae, in the elastic layers through which cells can pass. The media, composed of smooth muscle cells and extracellular matrix, subserves the contractile and elastic functions of the vessel. The elastic component, more prominent in large arteries (e.g., the aorta and its primary branches), stretches during the high pressure of systole and then recoils during diastole. This repetitive action propels blood forward throughout the cardiac cycle. The muscular component, more prominent in smaller arteries such as arterioles, constricts or relaxes to alter vessel resistance and therefore luminal blood flow

Figure 5.1. Schematic diagram of the arterial wall. The intima, the innermost layer, overlies the muscular media demarcated by the internal elastic lamina. The external elastic lamina separates the media from the outer layer, the adventitia.

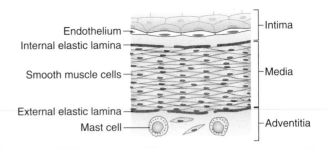

(flow = pressure/resistance, as will be described in Chapter 6). The adventitia contains blood vessels (vaso vasorum), nerves, and lymphatics that nourish the artery.

Atherosclerotic lesions develop and progress in association with dysfunction of elements in the vessel wall, most importantly endothelial cells, vascular smooth muscle cells, and their surrounding extracellular matrix.

Endothelial Cells

In a healthy artery, the endothelium serves structural, metabolic, and signaling functions that maintain the integrity of the vessel wall. The tightly adjoined endothelial cells form a barrier that contains circulating blood within the lumen of the vessel and limits the passage of large molecules from the circulation into the subendothelial space.

As blood traverses the vascular tree, it encounters antithrombotic molecules produced by the endothelium that prevent it from clotting. Some of these molecules reside on the endothelial surface (e.g., heparan sulfate, thrombomodulin, and plasminogen activators, as described in Chapter 7), while other antithrombotic substances are released into the circulation (e.g., prostacyclin and nitric oxide [NO], described in Chapter 6). The endothelium can also produce prothrombotic molecules, but in healthy arteries, a net anticoagulant state prevails.

In response to various stimuli, including the shear stress of blood flow or neurogenic signals, endothelial cells secrete substances that modulate contraction of smooth muscle cells in the underlying medial layer.

These substances can be vasodilating (e.g., nitric oxide, prostacyclin) or vasoconstricting (e.g., endothelin), influencing the resistance of the vessel and therefore luminal blood flow. In a normal artery, the predominance of vasodilator substances results in net smooth muscle relaxation.

Several of the aforementioned endothelial products (e.g., heparan sulfate, nitric oxide) additionally function within the vessel wall to inhibit migration of smooth muscle cells into the intimal layer and their subsequent proliferation. Such effects exemplify how endogenous mechanisms protect against atherosclerosis, as will be examined below.

Finally, endothelial cells play an important role in the immune response. For example, endothelial cells in post-capillary venules respond to local injury or infection by secreting chemicals known as chemokines, which attract circulating white blood cells to the area. At the same time, the endothelium increases production of cell-surface adhesion molecules, which allow mononuclear cells to bind to the endothelium and later move through the vessel to the site of tissue injury. In the absence of such pathologic stimulation, healthy arterial endothelial cells *resist* leukocyte adhesion and are therefore anti-inflammatory. However, under the adverse influences that are present during atherogenesis, they may abnormally *recruit* leukocytes to the vessel wall.

Thus, in its normal state, the intimal endothelial layer provides a protective non-thrombogenic surface with homeostatic vasodilator and anti-inflammatory properties (Table 5.1). It appears that nondenuding injury of the endothelium triggers the development of atherosclerotic lesions, as will be examined.

Vascular Smooth Muscle Cells

Smooth muscle cells within the vessel wall have both contractile and synthetic capabilities. Various vasoactive substances stimulate the smooth muscle cells to contract. Such agonists include circulating molecules (e.g., angiotensin II), those released from local nerve terminals (e.g., acetylcholine), or those originating from the overlying endothelium (e.g., endothelin, NO). When a vasoactive ligand binds to its specific receptor on the smooth muscle cell, myocyte contraction or relaxation follows, thus altering the diameter of the vessel's lumen.

Vascular smooth muscle cells also have synthetic functions. In healthy vessels, they produce the collagen, elastin, and proteoglycans that form the vascular extracellular matrix. Smooth muscle cells can also produce various vasoactive and inflammatory mediators. Such products include cytokines, particularly interleukin-6 (IL-6) and tumor necrosis factor-α (TNF-α), which can promote lymphocyte proliferation, induce endothelial expression of leukocyte

adhesion molecules, and propagate inflammatory responses. These synthetic functions of smooth muscle cells become more prominent in disease states such as atherosclerosis.

Extracellular Matrix

In healthy arteries, fibrillar collagen and elastin comprise the bulk of the extracellular matrix in the medial layer. Interstitial collagen fibrils, constructed from intertwining helical proteins, have great biomechanical strength. Elastin provides flexibility. Together these components maintain the structural integrity of the vessel despite high pressures within the lumen and, in the case of elastic arteries, store the kinetic energy of systole, which subsequently promotes diastolic flow. Recent evidence suggests that the extracellular matrix also regulates the growth of its resident cells. Native fibrillar collagen, in particular, can inhibit smooth muscle cell proliferation in vitro. In addition, matrix components influence cellular responses to stimuli: matrix-bound cells respond differently to growth factors and are less likely to undergo apoptosis (programmed cell death).

TABLE 5.1. Endothelial Cell Functions

Activity	Normal Endothelium	"Activated" (Dysfunctional) Endothelium
Barrier function	Forms tight barrier that restricts passage of large molecules and cells into subendothelial space	Demonstrates increased permeability
Antithrombotic activity	Resists thrombosis through actions of heparan sulfate, thrombomodulin, plasminogen activators, and secretion of platelet inhibitors (e.g., prostacyclin, NO)	Reduced antithrombotic properties (e.g., decreased secretion of prostacyclin and NO)
Effect on vascular tone	Promotes vasodilation through secretion of prostacyclin and NO	Promotes vasoconstriction due to impaired secretion of prostacyclin and NO
Effect on arterial smooth muscle cells	Inhibits smooth muscle cell migration and proliferation (via heparan sulfate and NO)	Promotes smooth muscle cell migration and proliferation (decreased secretion of NO, increased secretion of PDGF)
Immune function	Binds leukocytes appropriately in response to cell injury	Promotes leukocyte chemotaxis, adhesion, and penetration via increased cytokine production (e.g., M-CSF, MCP-1) and cellular adhesion molecules and selectins

NO, nitric oxide; PDGF, platelet-derived growth factor; M-CSF, macrophage colony stimulating factor; MCP-1, monocyte chemoattractant protein 1.

PATHOGENESIS OF ATHEROSCLEROSIS

Considerable evidence supports the view that atherogenesis is a chronic inflammatory process. Ongoing research has identified several key stimuli and components of this inflammatory response (Fig. 5.2). The steps include accumulation of lipids within the intima, recruitment of leukocytes and smooth muscle cells to the vessel wall, and deposition of extracellular matrix. This discussion provides a general framework, the specific details of which will likely undergo refinement as further knowledge evolves.

Endothelial Dysfunction

Many researchers believe that *"injury" to the arterial endothelium represents a primary event in atherogenesis.* Actual desquamative injury or sloughing of endothelial cells occurs later than the dysfunction or activation of these cells that occurs in the earliest stages of this disease.

Physical forces may cause endothelial dysfunction. For example, arterial branch points disturb laminar (i.e., smooth) blood flow. Normal laminar shear forces favor the endothelial expression of the enzyme that produces nitric oxide (which is beneficial as an endogenous vasodilator, inhibitor of platelet aggregation, and anti-inflammatory substance, as described in Chapter 6) and accentuates expression of the anti-oxidant enzyme superoxide dismutase. The disturbed flow at arterial branch points locally alters these normally atheroprotective functions of the endothelium. In fact, atherosclerotic lesions commonly develop around arterial branch points, and arteries with few branches (e.g., the internal mammary artery) show relative resistance to atherosclerosis.

Endothelial dysfunction may also result from exposure to a "toxic" chemical environment. For example, cigarette smoking, abnormal circulating lipid levels, or diabetes—all known risk factors for atherosclerosis—can promote endothelial dysfunction. Recent studies indicate that each of these states increases endothelial production of reactive oxygen species. These substances, primarily superoxide anion, interact with other intracellular

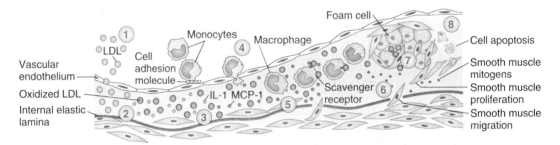

Figure 5.2. **Schematic diagram of the evolution of atherosclerotic plaque.** (1) Accumulation of lipoprotein particles in the intima. The darker color depicts modification of the lipoproteins (e.g., by oxidation or glycation). (2) Oxidative stress, including constituents of modified LDL (mLDL), induces local cytokine elaboration. (3) These cytokines induce increased expression of adhesion molecules that bind leukocytes and of chemoattractant molecules (e.g., monocyte chemoattractant protein 1 [MCP-1]) that direct leukocyte migration into the intima. (4) Blood monocytes, after entering the artery wall in response to chemoattractants, encounter stimuli such as macrophage colony stimulating factor (M-CSF) that augment their expression of scavenger receptors. (5) Scavenger receptors mediate the uptake of modified lipoprotein particles and promote the development of foam cells. Macrophage foam cells are a source of additional cytokines and effector molecules such as superoxide anion (O_2^-) and matrix metalloproteinases. (6) Smooth muscle cells migrate into the intima from the media. Note the increasing intimal thickness. (7) Intimal smooth muscle cells divide and elaborate extracellular matrix, promoting matrix accumulation in the growing atherosclerotic plaque. In this manner, the fatty streak can evolve into a fibrofatty lesion. (8) In later stages, calcification can occur (not depicted) and fibrosis continues, sometimes accompanied by smooth muscle cell death (including programmed cell death or apoptosis), yielding a relatively acellular fibrous capsule surrounding a lipid-rich core that may also contain dying or dead cells. LDL, low-density lipoprotein. IL-1, interleukin 1. (Modified from Braunwald E, Zipes D, Libby P, eds. Heart Disease: A Textbook of Cardiovascular Medicine. Philadelphia: WB Saunders, 2001:997.)

TABLE 5.2. Plasma Lipoproteins (In Order of Increasing Density)

Type	Source	Major Lipid Component	Associated Apoproteins
Chylomicrons	Gastrointestinal tract	Triglycerides	A-I, A-II, A-IV, B-48, C-1, C-II, C-III, E
VLDL	Liver	Triglycerides	B-100, C-I, C-II, C-III, E
IDL	Remnant of VLDL	Cholesterol	B-100, E
LDL	Metabolism of IDL	Cholesterol	B-100
HDL	Gastrointestinal tract, liver	Cholesterol	A-1, A-II, C-I, C-II, C-III, E

VLDL, very–low-density lipoprotein; *IDL,* intermediate-density lipoprotein; *LDL,* low-density lipoprotein; *HDL,* high-density lipoprotein.

molecules to influence the metabolic and synthetic functions of the endothelial cell.

Even before atherosclerotic lesions form, these physical and chemical factors can adversely affect endothelial functions, manifested by 1) impairment of the endothelium's role as a permeability barrier, 2) release of inflammatory cytokines, 3) increased transcription of cell-surface adhesion molecules, 4) altered release of vasoactive substances (e.g., prostacyclin and NO), and 5) interference with normal antithrombotic properties. These undesired effects of endothelial dysfunction (see Table 5.1) lay the groundwork for subsequent events in the development of atherosclerosis.

Lipoprotein Entry and Modification

Lipoproteins ferry water-insoluble fats through the bloodstream. These particles consist of a lipid core surrounded by more hydrophilic phospholipid, free cholesterol, and apolipoproteins (also called apoproteins). The apoproteins present on different classes of lipoprotein molecules serve to direct the particles to specific organ and tissue receptors. Five major classes of lipoproteins exist, distinguished by their densities, lipid constituents, and associated apoproteins (Table 5.2): chylomicrons, very–low-density lipoproteins (VLDL), intermediate-density lipoproteins (IDL), low-density lipoproteins (LDL), and high-density lipoproteins (HDL). Box 5.1 summarizes the major pathways of lipoprotein transport and metabolism. Of note, elevated LDL levels correlate closely with atherosclerosis development. Conversely, elevated HDL levels protect against athero-

sclerosis, thought to be related to HDL's ability to transport lipids away from peripheral tissues back to the liver for disposal.

When the endothelium becomes dysfunctional, it no longer serves as an effective barrier to the passage of circulating lipoproteins into the arterial wall. For example, increased endothelial permeability allows the entry of LDL into the intima, a process facilitated by an elevated circulating LDL concentration. Once within the intima, LDL accumulates in the subendothelial space by binding to components of the extracellular matrix known as proteoglycans. This "trapping" increases the residence time of LDL within the vessel wall, where the lipoprotein may undergo chemical modifications that appear critical to the development of atherosclerotic lesions. Hypertension, a major risk factor for atherosclerosis, may promote retention of lipoproteins in the intima by accentuating the production of LDL-binding proteoglycans by smooth muscle cells.

Oxidation is one type of modification that befalls LDL trapped in the subendothelial space. It can result from the local action of reactive oxygen species and pro-oxidant enzymes derived from activated endothelial or smooth muscle cells, or from macrophages that penetrate the vessel wall. In diabetics with sustained hyperglycemia, *glycation* of LDL also occurs, rendering LDL antigenic and ultimately pro-inflammatory.

These biochemical modifications of LDL have several major consequences: 1) modified LDL (mLDL) acts as a chemoattractant that recruits circulating monocytes to the vessel wall; 2) mLDL increases endothelial

---

Box 5.1. The Lipoprotein Transport System

The movement of lipids through the circulation serves critical biologic functions. Triglycerides are transported from the intestine and liver to muscles and adipose tissue, to be utilized or stored for energy. Cholesterol is ferried to peripheral tissues for membrane synthesis and steroid hormone production as well as to the liver for bile acid formation. The major circulating lipoprotein pathways are shown in the figure. The most important apolipoproteins (apo) responsible for directing the particles to specific tissue receptors are indicated in parentheses.

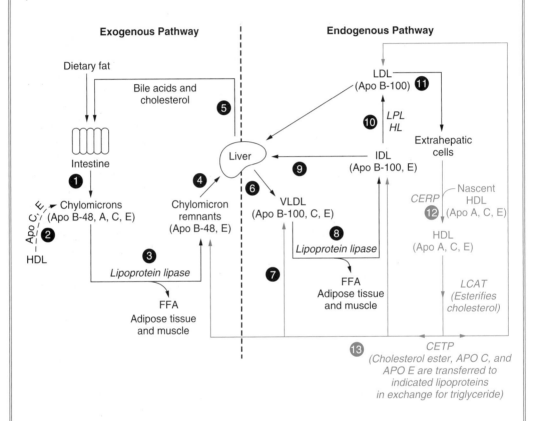

The "exogenous" lipoprotein pathway is indicated in the figure by the following numeric labels. (1) Dietary fats are absorbed by the gastrointestinal tract and repackaged as chylomicrons, accompanied by apo B-48. These large particles, which are particularly rich in triglycerides, enter the circulation via the lymphatic system. (2) Chylomicrons in the bloodstream interact with HDL particles (of gastrointestinal tract and liver origin), during which apo C and E are transferred to the chylomicrons. Apo C (subtype CII) enhances interactions of the chylomicron with lipoprotein lipase, while apo E binds hepatic receptors avidly. (3) *Lipoprotein lipase (LPL),* an enzyme present in capillary endothelial cells of adipose and muscle tissue, hydrolyzes the triglycerides within chylomi-

crons. Adipose tissue accepts and stores the resulting free fatty acids (FFA), while cardiac and skeletal muscle absorb the fatty acids for energy use. In muscle, such absorption requires the hormone insulin. In the setting of decreased insulin, or insulin-resistant states such as diabetes mellitus, unused free fatty acids persist in the bloodstream until returning to the liver, where they are repackaged as triglycerides. During lipolysis by LPL, some surface components (e.g., apo C and E) are transferred back to HDL particles.
(4) Chylomicron remnants are removed from the circulation by the liver, mediated by apo E. (5) One fate of cholesterol in the liver is incorporation into bile acids, which are exported to the intestine, completing the exogenous pathway.

The "endogenous" lipoprotein pathway is shown in the figure by the following numeric labels. (6) The liver packages cholesterol and triglycerides, along with apolipoproteins and phospholipid, into very–low-density lipoprotein (VLDL) particles. The predominant apolipoprotein of VLDL is apo B-100. Although the triglyceride content of VLDL is much higher than the cholesterol content, this is the main means by which the liver secretes cholesterol into the bloodstream.
(7) Like chylomicrons, VLDL interacts with HDL, mediated by the enzyme *cholesteryl ester transfer protein (CETP)*. In this process, VLDL exchanges some of its triglyceride for apo C, apo E, and cholesteryl esters from HDL particles (as described in #13 below). (8) The VLDL is then catabolized by lipoprotein lipase in capillary beds (similar to chylomicrons), releasing fatty acids to muscle and adipose tissue. (9) Approximately 50% of the VLDL remnants (termed "intermediate density lipoprotein (IDL)") are then cleared by the liver by hepatic receptors that recognize apo E. (10) The remaining IDL is catabolized further by LPL and hepatic lipases (HL), which remove additional triglyceride, apo E and apo C, forming low–density lipoprotein (LDL) particles. Essentially all circulating LDL is derived from IDL in this way. (11) Plasma clearance of LDL occurs primarily via LDL receptor-mediated endocytosis in the liver and peripheral cells, directed by LDL's apolipoprotein B-100.

Cholesterol in the liver can be incorporated into bile acids and excreted into the intestine (as described in #5 above) or packaged into VLDL and secreted into the bloodstream (#6 above). In nonhepatic tissues, the internalized cholesterol is directed to hormone production, membrane synthesis, or storage. Peripheral cells augment LDL receptor expression when intracellular cholesterol levels are low. (12) Under conditions of intracellular cholesterol excess, the cells increase transcription of *cholesterol efflux regulatory protein (CERP)*, which is the product of the ATP binding-cassette 1 gene (ABC A-1 gene). CERP facilitates cholesterol removal from the cell by circulating high–density lipoprotein (HDL) particles, which in turn deliver the cholesterol to the liver in a process known as *reverse cholesterol transport* (shown in blue color). As free cholesterol is acquired by nascent (immature) circulating HDL particles, it is esterified by *lecithin cholesterol acyltransferase (LCAT)*, an enzyme activated by apo A of HDL. The hydrophobic cholesterol esters move into the particle's core. (13) The majority of cholesterol esters in HDL can then be exchanged in the circulation (via the enzyme CETP) with any of the apo B containing lipoproteins (e.g., VLDL, IDL, LDL), which deliver the cholesterol back to the liver.

expression of genes encoding mediators of inflammation (e.g., monocyte colony stimulating factor [M-CSF], monocyte chemoattractant protein [MCP-1], and certain leukocyte adhesion molecules); and 3) unlike normal LDL particles, mLDL can be ingested by macrophages and other cells in large quantities because it is not regulated by "negative feedback inhibition." Normally, cells take up LDL via surface LDL receptors. When intracellular cholesterol content increases, the number of LDL receptors expressed on the cell surface decreases, such that further lipoprotein uptake is lessened. However, such receptors do not recognize LDL that has undergone chemical modification; therefore, mLDL cannot be internalized by that mechanism. Conversely, macrophages can ingest mLDL through scavenger receptors that, unlike classical LDL receptors, evade negative feedback inhibition and permit engorgement of the cell as it fills with the cholesterol-rich lipid. Such lipid-laden scavenger cells, also known as "foam cells," abound in early atherosclerotic lesions.

Recruitment of Leukocytes

Following the entry and biochemical modification of LDL, subsequent key steps in atherogenesis include the attraction and adherence of leukocytes, primarily monocytes and T lymphocytes, to the vessel wall. Several factors contribute to this process: 1) the chemoattractant properties ascribed to mLDL; 2) endothelial expression of specific cytokines (e.g., MCP-1 and interleukin-1 [IL-1]); and 3) the expression of leukocyte adhesion molecules on the luminal surface of the injured endothelial cells. Examples of adhesion molecule include vascular cell adhesion molecule-1 (VCAM-1) and intercellular adhesion molecules-1 (ICAM-1), members of the immunoglobulin gene superfamily that bind integrin molecules on white blood cells. Another class of adhesion molecules, the selectins, binds carbohydrate moieties on the leukocyte surface. Components of oxidatively modified LDL stimulate the expression of such endothelial-leukocyte adhesion molecules. Thus,

lipid accumulation within the intima directly promotes subsequent inflammation of the vessel wall.

After monocytes have adhered to the luminal surface of the intima, they may penetrate into the subendothelial space by slipping between the junctions of the endothelial monolayer. Once localized beneath the endothelium, monocytes differentiate into macrophages, the phagocytic cells capable of ingesting modified LDL in large quantities by the scavenger pathway described above. In this manner, macrophages become lipid-laden foam cells, the primary constituent of the atherosclerotic lesion known as the **fatty streak.**

Fatty streaks represent the earliest visible lesions of atherosclerosis. On gross inspection, they appear as areas of yellow discoloration on the artery's inner surface. Fatty streaks may occur as spots less than 1 mm in diameter or streaks 1- to 2-mm wide and up to 1 cm long (Fig. 5.3). They do not protrude into the arterial lumen and do not disturb blood flow. Surprisingly, fatty streaks exist in the aorta and coronary arteries of most individuals *by age 20.* They do not cause symptoms, and in some locations in the vasculature, they may regress over time. However, in other locations such as the coronary arteries, fatty streaks can develop into more ominous **fibrous plaques.**

T lymphocytes, the principal mediators of the cellular immune system, also arrive in the intima early during atherogenesis. T cells constitute a relatively small fraction of the cells within an atheromatous plaque, outnumbered by macrophages and smooth muscle cells. However, T cells become activated during atherogenesis and produce cytokines that likely modulate lesion formation.

Recruitment of Smooth Muscle Cells

The transition from fatty streak to fibrous plaque involves the migration of smooth muscle cells from the arterial media into the injured intima, proliferation of the smooth muscle cells within the intima, and leukocyte activation. The increase in the smooth muscle cell mass growing from the medial layer into the diseased intima, the accumulation of leukocytes and foam cells, and the development of a surrounding "fibrous cap" of extracellular matrix tissue with embedded smooth muscle cells characterize the fibrous plaque of advanced atherosclerotic disease.

Fibrous plaques appear to localize to the same sites where fatty streaks typically occur. Grossly, they form firm, pale gray, elevated lesions (Fig. 5.5). They may project into the arterial lumen and, if sufficiently large, constitute a clinically significant stenosis that reduces blood flow through the vessel. Fibrous plaques often contain a necrotic core of cell debris, which may result from the toxic effects of highly oxidized LDL and the accumulation of oxygen-derived free radicals and hydrolytic enzymes derived from activated macrophages and T cells. The necrotic core may also contain degenerating

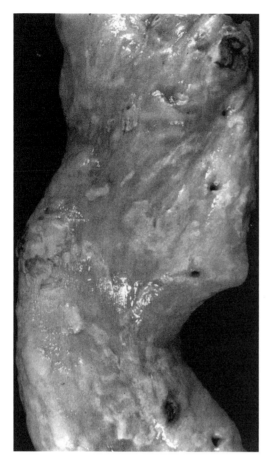

Figure 5.3. **Gross specimen of an aorta with extensive fatty streak formation.** (Courtesy of Dr. Frederick Schoen, Brigham & Women's Hospital, Boston, MA.)

secretion of connective tissue by the smooth muscle cells. Foam cells, activated platelets, and endothelial cells can all elaborate substances responsible for smooth muscle cell migration and proliferation (Fig. 5.4).

Foam cells produce several factors that contribute to smooth muscle cell recruitment. For example, they release platelet-derived growth factor (PDGF), which stimulates the migration of smooth muscle cells into the intimal subendothelial space, where they subsequently replicate. Foam cells also release cytokines and growth factors (e.g., TNF-α, IL-1, fibroblast growth factor, and transforming growth factor-β) that additionally modulate smooth muscle cell proliferation and synthesis of extracellular matrix proteins as well as stimulate

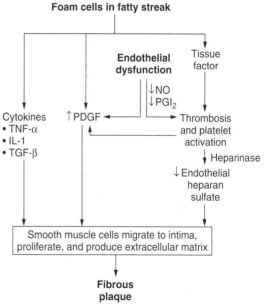

Figure 5.4. **The transition from fatty streak to fibrous plaque involves the migration and proliferation of smooth muscle cells and production of extracellular matrix.** Substances released from foam cells, dysfunctional endothelial cells, and platelets contribute to this process. TNF-α, tumor necrosis factor-α; IL-1, interleukin-1; TGF-β, transforming growth factor-β; PDGF-platelet-derived growth factor; NO, nitric oxide; PGI$_2$, prostacyclin.

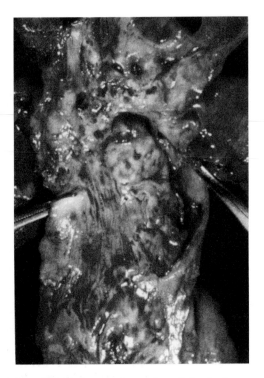

Figure 5.5. **Gross specimen of an abdominal aorta with extensive fibrous plaque formation.** (Courtesy of Dr. Frederick Schoen, Brigham & Women's Hospital, Boston, MA.)

foam cells, which in fibrous plaques are more likely derived from smooth muscle cells than from macrophages. These foam cells release cholesterol crystals, which may then become engulfed by new smooth muscle cells growing into the lesion.

The core of the fibrous plaque is excessively thrombogenic. Foam cells produce large amounts of tissue factor, which can activate the coagulation pathway when contact is made with components in blood. Since the atheromatous plaque is covered by a fibrous cap and endothelium, the thrombogenic core containing tissue factor is usually "hidden" from circulating blood. However, small breaches in the integrity of advanced atherosclerotic lesions may expose tissue factor, and microthrombi rich in platelets can then adhere to areas of the interrupted endothelium. The activated platelets within such microthrombi release potent factors that also contribute to smooth muscle cell migration and proliferation. These factors include PDGF (the ac-

tions of which are described above), and heparinase. The latter degrades heparan sulfate, a polysaccharide in the extracellular matrix that normally *inhibits* smooth muscle cell migration and proliferation.

Other alterations in vascular cell biology may contribute to atherogenesis as well. For example, the "monoclonal hypothesis" views autonomous smooth muscle proliferation in the intima induced by genetic, chemical, or viral stimuli as a key process in lesion formation. The finding that the cells within some human atherosclerotic plaques appear to descend from a single smooth muscle cell supports this view.

COMPLICATIONS OF ATHEROSCLEROSIS

Fibrous plaques are not homogeneously distributed throughout the vasculature. They usually develop first in the dorsal aspect of the abdominal aorta and proximal coronary arteries, followed by the popliteal arteries, descending thoracic aorta, internal carotid arteries, and renal arteries. Therefore, the regions perfused by these vessels are the ones that most commonly suffer the consequences of atherosclerosis.

Complications of fibrous plaques—including calcification, rupture, hemorrhage, and embolization—have dire clinical results, due to acute restriction of blood flow or alterations in vessel wall integrity. These complications, which are discussed in greater detail in later chapters, include:

1. Calcification of fibrous plaque, which imparts a pipe-like rigidity to the vessel wall and increases its fragility.
2. Rupture or ulceration of the fibrous plaque, which exposes thrombogenic material in the core to circulating blood, causing a thrombus to form at that site. Such thrombosis can occlude the vessel and result in infarction of the involved organ. Alternatively, the thrombus material can incorporate into the lesion and add to the bulk of the plaque.
3. Hemorrhage into the plaque from rupture of the fibrous cap or of the tiny capillaries that vascularize the plaque.

The resulting hematoma may further narrow the vessel lumen.

4. Embolization of fragments of disrupted atheroma to distal vascular sites.

5. Weakening of the vessel wall, as the fibrous plaque subjects the neighboring medial layer to increased pressure, which may provoke atrophy and loss of elastic tissue with subsequent dilatation of the artery, forming an aneurysm.

Atherosclerotic plaques usually grow gradually and attract attention only when a lesion sufficiently restricts blood flow to an organ, or alters the integrity of an artery, such that symptoms develop. The major clinical manifestations that arise from the complications of fibrous plaque are summarized in Table 5.3. For example, as described in Chapter 6, atherosclerotic lesions within the coronary arteries may impair perfusion to the myocardium and produce intermittent chest discomfort (angina pectoris), the classic symptom of coronary artery disease. In other instances, a fibrous plaque may become complicated by a superimposed thrombus that fully obstructs a coronary artery, resulting in a sudden acute myocardial infarction (as described in Chapter 7).

Recent studies have shown that the degree of coronary artery narrowing (as, for example, observed by coronary angiography) correlates poorly with the subsequent occurrence of myocardial infarction at that site. Such observations support the hypothesis that acute coronary events usually result from plaque rupture with superimposed thrombosis, rather than vessel occlusion due to gradual, progressive enlargement of fibrous plaque. The "culprit lesions" that lead to acute thrombosis and clinical events such as myocardial infarction often appear innocent (i.e., only mildly narrowed) angiographically.

One factor that contributes to a plaque's susceptibility to rupture is the thickness of the fibrous cap that separates the lesion's foam cells (which contain tissue factor, the powerful procoagulant) from circulating blood elements (Fig. 5.6). Whereas lesions with thick fibrous caps may cause pronounced arterial narrowing, they have less propensity to rupture. Conversely, "vulnerable" plaques have thinner caps, often appear minor angiographically, but are fragile and more likely to rupture, inciting thrombosis. Such vulnerable plaques often have a very rich lipid core and a high concentration of inflammatory cells (e.g., macrophages and T lymphocytes).

Gamma interferon, a T-lymphocyte–derived mediator elaborated in response to chronic inflammation within plaque, can inhibit collagen synthesis by smooth muscle cells, and impede the ability of these cells to maintain and repair the fibrous cap that protects the lesion from rupture. Gamma interferon can also activate local macrophages. The macrophages in athero-

TABLE 5.3. Complications of Atherosclerosis

Complication	Mechanism	Examples
Narrowing and calcification of vessel	Progressive development of fibrous plaque Organization of microthrombi within lesion	Myocardial ischemia (Chapter 6) Limb claudication (Chapter 15)
Thrombus formation with occlusion of lumen	Plaque ulceration or rupture Plaque hemorrhage with rupture	Myocardial infarction or unstable angina Thrombotic stroke (cerebral infarction)
Peripheral emboli	Fragmentation and passage of atheromatous material from large proximal vessel to smaller peripheral vessels	Embolic stroke Atheroembolic renal failure
Weakening of vessel wall	Pressure on neighboring medial layer promotes atrophy of muscle cells and loss of elastic tissue	Aortic aneurysms (Chapter 15)

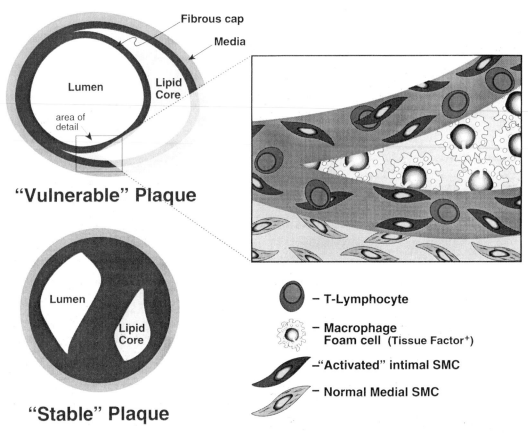

Figure 5.6. **Schematic diagram demonstrating characteristics of "vulnerable" and "stable" atherosclerotic plaques.** The vulnerable plaque usually has a substantial lipid core and a thin fibrous cap separating the thrombogenic macrophages (bearing tissue factor) from the blood. At sites of lesion disruption, smooth muscle cells (SMCs) are often activated. In contrast, the stable plaque has a thick fibrous cap protecting the lipid core from contact with the blood. Clinical data suggest that stable plaques more often show luminal narrowing detectable by angiography than do vulnerable plaques. (Reproduced with permission from Libby P. Molecular bases of the acute coronary syndromes. Circulation 1995;91:2844–2850, copyright 1995, American Heart Association.)

sclerotic lesions often localize at the borders of the plaque, abutting normal tissue (the "shoulder regions"), and release mediators of inflammation and enzymes (matrix metalloproteinases) that degrade collagen and elastin, thereby further weakening the fibrous cap and predisposing it to rupture.

RISK FACTORS FOR ATHEROSCLEROSIS AND PREVENTION STRATEGIES

Many population studies have identified several specific attributes that are associated with the development of atherosclerosis. For example, the Framingham Heart Study has provided longitudinal follow-up of a large cohort of individuals, examining the relationship between risk factors and cardiovascular outcomes. Another source of data, the Multiple Risk Factor Intervention Trial (MRFIT), screened more than 325,000 men to evaluate the relationship between risk factors and subsequent cardiovascular disease and mortality. Studies such as these have identified major, potentially modifiable risk factors for atherosclerosis including: 1) aberrant levels of circulating lipids ("dyslipidemia"), 2) hypertension, 3) cigarette smoking, and 4) diabetes mellitus.

Major "nonmodifiable" risk factors include advanced age, male gender, and a history of the development of coronary disease among family members at a young age (i.e., male family members younger than age 55 or female family members younger than age 65). Additional potentially modifiable risk factors include obesity and low levels of physical activity. Recently, certain markers have been associated with the development of atherosclerosis and are undergoing rigorous evaluation as "new" risk factors. These include elevated circulating levels of 1) the amino acid metabolite homocysteine, 2) the special lipoprotein particle Lp(a), and 3) certain markers of inflammation including the acute-phase reactant C-reactive protein.

Dyslipidemia

A large and consistent body of evidence establishes abnormal circulating lipid levels as a major risk factor for the development of atherosclerosis. Observational studies have shown that compared with countries with traditionally low saturated fat intake and low serum cholesterol levels (e.g., Japan and certain Mediterranean states), the United States and other societies with higher consumption of saturated fat and cholesterol levels have higher mortality rates due to coronary disease.

Similarly, data from the Framingham Study and other trials have shown that the risk of ischemic heart disease increases with higher total serum cholesterol levels. The coronary risk is approximately twice as high for an individual with a total cholesterol level of 240 mg/dL than for one with a cholesterol level of 200 mg/dL.

However, not *all* lipoproteins bearing cholesterol are harmful. In fact, cholesterol has a variety of critical functions in normal physiology. All cells require cholesterol to form membranes and maintain fluidity of the phospholipid bilayer. Some cells use cholesterol to synthesize specialized products, such as steroid hormones and bile salts.

Normally, intracellular cholesterol content is maintained by the tight regulation of cholesterol uptake, de novo synthesis, storage, and its efflux from the cell. The enzyme HMG CoA reductase is the rate-limiting step of intracellular cholesterol biosynthesis. Cellular uptake of cholesterol is con-

trolled by receptor-mediated endocytosis of circulating LDL particles. High intracellular cholesterol levels *inhibit* the enzyme HMG CoA reductase and signal the cell to decrease production of LDL receptors. A sufficient quantity of intracellular cholesterol in peripheral cells also triggers increased production of cholesterol efflux regulatory protein (CERP), a product of the recently identified ATP binding cassette 1 (ABC A-1) gene. CERP mediates the transfer of membrane cholesterol to HDL particles, which transport the excess cholesterol back to the liver in a process known as reverse cholesterol transport (see Box 5.1). Due to its ability to remove intracellular lipids, HDL protects against lipid accumulation, and serum HDL levels correlate *inversely* with the presence of atherosclerotic disease. Thus HDL is often termed "good cholesterol."

Conversely, high levels of LDL correlate with an *increased* incidence of atherosclerosis and coronary artery disease. When present in excess, LDL can accumulate in the subendothelial space and undergo the chemical modifications that further damage the intima as described above, inciting or enhancing the development of atherosclerotic lesions. LDL is thus commonly known as "bad cholesterol."

Elevated serum LDL may persist for many reasons, including a high-fat diet or because of defects in the LDL-receptor clearance mechanism. Patients with genetic defects in the LDL receptor (usually heterozygotes with one normal and one defective gene coding for the receptor) cannot remove LDL from the circulation efficiently. This condition is called *familial hypercholesterolemia,* and such individuals have high plasma LDL levels and develop premature atherosclerosis. Homozygotes who *totally* lack functional LDL receptors may sustain a myocardial infarction as early as the first decade of life.

Recently, subclasses of circulating LDL have been identified based on the buoyant densities of the particles. Researchers have examined whether smaller, dense LDL particles are more likely than large LDL particles to increase the risk of myocardial infarction, with conflicting results. Although the presence of abundant circulating small LDL does correlate with coronary disease, it may simply serve as a marker for other lipid abnormalities. Clinically, measurement of LDL particle size has limited use, since a high triglyceride value and a low level of HDL correlate with the presence of small, dense LDL particles.

Increasing evidence implicates triglyceride-rich lipoproteins, such as VLDL and IDL, in the development of atherosclerosis. It is not yet clear if these particles participate directly in atherogenesis or simply keep company with low levels of HDL cholesterol. Of note, poorly controlled type II diabetes mellitus is often associated with hypertriglyceridemia and low HDL levels, frequently accompanied by central obesity (increased abdominal girth) and hypertension. This clustering of risk factors, known as the **metabolic syndrome,** may relate to a state of insulin resistance (described in Chapter 13) and is particularly atherogenic. Other secondary causes of abnormal serum lipid levels include thyroid, renal, and liver disease as well as certain medications, such as immunosuppressive and antiretroviral therapies.

Lipid-Altering Therapy

Strategies that improve abnormal lipid levels can limit atherosclerosis and its clinical complications. Many large studies of patients with coronary disease show that dietary or pharmacologic reduction of serum cholesterol can prevent progression—and in some cases induce modest regression—of coronary atherosclerotic lesions. Such studies form the basis of current screening guidelines, devised by the third National Cholesterol Education Program panel, which recommends a fasting lipid profile every 5 years for all adults. These guidelines identify an "optimal" LDL cholesterol level as <100 mg/dL. Patients with established atherosclerosis or those who have equivalent risk should be treated to attain this goal.

Diet and exercise are two important components of the lipid-lowering arsenal. For example, the Lyon Heart Study demonstrated that patients with heart disease who reduced saturated fat intake substantially decreased their risk of recurrent cardiac events. The Mediterranean-style diet implemented in this study replaced saturated fats with polyunsaturated fats. In vitro evidence indicates that polyunsaturated fats may activate a transcription factor (peroxisomal proliferation activating receptor-α [PPAR-α]), which increases expression of the major HDL apoprotein (A1) and of the enzyme lipoprotein lipase as well as inhibits cytokine-induced expression of leukocyte adhesion molecules on endothelial cells. These actions are potentially antiatherogenic. Physical activity and loss of excessive weight are other ways to nonpharmacologically improve the lipid profile.

When lifestyle modifications fail to achieve target values, a variety of drugs can be used to treat abnormal lipid levels. The major groups of lipid-altering agents are described in Chapter 17 and include HMG CoA reductase inhibitors, bile-acid binding agents, niacin, and fibric acid derivatives. The most effective LDL-lowering agents are the HMG CoA reductase inhibitors (also known as "statins"). As detailed in Chapter 17, statins inhibit the rate-limiting enzyme responsible for cholesterol biosynthesis. The resultant low intracellular cholesterol concentrations lead to increased LDL-receptor expression and thus augmented clearance of LDL particles from the bloodstream. Statins also lower the rate of VLDL synthesis by the liver, and by an unknown mechanism, raise HDL levels.

Major clinical trials evaluating statin therapy have consistently demonstrated striking reductions in ischemic cardiac events, the occurrence of strokes, and (in many cases) mortality rates (Table 5.4). Such studies have included individuals with broad ranges of LDL levels and cardiac risk, with or without known preexisting atherosclerotic disease, and the benefits of statins extend widely to each of these groups.

The impressive benefits of statins likely derive from several mechanisms. The combination of lowering LDL and elevating

TABLE 5.4. Randomized, Double-Blind, Placebo-Controlled Clinical Trials of Statin Therapy

Trial	n	Baseline Lipids	Known CAD?	Follow-up (yr)	ΔTotal Cholesterol[a]	ΔLDL[a]	ΔHDL[a]	ΔCoronary Events[b]	ΔCardiovascular Mortality[b]
4S[c]	4444	High LDL	Yes	5.4	−25%	−35%	+8%	−34%	−30%
WOSCOPS[d]	6595	High LDL	No	4.9	−20%	−26%	+5%	−31%	−32%
CARE[e]	4159	Average LDL	Yes	5.0	−20%	−28%	+5%	−24%	—
LIPID[f]	9014	Average-high LDL	Yes	6.1	−18%	−25%	+5%	—	−24%
AFCAPS/TexCAPS[g]	6605	Average total and LDL; low HDL	No	5.2	−18%	−25%	+6%	−37%	—
HPS[h]	20,000	Total cholesterol >135 mg/dL	±	5.5	—	−30%	—	−26%	−18%

[a]Change in lipid levels with statin therapy.
[b]Outcomes in patients randomized to statin therapy versus patients randomized to placebo.
[c]Scandinavian Simvastatin Survival Study. Lancet 1994;344:1383–1389.
[d]West of Scotland Coronary Primary Prevention Study. N Engl J Med 1995;333:1301–1307.
[e]Cholesterol and Recurrent Events. N Engl J Med 1996;335:1001–1009.
[f]The Long-term Intervention with Pravastatin in Ischaemic Disease. N Engl J Med 1998;339:1349–1357.
[g]The Air Force/Texas Coronary Atherosclerosis Prevention Study. JAMA 1998;279:1615–1622.
[h]Heart Protection Study. Presented at the American College of Cardiology annual meeting, March 2002 Atlanta, GA.
CAD, coronary artery disease; LDL, low-density lipoprotein; HDL, high-density lipoprotein.

HDL may reduce the lipid content of atherosclerotic plaques and thus favorably affect their biologic activity. Other potential actions include increased NO synthesis, enhanced fibrinolytic activity, inhibition of smooth muscle proliferation and monocyte recruitment, and a reduction in macrophage production of matrix-degrading enzymes. In vitro studies suggest that statins may also reduce inflammation by inhibiting the macrophage cytokines TNF-α, IL-1, and IL-6 or by augmenting peroxisome proliferator-activated receptor-α (PPAR-α), thereby reducing endothelial expression of leukocyte adhesion molecules and macrophage tissue factor production. Clinical trials have corroborated an anti-inflammatory action of statins (e.g., they reduce plasma levels of C-reactive protein, a marker of inflammation described below).

Tobacco Smoking

Numerous studies have shown that cigarette smoking increases the risk of atherosclerosis and ischemic heart disease. Even minimal smoking increases the risk, and the heaviest smokers are at the greatest danger of cardiovascular events. Studies indicate that low-tar and low-nicotine cigarettes do not significantly decrease the occurrence of myocardial infarction compared with regular cigarettes.

Cigarette smoking could lead to atherosclerotic disease in a variety of ways, including enhanced oxidative modification of LDL, decreased circulating HDL levels, endothelial dysfunction due to tissue hypoxia and increased oxidant stress, increased platelet adhesiveness, increased soluble leukocyte adhesion molecules and other markers of inflammation, inappropriate stimulation of the sympathetic nervous system by nicotine, and displacement of oxygen by carbon monoxide from hemoglobin. Extrapolation from animal experiments suggests that smoking may contribute to complications of atherosclerosis as much from a prothrombotic effect as from accelerating atherogenesis.

Fortunately, smoking cessation can reverse some of the adverse effect. Epidemiologic studies have shown that people who stop smoking greatly reduce their likelihood of coronary heart disease compared with those who continue to smoke. In one study, after 3 years of cessation, the risk of coronary artery disease became similar to subjects who never smoked.

Hypertension

Elevated blood pressure (either systolic or diastolic) augments the risk of developing atherosclerosis, coronary heart disease, and stroke (as described in more detail in Chapter 13). The association of elevated blood pressure with cardiovascular disease does not appear to have a specific threshold. Rather, risk increases continuously with progressively higher values. Systolic pressure predicts adverse outcomes more reliably than diastolic pressure, particularly in the increasing elderly population.

Hypertension may accelerate atherosclerosis in several ways. Animal studies have shown that elevated blood pressure injures vascular endothelium and may increase the permeability of the vessel wall to lipoproteins. In addition to causing direct endothelial damage, increased hemodynamic stress has also been shown to increase the number of scavenger receptors on macrophages, thus enhancing the development of foam cells. Cyclic circumferential strain, increased in hypertensive arteries, can augment the production by smooth muscle cells of proteoglycans that bind and retain LDL particles, promoting their accumulation in the intima and facilitating their oxidative modification. Angiotensin II, a mediator of hypertension, acts not only as a vasoconstrictor but also as a pro-inflammatory cytokine. Thus, hypertension may also promote atherogenesis by contributing to inflammation.

Antihypertensive Therapy

Like dyslipidemias, treatment of hypertension should start with lifestyle modifications but often requires pharmacologic intervention. The Dietary Approaches to Stop Hypertension (DASH) studies demonstrated that a diet high in fruits and vegetables, with dairy products low in fat, and an overall reduced sodium content can significantly improve systolic and diastolic blood pressures. Regular exercise can also reduce resting blood pressure levels.

Many medications are available to lower blood pressure, including diuretics, beta-adrenergic receptor antagonists, drugs that interfere with the renin-angiotensin system, calcium channel blockers, and alpha-adrenergic inhibitors. The benefits and limitations of such therapies are described in Chapters 13 and 17.

Diabetes Mellitus

Diabetes increases the risk of atherosclerosis, and diabetics have a three- to five-fold increased likelihood of suffering cardiovascular events. The mechanism may relate in part to the non-enzymatic glycation of lipoproteins in diabetic patients (which may enhance uptake of cholesterol by scavenger macrophages, as discussed above) or to a prothrombotic tendency and anti-fibrinolytic state that may prevail in patients with this condition. Diabetic individuals frequently have impaired endothelial function, gauged by the reduced bioavailability of NO and increased leukocyte adhesion. Tight control of serum glucose levels in diabetic patients reduces the risk of *microvascular* complications such as retinopathy and nephropathy, but studies thus far have not demonstrated fewer *macrovascular* outcomes such as myocardial infarction and stroke. However, the control of hypertension and dyslipidemia in diabetics *does* profoundly reduce risk of cardiac and cerebrovascular complications.

Adult onset (type II) diabetes is often part of the "metabolic syndrome," as described above, in association with hypertension, abnormal lipid levels (hypertriglyceridemia, reduced HDL, and a predominance of small, dense LDL particles), and increased abdominal girth. Central to this syndrome is the presence of insulin resistance in peripheral cells. In fact, the presence of insulin resistance appears to promote atherosclerosis long before affected patients are found to be overtly diabetic.

Physical Activity

Exercise may mitigate atherogenesis in several ways. In addition to beneficial effects on the lipid profile and blood pressure, exercise *enhances* insulin sensitivity and the endothelial production of NO. Long-term prospective studies of both men and women indicate that even modest activities, such as brisk walking, can protect against cardiovascular mortality. Although no randomized primary prevention trials have examined the effects of exercise on cardiac event rates, the proven benefits on the cardiovascular risk profile should promote increased physical activity to all individuals at risk of developing atherosclerotic disease.

Estrogen Status

Before menopause, women have a lower incidence of coronary events than men. After menopause, however, the coronary risks are similar in men and women. Indeed, cardiovascular events outstrip by far other causes of mortality in women, including breast and other cancers. This observation suggests that estrogen (the levels of which decline after menopause) may have atheroprotective properties. Physiologic estrogen levels in premenopausal women lower LDL and lipoprotein (a) (described below) and raise HDL levels. Experimentally, estrogen demonstrates potentially beneficial antioxidant and antiplatelet actions as well as improves endothelium-dependent vasodilation.

Observational studies indicate that postmenopausal women who receive hormone replacement therapy have a reduced risk of coronary disease. Surprisingly, however, data from the Heart and Estrogen/progestin Replacement Study (HERS), a major randomized controlled trial of hormone replacement in women with preexisting coronary disease, actually demonstrated an early *increased* vascular risk associated with hormone use. It currently remains unclear, then, whether cardioprotection in premenopausal women results from estrogen itself, or if other factors contribute. Results from ongoing prospective trials will help clarify this very important issue.

Emerging Risk Factors

In addition to the well-established risk factors described above, a number of novel markers of atherosclerotic risk have recently emerged.

Homocysteinemia

Several studies have shown a significant relationship between circulating levels of the amino acid homocysteine and the incidence of coronary, cerebral, and peripheral artery disease. The mechanism by which homocysteine might increase atherosclerotic risk is not known, but current evidence suggests that abnormally high amounts of this substance may promote thrombosis. Hyperhomocysteinemia can result from genetic defects in methionine metabolism or insufficient dietary intake of folic acid, a cofactor in the methionine pathway. Although folic acid and other B-vitamin supplements reduce high serum homocysteine levels, there is currently no proof that such therapy actually reduces atherosclerotic disease.

Lipoprotein (a)

Some studies have identified lipoprotein (a) [referred to as Lp(a), and pronounced "L-P-little-A"] as an independent risk factor for coronary artery disease. Lp(a) is a special form of LDL, whose major apolipoprotein (apo-B-100) is linked by a disulfide bridge to another protein, known as apo(a). Apo(a) structurally resembles plasminogen, a plasma protein that is important for the endogenous lysis of fibrin clots (see Chapter 7). Thus, the detrimental effect attributed to Lp (a) may relate to competition with normal plasminogen activity. Like homocysteine, not all population studies support a link between Lp(a) and cardiovascular events, although individuals with the highest Lp(a) levels do in fact appear to be at increased risk.

An individual's Lp(a) level is primarily determined by inheritance and has a skewed distribution, with higher levels among blacks. Diet and exercise have little influence on Lp(a), and drugs designed to specifically lower its level do not exist. However, nicotinic acid is one agent that reduces Lp(a) as one of its multiple beneficial lipid effects. Thus far, it has not been shown that specifically targeting Lp(a) by drug therapy improves cardiovascular outcomes.

C-Reactive Protein and Other Markers of Inflammation

As described above, the pathogenesis of atherosclerosis involves inflammation at every stage; thus, markers of inflammation are being investigated as predictors of cardiac risk. Recall that lipoprotein entry and modification in the vessel wall trigger the release of cytokines, followed by leukocyte infiltration, more cytokine release, and smooth muscle migration and proliferation in the intima. Cytokines (e.g., IL-6) travel to the liver and incite increased production of "acute phase reactants," including fibrinogen, C-reactive protein, and serum amyloid A.

Of these molecules, elevated serum levels of C-reactive protein (CRP) have shown the greatest promise as a marker of low-grade systemic inflammation associated with atherosclerotic disease. Large studies of apparently healthy men and women indicate that those with high CRP levels, measured by a readily available high-sensitivity assay, have a greatly increased risk of adverse cardiovascular outcomes compared to those with low serum levels. Thus, measurement of CRP may prove useful as a screening tool in assessing cardiovascular risk and targeting therapy to select individuals for primary prevention of vascular disease. However, this hypothesis has not yet undergone rigorous prospective testing.

In addition to being a marker of risk, CRP may actually participate as a *mediator* of atherogenesis. For example, CRP can activate complement, thus contributing to a sustained inflammatory state. The lipid-lowering HMG CoA reductase inhibitors (statins) decrease CRP levels, but evidence does not yet affirm that therapy should specifically target CRP lowering.

Infection

Several studies have identified certain infectious agents (e.g., herpes viruses, *Chlamydia pneumoniae*) in some atherosclerotic lesions, raising the question of their potential role in atherogenesis. Such studies have generated substantial controversy, and definite proof of a causal role is lacking. Although it is uncertain if such infections truly play a role in atherogenesis, there are theoretical reasons to investigate this possibility. For example, Chlamydia species produce a protein, heat shock protein 60 (HSP-60), that activates macrophages and stimulates the production of enzymes (matrix metalloproteinases) that can impair the stability of the atherosclerotic plaque's fibrous cap. Other possible atherogenic properties of chlamydial HSP-60 or bacterial endotoxins include induction of foam cell formation, lipoprotein oxidation, and increased procoagulant activity. Although the pathogenic relationships remain unproven, some researchers believe that infectious agents furnish an additional source of endothelial injury and inflammation that could initiate or exacerbate atherogenesis. To date, well-powered trials have *not* shown that antibiotic treatment directed against such putative infections reduces the risk of future cardiac events in survivors of myocardial infarction.

SUMMARY

1. The arterial wall consists of three layers: the intima, media, and adventitia. Metabolically active endothelial cells comprise the intima. The media contains mostly smooth muscle cells and extracellular matrix. The adventitia includes microvessels, nerves, and lymphatics that serve the artery. Atherosclerotic lesions develop and progress due to dys-

function of components of the arterial wall as they interact with additional external factors.

2. In health, the endothelial layer of the intima provides a protective nonthrombogenic surface with vasomotor and anti-inflammatory roles. Activation of the endothelium, particularly by inflammation, occurs early in the development of atherosclerotic lesions.

3. Atherogenesis involves accumulation of lipids within the intima with subsequent chemical modification of lipoprotein constituents, recruitment of leukocytes and smooth muscle cells, and deposition of extracellular matrix. Cytokines and growth factors produced by dysfunctional vascular cells and activated leukocytes mediate these processes. Eventually, the pathologic lesions of atherosclerosis, the fatty streak first and the fibrous plaque later, become visible on gross inspection.

4. Clinical manifestations of atherosclerosis result from narrowing of the lumen, calcification of the vessel wall, and plaque disruption that leads to superimposed thrombus formation. Common manifestations include angina pectoris, myocardial infarction, stroke, and peripheral arterial disease. Weakening of the arterial wall can result in an aneurysm.

5. Major modifiable risk factors for atherosclerosis include dyslipidemia (high LDL or low HDL), hypertension, smoking, and diabetes. Aggressive recognition and correction of modifiable risk factors through lifestyle improvements and pharmacologic therapy reduce cardiovascular morbidity and mortality.

One of the most common clinical manifestations of atherosclerosis is coronary artery disease, which is the subject of the next chapter.

Acknowledgments   Contributors to the previous editions of this chapter were Rushika Fernandopulle, MD; Gopa Bhattacharyya, MD; Joseph Loscalzo, MD, PhD; and Peter Libby, MD.

Additional Reading

Beckman JA, Creager MA, Libby P. Diabetes and atherosclerosis. JAMA, 2002; 287:2570-81.

Executive summary of the Third Report of the National Cholesterol Education Project Expert Panel on Detection, Evaluation, and Treatment of High Blood Cholesterol in Adults. JAMA 2001;285: 2486–2496.

Knopp RH. Drug treatment of lipid disorders. N Engl J Med 1999;341:498–508.

Libby P. Current concepts of the pathogenesis of the acute coronary syndromes. Circulation 2001;104: 365–372.

Libby P, Ridker PM, Maseri A. Inflammation and atherosclerosis. Circulation 2002;105:1135–1143.

Pearson TA. New tools for coronary risk assessment—what are their advantages and limitations? Circulation 2002;105:886–892.

Ridker PM, Genest J, Libby P. Risk factors for atherosclerotic disease. In: Braunwald E, ed. Heart Disease: A Textbook of Cardiovascular Medicine. Philadelphia: WB Saunders, 2001: 1010–1039.

Smith SC, Blair SN, Bonow RO, et al. AHA/ACC guidelines for preventing heart attack and death in patients with atherosclerotic cardiovascular disease: 2001 update. A statement for healthcare professionals from the American Heart Association and the American College of Cardiology. J Am Coll Cardiol 2001;38:1581–1583.

Von Eckardstein A, Nofer JR, Assmann G. High density lipoproteins and arteriosclerosis: role of cholesterol efflux and reverse cholesterol transport. Arterioscler Thromb Vasc Biol 2001;21:13–27.

Ischemic Heart Disease

*Anurag Gupta, Marc S. Sabatine,
and Leonard S. Lilly*

Chapter

6

**Determinants of Myocardial Oxygen Supply
and Demand**
  Myocardial Oxygen Supply
  Myocardial Oxygen Demand
Pathophysiology of Ischemia
  Fixed Vessel Narrowing
  Endothelial Cell Dysfunction
  Other Causes of Myocardial Ischemia
Consequences of Ischemia
  Ischemic Syndromes

Clinical Features of Chronic Stable Angina
  History
  Physical Examination
  Diagnostic Studies
  Natural History
Treatment
  Medical Treatment of an Acute Episode of Angina
  Medical Treatment to Prevent Recurrent Ischemic
  Episodes
  Medical Treatment to Prevent MI and Death
  Revascularization
  Medical Versus Revascularization Therapy

In 1772, the British physician William Heberden reported a disorder in which patients developed an uncomfortable sensation in the chest when walking. Labeling it "angina pectoris," Heberden noted that this discomfort would disappear soon after the patient stood still but would worsen again with exertion. Although he did not know the cause of this sensation, it is likely that his report was the first to describe the symptoms of ischemic heart disease, a condition of insufficient myocardial perfusion, that now afflicts millions of Americans and is the leading cause of death in industrialized nations.

The clinical presentation of ischemic heart disease can be highly variable and forms a spectrum of syndromes (Table 6.1). For example, ischemia may be accompanied by the exertional symptoms originally described by Heberden, still known as angina pectoris. In other cases, it may occur without any symptoms at all, a condition termed "silent" ischemia. This chapter describes the causes and consequences of chronic ischemic heart disease and provides a framework for the diagnosis and treatment of affected patients.

DETERMINANTS OF MYOCARDIAL OXYGEN SUPPLY AND DEMAND

The most common manifestation of ischemic heart disease, angina pectoris, literally means "strangling in the chest." Although other diseases may lead to similar chest discomfort, angina refers to the condition that arises from an imbalance between myocardial oxygen supply and demand. By far, the leading cause of that imbalance is coronary artery disease (CAD), in which a reduction in oxygen supply is due to atherosclerotic narrowings in one or more of the coronary arteries.

In the normal heart, there is a continuous match between the oxygen requirements of the myocardium and coronary arterial supply. Even during vigorous exercise, when the heart's metabolic needs increase, so does the delivery of oxygen to the myocardial cells, so that the balance is maintained. The following sections describe the key determinants of myocardial oxygen supply and demand in normal individuals (Fig. 6.1) and how they are altered by the presence of CAD.

TABLE 6.1. Clinical Definitions

Syndrome	Description
Ischemic heart disease	Condition in which imbalance between myocardial oxygen supply and demand results in myocardial hypoxia and accumulation of waste metabolites; most often due to atherosclerotic disease of the coronary arteries ("coronary artery disease")
Angina pectoris	Uncomfortable sensation in the chest and neighboring anatomic structures produced by myocardial ischemia
Stable angina	Chronic pattern of transient angina pectoris, precipitated by physical activity or emotional upset, relieved by rest within a few minutes; episodes often associated with temporary depression of the ST segment, but permanent myocardial damage does not result
Variant angina	Typical anginal discomfort, usually *at rest*, which develops because of coronary artery spasm, rather than an increase of myocardial oxygen demand; episodes often associated with transient shifts of the ST segment (usually ST elevation)
Unstable angina	Pattern of increased frequency and duration of angina episodes, produced by less exertion, or at rest; high frequency of progression to myocardial infarction if untreated
Silent ischemia	Asymptomatic episodes of myocardial ischemia; can be detected by ECG and other laboratory techniques
Myocardial infarction	Region of myocardial necrosis usually due to prolonged cessation of blood supply; most often results from acute thrombus at site of coronary atherosclerotic stenosis; may be first clinical manifestation of ischemic heart disease, or there may be a history of angina pectoris

Myocardial Oxygen Supply

The supply of oxygen to the myocardium depends on the **oxygen-carrying capacity** of the blood and the rate of **coronary blood flow.** The oxygen-carrying capacity is determined by the hemoglobin content of blood and systemic oxygenation. In the absence of anemia or lung disease, oxygen-carrying capacity remains fairly constant. However, coronary blood flow is much more dynamic, and regulation of that flow is responsible for matching the oxygen supply with metabolic requirements.

As in all blood vessels, coronary artery flow (Q) is directly proportional to the vessel's perfusion pressure (P) and is inversely proportional to coronary vascular resistance (R). This is expressed as $Q \propto P/R$.

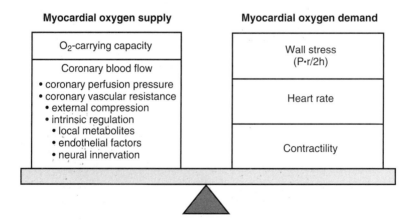

Figure 6.1. Major determinants of myocardial oxygen supply and demand. P, ventricular pressure; r, ventricular radius; h, ventricular wall thickness.

However, unlike other arterial systems in which the greatest blood flow occurs during systole, *the predominance of coronary perfusion takes place during diastole.* This is so because systolic flow is obstructed by compression of the small coronary branches as they course through the contracting myocardium.

Coronary flow is unimpaired in diastole, because the relaxed myocardium does not compress the coronary vasculature. Thus, in the case of the coronaries, **perfusion pressure** can be approximated by the aortic diastolic pressure. Conditions that decrease aortic diastolic pressure (such as hypotension or aortic regurgitation) decrease coronary artery perfusion pressure and may impair myocardial oxygen supply.

Coronary vascular resistance is the other major determinant of coronary blood flow. In the normal artery, this resistance is dynamically modulated by 1) forces that externally compress the coronary arteries, and 2) factors that alter intrinsic coronary tone.

External Compression

External compression is exerted on the coronary vessels during the cardiac cycle by contraction of the surrounding myocardium. The degree of compression is directly related to intramyocardial pressure and is therefore greatest during systole, as described in the previous section. Moreover, when the myocardium contracts, the subendocardium, adjacent to the high intraventricular pressure, is subjected to greater force than the outer muscle layers. This is one reason why the subendocardium is the region most vulnerable to ischemic damage.

Intrinsic Control of Coronary Tone

Unlike most tissues, the heart cannot increase oxygen extraction on demand because in its basal state it removes nearly as much oxygen as possible from its blood supply. Thus, *any additional oxygen requirement must be met by an increase in blood flow,* and autoregulation of coronary vascular resistance is the most important mediator of this process. Factors that participate in the

regulation of coronary vascular resistance include the accumulation of local metabolites, endothelium-derived substances, and neural innervation.

Metabolic Factors

The accumulation of local metabolites significantly affects coronary vascular tone and acts to modulate myocardial oxygen supply to meet changing metabolic demands. During states of hypoxemia, aerobic metabolism and oxidative phosphorylation in the mitochondria are inhibited. High-energy phosphates, including adenosine triphosphate (ATP), cannot be regenerated. Consequently, adenosine diphosphate (ADP) and monophosphate (AMP) accumulate and are subsequently degraded to adenosine. Adenosine is a potent vasodilator and is thought to be the prime metabolic mediator of vascular tone. By binding to receptors on vascular smooth muscle, adenosine decreases calcium entry into cells, which leads to relaxation, vasodilatation, and increased coronary blood flow. Other metabolites that act locally as vasodilators include lactate, acetate, hydrogen ions, and carbon dioxide.

Endothelial Factors

Endothelial cells of the arterial wall produce a number of vasoactive substances that contribute to the regulation of vascular tone. *Vasodilators* produced by the endothelium include nitric oxide (formerly termed "endothelium-derived relaxing factor"), prostacyclin, and endothelium-derived hyperpolarizing factor (EDHF). Endothelin-1 is an example of a natural endothelium-derived *vasoconstrictor.*

The identification and important actions of endothelium-derived **nitric oxide** (NO) are described in Box 6.1. NO regulates vascular tone by diffusing into and then relaxing neighboring arterial smooth muscle by a cyclic guanosine monophosphate (cGMP)-dependent mechanism. The production of NO by normal endothelium occurs in the basal state and is additionally stimulated by many substances and conditions. For exam-

Box 6.1. Endothelium-Derived Relaxing Factor, Nitric Oxide, and the Nobel Prize

Normal arterial endothelial cells synthesize potent vasodilator substances that contribute to the modulation of vascular tone. Among the first of these to be identified were prostacyclin (an arachidonic acid metabolite) and endothelium-derived relaxing factor (EDRF).

EDRF was first studied in the 1970s. In experimental preparations, it was shown that acetylcholine (ACh) has two opposite actions on blood vessels. Its direct effect on vascular smooth muscle cells is to cause vasoconstriction, but when an intact endothelial lining overlies the smooth muscle cells, vasodilation occurs instead. Subsequent experiments showed that ACh causes the endothelial cells to release a chemical mediator (that was termed EDRF) that quickly diffuses to the adjacent smooth muscle cells and results in their relaxation with subsequent vasodilation of the vessel.

More recent research has demonstrated that the mysterious EDRF is actually the *nitric oxide* (NO) radical. When ACh (or other endothelial-dependent vasodilators such as serotonin or histamine) binds to endothelial cells, intracellular free calcium increases, which activates the enzyme nitric oxide synthase (NOS). NOS catalyzes the formation of NO from the amino acid L-arginine (see figure). NO diffuses from the endothelium to the adjacent vascular smooth muscle, where it activates guanylyl cyclase (G-cyclase). G-cyclase in turn forms cyclic guanosine monophosphate (cGMP) from guanosine triphosphate (GTP). The increased intracellular cGMP results in smooth muscle cell relaxation through mechanisms that involve a reduction in cytosolic Ca^{++}. The increase in cGMP is also associated with beneficial antimigratory effects of the smooth muscle cells.

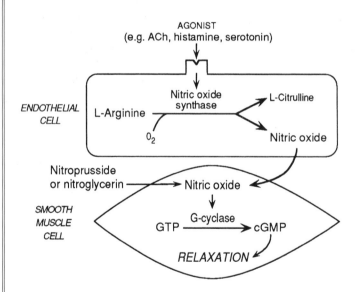

In distinction to the endothelial-dependent vasodilators, some agents cause smooth muscle relaxation *independent* of the presence of endothelial cells. For example, the drugs sodium nitroprusside and nitroglycerin result in vasodilation by providing an exogenous source of NO to vascular smooth muscle cells, thereby activating G-cyclase and forming cGMP without endothelial cell participation.

In the cardiac catheterization laboratory, the intracoronary administration of ACh in a normal individual causes vasodilation of the vessel, presumably through the release of NO. However, in conditions of endothelial dysfunction, such as atherosclerosis, intracoronary ACh administration results in paradoxical *vasoconstriction* in-

(Modified from Furchgott RF. The discovery of endothelium-derived relaxing factor and its importance in the identification of nitric oxide. JAMA 1996; 276:1186–1188.)

stead. This likely reflects reduced production of NO by the dysfunctional endothelial cells, such that there is unopposed direct vasoconstriction of the smooth muscle by ACh. Of particular interest is that the loss of vasodilatory response to infused ACh is evident in individuals with certain cardiac risk factors (e.g., elevated LDL cholesterol, hypertension, cigarette smoking) even before the physical appearance of atheromatous plaque. Thus, the impaired release of NO may be an early and sensitive predictor for the later development of atherosclerotic lesions.

The significance of these discoveries was highlighted in 1998, when the Nobel Prize in Medicine was awarded to the scientists who discovered the critical role of NO as a cardiovascular signaling molecule.

ple, its release is augmented when the endothelium is exposed to acetylcholine (ACh), thrombin, products of aggregating platelets (e.g., serotonin and ADP), or even the shear stress of blood flow. Although the *direct* effect of many of these substances on vascular smooth muscle is to cause *vasoconstriction,* the induced release of NO from the normal endothelium results in *vasodilatation* instead (Fig. 6.2).

Prostacyclin, an arachidonic acid metabolite, has vasodilator properties that are similar to those of NO (see Fig. 6.2). It is released from endothelial cells in response to many stimuli, including hypoxia, shear stress, acetylcholine, and platelet products (such as serotonin). It causes relaxation of vascular smooth muscle by a cyclic AMP-dependent mechanism.

Endothelium-derived hyperpolarizing factor (EDHF) also appears to have important vasodilatory properties. Like endothelial-derived NO it is believed to be a diffusible substance released by the endothelium, which hyperpolarizes (and therefore relaxes) neighboring vascular smooth muscle cells. This factor(s) is not yet well-characterized, although its action does not appear to involve increases in the cyclic nucleotides (cGMP or cAMP) in the smooth muscle cell.

Endothelin-1 is a potent vasoconstrictor produced by endothelial cells and partially counteracts the vasodilating properties of

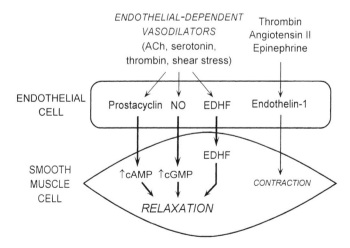

Figure 6.2. **Endothelium-derived vasoactive substances and their regulators.** Endothelium-derived vasodilators are shown on the left and include nitric oxide (NO), prostacyclin, and endothelium-derived hyperpolarizing factor (EDHF). Endothelin-1 is an endothelium-derived vasoconstrictor. In the normal state, the vasodilator influence predominates over that of vasoconstriction. ACh, acetylcholine.

NO and prostacyclin. Its expression is stimulated by several factors including thrombin, angiotensin II, epinephrine, and the shear stress of blood flow.

Under normal circumstances, the healthy endothelium promotes vascular smooth muscle *relaxation* (vasodilatation) through elaboration of substances such as NO and prostacyclin, the influences of which predominate over the endothelial vasoconstrictors (see Fig. 6.2). As shall be seen, however, dysfunctional endothelium (as in atherosclerotic vessels) secretes reduced amounts of vasodilators, such that the balance shifts toward vasoconstriction instead.

Neural Factors

The neural control of vascular resistance has both sympathetic and parasympathetic components. Under normal circumstances, the contribution of the parasympathetic nervous system appears minor, but *sympathetic receptors* play an important role. Coronary vessels contain both α-adrenergic and β$_2$-adrenergic receptors. Stimulation of α-adrenergic receptors results in vasoconstriction. Conversely, β$_2$-receptor stimulation promotes vasodilatation.

It is the interplay among the metabolic, endothelial, and neural regulating factors that determines the net impact on coronary vascular tone. For example, catecholamine stimulation of the heart may initially cause coronary *vasoconstriction* via the α-adrenergic receptor neural effect. However, catecholamine stimulation also increases myocardial oxygen consumption through increased heart rate and contractility (β$_1$-adrenergic effect), and the resulting increased production of local metabolites induces net coronary *dilatation* instead.

Myocardial Oxygen Demand

There are three major determinants of myocardial oxygen demand: 1) ventricular wall stress, 2) heart rate, and 3) contractility (also termed the inotropic state). Additionally, very small amounts of oxygen are consumed to provide energy for basal cardiac metabolism and electrical depolarization.

Ventricular **wall stress (σ)** is the tangential force acting on the myocardial fibers, tending to pull them apart, and energy is expended in opposing that force. Wall stress is related to intraventricular pressure (P), the radius of the ventricle (r), and ventricular wall thickness (h). Approximated by LaPlace's relationship,

$$\sigma = \frac{P \cdot r}{2h}$$

Thus, wall stress is directly proportional to the radius of the left ventricle. Conditions that augment left ventricular (LV) filling (e.g., mitral or aortic regurgitation) increase the ventricular radius and raise wall stress and oxygen consumption. Conversely, any physiologic or pharmacologic maneuver that decreases LV filling and size (such as nitrate therapy) decreases wall stress and myocardial oxygen consumption.

Wall stress is also proportional to systolic ventricular pressure. Circumstances that increase pressure development in the left ventricle, such as aortic stenosis or hypertension, increase the wall stress and myocardial oxygen consumption. Conditions that decrease ventricular pressure, such as antihypertensive therapy, reduce myocardial oxygen consumption.

Finally, wall stress is *inversely* proportional to ventricular wall thickness, since the force is spread out among a greater muscle mass. A hypertrophied heart has lower wall stress and oxygen consumption per gram of tissue than a thinned-wall heart. Thus, when hypertrophy develops in conditions of chronic pressure overload, such as aortic stenosis, it serves a compensatory role in reducing oxygen consumption.

The second major determinant of myocardial oxygen demand is **heart rate.** If the heart rate accelerates, the number of contractions and the amount of ATP consumed per minute increases and oxygen requirements rise. Conversely, slowing the heart rate (e.g., using a β-blocker drug) decreases ATP utilization and oxygen consumption.

The third major determinant of oxygen demand is myocardial **contractility,** a measure of the force of contraction (described in Chapter 9). Circulating catecholamines, or the administration of positive inotropic drugs, directly increases the force of contraction and increases oxygen utilization. Conversely, negative inotropic effectors, such as β-adrenergic blocking drugs, decrease myocardial oxygen consumption.

In the normal state, autoregulatory mechanisms adjust coronary tone to match myocardial oxygen supply with oxygen requirements. In the absence of obstructive coronary disease, the autoregulatory mechanisms maintain a fairly constant rate of coronary flow, as long as the aortic perfusion pressure is approximately 60 mm Hg or greater. In the setting of advanced coronary atherosclerosis, however, the fall in perfusion pressure distal to the arterial stenosis, and dysfunction of the endothelium of the involved segment, set the stage for a mismatch between the available blood supply and myocardial metabolic demands.

PATHOPHYSIOLOGY OF ISCHEMIA

The traditional view has been that myocardial ischemia in CAD results from fixed atherosclerotic plaques that narrow the vessel's lumen and limit myocardial blood supply. However, recent research has demonstrated that the reduction of blood flow results from the *combination* of fixed vessel narrowing *and* abnormal vascular tone, contributed to by atherosclerosis-induced endothelial cell dysfunction.

Fixed Vessel Narrowing

The hemodynamic significance of atherosclerotic coronary artery stenoses relates to both the fluid mechanics and the anatomy of the vascular supply.

Fluid Mechanics

Poiseuille's law states that for flow through a vessel,

$$Q = \frac{\Delta P \pi r^4}{8 \eta L}$$

in which Q is flow, ΔP is the pressure difference between the points being measured, r is the vessel radius, η is the fluid viscosity,

and L is the vessel length. By analogy to Ohm's law, flow is also equal to the pressure difference divided by the resistance (R) to flow:

$$Q = \frac{\Delta P}{R}$$

By combining these two formulas, resistance to blood flow in a vessel can be expressed as:

$$R = \frac{8 \eta L}{\pi r^4}$$

Thus, vascular resistance is governed, in part, by the geometric component L/r^4. That is, the hemodynamic significance of a stenotic lesion depends on its length and, far more importantly, on the degree of vessel narrowing (i.e., the reduction of r) that it causes.

Anatomy

The coronary arteries consist of large, proximal epicardial segments and smaller, distal resistance vessels. The proximal vessels are subject to overt atherosclerosis that results in stenotic plaques. The distal vessels are usually free of flow-limiting plaques and can adjust their vasomotor tone in response to metabolic needs. These resistance vessels serve as a reserve, increasing their diameter with exertion to meet increasing oxygen demand and dilating, even at rest, if a proximal stenosis is sufficiently severe.

The hemodynamic significance of coronary artery narrowing depends on both the degree of stenosis of the epicardial portion of the vessel and the amount of *compensatory vasodilatation* the distal resistance vessels are able to achieve (Fig. 6.3). If a stenosis narrows the lumen diameter by less than 60%, the maximal potential blood flow through the artery is not significantly altered and, in response to exertion, the resistance vessels can dilate to provide adequate blood flow. When a stenosis narrows the diameter by more than approximately 70%, resting blood flow is normal, but maximal blood flow is reduced even with full dilatation of the resistance vessels. In this situa-

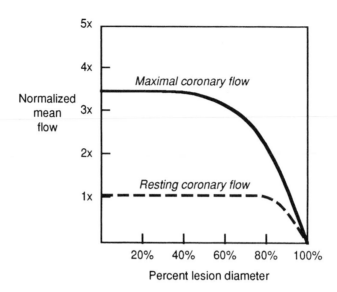

Figure 6.3. Resting and maximal coronary blood flow are affected by the magnitude of proximal arterial stenosis (percent lesion diameter). The dotted line indicates resting blood flow, and the solid line represents maximal blood flow (i.e., when there is full dilatation of the distal resistance vessels). Compromise of maximal blood flow is evident when the proximal stenosis reduces the coronary lumen diameter by more than ~70%. Resting flow may be compromised if the stenosis exceeds ~90%. (Modified from Gould KL, Lipscomb K. Effects of coronary stenoses on coronary flow reserve and resistance. Am J Cardiol 1974;34:50.)

tion, when oxygen demand increases (e.g., from the elevated heart rate and force of contraction during physical exertion), coronary flow reserve is inadequate, oxygen demand exceeds supply, and myocardial ischemia results. If the stenosis compromises the vessel lumen by more than approximately 90%, then even with maximal dilatation of the resistance vessels, blood flow may be inadequate to meet basal requirements and ischemia can develop *at rest.*

Although collateral channels (see Chapter 1) may become apparent between nonobstructed coronaries and sites distal to atherosclerotic stenoses, and such flow can buffer the fall in myocardial oxygen supply, it is usually not sufficient to prevent ischemia during exertion in critically narrowed vessels.

Endothelial Cell Dysfunction

In addition to fixed vessel narrowing, the other major contributor to reduced myocardial oxygen supply in chronic CAD is endothelial dysfunction. Abnormal endothelial cell function can contribute to the pathophysiology of ischemia in two ways:

1) by inappropriate vasoconstriction of coronary arteries, and 2) through loss of normal antithrombotic properties.

Inappropriate Vasoconstriction

In normal individuals, physical activity or mental stress result in measurable coronary artery *vasodilatation.* This effect is thought to be regulated by activation of the sympathetic nervous system, with increased blood flow and shear stress stimulating the release of endothelial-derived vasodilators, such as NO. It is postulated that in normal individuals, the relaxation effect of NO outweighs the direct α-adrenergic constrictor effect of catecholamines on arterial smooth muscle, such that vasodilatation results. However, in patients with dysfunctional endothelium (e.g., atherosclerosis), an *impaired release of endothelial vasodilators* leaves the direct catecholamine effect unopposed, such that relative *vasoconstriction* occurs instead. The resultant decrease in coronary blood flow contributes to ischemia. Even the vasodilatory effect of local metabolites (such as adenosine) is attenuated in patients with dysfunctional endothelium, further uncoupling the regulation of vascular tone from metabolic demands.

In patients with risk factors for CAD such as hypercholesterolemia, diabetes mellitus, hypertension, and cigarette smoking, impaired endothelial-dependent vasodilation is noted even before visible atherosclerotic lesions have developed. This suggests that endothelial dysfunction occurs very early in the atherosclerotic process in epicardial arteries.

Inappropriate vasoconstriction also appears to be important in acute coronary syndromes (i.e., unstable angina and myocardial infarction [MI]). As will be dis-

cussed in greater detail in Chapter 7, the usual cause of acute coronary syndromes is disruption of atherosclerotic plaque, with superimposed platelet aggregation and thrombus formation. In normal individuals, the products of platelet aggregation in a developing clot (e.g., serotonin, ADP) result in vasodilatation because they stimulate the endothelial release of NO. However, with dysfunctional endothelium, the direct *vaso-constricting* actions of platelet products predominate and constriction occurs instead (Fig. 6.4), further compromising flow through the arterial lumen.

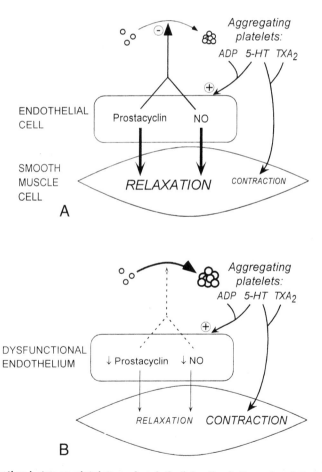

Figure 6.4. **The interaction between platelets and endothelial cells. A.** Normal endothelium. Aggregating platelets release thromboxane (TXA_2) and serotonin (5-HT), the direct vascular effects of which cause contraction of vascular smooth muscle and vasoconstriction. However, platelet products (e.g., ADP, 5-HT) also stimulate the endothelial release of the potent vasodilators nitric oxide (NO) and prostacyclin, such that the net effect is smooth muscle relaxation instead. Endothelial production of NO and prostacyclin also serves antithrombotic roles, which limit further platelet aggregation. **B.** Dysfunctional endothelium demonstrates impaired release of the vasodilator substances, such that net smooth muscle *contraction* and *vasoconstriction* supervene. The reduced endothelial release of NO and prostacyclin diminishes their antiplatelet effect, such that thrombosis proceeds unchecked.

Platelet Aggregation

In addition to their vasodilatory actions, factors released from endothelial cells (including NO and prostacyclin) also exert antithrombotic properties by interfering with platelet aggregation (see Fig. 6.4). However, in states of endothelial cell dysfunction, there is reduced release of these substances; therefore, the antithrombotic effect is attenuated. Thus, in syndromes characterized by thrombosis (i.e., the acute coronary syndromes discussed in Chapter 7) , the impaired release of NO and prostacyclin allows platelets to aggregate and to secrete their potentially harmful procoagulants and vasoconstrictors.

Other Causes of Myocardial Ischemia

In addition to atherosclerotic CAD, other conditions may result in an imbalance between myocardial oxygen supply and demand and result in ischemia. Causes of decreased myocardial oxygen supply include 1) decreased aortic perfusion pressure (e.g., due to hypotension or aortic regurgitation), and 2) a severe decrease in blood oxygen-carrying capacity (e.g., significant anemia or hypoxemia). For example, a patient with massive bleeding from the gastrointestinal tract may develop myocardial ischemia and angina pectoris, even in the absence of atherosclerotic coronary disease, because of a reduction in tissue oxygen delivery (i.e., the loss of hemoglobin).

On the other side of the balance, a profound increase in myocardial oxygen demand can cause ischemia, even in the absence of coronary atherosclerosis or otherwise impaired myocardial oxygen supply. This can occur, for example, with severe aortic stenosis, in which there is significantly increased wall stress due to the greatly elevated LV systolic pressure.

CONSEQUENCES OF ISCHEMIA

The consequences of ischemia reflect the inadequate myocardial oxygenation and local accumulation of metabolic waste products. For example, during ischemia, the myocytes convert from aerobic to anaerobic metabolic pathways. The reduced generation of ATP impairs the interaction of the contractile proteins and results in a transient reduction of both ventricular systolic contraction and diastolic relaxation. The consequent elevation of LV diastolic pressure is transmitted (via the left atrium and pulmonary veins) to the pulmonary capillaries and can precipitate pulmonary congestion and the symptom of dyspnea. In addition, metabolic products such as lactate, serotonin, and adenosine accumulate locally. It is suspected that one or more of these compounds activate peripheral pain receptors in the C7 through T4 distribution and may be the mechanism by which the discomfort of angina is produced. The accumulation of local metabolites and transient abnormalities of myocyte ion transport may also precipitate dangerous arrhythmias (as described in Chapter 11).

The ultimate fate of myocardium subjected to ischemia depends on the severity and duration of the imbalance between oxygen supply and demand. It was previously thought that ischemic cardiac injury results in either irreversible myocardial necrosis (i.e., MI) or rapid and full recovery of myocyte function (e.g., after a brief episode of typical angina). It is now known that in addition to those outcomes, ischemic insults can sometimes result in a period of *prolonged* contractile dysfunction *without* myocyte necrosis, and recovery of normal function may ultimately follow.

For example, **stunned myocardium** refers to tissue that, after suffering a period of severe ischemia (but not necrosis), demonstrates prolonged systolic dysfunction even after the return of normal myocardial blood flow. In this setting, the functional, biochemical, and ultrastructural abnormalities following ischemia are reversible and contractile function gradually recovers. The mechanism responsible for this delayed recovery of function is not known but may involve myocyte calcium overload or the accumulation of oxygen-derived free radicals during ischemia. In general, the magnitude of stunning is proportional to the degree of the preceding ischemia, and this state is likely the pathophysiologic response to an ischemic insult that just falls short of causing irreversible necrosis.

In distinction, **hibernating myocardium** refers to tissue that manifests *chronic* ventricular contractile dysfunction in the face of a persistently reduced blood supply, usually because of multivessel CAD. In this situation, irreversible damage has not occurred and ventricular function can *promptly* improve if appropriate blood flow is restored (e.g., by coronary angioplasty or bypass surgery).

The concepts of stunned and hibernating myocardium are important in the clinical setting. Such regions of myocardium contract poorly when imaged (e.g., by echocardiography or contrast angiography) and can appear indistinguishable from irreversibly infarcted heart muscle. However, they can be differentiated from necrotic regions by special imaging studies (e.g., dobutamine echocardiography, thallium-201 viability study or positron emission tomography [PET] scan, described in Chapter 3). That distinction often influences the decision of whether to undertake angioplasty or coronary bypass procedures, since stunned or hibernating myocardium would be expected to improve with mechanical revascularization, whereas truly infarcted myocardium would not.

Ischemic Syndromes

Myocardial ischemia occurs when there is a mismatch between myocardial oxygen supply and demand. Nevertheless, depending on the underlying pathophysiologic processes and the timing and severity of the ischemic insult, a spectrum of different clinical syndromes may be manifest (Fig. 6.5).

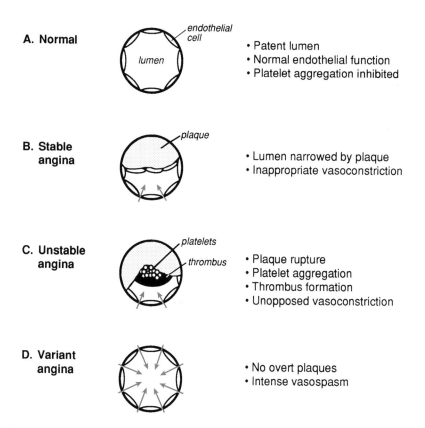

Figure 6.5. Pathophysiologic findings in anginal syndromes. A. Normal coronary arteries are widely patent, and the endothelium functions normally. **B.** In stable angina, atherosclerotic plaque and inappropriate vasoconstriction (due to dysfunctional endothelium) reduce the vessel lumen's size and coronary blood flow. **C.** In unstable angina, disruption of the plaque triggers platelet aggregation, thrombus formation, and vasoconstriction, all of which contribute to reduced coronary blood supply. **D.** In variant angina, atherosclerotic plaques are absent; rather, ischemia is due to intense vasospasm that reduces myocardial oxygen supply.

Stable Angina (see Fig. 6.5B)

Chronic stable angina is generally due to fixed, obstructive atheromatous plaque in one or more coronary arteries. The pattern of symptoms is usually related to the degree of stenosis. As described in the pathophysiology section above, when atherosclerotic stenoses narrow a coronary artery lumen diameter by more than approximately 70%, the reduced flow capacity may be sufficient to serve the low cardiac oxygen needs at rest, but is insufficient to compensate for any significant increase in oxygen demand (see Fig. 6.3). During physical exertion, for example, activation of the sympathetic nervous system results in increased heart rate, blood pressure, and contractility, all of which contribute to augmented myocardial oxygen consumption. During the period that oxygen demand exceeds available supply, myocardial ischemia results, often accompanied by the chest discomfort of angina pectoris. The ischemia and symptoms persist until the increased demand is alleviated and oxygen balance is restored. A pattern of chronic, predictable transient angina during exertion or emotional stress is termed "stable angina."

Potentially contributing to the inadequate oxygen supply in stable angina is inappropriate coronary vasoconstriction due, at least in part, to atherosclerosis-associated endothelial dysfunction. In a normal individual, the increased myocardial oxygen demand during exertion is balanced by an increased supply of blood as the accumulation of local metabolites induces vasodilatation. With endothelial cell dysfunction, however, vasodilatation is impaired and the vessels may paradoxically vasoconstrict in response to exercise-induced catecholamine stimulation of α-adrenergic receptors on the smooth muscle cells of coronary arteries.

As a result, the extent of coronary artery narrowing in patients with atherosclerosis is not necessarily constant. Rather, it can vary from moment to moment because of changes in the superimposed coronary vascular tone. For some patients with stable angina, alterations in tone play a minimal role in the decreased myocardial oxygen supply, and the level of physical activity required to precipitate angina is fairly constant. These patients have "fixed-threshold" angina. In other cases, the degree of dynamic obstruction caused by vasoconstriction or vasospasm plays a more prominent role, and such patients may have "variable-threshold" angina. For example, on a given day, such a patient can exert herself or himself without chest discomfort, but on another day, the same degree of myocardial oxygen demand *does* produce symptoms—the difference reflects alterations in vascular tone over the sites of fixed stenosis. Other clinical features of chronic stable angina are described in greater detail later in this chapter.

Unstable Angina

A patient with chronic, stable angina may experience a sudden increase in the tempo and duration of ischemic episodes, occurring with lesser degrees of exertion and even at rest. This acceleration of symptoms is known as unstable angina and is often a precursor to acute MI. Unstable angina and acute MI are also known as acute coronary syndromes and result from distinct pathophysiologic mechanisms, most commonly rupture of an unstable atherosclerotic plaque with subsequent platelet aggregation and thrombosis (see Fig. 6.5C). Acute coronary syndromes are described in Chapter 7.

Variant Angina

A small minority of patients manifest episodes of focal *coronary artery spasm* in the absence of overt atherosclerotic lesions, and this syndrome is known as "variant" or "Prinzmetal's" angina. In this case, intense vasospasm alone reduces coronary oxygen supply and results in angina (see Fig. 6.5D). The mechanism by which such profound spasm develops is not known. It is thought that many patients with this disorder may actually have early atherosclerosis manifested only by a dysfunctional endothelium, as the response to endothelium-dependent vasodilators (e.g., ACh and serotonin) is often abnormal.

Variant angina often occurs at rest because ischemia in this case is due to transient reduction of the coronary oxygen supply, rather than an increase in myocardial oxygen demand.

Silent Ischemia

Episodes of cardiac ischemia sometimes occur in the absence of perceptible discomfort or pain, and such instances are referred to as "silent ischemia." These asymptomatic episodes can occur in patients who on other occasions experience typical *symptomatic* angina. Conversely, in some individuals, silent ischemia may be the *only* manifestation of CAD. As can be imagined, it may be difficult to diagnose silent ischemia, but its presence can be detected by laboratory techniques such as continuous ambulatory electrocardiography or elicited by exercise stress testing (described below). One study estimated that silent ischemic episodes occur in 40% of patients with stable symptomatic angina and in 2.5–10% of asymptomatic middle-aged men. When considering the importance of anginal discomfort as a physiologic warning signal, the asymptomatic nature of silent ischemia becomes all the more alarming.

The reason why some episodes of ischemia are "silent" whereas others are symptomatic has not been elucidated. The degree of ischemia cannot fully explain the disparity, as even MI may present without symptoms in some patients. However, silent ischemia is particularly common among diabetics, suggesting the possibility of impaired pain sensation due to peripheral neuropathy.

Syndrome X

This term refers to patients with typical symptoms of angina pectoris who have no evidence of significant atherosclerotic coronary stenoses on coronary angiograms. Some of these patients may show definite laboratory signs of ischemia during exer-

cise testing. The pathogenesis of ischemia in this situation may be related to inadequate vasodilator reserve of the coronary resistance vessels. It is thought that the resistance vessels (which are too small to be visualized by coronary angiography) in this disorder may not dilate appropriately during periods of increased myocardial oxygen demand. Microvascular dysfunction, or vasospasm, and abnormal pain perception with hypersensitivity may also contribute to this syndrome. Patients with syndrome X have a better prognosis than those with overt atherosclerotic disease.

CLINICAL FEATURES OF CHRONIC STABLE ANGINA

History

The most important part of the clinical evaluation of ischemic heart disease is the history described by the patient. Because chest pain is such a common complaint, it is important to focus on those characteristics that help distinguish myocardial ischemia from other causes of discomfort. From a diagnostic standpoint, it would be ideal to interview and examine a patient during an actual episode of angina, but most individuals are asymptomatic during the routine office or clinic examination. Therefore, a careful history probing several features of the discomfort should be elicited.

Quality

Angina is most often described as a "pressure," "discomfort," "tightness," "heaviness," or "constriction" in the chest. It is rare that the sensation is actually described as a *pain,* and often a patient will correct the physician who refers to the anginal symptom as such. Anginal discomfort is neither sharp nor stabbing, and it does not vary significantly with inspiration or movement of the chest wall. It is a steady discomfort that lasts a few minutes, yet rarely more than 5–10 minutes. It *always* lasts more than a second or two, and this helps to differentiate it from sharper musculoskeletal pains. Occasionally, a patient likens the sensation to "an elephant sitting on my chest."

While describing angina, the patient may place a clenched fist over his or her sternum, referred to as **Levine's sign,** as if defining the constricting discomfort by that tight grip.

Location

Anginal discomfort is usually *diffuse* rather than localized to a single point. It is most often located retrosternally or in the left precordium, but may occur anywhere in the chest, back, arms, neck, lower face, or upper abdomen. It often radiates to the shoulders and inner aspect of the arms, especially on the left side.

Accompanying Symptoms

During the discomfort of an acute anginal attack, generalized sympathetic and parasympathetic stimulation may result in *tachycardia, diaphoresis,* and *nausea.* Ischemia also results in transient dysfunction of LV systolic contraction and diastolic relaxation. The resultant elevation of LV diastolic pressure is transmitted to the pulmonary vasculature and often causes shortness of breath (*dyspnea*) during the episode. Transient *fatigue* and *weakness* are also common, particularly in elderly patients.

Precipitants

Angina, when not due to pure vasospasm, is precipitated by conditions that increase myocardial oxygen demand (e.g., increased heart rate, contractility, or wall stress). These include physical exertion, anger, and other emotional excitement. Other factors that increase myocardial oxygen demand and precipitate anginal discomfort in patients with CAD include a large meal or cold weather. The latter induces peripheral vasoconstriction, which in turn augments myocardial wall stress as the left ventricle contracts against the increased resistance.

Angina is generally relieved within minutes after the cessation of the activity that precipitated it and even more quickly (within 3–5 minutes) by sublingual nitroglycerin. This response can help differentiate myocardial ischemia from many of the other conditions that produce chest discomfort.

Patients who experience angina primarily due to increased coronary artery tone or vasospasm often develop symptoms at rest, independent of those activities that increase myocardial oxygen demand.

Frequency

Although the level of exertion necessary to precipitate angina may remain fairly constant, the frequency of episodes varies considerably because patients quickly learn which activities cause their discomfort and avoid them. It is thus important to inquire about reductions in activities of daily living when taking the history.

Risk Factors

In addition to the description of chest discomfort, a careful history should uncover risk factors that predispose to atherosclerosis and CAD, including cigarette smoking, hypercholesterolemia, hypertension, diabetes, and a family history of premature coronary disease (see Chapter 5).

Differential Diagnosis

Several conditions can mimic angina pectoris, including gastroesophageal reflux, esophageal spasm, biliary pain, pericarditis, and musculoskeletal conditions such as chest wall pain, spinal osteoarthritis, and cervical radiculitis. The history remains of paramount importance in distinguishing myocardial ischemia from these disorders. In contrast to angina pectoris, gastrointestinal causes of recurrent chest pain are often precipitated by certain foods and are unrelated to exertion. Musculoskeletal causes of chest discomfort tend to be more superficial or can be localized to a discrete spot (i.e., the patient can point to the pain with one finger) and often vary with changes in position. Similarly, the presence of pleuritic pain (sharp pain aggravated by respiratory movements) argues against angina as the cause—this symptom is more likely due to pericarditis (or pulmonary conditions such as pleuritis, pneumonia, or pulmonary embolism). Useful differentiating features are listed in Table 6.2.

Physical Examination

If it is possible to examine a patient *during* an anginal attack, several transient physical signs may be detected (Fig. 6.6). An increased heart rate and blood pressure are common because of the augmented sympathetic response. Myocardial ischemia may lead to papillary muscle dysfunction and therefore mitral regurgitation. Ischemia-induced regional ventricular contractile abnormalities can sometimes be detected as an abnormal bulging impulse on palpation of the left chest. Ischemia de-

creases ventricular compliance, producing a stiffened ventricle and therefore an S_4 gallop on physical examination during atrial contraction (see Chapter 2). However, if the patient is free of chest discomfort during the examination, there may be *no* abnormal physical findings.

Diagnostic Studies

Once angina is suspected, several diagnostic tests may be helpful in confirming myocardial ischemia as the cause. Many of these tests are costly, so that it is important to choose the appropriate studies for each patient.

Electrocardiogram (ECG)

One of the most useful tools is an ECG obtained during an anginal episode. Al-

TABLE 6.2. Causes of Recurrent Chest Pain

Condition	Differentiating Features
Cardiac	
Myocardial ischemia	• Retrosternal tightness or pressure; typically radiates to neck, jaw, or left shoulder and arm • Lasts a few minutes (usually < 10 min) • Brought on by exertion, relieved by rest • Relieved by nitroglycerin • ECG: transient ST depressions or elevations
Pericarditis	• Sharp, pleuritic pain that varies with position; friction rub on auscultation • Can last for hours to days • ECG: diffuse ST elevations and PR depression
Gastrointestinal	
Gastroesophageal reflux	• Retrosternal burning • Precipitated by certain foods, worsened by supine position, unaffected by exertion • Relieved by antacids, not by nitroglycerin
Peptic ulcer disease	• Epigastric ache or burning • Occurs after meals, unaffected by exertion • Relieved by antacids, not by nitroglycerin
Esophageal spasm	• Retrosternal pain accompanied by dysphagia • Precipitated by meals, unaffected by exertion • May be relieved by nitroglycerin
Biliary colic	• Constant, deep right upper quadrant pain; can last hours • Brought on by fatty foods, unaffected by exertion • Not relieved by antacids or nitroglycerin
Musculoskeletal	
Costochondral syndrome	• Sternal pain worsened by chest movement • Costochondral junctions tender to palpation • Relieved by antiinflammatory drugs, not by nitroglycerin
Cervical radiculitis	• Constant ache or shooting pains, may be in a dermatomal distribution • Worsened by neck motion

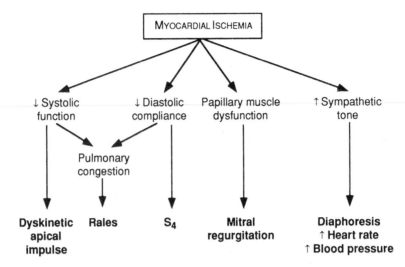

Figure 6.6. **Pathophysiology of physical signs during acute myocardial ischemia.**

though this is easy to arrange when symptoms occur in hospitalized patients, it may not be possible to "catch" episodes in individuals seen on an outpatient basis. During myocardial ischemia, ST segment and T wave changes often appear (Fig. 6.7). Acute ischemia usually results in transient horizontal or downsloping ST segment depressions and T wave flattening or inversions. Occasionally, ST segment *elevations* are seen; this is suggestive of more severe transmural myocardial ischemia and can also be seen during the intense vasospasm of "variant" angina. In distinction to an acute MI, these ST deviations quickly normalize with resolution of the patient's

symptoms. In fact, ECGs obtained during periods free of ischemia are completely normal in approximately half of patients with stable angina. In others, chronic "nondiagnostic" ST and T wave deviations may be present. Evidence of a previous MI (e.g., pathologic Q waves) on the ECG also points to the presence of underlying coronary disease.

Exercise Stress Test

Since an ECG obtained during or between episodes of chest discomfort may be normal, such tracings do not rule out the diagnosis of ischemic heart disease. For this

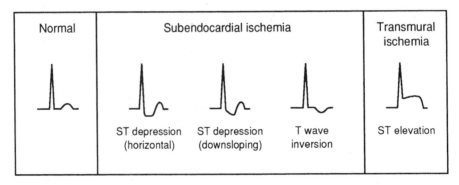

Figure 6.7. **Common transient ECG abnormalities during ischemia.** Subendocardial ischemia causes ST segment depressions and/or T wave flattening or inversions. Severe transient transmural ischemia can result in ST segment *elevations*, similar to the early changes in acute myocardial infarction. When transient ischemia resolves, so do the electrocardiographic changes.

reason, an **exercise stress test** (also termed exercise tolerance test) is a valuable diagnostic and prognostic aid. During this test, the patient exercises on a treadmill or a stationary bicycle to progressively higher workloads. He or she is observed for chest discomfort or inordinate dyspnea. Heart rate and ECG tracings are continuously recorded, and blood pressure is checked at regular intervals. The test is continued until angina develops, signs of myocardial ischemia appear on the ECG, a target heart rate is achieved, or the patient becomes too fatigued to continue.

The test is considered *positive* for ischemic heart disease if the patient's typical chest discomfort is reproduced or if ECG abnormalities consistent with ischemia develop (i.e., ≥1 mm horizontal or downsloping ST segment depressions). By these criteria, the test has approximately 65–70% sensitivity and 75–80% specificity in detecting patients with anatomically significant coronary disease. The stress test is considered *markedly positive* if one or more of the following signs of severe ischemic heart disease occur: 1) the ischemic ECG changes develop in the first 3 minutes of exercise or persist 5 minutes after exercise has stopped, 2) the magnitude of the ST segment depressions is ≥2 mm, 3) the systolic blood pressure decreases during exercise (i.e., due to ischemia-induced impairment of contractile function), 4) high-grade ventricular arrhythmias develop, or 5) the patient cannot exercise for at least 2 minutes because of cardiopulmonary limitations. Patients with markedly positive tests are more likely to have severe, multivessel coronary disease.

The utility of a stress test may be affected by the patient's medications. For example, β-blockers or certain calcium channel blockers may blunt the ability to achieve the target heart rate. In these situations, one must consider the purpose of the stress test. If it is to determine whether ischemic heart disease is present, then those medications are typically withheld for 24–48 hours before the test. On the other hand, if the patient has known ischemic heart disease and the purpose of the test is to assess the efficacy of the current medical regimen, then

testing should be performed while the patient takes his or her usual antianginal medications.

Nuclear Exercise Studies

As the standard exercise stress test relies on ischemia-related changes on the ECG, the test is less useful in patients with baseline abnormalities of the ST segments (e.g., as seen in left bundle branch block or LV hypertrophy). In addition, the standard exercise stress test sometimes yields equivocal results in patients for whom the clinical suspicion of ischemic heart disease is high. In these situations, radionuclide imaging can be combined with exercise stress testing to overcome these limitations and to increase the sensitivity and specificity of the test.

During myocardial perfusion scintigraphy (described in Chapter 3), a radionuclide (usually either thallium-201 or technetium-99m-labeled compounds) is injected intravenously at peak exercise and immediate imaging is performed. The radionuclide accumulates in proportion to the degree of perfusion of viable myocardial cells. Therefore, areas of poor perfusion (i.e., regions of ischemia) during exercise do not accumulate radionuclide and will appear as "cold spots" on the image. However, irreversibly infarcted areas also do not take up the radionuclide, and they too will appear as cold spots. To differentiate between transient ischemia and infarcted tissue, repeat imaging is performed several hours later. If the cold spot fills in, a region of *transient ischemia* has been identified. If the cold spot remains unchanged, then a region of irreversible *infarction* is likely.

Radionuclide exercise tests are 80–90% sensitive and 80–90% specific for the presence of clinically significant CAD. Because these techniques are expensive, their use in screening for CAD should be reserved for 1) patients in whom baseline ECG abnormalities preclude interpretation of a standard exercise test, or 2) the improvement of testing sensitivity when standard stress test results are discordant with the clinical suspicion of coronary disease.

Exercise Echocardiography

At many centers, exercise testing with *echocardiographic* imaging is an alternative technique used to diagnose myocardial ischemia in patients with baseline ST or T wave abnormalities or in those with equivocal standard stress tests. In this technique, LV contractile function is assessed by echocardiography at baseline and immediately after treadmill or bicycle exercise. The test indicates inducible myocardial ischemia if ventricular contractile abnormalities develop with exertion.

Pharmacologic Stress Tests

For patients unable to exercise (e.g., patients with severe arthritis), *pharmacologic* stress testing can be performed using various agents, including the inotrope *dobutamine* (which increases myocardial oxygen demand by stimulating the heart rate and force of contraction) or the vasodilators *dipyridamole or adenosine.* Dipyridamole blocks the cellular uptake of adenosine and thereby increases its circulating concentration. When adenosine binds to its vascular receptors, coronary vasodilatation results. As ischemic regions are already maximally dilated (in compensation for the epicardial coronary stenoses), the drug-induced vasodilatation increases flow to the myocardium perfused by healthy coronary arteries and thus "steals" blood away from the diseased segments. As a result, nuclear perfusion imaging (using thallium-201 or technetium-99m-labeled compounds) performed right after adenosine or dipyridamole administration displays ischemic myocardium as regions of relatively decreased perfusion ("cold spots"). Alternatively, pharmacologic stress testing can be performed with echocardiography in place of nuclear imaging.

Coronary Angiography

A more direct means to identify coronary artery stenoses is by coronary angiography, in which atherosclerotic lesions are visualized radiographically following the injection of radiopaque contrast material into the artery (Fig. 6.8; also see Chapter 3). The risk of this procedure is low, but significantly greater than that of the noninvasive studies described above.

The diagnosis of CAD can be made in most patients from the history supplemented by noninvasive studies. If, however, the diagnosis is unclear, symptoms do not respond to medical therapy, the patient has an unstable presentation, or the results of noninvasive tests are so abnormal that severe CAD warranting revascularization is likely, then cardiac catheterization and angiography are undertaken.

Although coronary angiography is considered the "gold standard" for the diagnosis of CAD, it should be noted that it provides only anatomic information. The clinical significance of lesions detected by angiography depends not only on the degree of narrowing, but also on the physiologic consequences. Therefore, treatment decisions are made not only on the finding of such stenoses, but even more so on their functional effects, manifest by the patient's

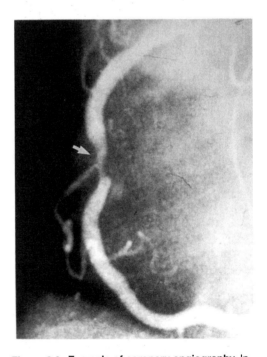

Figure 6.8. Example of coronary angiography. Injection of the right coronary artery demonstrates a stenosis in the midportion of the vessel, indicated by the arrow. (Courtesy of Dr. William Daley.)

symptoms, the viability of the myocardium segment served by stenotic vessels, and the degree of ventricular contractile dysfunction (see below). Furthermore, standard arteriography does not reveal the composition of the atherosclerotic plaque or its vulnerability to rupture (see Chapter 5).

New *noninvasive* techniques to visualize coronary anatomy (e.g., magnetic resonance angiography) are under study and are described in Chapter 3.

Natural History

The patient with chronic angina may show no change in the stable pattern of ischemia for many years. In some individuals, however, the course may be punctuated at any time by the occurrence of unstable angina, MI, or sudden ischemic death. These complications are often related to acute thrombosis at the site of disrupted atherosclerotic plaque (as will be described in Chapter 7). Why some individuals but not others sustain these complications remains a subject of intense clinical and basic science investigation, and may relate to the vulnerability of plaque to rupture.

Before the current era of sophisticated pharmacotherapy, coronary angioplasty, and surgical procedures, studies showed that the annual mortality rate of patients with CAD corresponded to the number of vessels containing significant stenoses (Table 6.3). For example, patients with advanced stenoses within a single coronary vessel could expect an annual mortality rate of <4%. Those with two involved vessels had an annual mortality rate of 7–10%, and those with advanced, three-vessel disease showed a 10–12% mortality rate. If the left main artery was significantly stenosed, the mortality rate was significantly increased (15–25%). These outcomes were worse in corresponding patients with subnormal ventricular contractile function.

More recent studies have continued to show that the location and extent of coronary stenoses are important, but that other critical predictors of mortality include 1) the degree of impaired LV contractile function, 2) poor exercise capacity, and 3) the

TABLE 6.3. Natural History of Angina Pectoris (Before Current Aggressive Medical/Surgical Era)

No. of Stenosed Vessels	Annual Mortality (%)
1	<4
2	7–10
3	10–12
Left main stenosis	15–25

Prognosis is worse in patients with impaired left ventricular function.
Reprinted with permission from Humphries JO. Expected course of patients with coronary artery disease. In: Rahimtoola SH, ed. Coronary Bypass Surgery. Philadelphia: FA Davis, 1977.

magnitude of clinical anginal symptoms. These predictors are taken into account when contemplating treatment decisions.

The mortality associated with CAD has declined significantly over the past three decades: the age-adjusted death rate has fallen by more than 50%. This is likely related to the following: 1) atherosclerotic risk reduction through improved lifestyle changes (e.g., less tobacco use, less dietary fat consumption, and more exercise), 2) improved therapeutic strategies and longevity following acute MI (see Chapter 7), and 3) advances in the medical and surgical therapies of chronic CAD.

TREATMENT

The goals of therapy in chronic ischemic heart disease are to decrease the frequency of anginal attacks, to prevent MI, and to prolong survival. A long-term crucial step is to address those risk factors that led to the development of atherosclerotic coronary disease in the first place. Recent data convincingly demonstrate the benefit of smoking cessation, cholesterol reduction, and blood pressure control in lowering the risk of coronary disease events. Improvements in other risk factors for CAD, including diabetes mellitus, obesity, and physical inactivity, are also likely to reduce the risk of adverse outcomes, although the benefits of these interventions are less well documented.

The strategy underlying current therapy of stable angina is to restore the balance between myocardial oxygen supply and demand and to prevent the complications of ischemic heart disease. The following sections describe medical and surgical strategies to 1) reduce ischemia and its symptoms, and 2) prevent MI and death in patients with chronic stable angina.

Medical Treatment of an Acute Episode of Angina

When experiencing angina, the patient should cease physical activity. Sublingual nitroglycerin, an organic nitrate, is the drug of choice in this situation. Placed under the tongue, this medication produces a slight burning sensation as the nitroglycerin is absorbed through the mucosa, and the drug begins to take effect in 1–2 minutes. Nitrates relieve ischemia primarily through vascular smooth muscle relaxation, particularly venodilatation. Venodilatation reduces venous return to the heart, with a subsequent decline in LV volume (a determinant of wall stress), which causes myocardial oxygen consumption to fall.

A second action of nitrates is to dilate the coronary vasculature, with subsequent augmentation of coronary blood flow. This effect may be of minimal value in the common individual with angina in whom maximal coronary dilatation has already resulted from the accumulation of local metabolites. However, when coronary vasospasm plays a role in the development of ischemia, nitrate-induced coronary vasodilatation may be particularly beneficial.

Medical Treatment to Prevent Recurrent Ischemic Episodes

Pharmacologic agents are also the first line of defense in the *prevention* of anginal attacks. The goal of these agents is to decrease the cardiac workload (i.e., reduce myocardial oxygen demand) and to increase myocardial perfusion. The three classes of medications typically used are the organic nitrates, β-adrenergic blockers, and calcium channel blockers (Table 6.4).

Organic nitrates (e.g., nitroglycerin, isosorbide dinitrate, isosorbide mononitrate), as discussed above, relieve ischemia primarily through venodilatation (i.e., lower wall stress results from a smaller ven-

---

TABLE 6.4. Pharmacologic Agents in the Treatment of Angina

Drug Class	Mechanism of Action	Adverse Effects

Organic nitrates	↓ *Myocardial O₂ demand*
	  ↓ Preload (venodilatation)
	
	↑ *O₂ supply*
	  ↑ Coronary perfusion
	  ↓ Coronary vasospasm
		• Headache
		• Hypotension
		• Reflex tachycardia

β-blockers	↓ *Myocardial O₂ demand*
	  ↓ Contractility
	  ↓ Heart rate
		• Excessive bradycardia
		• ↓ LV contractile function
		• Bronchoconstriction
		• May worsen diabetic control
		• Fatigue

Calcium channel blockers (agent specific—see key)	↓ *Myocardial O₂ demand*
	  ↓ Preload (venodilatation)
	  ↓ Wall stress (↓BP)
	  ↓ Contractility (V, D)
	  ↓ Heart rate (V, D)
	↑ *O₂ supply*
	  ↑ Coronary perfusion
	  ↓ Coronary vasospasm
		• Headache, flushing
		• ↓ LV contraction (V, D)
		• Marked bradycardia (V, D)
		• Edema (especially N, D)
		• Constipation (especially V)

Aspirin	↓ *Platelet aggregation*	• Gastrointestinal irritation or bleeding

LV, left ventricular; *BP*, blood pressure; *V*, verapamil; *D*, diltiazem; *N*, nifedipine and other dihydropyridine Ca⁺⁺ channel antagonists.

tricular radius) and possibly through coronary vasodilatation. The organic nitrates are the oldest of antianginal drugs and come in several preparations. Sublingual nitroglycerin tablets or spray are the forms used in the treatment of acute attacks because of their rapid onset of action. In addition, by taking a dose immediately before engaging in those activities known to provoke angina, these rapidly acting nitrates are useful as *prophylaxis* against anginal attacks.

Longer-acting anginal prevention can be achieved through a variety of nitrate preparations, including oral tablets of isosorbide dinitrate (or mononitrate) or a transdermal nitroglycerin patch, which is applied once a day. A limitation to chronic nitrate therapy is the development of drug tolerance (i.e., decreased effectiveness of the drug during continued administration), which occurs to some degree in most patients. This undesired effect can be overcome by providing a nitrate-free interval for several hours each day, usually while the patient sleeps.

There is no evidence that nitrates improve survival or prevent infarctions in patients with chronic CAD, and they are used purely for symptomatic relief. Common side effects include headache, lightheadedness, and palpitations induced by reflex sinus tachycardia. The latter can be prevented by combining a β-blocker with the nitrate regimen.

β-blockers (described further in Chapter 17) exert their antianginal effect primarily by reducing myocardial oxygen demand. They are directed against β-receptors, of which there are two classes. β_2-adrenergic receptors are located throughout peripheral blood vessels and the bronchial tree, and β_1-adrenergic receptors are restricted to the myocardium. The stimulation of β_1 receptors by catecholamines and sympathomimetic drugs increases heart rate and contractility. Consequently, β-adrenergic *antagonists* decrease the force of ventricular contraction and heart rate, thereby relieving ischemia by reducing myocardial oxygen demand. In addition, slowing the heart rate may benefit myocardial oxygen supply by augmenting the time spent in diastole,

the phase when coronary perfusion primarily occurs.

In addition to suppressing angina, several recent studies have shown that β-blockers decrease the rates of recurrent infarction and mortality following an acute MI (see Chapter 7). Moreover, they have been shown to reduce the likelihood of a first MI in patients with hypertension. Thus, β-blockers are considered first-line therapy in the treatment of CAD.

Beta-blockers are generally well-tolerated but have several potential side effects. For example, they may precipitate bronchospasm in patients with underlying asthma by antagonizing β_2 receptors in the bronchial tree. Although β_1-*selective* blockers are theoretically less likely to exacerbate bronchospasm in such patients, drug selectivity for the β_1 receptor is not complete, and in general, all beta-blockers should be avoided in patients with obstructive airway disease.

Beta-blockers are also generally not used in patients with *decompensated* LV dysfunction because they could intensify heart failure symptoms by further reducing inotropy. (However, as described in Chapter 9, β-blockers actually *improve* outcomes in patients with stable heart failure conditions.) Beta-blockers are also relatively contraindicated in patients with marked bradycardia or certain types of heart block, to avoid additional impairment of electrical conduction.

Beta-blockers sometimes cause fatigue and sexual dysfunction. They should be used with caution in insulin-treated diabetics, as they can mask tachycardia and other catecholamine-mediated responses that can warn of hypoglycemia. One might also expect that β-blockers would decrease myocardial blood perfusion by blocking the vasodilating β_2-adrenergic receptors on the coronary arteries. However, this effect is usually attenuated by autoregulation and vasodilation of the coronary vessel owing to the accumulation of local metabolites.

Calcium channel blockers (see Chapter 17) antagonize voltage-gated L-type calcium channels, but the actions of the individual drugs of this group vary. The dihydropyridines (e.g., nifedipine and amlodip-ine) are potent vasodilators. They relieve myocardial ischemia by 1) decreasing oxy-gen demand (*venodilatation* reduces ventric-ular filling and size; *arterial dilatation* re-duces the resistance against which the left ventricle contracts—both actions reduce wall stress), and 2) increasing myocardial oxygen supply via coronary dilatation. By the latter mechanism, they are also potent agents for the relief of coronary artery vasospasm.

Nondihydropyridine calcium channel blockers (verapamil and diltiazem) also act as vasodilators but are not as potent in this regard as the dihydropyridines. However, these agents have additional beneficial an-tianginal effects stemming from their more potent cardiac depressant effects: they re-duce the force of ventricular contraction (inotropy) and slow the heart rate. Accord-ingly, verapamil and diltiazem also de-crease myocardial oxygen demand by these mechanisms.

Questions have been raised about the safety of *short-acting* calcium channel block-ing drugs in the treatment of ischemic heart disease. In meta-analyses of randomized trials, these drugs have been associated with an *increased* incidence of MI and mor-tality. The adverse effect may relate to the rapid hemodynamic effects and blood pres-sure swings induced by the short-acting agents. Therefore, only *long-acting* calcium-channel blocking drugs are recommended in the treatment of chronic angina, gener-ally as second-line drugs, if symptoms are not controlled by β-blockers and nitrates.

The three groups of antianginal drugs can be used alone or in combination. How-ever, care should be taken in combining a β-blocker with a nondihydropyridine calcium channel blocker (verapamil or diltiazem) because the additive negative chronotropic effect can cause excessive bradycardia, and the combined negative inotropic effect could precipitate heart failure in patients with LV contractile dysfunction.

Although useful in controlling symptoms of angina, none of the antianginal drug groups has been shown to slow or reverse the atherosclerotic process responsible for the arterial lesions of chronic CAD. More-over, although β-blockers have demon-strated mortality benefits in patients after MI (see Chapter 7), none of the antianginal agents has been proved to improve survival in patients with chronic stable angina and preserved LV function.

Medical Treatment to Prevent MI and Death

Antiplatelet therapy with aspirin re-duces the risk of MI in patients with chronic angina and should be a standard addition to the regimen of drugs used to treat CAD. Platelet aggregation and thrombosis are key elements in the pathophysiology of acute MI and unstable angina (see Chapter 7). Aspirin has antithrombotic actions through inhibition of platelet aggregation (and therefore reduces the release of platelet-derived procoagulants and vaso-constrictors) as well as antiinflammatory properties that may be important in stabi-lizing atheromatous plaque. Unless con-traindications are present (e.g., allergy or gastric irritation), aspirin should be contin-ued indefinitely in all patients with CAD. Other drugs that inhibit platelet aggrega-tion and thrombosis, such as clopidogrel (see Chapter 17), should be considered for aspirin-allergic patients.

Lipid-lowering therapy also reduces cardiovascular clinical events. In particular, HMG CoA reductase inhibitors ("statins") lower MI and death rates in patients with established coronary disease and in those at high risk of developing CAD. The benefits of statin therapy are believed to go beyond their lipid-lowering effects, as there is evi-dence that they improve endothelial cell dysfunction and may help stabilize athero-sclerotic plaques. Current guidelines rec-ommend that LDL cholesterol be main-tained at <100 mg/dL in patients with atherosclerotic disease (see Chapter 5).

Angiotensin-converting enzyme (ACE) inhibitors, conventionally used to treat hy-pertension and heart failure, benefit pa-tients with coronary disease as well. As dis-cussed in Chapter 7, ACE inhibitors reduce mortality and the risk of reinfarction after an MI. More recently, the Heart Outcomes Prevention Evaluation study showed that ACE inhibition also reduces the risk of MI and death in patients with chronic vascular disease, including those with CAD. The likely beneficial mechanisms of ACE inhibitors in this regard include reductions in LV hypertrophy, improvements in ventricular function, and possibly antithrombotic and endothelial effects. Thus, cardiologists now frequently recommend that an ACE inhibitor be included in the medical regimen of patients with chronic CAD.

Revascularization

Patients with angina that becomes asymptomatic during pharmacologic therapy are usually followed by their physicians with continued emphasis on reducing cardiac risk factors. However, more aggressive **mechanical revascularization** is pursued if 1) the patient's symptoms of angina do not respond adequately to anti-anginal drug therapy, 2) unacceptable side effects of medications occur, or 3) the patient is found to have a specific type of high-risk coronary disease for which surgical revascularization is known to improve survival (described below). The two techniques used to accomplish mechanical revascularization are percutaneous coronary intervention and coronary artery bypass graft surgery.

Percutaneous coronary interventions (PCI) include percutaneous transluminal coronary angioplasty (PTCA), a procedure performed under fluoroscopy in which a balloon-tipped catheter is inserted through a peripheral artery (usually femoral, brachial, or radial) and maneuvered into the stenotic segment of a coronary vessel. The balloon at the end of the catheter is then inflated under high pressure to dilate the stenosis, after which the balloon is deflated and the catheter is removed from the body. The improvement in the size of the coronary lumen increases coronary perfusion and myocardial oxygen supply. Effective dilatation of the stenosis results from compression of the atherosclerotic plaque and often by creating a fracture within the lesion and stretching the underlying media.

Many types of coronary stenoses are amenable to balloon dilation, and complications are infrequent. The risk of a Q-wave MI during the procedure is less than 1.5%, and mortality is less than 1%. Unfortunately, approximately one-third of patients who undergo standard PTCA develop recurrent symptoms within 6 months, due to restenosis of the dilated artery, and require additional coronary interventions. In rigorous angiographic studies, the incidence of restenosis after PTCA has been found to be even greater—as high as 50%.

Fortunately, the past decade has witnessed major advances in percutaneous techniques, most notably the development of *coronary stents* that can be placed at the time of PCI and significantly reduce the rate of restenosis. Coronary stents are slender, cage-like, stainless-steel support devices that in their collapsed configuration can be threaded into the region of stenosis by a catheter. Once in position, the stent is expanded into its open position by inflating a high-pressure balloon in its interior. The balloon and attached catheter are then removed, but the stent is left permanently in place to serve as a scaffold to maintain arterial patency. Because stents are thrombogenic, a combination of oral antiplatelet agents (typically aspirin plus clopidogrel) is crucial for at least 4 weeks after stent implantation.

Compared with conventional PTCA, stent implantation results in larger luminal diameters, decreased restenosis rates, and reduced need for repeat angioplasty procedures. Although restenosis due to vessel elastic recoil is greatly diminished by stent placement, neointimal proliferation (i.e., migration and stimulation of smooth muscle cells and production of extracellular matrix) is not. It is an important cause of in-stent restenosis and recurrent symptoms. Strategies to address the latter problem include intracoronary radiation therapy (brachytherapy) and most recently antiproliferative drug eluting stents, which have shown great promise in preventing neointimal proliferation.

In addition to balloon angioplasty and stents, other percutaneous coronary interventions are sometimes used to improve coronary patency. *Directional coronary atherectomy* involves positioning a windowed cylindrical housing against a stenosis as an attached balloon is inflated against the opposite wall. A rotating metal blade is then advanced within the housing and used to shave plaque from the vessel wall and extract the fragments through the catheter tip. *Rotational atherectomy* uses a rapidly spinning burr to penetrate calcified or fibrotic plaque. Neither of these techniques has proved superior to standard balloon angioplasty at maintaining vessel patency over the long term, but they can be used to remove intracoronary plaque burden before stenting.

Although percutaneous revascularization techniques are, in general, superior to standard medical therapy for relief of angina, they have not been shown to reduce the risk of MI or death due to coronary disease.

Coronary artery bypass graft (CABG) surgery entails grafting portions of a patient's native blood vessels to bypass obstructed coronary arteries. Two types of surgical grafts are used (Fig. 6.9). The first employs native veins, typically a section of the saphenous vein (a "superfluous" vessel removed from the leg) which is sutured from the base of the aorta to a coronary segment downstream from the region of stenosis. In the second method, *arterial* grafts are used, most commonly an internal mammary artery (a "superfluous" branch of each subclavian artery) which can be directly anastomosed distal to a stenotic coronary site. Vein grafts have a patency rate of up to 80% at 12 months but are vulnerable to accelerated atherosclerosis; by 10 years following surgery more than 50% have occluded. In contrast, internal mammary artery (IMA) grafts are more resistant to atherosclerosis with a patency rate of 90% at 10 years. Therefore, IMA grafts are often used to perfuse sites of critical flow such as the left anterior descending artery. Recent evidence supports the use of aggressive lipid-lowering drug therapy after CABG to improve the long-term patency rates of bypass grafts.

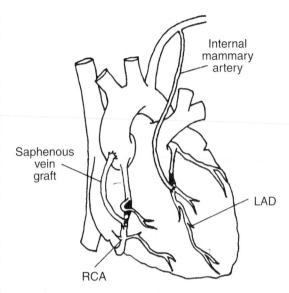

Figure 6.9. **Coronary artery bypass surgery. A.** The left internal mammary artery originates from the left subclavian artery, and in this schematic, is anastomosed to the left anterior descending (LAD) coronary artery distal to a tight stenosis (black segment). **B.** One end of a saphenous vein graft is sutured to the proximal aorta and the other end to the right coronary artery (RCA) distal to a stenotic segment.

Medical Versus Revascularization Therapy

Many patients with chronic, stable angina can be successfully managed with pharmacologic therapy alone. However, if anginal symptoms prove refractory to a good pharmacologic program, or if intolerable drug side effects develop, coronary angiography is usually recommended for further therapeutic planning. For patients whose angina *is* controlled by medications, it is standard to perform noninvasive testing (e.g., exercise testing, echocardiography) to identify those with high-risk disease, as the long-term prognosis for such patients can be improved by coronary revascularization.

Once coronary angiography is obtained, the decision of whether to proceed with percutaneous intervention versus bypass graft surgery depends on several considerations, including those listed in Table 6.5. In general, patients with persistent episodes of angina and significant stenoses in one to two coronary arteries are good candidates

TABLE 6.5. Relative Benefits of PCI and CABG

Percutaneous Coronary Interventions (PCI)	Coronary Artery Bypass Graft Surgery (CABG)
Less invasive than CABG	More effective for long-term relief of angina than PCI or pharmacologic therapy
Shorter hospital stay and easier recuperation than CABG	Most complete revascularization
Superior to pharmacologic therapy for relief of angina (but does not reduce risk of MI or death)	Improved survival in patients with: > 50% left main stenosis Three-vessel CAD, especially if LV contractile function is impaired Two-vessel disease with tight (> 75%) LAD stenosis Diabetes and two- to three-vessel disease

MI, myocardial infarction; CAD, coronary artery disease; LV, left ventricle; LAD, left anterior descending coronary artery.

for PCI, as are select lower-risk patients with three-vessel disease. Conversely, patients who fare better over the long-term with CABG include those with significant (>50%) stenosis of the left main coronary, and patients with two- to three-vessel disease who also have reduced LV contractile function or diabetes.

Each of the above described approaches for the treatment of coronary disease is benefiting from rapidly developing research advancements. New surgical techniques (increased use of various arterial grafts, less invasive operations), novel adjuncts to stenting (potent antithrombotic drugs, advanced approaches to prevent in-stent restenosis), and progress in pharmacologic management (aggressive use of statins and ACE inhibitors) will likely further improve outcomes and better define the best therapeutic approaches for specific subsets of patients with chronic CAD.

SUMMARY

1. Cardiac ischemia results from an imbalance between myocardial oxygen supply and demand. Myocardial oxygen supply is determined by the oxygen-carrying capacity of the blood and coronary blood flow. The latter is dependent on the coronary perfusion pressure and coronary vascular resistance. Key regulators of myocardial oxygen demand include myocardial wall stress, heart rate, and contractility.

2. In the presence of atherosclerotic disease, myocardial oxygen supply is compromised. Atherosclerotic plaques cause vascular lumen narrowing and reduce coronary blood flow. In addition, atherosclerosis-associated endothelial cell dysfunction causes inappropriate vasoconstriction of the coronary resistance vessels.

3. Angina pectoris is the most frequent symptom of intermittent ischemia, and its diagnosis relies heavily on the patient's description of the discomfort. Angina may be accompanied by signs and symptoms of adrenergic stimulation, pulmonary congestion, and transient LV systolic and diastolic dysfunction.

4. Laboratory studies useful in the diagnosis of angina include the electrocardiogram (ST segment and T wave abnormalities), exercise (or pharmacologic) stress testing, and coronary angiography.

5. Standard pharmacologic therapy for the treatment of chronic angina includes agents to prevent ischemia and relieve symptoms (organic nitrates, β-blockers, and calcium channel antagonists, alone or in combination) as well as agents that reduce the risk of MI and death (aspirin, anticholesterol therapy, and consideration of ACE inhibitors). Modifiable risk factors for atherosclerosis should be corrected.

6. Revascularization with PCI or CABG surgery may provide relief from ische-

mia in patients with chronic angina who are refractory to, or unable to tolerate, medical therapy. CABG confers improved survival rates to certain high-risk groups.

Acknowledgments   Contributors to the previous editions of this chapter were Christopher P. Chiodo, MD; Carey Farquhar, MD; Rainu Kaushal, MD; William Carlson, MD; Michael E. Mendelsohn, MD; Marc S. Sabatine, MD; Patrick T. O'Gara, MD; and Leonard S. Lilly, MD.

ADDITIONAL READING

Bittl JA. Advances in coronary angioplasty. N Engl J Med 1996;335:1290–1302.

Bypass Angioplasty Revascularization Investigation (BARI) Investigators. Comparison of coronary bypass surgery with angioplasty in patients with multivessel disease. N Engl J Med 1996;335:217–225.

CAPRIE Steering Committee. A randomised, blinded, trial of clopidogrel versus aspirin in patients at risk of ischemic events (CAPRIE). Lancet 1996;348:1329–1339.

CASS Principal Investigators and Their Associates. Coronary Artery Surgery Study (CASS): a randomized trial of coronary artery bypass surgery: survival data. Circulation 1983;68:939–950.

Cooper HA, Braunwald E. Clinical importance of stunned and hibernating myocardium. Coron Artery Dis 2001;12:387–392.

Detre KM, Holubkov R. Coronary revascularization on balance: Robert L. Frye lecture. Mayo Clin Proc 2002;77:72–82.

Douglas PS, Ginsburg GS. Current concepts: the evaluation of chest pain in women. N Engl J Med 1996;334:1311–1315.

Eagle KA, Guyton RA, Davidoff R, et al. ACC/AHA guidelines for coronary artery bypass graft surgery: executive summary and recommendations: a report of the American College of Cardiology/American Heart Association task force on practice guidelines. Circulation 1999;100:1464–1480.

Feletou M, Vanhoutte PM. The alternative: EDHF. J Mol Cell Cardiol 1999;31:15–22.

Fuster V, Badimon L, Badimon JJ, et al. The pathogenesis of coronary artery disease and the acute coronary syndromes. N Engl J Med 1992;326:242–250, 310–318.

Gibbons RJ, Chatterjee K, Daley J, et al. ACC/AHA/ACP-AISM guidelines for the management of patients with chronic stable angina: executive summary and recommendations: a report of the American College of Cardiology/American Heart Association Task Force on Practice Guidelines. Circulation 1999;99:2829–2848.

Heart Outcomes Prevention Evaluation (HOPE) Study Investigators. Effects of an angiotensin-converting-enzyme inhibitor, ramipril, on cardiovascular events in high-risk patients. N Engl J Med 2000;342:145–153.

Pitt B, Waters D, Brown WV, et al., for the Atorvastatin Versus Revascularization Treatment Investigators. Aggressive lipid-lowering therapy compared with angioplasty in stable coronary artery disease. N Engl J Med 1999;341:70–76.

Post Coronary Artery Bypass Graft Trial Investigators. The effect of aggressive lowering of low-density lipoprotein cholesterol levels and low-dose anticoagulation on obstructive changes in saphenous-vein coronary artery bypass grafts. N Engl J Med. 1997;336:153–162.

RITA Trial Participants. Coronary angioplasty versus coronary artery bypass surgery: the Randomised Intervention Treatment of Angina (RITA) trial. Lancet 1993;341:573–580.

RITA-2 Trial Participants. Coronary angioplasty versus medical therapy for angina: the second Randomized Intervention Treatment of Angina (Rita-2) trial. Lancet 1997;350:461-468.

Scanlon PJ, Faxon DP, Audet A-M, et al. ACC/AHA guidelines for coronary angiography: executive summary and recommendations: a report of the American College of Cardiology/American Heart Association Task Force on Practice Guidelines. Circulation 1999;99:2345–2357.

Smith SC Jr, Dove JT, Jacobs AK, et al. ACC/AHA guidelines of percutaneous coronary interventions—executive summary: a report of the American College of Cardiology/American Heart Association Task Force on Practice Guidelines. J Am Coll Cardiol 2001;37:2215–2238.

Treasure CB, Klein JL, Weintraub WS, et al. Beneficial effects of cholesterol-lowering therapy on the coronary endothelium in patients with coronary artery disease. N Engl J Med 1995;332:481–487.

Williams SV, Fihn SD, Gibbons RJ. Guidelines for the management of patients with chronic stable angina: diagnosis and risk stratification. Ann Intern Med 2001;135:530–547.

Acute Coronary Syndromes

Anurag Gupta, Marc S. Sabatine, Patrick T. O'Gara, and Leonard S. Lilly

Chapter 7

Pathogenesis of Acute Coronary Syndromes
Normal Hemostasis
Endogenous Antithrombotic Mechanisms
Pathogenesis of Coronary Thrombosis
Nonatherosclerotic Causes of Acute Coronary
  Syndromes
Pathology and Pathophysiology
Early Changes
Late Changes
Functional Changes
Clinical Features of Acute Coronary Syndromes
Clinical Presentation
Diagnosis of Acute Coronary Syndromes

Treatment of Acute Coronary Syndromes
Acute Treatment of Unstable Angina/Non-ST-
  Elevation MI
Acute Treatment of ST-Elevation MI
Complications
Recurrent Ischemia
Arrhythmias
Myocardial Dysfunction
Right Ventricular Infarction
Mechanical Complications
Pericarditis
Thromboembolism
Post-MI Risk Stratification and Management

Acute coronary syndromes (ACS) are life-threatening conditions that can punctuate the course of patients with coronary artery disease at any time. These syndromes encompass a continuum that ranges from an unstable pattern of angina to the most severe form of acute myocardial infarction (MI), the condition of irreversible necrosis of heart muscle (Fig. 7.1). All acute syndromes share a common initiating pathophysiologic mechanism, as will be examined.

The frequency of ACS is staggering: more than 1.6 million people are admitted to the hospital in the United States each year with one of these conditions. However, despite that daunting statistic, there has been a substantial and continuous decline in the mortality rate associated with ACS in recent decades, due to important therapeutic and preventive advances. This chapter considers the events that lead to ACS, the pathologic and functional changes that follow, and therapeutic approaches that ameliorate the aberrant pathophysiology.

PATHOGENESIS OF ACS

The vast majority (>90%) of ACS result from disruption of an atherosclerotic plaque with subsequent platelet aggregation and formation of an intracoronary thrombus. The thrombus transforms a region of plaque narrowing to one of severe or complete occlusion, and the impaired blood flow through the involved artery causes a severe imbalance between myocardial oxygen supply and demand. The form of ACS that results depends on the degree of coronary obstruction and associated ischemia (see Fig. 7.1). A *partially* occlusive thrombus is the typical cause of the closely related syndromes **unstable angina** (UA) and **non-ST-segment elevation myocardial infarction** (NSTEMI, also referred to as "non–Q-wave MI"), with the latter being distinguished from the former by the presence of myocardial necrosis. If the coronary thrombus *completely* obstructs the coronary artery, then more severe ischemia results with accompanying necrosis, most often

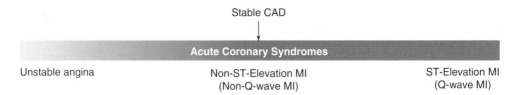

Figure 7.1. **The continuum of acute coronary syndromes ranges from unstable angina, through non-ST-elevation myocardial infarction (also referred to as "non-Q-wave" myocardial infarction [MI]), to ST-elevation MI (also referred to as "Q-wave" MI).**

causing an ACS at the other end of the spectrum: an **ST-segment elevation myocardial infarction** (STEMI; also referred to as "Q-wave MI").

The responsible thrombus in ACS appears to be generated by interactions among the atherosclerotic plaque, the coronary endothelium, circulating platelets, and the dynamic vasomotor tone of the vessel wall, all of which overwhelm natural protective mechanisms, as is now reviewed.

Normal Hemostasis

When a normal blood vessel is injured, the endothelial surface becomes disrupted and thrombogenic connective tissue is exposed. *Primary hemostasis* is the first line of defense against bleeding. This process begins within seconds of vessel injury and is mediated by circulating platelets, which adhere to collagen in the vascular subendothelium and aggregate to form a "platelet plug." While the primary hemostatic plug forms, the exposure of subendothelial tissue factor activates the plasma coagulation cascade, initiating the process of *secondary hemostasis.* The plasma coagulation proteins involved in secondary hemostasis are sequentially activated at the site of injury and ultimately form a fibrin clot by the action of thrombin. The resulting clot stabilizes and strengthens the platelet plug.

The normal hemostatic system minimizes blood loss from injured vessels, but there is little difference between this physiologic response and the pathologic process of coronary thrombosis triggered by disruption of atherosclerotic plaques.

Endogenous Antithrombotic Mechanisms

Normal blood vessels, including the coronary arteries, are replete with safeguards that prevent spontaneous thrombosis and occlusion, some examples of which are shown in Figure 7.2.

Inactivation of Clotting Factors

Several natural inhibitors tightly regulate the coagulation process to oppose clot formation and maintain blood fluidity. The most important of these are antithrombin III, proteins C and S, and tissue factor pathway inhibitor.

Antithrombin III (ATIII) is a plasma protein that irreversibly binds to thrombin and other clotting factors, inactivating them and facilitating their clearance from the circulation (see mechanism 1 in Fig. 7.2). The effectiveness of ATIII is increased a thousand-fold by binding to heparan sulfate, a heparin-like molecule normally present on the luminal surface of endothelial cells.

Protein C/protein S/thrombomodulin is a natural anticoagulant system that inactivates the "acceleration" factors of the coagulation pathway (i.e., factors Va and VIIIa). Protein C is synthesized in the liver and circulates in an inactive form. Thrombomodulin is a thrombin-binding receptor normally present on endothelial cells. Thrombin that is bound to thrombomodulin cannot convert fibrinogen to fibrin (the final reaction in clot formation). Instead, the thrombin-thrombomodulin complex activates protein C. Activated protein C degrades factors Va and VIIIa (see mechanism 2 in Fig. 7.2), thereby inhibiting coagulation. The presence of protein S in the circulation enhances the inhibitory function of protein C.

Tissue factor pathway inhibitor (TFPI) is a plasma serine protease inhibitor that is activated by coagulation factor Xa. The factor Xa/TFPI complex binds to and inactivates the complex of tissue factor with factor VIIa that normally triggers the "extrinsic" coagulation pathway (see mechanism 3 in Fig. 7.2). Thus, TFPI serves as a negative feedback inhibitor that interferes with coagulation.

Lysis of Fibrin Clots

Tissue plasminogen activator (tPA) is a protein secreted by endothelial cells in response to many triggers of clot formation. tPA cleaves the protein plasminogen to

form active plasmin, which in turn enzymatically degrades fibrin clots (mechanism 4 in Fig. 7.2). When tPA binds to fibrin in a forming clot, its ability to convert plasminogen to plasmin is greatly enhanced.

Endogenous Platelet Inhibition and Vasodilatation

Prostacyclin is synthesized and secreted by endothelial cells, as described in Chapter 6. It increases platelet levels of cyclic AMP and thereby strongly inhibits platelet activation and aggregation (see mechanism 5 in Fig. 7.2). Prostacyclin also *indirectly* inhibits coagulation via its potent vasodilating properties. Vasodilatation helps guard against thrombosis by augmenting blood flow (which minimizes contact between

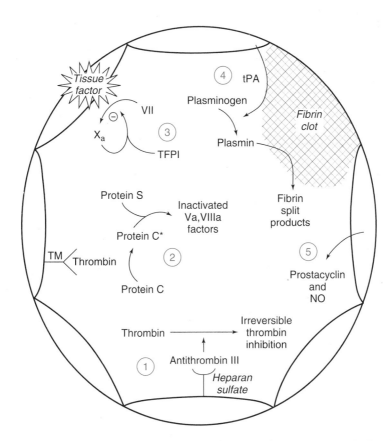

Figure 7.2. **Endogenous protective mechanisms against thrombosis and vessel occlusion. 1.** Inactivation of thrombin by antithrombin III (ATIII), the effectiveness of which is enhanced by binding of ATIII to heparan sulfate. **2.** Inactivation of clotting factors Va and VIIIa by activated protein C (protein C*), an action that is enhanced by protein S. Protein C is activated by the thrombomodulin (TM)-thrombin complex. **3.** Inactivation of factor VII/tissue factor complex by tissue factor pathway inhibitor (TFPI). **4.** Lysis of fibrin clots by tissue plasminogen activator (tPA). **5.** Inhibition of platelet activation by prostacyclin and NO.

procoagulant factors) and by reducing shear stress (an inducer of platelet activation).

Nitric oxide (NO) is also secreted by endothelial cells as described in Chapter 6. It acts locally to inhibit platelet activation (see mechanism 5 in Fig. 7.2), and it too serves as a potent vasodilator.

Pathogenesis of Coronary Thrombosis

Normally, the above mechanisms serve to prevent spontaneous intravascular thrombus formation. However, abnormalities associated with atherosclerotic lesions may overwhelm these defenses and result in coronary thrombosis and vessel occlusion (Fig. 7.3). Atherosclerosis contributes to thrombus formation by: 1) plaque rupture, which exposes the circulating blood elements to thrombogenic substances, and 2) endothelial dysfunction with the loss of normal protective antithrombotic and vasodilatory properties.

Atherosclerotic **plaque rupture** is considered to be the major trigger of coronary thrombosis. The underlying causes of plaque disruption are likely multifactorial, as delineated in Chapter 5, and include 1) chemical factors, including inflammatory cytokines, that increase the vulnerability of plaque to rupture, and 2) physical stresses to which the atherosclerotic lesions are subjected. Plaques consist of a fibrous external cap that surrounds a lipid-laden and necrotic core. There is evidence that substances released from leukocytes within the plaque can compromise the integrity of the fibrous cap. For example, T lymphocytes elaborate gamma interferon, which inhibits collagen synthesis by smooth muscle cells and thereby interferes with the usual strength of the fibrous cap. Additionally, cells within atherosclerotic lesions produce enzymes (e.g., collagenases and gelatinases) that degrade the interstitial matrix, further compromising the stable structure of the plaque. A weakened or thin-capped

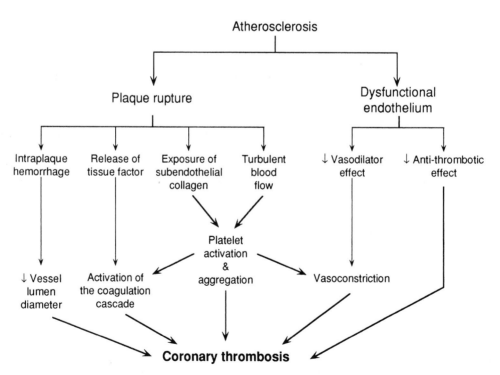

Figure 7.3. Mechanisms of coronary thrombus formation. Factors that contribute to this process include plaque disruption (e.g., rupture), activation of platelets and the clotting cascade, and inappropriate vasoconstriction and loss of normal antithrombotic defenses because of dysfunctional endothelium.

plaque is subject to rupture, particularly in its "shoulder" region (the border with the normal arterial wall that is subjected to high circumferential stress) either spontaneously or by physical forces, such as intraluminal blood pressure and torsion from the beating myocardium. The hypothesis that inflammation plays a critical role in destabilizing plaque in the etiology of ACS is described further in Chapter 5.

ACS sometimes occur in the setting of certain triggers, such as strenuous physical activity or emotional stress. The activation of the sympathetic nervous system in these situations increases the blood pressure, heart rate, and force of ventricular contraction, actions that may stress the atherosclerotic lesion, thereby causing the plaque to fissure or rupture. In addition, myocardial infarction (MI) is most likely to occur in the early morning hours. This observation may relate to the fact that key physiologic stressors (such as systolic blood pressure, blood viscosity, and plasma epinephrine levels) tend to be most elevated at that time of day, and these factors subject vulnerable plaques to rupture.

Following plaque rupture, thrombus formation is triggered via multiple mechanisms (see Fig. 7.3). The *exposure of tissue factor* from the atheromatous core triggers the coagulation pathway, while the exposure of subendothelial collagen activates platelets. Activated platelets release the contents of their granules, which include facilitators of *platelet aggregation* (e.g., adenosine diphosphate [ADP], fibrinogen), *activators of the coagulation cascade* (e.g., factor Va), and *vasoconstrictors* (e.g., thromboxane and serotonin). The developing intracoronary thrombus, intraplaque hemorrhage, and vasoconstriction all contribute to narrowing the vessel lumen, creating *turbulent blood flow* that contributes to shear stress and further platelet activation.

Dysfunctional endothelium, which is apparent even in mild atherosclerotic coronary disease, also increases the likelihood of thrombus formation. In the setting of dysfunctional endothelium, reduced amounts of vasodilators (e.g., NO and prostacyclin) are released and inhibition of platelet aggregation by these factors is impaired, such that a key defense against thrombosis is lost.

Not only is dysfunctional endothelium less equipped to prevent platelet aggregation, but it is also less able to counteract the vasoconstricting products of platelets. During thrombus formation, vasoconstriction is promoted both by platelet products (thromboxane and serotonin) and by thrombin within the developing clot. The *normal* platelet-associated vascular response is vasodilatation, because platelet products stimulate endothelial NO and prostacyclin release, the influences of which predominate over direct platelet-derived vasoconstrictors (see Fig. 6.4). However, reduced secretion of endothelial vasodilators in atherosclerosis allows vasoconstriction to proceed unchecked. Similarly, thrombin in a forming clot is a potent vascular smooth muscle constrictor in the setting of dysfunctional endothelium. Vasoconstriction causes torsional stresses that can contribute to plaque rupture or can transiently occlude the stenotic vessel through heightened arterial tone. The reduction in coronary blood flow caused by vasoconstriction also reduces the washout of coagulation proteins, such that thrombogenicity is enhanced.

Significance of Coronary Thrombosis

The formation of an intracoronary thrombus results in one of several potential outcomes (Fig. 7.4). For example, plaque rupture is sometimes superficial, minor, and self-limited, such that only a small, nonocclusive thrombus forms. In this case, the small thrombus may simply become incorporated into the growing atheromatous lesion through fibrotic organization or lysed by natural fibrinolytic mechanisms. Recurrent asymptomatic plaque ruptures of this type may cause gradual progressive enlargement of the coronary stenosis.

However, deeper plaque rupture may result in greater exposure of subendothelial collagen and tissue factor, with formation of a larger thrombus that more substantially occludes the vessel's lumen. Such obstruction may cause prolonged severe ischemia and the development of an

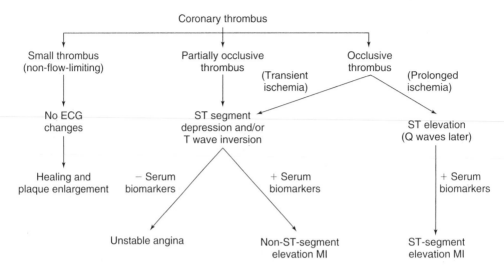

Figure 7.4. Consequences of coronary thrombosis. A small thrombus formed on superficial plaque rupture may not result in symptoms or ECG abnormalities, but healing and fibrous organization may incorporate the thrombus into the plaque, causing the atherosclerotic lesion to enlarge. A partially occlusive thrombus (with or without superimposed vasospasm) narrows the arterial lumen, restricts blood flow, and can cause unstable angina or a non-ST-elevation MI, either of which may result in ST depression and/or T wave inversion on the ECG. A totally occlusive thrombus with prolonged ischemia is the most common cause of ST-elevation MI, in which the ECG initially shows ST segment elevation, followed by Q wave development. An occlusive thrombus that recanalizes, or one that develops in a region served by adequate collateral blood flow, may result in less prolonged ischemia and a non-ST-elevation MI instead. Markers of myocardial necrosis include cardiac-specific troponins and creatine kinase MB isoenzyme.

acute coronary syndrome. If the intraluminal thrombus at the site of plaque disruption *totally* occludes the vessel, blood flow beyond the obstruction will cease, prolonged ischemia will occur, and an MI (usually an ST-elevation MI) will result. Conversely, if the thrombus *partially* occludes the vessel (or if it totally occludes the vessel, but only transiently, because of spontaneous recanalization, or by relief of superimposed vasospasm), the severity

and duration of ischemia will be less, and a smaller non-ST-elevation MI or UA are the more likely outcomes. The distinction between a non-ST-elevation MI and UA is based on the degree of the ischemia and whether the event is severe enough to cause necrosis, indicated by the presence of certain serum biomarkers (see Fig. 7.4). Nonetheless, UA and NSTEMI act quite alike and the management of these entities is similar.

Occasionally, a non-ST-elevation infarct may result from total coronary occlusion. In this case, it is likely that a substantial collateral blood supply limits the extent of necrosis, such that a larger ST-elevation MI is prevented.

Nonatherosclerotic Causes of Acute Coronary Syndromes

Rarely, mechanisms other than acute coronary thrombus formation can precipitate an acute coronary syndrome (Table 7.1). These should be suspected when an ischemic syndrome occurs in young indi-

TABLE 7.1. Causes of Acute Coronary Syndromes

Atherosclerosis with superimposed thrombus
Vasculitic syndromes (see Chapter 15)
Coronary emboli (e.g., from endocarditis, artificial valves)
Congenital anomalies of the coronary arteries
Coronary trauma or aneurysm
Severe coronary artery spasm (primary or cocaine-induced)
Increased blood viscosity (e.g., polycythemia vera, thrombocytosis)
Significantly increased myocardial oxygen demand (e.g., aortic stenosis)

viduals or those without coronary risk factors. For example, coronary emboli from mechanical or infected cardiac valves can lodge in the coronary circulation, or inflammation from acute vasculitis can initiate coronary occlusion. Occasionally, intense transient coronary spasm can sufficiently reduce myocardial blood supply to result in UA or infarction.

A very unfortunate cause of ACS is cocaine abuse. Cocaine increases sympathetic tone by blocking the presynaptic reuptake of norepinephrine and by enhancing the release of adrenal catecholamines, which can lead to vasospasm and therefore decreased myocardial oxygen supply. An acute coronary syndrome may ensue as a result of increased myocardial oxygen demand associated with cocaine-associated sympathetic myocardial stimulation (increased heart rate and blood pressure) in the face of the decreased oxygen supply.

PATHOLOGY AND PATHOPHYSIOLOGY

MI (both STEMI and NSTEMI) results when myocardial ischemia is sufficiently severe to cause myocyte necrosis. Although by definition UA does not result in necrosis, MI may subsequently ensue if the underlying pathophysiology of that condition is not promptly corrected.

In addition to their clinical descriptions, infarctions can be described pathologically by the extent of necrosis they produce within the myocardial wall. **Transmural infarcts** span the entire thickness of the myocardium and result from total, prolonged occlusion of an epicardial coronary artery. Conversely, **subendocardial infarcts** exclusively involve the innermost layers of the myocardium. The subendocardium is particularly susceptible to ischemia because it is the zone subjected to the highest pressure from the ventricular chamber, has few collateral vessels that supply it, and is perfused by vessels that must pass through layers of contracting myocardium.

Infarction represents the culmination of a disastrous cascade of events initiated by ischemia that has progressed from a potentially reversible phase to irreversible cell death. Myocardium that is supplied directly by an occluded vessel may die quickly. The adjacent tissue may not necrose immediately, because it may also be perfused by nearby patent vessels. The neighboring cells may become increasingly ischemic over time, however, as demand for oxygen continues in the face of decreased oxygen supply. Thus, the region of infarction may subsequently extend outward. The extent of tissue that ultimately succumbs to infarction therefore relates to 1) the mass of myocardium perfused by the occluded vessel, 2) the magnitude and duration of coronary blood flow limitation, 3) the oxygen demand of the affected region, 4) the adequacy of collateral vessels that provide blood flow from neighboring nonoccluded coronary arteries, and 5) the degree of tissue response that modifies the ischemic process.

The pathophysiologic events that transpire during MI predict efficacious therapies and possible complications. Generally, these events occur in two stages: early changes at the time of acute infarction, and late changes during myocardial healing and remodeling.

Early Changes

Early changes include the histologic evolution of the infarct and the functional impact of oxygen deprivation on myocardial contractility. These changes culminate in coagulative necrosis of the myocardium in 2–4 days.

Cellular Changes

As oxygen levels fall in the myocardium supplied by an abruptly occluded coronary vessel, there is a rapid shift from aerobic to anaerobic glycolytic metabolism (Fig. 7.5). Because mitochondria can no longer oxidize fats or products of glycolysis, high-energy phosphate production drops dramatically and anaerobic glycolysis leads to the accumulation of lactic acid. This results in a lowered pH.

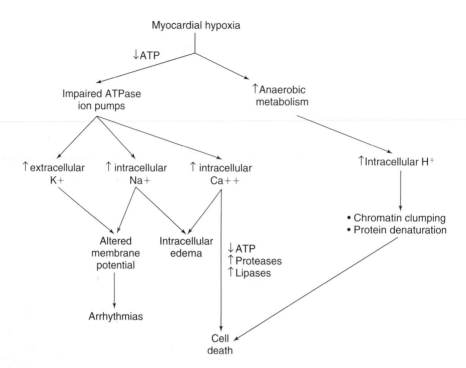

Figure 7.5. **Mechanisms of cell death in myocardial infarction.** Acute ischemia rapidly depletes the intracellular supply of ATP as aerobic metabolism fails. Subsequent intracellular acidosis and impairment of ATP-dependent processes culminate in intracellular calcium accumulation, edema, and cell death.

Furthermore, the paucity of high-energy phosphates such as adenosine triphosphate (ATP) interferes with the transmembrane Na^+/K^+ ATPase, with resultant elevation in intracellular $[Na^+]$ and extracellular $[K^+]$. Rising $[Na^+]$ contributes to cellular edema. Membrane leak and rising extracellular K^+ concentration contributes to alterations in the transmembrane electrical potential, predisposing the myocardium to lethal arrhythmias.

Intracellular Ca^{++} accumulates in the damaged myocytes and is thought to contribute to the final common pathway of cell destruction through the activation of degradative lipases and proteases.

Collectively, these metabolic changes decrease myocardial function as early as 2 minutes following occlusive thrombosis. Without intervention, *irreversible* cell injury ensues in 20 minutes and is best marked by the development of membrane defects. As proteolytic enzymes leak across the myocyte's altered membrane, they damage adjacent myocardium, and the release of specific macromolecules into the circulation serves as a clinical marker of acute infarction.

Edema of the myocardium develops within 4–12 hours, as vascular permeability increases and interstitial oncotic pressure rises (because of the leak of intracellular proteins). The earliest histologic changes of irreversible injury are **wavy myofibers,** which appear as intercellular edema separates the myocardial cells that are tugged about by the surrounding, functional myocardium (Fig. 7.6). **Contraction bands** can often be seen near the borders of the infarct: sarcomeres are contracted and consolidated and appear as bright eosinophilic belts.

An acute inflammatory response, with infiltration of neutrophils, begins after approximately 4 hours and incites further tissue damage. Within 18–24 hours, **coagulation necrosis** is evident with pyknotic nuclei and bland eosinophilic cytoplasm, seen by light microscopy. These early changes are demonstrated in Figure 7.6 and summarized in Table 7.2.

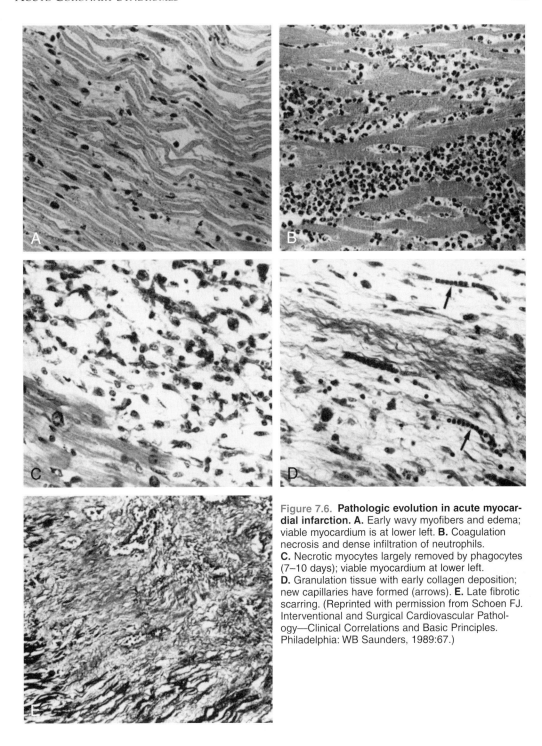

Figure 7.6. **Pathologic evolution in acute myocardial infarction. A.** Early wavy myofibers and edema; viable myocardium is at lower left. **B.** Coagulation necrosis and dense infiltration of neutrophils. **C.** Necrotic myocytes largely removed by phagocytes (7–10 days); viable myocardium at lower left. **D.** Granulation tissue with early collagen deposition; new capillaries have formed (arrows). **E.** Late fibrotic scarring. (Reprinted with permission from Schoen FJ. Interventional and Surgical Cardiovascular Pathology—Clinical Correlations and Basic Principles. Philadelphia: WB Saunders, 1989:67.)

Gross Changes

Gross morphologic changes do not appear until 18–24 hours after coronary occlusion, although certain staining techniques (e.g., tetrazolium) permit the pathologist to identify regions of infarction earlier. Most often, ischemia and infarction begin in the subendocardium and then extend laterally and outward toward the epicardium.

Late Changes

Late pathologic changes in the course of acute MI (see Table 7.2) include 1) the clearing of necrotic myocardium by macrophages, and 2) the deposition of collagen to form scar tissue.

Irreversibly injured myocytes do not regenerate; rather, the cells are removed and replaced by fibrous tissue. Macrophages invade the inflamed myocardium shortly after neutrophil infiltration and remove necrotic tissue. This period of tissue resorption is termed **yellow-softening,** as connective tissue elements are destroyed and removed along with dead myocardial cells. This phagocytic clearing, combined with thinning and dilation of the infarcted zone, results in structural weakness of the ventricular wall and the possibility of myocardial wall rupture at this stage. **Fibrosis** subsequently ensues, and scarring is complete by 7 weeks after infarction (see Fig. 7.6).

Functional Changes

Impaired Contractility and Compliance

Infarction quickly leads to impaired contractile function of the ventricle (**systolic dysfunction**). Ventricular output is further compromised because *synchronous* contraction of myocytes is lost. When infarction results in an area of decreased contractility, that region is termed "hypokinetic"; segments that do not contract at all are called "akinetic"; and "dyskinetic" regions are those that bulge outward during systolic ventricular contraction.

During infarction, the left ventricle is also adversely compromised by **diastolic dysfunction.** Ischemia and/or infarction impair diastolic relaxation (an energy-dependent process as described in Chapter 1), which reduces ventricular compliance and contributes to elevated ventricular filling pressures.

Stunned Myocardium

Sometimes transient myocardial ischemia can result in a very prolonged but gradually reversible period of contractile

TABLE 7.2. Pathologic Time Line in Transmural Infarction

Time	Event
Early changes	
1–2 min	ATP levels fall; cessation of contractility
10 min	50% depletion of ATP; cellular edema, decreased membrane potential and susceptibility to arrhythmias
20–24 min	Irreversible cell injury
1–3 hours	Wavy myofibers
4–12 hours	Hemorrhage, edema, PMN infiltration begins
18–24 hours	Coagulation necrosis (pyknotic nuclei with eosinophilic cytoplasm), edema
2–4 days	Total coagulation necrosis (no nuclei or striations, rimmed by hyperemic tissue); monocytes appear; PMN infiltration peaks
Late Changes	
5–7 days	Yellow-softening from resorption of dead tissue by macrophages
7+ days	Ventricular remodeling
7 weeks	Fibrosis and scarring complete

ATP, adenosine triphosphate; *PMN*, polymorphonuclear leukocyte.

dysfunction. For example, as discussed in Chapter 6, **stunned myocardium** refers to tissue that demonstrates prolonged systolic dysfunction after a discrete episode of severe ischemia, despite restoration of adequate blood flow, that *gradually* regains contractile force later. Stunning may play an important role in patients with UA or in myocardium adjacent to the region of an acute MI. In both instances, prolonged contractile dysfunction of affected ventricular segments may be evident after the event, simulating infarcted tissue, despite restoration of coronary blood flow (spontaneously or via mechanical revascularization). However, if the tissue is simply stunned rather than necrotic, its function will recover over time.

Ischemic Preconditioning

Brief ischemic insults to a region of myocardium may render that tissue more resistant to subsequent episodes of ischemia, a phenomenon termed **ischemic precondi-**

tioning. The clinical relevance is that patients who sustain an MI in the context of recent angina experience less morbidity and mortality than those without preceding anginal episodes. The mechanism of this phenomenon is unknown but appears to involve ischemia-related activation of adenosine receptors.

Ventricular Remodeling

Following an MI, changes occur in the geometry of both the infarcted and noninfarcted ventricular muscle. Such alterations in chamber size and wall thickness affect long-term ventricular function and prognosis.

In the early post-MI period, infarct *expansion* may occur, in which the affected ventricular segment enlarges without additional myocyte necrosis. Infarct expansion represents thinning and dilatation of the necrotic zone of tissue, likely because of "slippage" between the muscle fibers, resulting in a decreased volume of myocytes in the region of the infarct. Infarct expansion can be detrimental because it increases ventricular size, which 1) augments wall stress, 2) impairs systolic contractile function, and 3) increases the likelihood of aneurysm formation.

In addition to early expansion of the infarcted territory, remodeling of the ventricle may also involve dilatation of the overworked *noninfarcted* segments, which are subjected to increased wall stress. This dilatation begins in the early post-infarct period and continues over the ensuing weeks and months. Initially, chamber dilatation serves a compensatory role since it increases cardiac output via the Frank-Starling mechanism (see Chapter 9), but progressive enlargement may ultimately lead to heart failure and also predisposes to ventricular arrhythmias.

Adverse ventricular remodeling can be beneficially modified by certain interventions. At the time of infarction, for example, reperfusion therapies limit infarct size and therefore decrease the likelihood of infarct expansion. In addition, the use of angiotensin-converting enzyme inhibitors has been shown to attenuate progressive remodeling and also reduces short- and long-term post-MI mortality (see below).

CLINICAL FEATURES OF ACUTE CORONARY SYNDROMES

Since ACS represent disorders along a continuum, there is overlap in their clinical features. In general, the severity of symptoms and associated laboratory findings progress from UA on one side of the continuum, through NSTEMI, to STEMI on the other end of the continuum (see Fig. 7.1). The distinction between these syndromes is made on the basis of the clinical presentation, the electrocardiographic findings, and serum biomarkers of myocardial damage. To institute appropriate immediate therapy, the most important distinction to make is between ACS that causes ST segment elevation on the ECG (STEMI) from those acute syndromes that do not (UA and NSTEMI).

Historically, MIs have been classified as "Q-wave" or "non–Q-wave" infarctions. Dogma held that transmural infarcts produce Q waves (after initial ST elevation) on the ECG, whereas subendocardial infarcts generate ST depressions without Q wave development. However, it is now known that these ECG findings do not reliably correlate with the pathologic findings and that there is much overlap between these types of infarction. Moreover, the use of Q waves to classify ACS is now less clinically important, because Q waves, unlike ST changes, may take hours or longer to develop and cannot be used to make early therapeutic decisions. Thus, for the remainder of this chapter, the terms STEMI and NSTEMI will be used instead of Q-wave and non–Q-wave MI, respectively.

Clinical Presentation

Unstable Angina

UA presents as an acceleration of ischemic symptoms in one of three ways: 1) a crescendo pattern in which a patient with chronic, stable angina experiences a sudden increase in the frequency, duration, and/or intensity of ischemic episodes; 2) angina that occurs at rest, without provocation; or 3) the new onset of angina, described as severe, in a patient without previous symptoms of coronary artery disease. Patients with UA may progress further along the continuum of ACS and develop evidence of necrosis (i.e., an acute MI) unless the condition is recognized and promptly treated.

Acute Myocardial Infarction

The symptoms and physical findings of acute MI (both STEMI and NSTEMI) can be predicted from the pathophysiology described earlier in this chapter and are summarized in Table 7.3. The pain experienced during an MI resembles anginal discomfort qualitatively but is usually more severe, lasts longer, and may radiate more widely. Like angina, the pain may result from the release of mediators such as adenosine and lactate from ischemic myocardial cells onto local nerve endings. Because ischemia in acute MI persists and proceeds to necrosis, these provocative substances continue to accumulate and activate afferent nerves for longer periods. The pain of infarction is often referred to other regions of the C7–T4 dermatomes, including the neck, shoulders, and arms. The pain of MI is rapid in onset and often briskly crescendos to leave its victims discomfited with profound "feelings of doom." Unlike a transient attack of angina, the pain does not wane with rest,

and there may be little response to the administration of sublingual nitroglycerin.

Although the chest discomfort in acute MI may be severe, that is not always the case. In fact, up to 25% of patients who sustain an MI are *asymptomatic* during the acute event, and the diagnosis is made only in retrospect. This is particularly common among diabetic patients who may not experience pain because of peripheral neuropathy. In addition, occasional patients who present with MI complicated by acute pericarditis may feel more of a sharp, pleuritic-type pain (see Chapter 14), rather than the typical MI symptoms.

The combination of pain and baroreceptor unloading (if hypotension is present) may trigger a dramatic sympathetic nervous system response. Systemic signs of catecholamine release include diaphoresis (sweating), tachycardia, and cool and clammy skin due to vasoconstriction.

As reduced LV contractility (systolic dysfunction) decreases the stroke volume, the diastolic volume and pressure within that chamber rise. The increase in LV pressure, compounded by the ischemia-induced stiffness of the chamber (*diastolic* dysfunction), is conveyed to the left atrium and pulmonary veins. The resultant pulmonary congestion decreases lung compliance and stimulates juxtacapillary receptors. These "J receptors" effect a reflex that results in rapid, shallow breathing and evokes the subjective feeling of dyspnea. Transudation

---

TABLE 7.3. Signs and Symptoms of Myocardial Infarction

1. Characteristic pain	
2. Sympathetic effect	• Diaphoresis • Cool and clammy skin
3. Parasympathetic (vagal effect)	• Nausea, vomiting • Weakness
4. Inflammatory response	• Mild fever
5. Cardiac findings	• S_4 (and S_3 if CHF present) gallop • Dyskinetic bulge (in anterior wall MI) • Pericardial friction rub (if pericarditis present) • Systolic murmur (if mitral regurgitation or VSD)
6. Other	• Pulmonary rales (if CHF present) • Jugular venous distention (if right ventricular MI)

CHF, congestive heart failure; *MI*, myocardial infarction; *VSD*, ventricular septal defect.

of fluid into the alveoli exacerbates this symptom.

Physical findings can be apparent on auscultation during an acute MI but depend on the location and extent of the infarct. The S_4 sound, indicative of atrial contraction into a noncompliant left ventricle, is frequently present. An S_3 sound is heard in the presence of failing LV systolic function. Pericardial friction rubs may be present over the heart if inflammation has extended to the pericardium. Finally, systolic murmurs appear when papillary muscle dysfunction or infarction causes mitral valvular insufficiency or when infarcts rupture through the interventricular septum to create a ventricular septal defect.

Myocardial necrosis also activates systemic responses to inflammation. Cytokines such as interleukin-1 and tumor necrosis factor are released from macrophages and vascular endothelium in response to tissue injury. These mediators evoke an array of clinical responses including low-grade fever and leukocytosis.

Not all patients with severe chest pain are in the midst of MI or UA. Table 7.4 lists other conditions that cause acute chest pain and features to differentiate them from an acute coronary syndrome.

Diagnosis of Acute Coronary Syndromes

The diagnosis of, and distinction between, ACS is made on the basis of 1) the patient's presenting symptoms, 2) typical acute ECG abnormalities, and 3) detection or absence of specific serum markers of myocardial necrosis (see Fig. 7.4 and Table 7.5). Specifically, UA is a clinical diagnosis that is supported by the patient's symptoms, transient ST abnormalities on the ECG (usually ST depres-

TABLE 7.4. Conditions That may be Confused With Acute Coronary Syndromes

Condition	Differentiating Features
Cardiac	
Acute coronary syndrome	• Retrosternal pressure, radiating to neck, jaw, or left shoulder and arm; more severe and lasts longer than previous anginal attacks • ECG: localized ST elevations or depressions
Pericarditis	• Sharp pleuritic pain (worsens with inspiration) • Pain varies with position (relieved by sitting) • Friction rub auscultated over precordium • ECG: diffuse ST elevations (see Chapter 14)
Aortic dissection	• Tearing, ripping pain that migrates over time (chest and back) • Asymmetry of arm blood pressures • Widened mediastinum on chest radiograph
Pulmonary	
Pulmonary embolism	• Localized pleuritic pain, accompanied by dyspnea • Pleural friction rub may be present • Predisposing conditions for venous thrombosis
Pneumonia	• Pleuritic chest pain • Cough and sputum production • Abnormal lung auscultation and percussion (i.e., consolidation) • Infiltrate on chest radiograph
Pneumothorax	• Sudden sharp, pleuritic unilateral chest pain • Decreased breath sounds and hyperresonance of affected side • Chest radiograph: increased lucency and absence of pulmonary markings
Gastrointestinal	
Esophageal spasm	• Retrosternal pain, worsened by swallowing • History of dysphagia
Acute cholecystitis	• Right upper quadrant abdominal tenderness • Often accompanied by nausea • History of fatty food intolerance

TABLE 7.5. Distinguishing Features of Acute Coronary Syndromes

	Unstable Angina	Myocardial Infarction	
		NSTEMI	STEMI
Typical symptoms	Crescendo, rest, or new onset severe angina	Prolonged "crushing" chest pain, more severe and wider radiation than usual angina	
Serum biomarkers	No	Yes	Yes
ECG initial findings	ST depression and/or T wave inversion	ST depression and/ or T wave inversion	ST elevation (and Q waves later)

NSTEMI, non-ST-elevation myocardial infarction (MI); *STEMI*, ST-elevation MI.

sion and/or T wave inversion), and the absence of serum biomarkers of myocardial necrosis. Non-ST-segment elevation MI is distinguished from UA by the detection of serum markers of necrosis and often more persistent ST-T wave abnormalities. The hallmark of ST-segment elevation MI is an appropriate clinical history coupled with ST-segment elevations on the presenting ECG plus serum markers of myocardial necrosis.

ECG Abnormalities

ECG abnormalities, which reflect abnormal electrical currents during ACS, are usually manifest in characteristic ways. In UA or NSTEMI, ST segment depression and/or T wave inversions are most common (Fig. 7.7). These abnormalities may be transient, occurring just during chest pain episodes in UA, or they may be more persistent in many patients with NSTEMI. In distinction, as described in Chapter 4, STEMI presents with a temporal sequence of abnormalities: initial ST segment elevation, followed over the next day by inversion of the T wave and Q wave development (Fig. 7.8). Note that these characteristic patterns of ECG abnormalities in ACS can often be minimized or aborted by early therapeutic interventions.

Serum Markers of Infarction

Necrosis of myocardial tissue causes disruption of the sarcolemma, so that intracellular macromolecules leak into the cardiac

Unstable Angina/Non-ST-elevation Myocardial Infarction

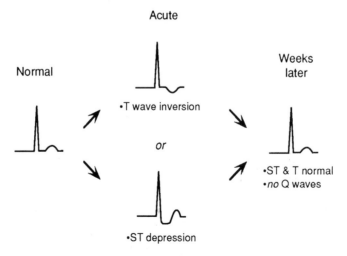

Figure 7.7. ECG abnormalities in unstable angina and non-ST-elevation myocardial infarction.

ST-Elevation Myocardial Infarction

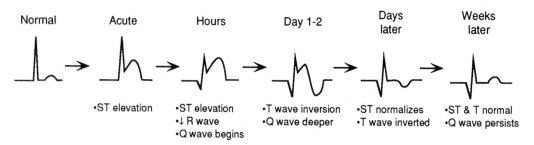

Figure 7.8. **ECG evolution during ST-elevation myocardial infarction.**

interstitium and ultimately into the bloodstream (Fig. 7.9). Detection of such molecules in the serum, particularly cardiac-specific troponins and creatine kinase-MB isoenzyme, serves important diagnostic and prognostic roles. In patients with STEMI or NSTEMI, these markers rise above a threshold level in a specific temporal sequence.

Cardiac-Specific Troponins

Troponin (Tn) is a regulatory protein in muscle cells that controls interactions between myosin and actin (see Chapter 1). It consists of three subunits, TnC, TnI and TnT. Although these subunits are found both in skeletal and cardiac muscle, the genes encoding for cardiac troponin I (cTnI) and troponin T (cTnT) are unique, and highly specific assays for their detection in the serum have been developed. Because serum levels of these components are virtually absent in healthy persons, the presence of even minor elevations of cTnI or cTnT serves as a sensitive and powerful marker of myocyte damage.

Cardiac troponins begin to rise 3–4 hours following an MI, peak between 18 and 36

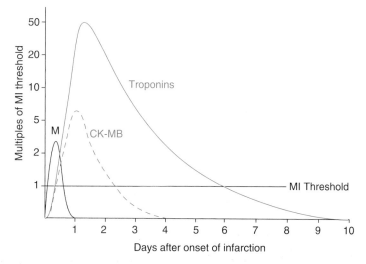

Figure 7.9. **Evolution of serum biomarkers in acute myocardial infarction (MI).** Curve "M" indicates the detection of myoglobin in the serum before other biomarkers. Serum CK (or **CK-MB** isoenzyme) begins to rise 3–8 hours after the onset of the acute infarct and peaks at 24 hours. Cardiac **troponins** are highly sensitive for myocardial injury and remain detectable in the serum for many days after the acute infarct. (Modified from Wu AH, Apple FS, Gibler WB, et al. National Academy of Clinical Biochemistry Standards of Laboratory Practice: Recommendations for the use of cardiac markers in coronary artery diseases. Clin Chem 1999;45:1104–1121.)

hours, then slowly decline, but persist for up to 10–14 days. Thus, they may be helpful for detection of MI for nearly 2 weeks after the event occurs. Given their high sensitivity and specificity, cardiac troponins are now the preferred serum biomarkers to detect myocardial necrosis.

Creatine Kinase

The enzyme creatine kinase (CK) reversibly transfers a phosphate group from creatine phosphate, the endogenous storage form of high-energy phosphate bonds, to ADP, producing ATP. Because creatine kinase is found in heart, skeletal muscle, brain, and many other organs, serum concentrations of this enzyme may become elevated following injury to any of these tissues.

There are, however, three *isoenzymes* of CK that improve diagnostic specificity for a myocardial source: CK-MM (found mainly in skeletal muscle), CK-BB (located predominantly in the brain), and **CK-MB** (localized mainly in the heart). Small amounts of CK-MB are found in other tissues, including the uterus, prostate, gut, diaphragm, and tongue. In the absence of trauma to these other organs, elevation of CK-MB is highly suggestive of myocardial injury. Since CK-MB makes up 1–3% of the CK in skeletal muscle, muscle trauma or intramuscular injections could also cause the appearance of this isoenzyme in the circulation. Therefore, to facilitate the diagnosis of MI, it is common to calculate the ratio of CK-MB/total CK. When using the sensitive monoclonal ("mass") assay for CK-MB, this ratio is usually >2.5% in the setting of myocardial injury and less than that when due to pure skeletal muscle injury.

The serum level of CK-MB starts to rise 3–8 hours following infarction, peaks at 24 hours, and returns to normal within 48–72 hours (see Fig. 7.9). This temporal sequence is important because other potential sources of CK-MB (e.g., skeletal muscle injury), or other non-MI cardiac conditions that raise serum levels of the isoenzyme

(e.g., myocarditis), do not usually show this delayed peaking pattern. Reperfusion procedures (such as thrombolytic therapy) during an MI result in a washout effect with an *earlier* than usual peak of the CK and CK-MB serum levels, as described below.

The detection of cardiac troponins in the serum is a much more sensitive marker for myocardial necrosis than CK-MB. As a result, many patients with ACS are found to have small elevations of cardiac troponins but "negative" CK-MB test results. Before the advent of troponin assays, such occurrences would have been labeled as UA (because of the absence of the CK-MB biomarker), but are now more accurately classified as "microinfarctions."

Since troponin and CK-MB levels do not become elevated in the serum until at least a few hours after the onset of MI symptoms, a single normal value drawn early in the course of treatment (e.g., in the hospital emergency department) does not rule out an acute MI; thus, their diagnostic utility is limited in that critical period. Consequently, other serum markers have been evaluated for earlier diagnosis of infarction. For example, **myoglobin**, a heme protein, is released into the circulation after myocardial injury and can be detected in the serum 1–4 hours after the onset of an MI, earlier than elevations of serum CK-MB or troponins. However, the rapid renal clearance of this molecule and its low specificity for myocardial damage limit its diagnostic value.

Another serum marker that may be encountered in the context of acute MI is **lactate dehydrogenase (LDH).** This enzyme catalyzes the reversible formation of lactate from pyruvate and is a nonspecific marker for myocardial necrosis that exhibits peak serum levels 3–5 days after an MI.

Sometimes the diagnosis of MI can remain uncertain even after careful evaluation of the patient's history, ECG, and serum biomarkers. In such a situation, an additional diagnostic study that may be useful is *echocardiography,* which typically reveals abnormalities of ventricular contraction in the region of ischemia or infarction.

TREATMENT OF ACUTE CORONARY SYNDROMES

The appropriate management of ACS requires rapid initiation of therapy to limit myocardial damage and minimize complications. Therapy must address the intracoronary thrombus that incited the syndrome and provide anti-ischemic measures to restore the balance between myocardial oxygen supply and demand. Although certain therapeutic aspects are common to all ACS, there is a critical difference in the approach to patients who present with ST-segment elevation (i.e., STEMI) compared with those without ST elevation (i.e., UA and NSTEMI). Patients with the former benefit from immediate aggressive thrombolytic medications, and the latter do not (Fig. 7.10 and as discussed below).

General in-hospital measures for patients with ACS include admitting the patient to an intensive care setting where continuous ECG monitoring for arrhythmias is undertaken. The patient is initially maintained at **bedrest** to minimize myocardial oxygen demand, while supplemental **oxygen** is administered (by face mask or nasal canula), if there is any degree of hypoxemia, to improve oxygen supply. Analgesics, such as **morphine,** are administered to reduce chest pain and anxiety, to further reduce myocardial oxygen needs.

Acute Treatment of Unstable Angina/Non-ST-Elevation MI

The management of UA and NSTEMI is essentially the same and therefore discussed together as one entity, whereas the unique approach to STEMI is discussed later. The primary focus of treatment for UA and NSTEMI consists of *antithrombotic* therapy aimed at stabilizing the underlying coronary thrombus and *anti-ischemic* medications to improve the balance between myocardial oxygen supply and demand.

Antithrombotic Therapy

The purpose of antithrombotic therapy, including anti-platelet and anticoagulant medications, is to prevent further propagation of the partially occlusive intracoronary thrombus while facilitating its dissolution by endogenous mechanisms. **Aspirin** inhibits platelet synthesis of thromboxane A_2, a potent mediator of platelet activation, and is one of the most important interventions to reduce mortality in patients with all forms of ACS. It should be administered immediately on presentation and continued indefinitely in patients without con-

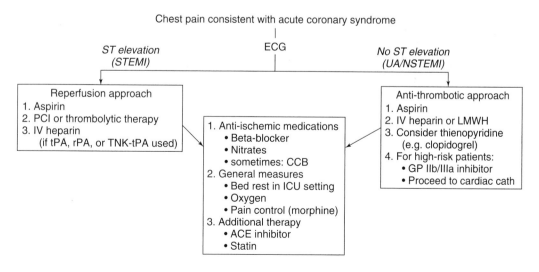

Chest pain consistent with acute coronary syndrome

ECG

ST elevation (STEMI)

No ST elevation (UA/NSTEMI)

Reperfusion approach
1. Aspirin
2. PCI or thrombolytic therapy
3. IV heparin
   (if tPA, rPA, or TNK-tPA used)

1. Anti-ischemic medications
   • Beta-blocker
   • Nitrates
   • sometimes: CCB
2. General measures
   • Bed rest in ICU setting
   • Oxygen
   • Pain control (morphine)
3. Additional therapy
   • ACE inhibitor
   • Statin

Anti-thrombotic approach
1. Aspirin
2. IV heparin or LMWH
3. Consider thienopyridine
   (e.g. clopidogrel)
4. For high-risk patients:
   • GP IIb/IIIa inhibitor
   • Proceed to cardiac cath

Figure 7.10. Management strategies in acute coronary syndromes. PCI, percutaneous coronary intervention. LMWH, low molecular weight heparin.

traindications to its use (e.g., allergy or underlying bleeding disorder).

Because aspirin blocks only one pathway of platelet activation and aggregation (as reviewed in Chapter 17), other antiplatelet agents have also been studied. The **thienopyridines** (e.g., ticlopidine and clopidogrel) inhibit ADP-mediated activation of platelets. A recent study of patients with UA/NSTEMI showed that the combination of aspirin plus clopidogrel was superior to aspirin alone in reducing cardiovascular mortality, and ongoing trials will help determine which subgroups of patients are most likely to benefit from that combination. A thienopyridine is also often used as a *substitute* for aspirin in patients who are allergic to aspirin.

Intravenous unfractionated heparin (UFH), an anticoagulant, is also standard therapy for UA/NSTEMI. It binds to ATIII, which greatly increases the potency of ATIII to inactivate clot-forming thrombin. UFH additionally inhibits coagulation factor Xa, slowing thrombin formation and thereby further impeding clot development. In patients with UA or NSTEMI, UFH improves cardiovascular outcomes and reduces the likelihood of progression from UA to MI. It is administered as a weight-based bolus, followed by continuous infusion, with adjustment in its dosage determined by frequent measurements of the serum activated partial thromboplastin time (aPTT). More recently, **low molecular weight heparins** (LMWH) have been developed, which are equally effective or superior to UFH in improving outcomes of patients with UA/NSTEMI. Like UFH, LMWH also interact with ATIII, but preferentially inhibit coagulation factor Xa. The pharmacologic properties of LMWH confer important advantages over UFH, including greater efficacy as an anticoagulant and more predictable bioavailability. As a result, LMWH therapy is easier to use, prescribed as one to two daily subcutaneous injections based on the patient's weight. Unlike UFH, repeated monitoring of blood tests and dosage adjustment are not necessary. Other advantages of LMWH are discussed in Chapter 17.

The **glycoprotein (GP) IIb/IIIa receptor antagonists** are another type of antithrombotic drug that have been shown to reduce mortality rates in high-risk patients with UA/NSTEMI (e.g., patients with ST segment deviations on ECG at time of presentation, the presence of serum biomarkers of myocardial necrosis, individuals with recurrent episodes of chest pain or for whom urgent cardiac catheterization is planned). These drugs (which include eptifibatide, tirofiban, and abciximab) are potent antiplatelet agents that block the final common pathway of platelet aggregation and are discussed further in Chapter 17.

Anti-Ischemic Therapy

The same pharmacologic agents used to decrease myocardial oxygen demand in chronic stable angina are used in UA/NSTEMI but are often administered more aggressively. **Nitrates** help bring about anginal relief through venodilatation, which lowers myocardial oxygen demand by diminishing venous return to the heart (reduced preload and therefore less wall stress). Nitrates may also improve coronary flow and prevent vasospasm through coronary vasodilatation. In UA/NSTEMI, nitroglycerin is often initially administered by the sublingual route, followed by a continuous intravenous infusion. In addition to providing symptomatic relief of angina, intravenous nitroglycerin is useful as a vasodilator in patients with ACS accompanied by heart failure or severe hypertension.

β-Blockers decrease sympathetic drive to the myocardium, thus reducing oxygen demand, and contribute to electrical stability. This group of drugs reduces the likelihood of progression from UA to MI and reduces mortality rates in patients who present with MI. In the absence of contraindications (e.g., significant bradycardia, bronchospasm, uncontrolled heart failure, or hypotension), a β-blocker is initially administered intravenously to achieve a heart rate of <70 bpm and then converted to an oral regimen. Such therapy is usually continued indefinitely after hospitalization because of proven long-term mortality benefits following an MI.

Non-dihydropyridine calcium channel antagonists (i.e., verapamil and diltiazem) exert anti-ischemic effects by decreasing heart rate and contractility and also through their vasodilatory properties (see Chapter 6). These agents do *not* confer mortality benefit to patients with ACS and are reserved for those in whom ischemia persists despite β-blocker and nitrate therapy, or for those with contraindications to β-blocker use. They should *not* be prescribed to patients with left ventricular (LV) systolic dysfunction, as clinical trials have shown adverse outcomes in such individuals.

Conservative Versus Early Invasive Management of UA/NSTEMI

The aggressiveness of therapy in UA/NSTEMI may be approached in two manners: 1) an "early invasive" approach, in which urgent cardiac catheterization is performed and coronary revascularization undertaken as needed, or 2) a "conservative" approach, in which patients are managed with medications (as detailed in the above section) and undergo angiography only if ischemic episodes recur, or if the results of a subsequent stress test indicate the need. A conservative approach offers the advantage of avoiding costly and potentially risky invasive procedures. On the other hand, an early invasive strategy allows rapid identification and definitive treatment (i.e., revascularization) of patients with critical coronary disease.

Although early randomized trials comparing these two approaches suggested that both strategies lead to comparable outcomes, more recent data (in the era of coronary stents and platelet GP IIb/IIIa inhibitors) indicate that an early invasive approach leads to improved outcomes and reduced mortality rates. An early invasive approach is most beneficial in patients with high-risk features, such as those with ST-segment deviations at the time of presentation, elevated serum biomarkers, and those with multiple cardiac risk factors.

Acute Treatment of ST-Elevation MI

The focus of treatment in STEMI is to quickly salvage jeopardized myocardium by restoring blood flow through the occluded coronary artery. One of the major medical advances of the later 20th century was the development of reperfusion therapies, namely thrombolytic drugs and percutaneous coronary interventions, to restore such flow, which in turn reduces the extent of myocardial necrosis and greatly improves survival. To be effective, these interventions must be undertaken as soon as feasible—the earlier the intervention occurs, the more myocardium can be salvaged. Decisions about therapy must be made within minutes of a patient's evaluation, based on the history and electrocardiographic findings, often before serum markers of necrosis would be expected to rise.

Thrombolytic Therapy

The goal of thrombolytic drugs is to accelerate lysis of the intracoronary thrombus to restore blood flow and limit myocardial damage. Be aware that this discussion does not pertain to patients with UA or non-ST-elevation MI—such individuals *do not* benefit from, and can be harmed by, thrombolytic therapy.

Currently used thrombolytic agents (more accurately termed *fibrinolytic* agents) include streptokinase, recombinant tissue-type plasminogen activator (alteplase, tPA), reteplase (rPA), and tenecteplase (TNK-tPA). Each of these agents functions by stimulating the natural fibrinolytic system: they transform the inactive precursor plasminogen into the active protease plasmin, which lyses fibrin clots (Fig. 7.11). Although the intracoronary thrombus responsible for the STEMI is the target, plasmin has poor substrate specificity and can degrade other proteins, including fibrinogen. As a result, bleeding is the most common complication of thrombolytic drugs. However, unlike the older thrombolytic streptokinase, newer agents (e.g., tPA, rPA, and TNK-tPA) bind preferentially to fibrin in a formed throm-

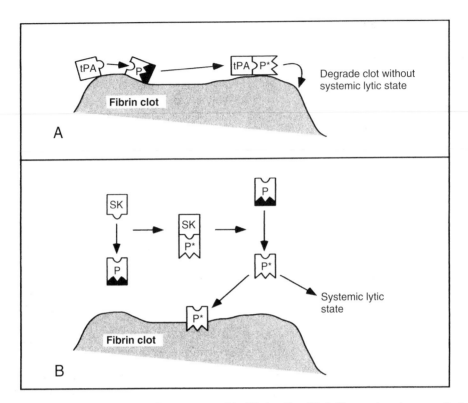

Figure 7.11. **Examples of thrombolytic agents used in ST-elevation MI. A.** Tissue plasminogen activator (tPA) cleaves fibrin-bound plasminogen (P) to form active plasmin (P*), which degrades the fibrin clot. The selectivity of tPA for fibrin-bound P results in localized thrombolysis and minimizes generalized systemic fibrinolysis. **B.** Streptokinase (SK) combines with fibrin-bound and circulating plasminogen to form an active complex, which in turn activates additional plasminogen molecules. The lack of selectivity for fibrin-bound plasminogen results in more of a systemic lytic state. TNK-tPA and rPA (see text) act similarly to tPA but can be administered as boluses, thus simplifying drug administration.

bus (i.e., the intracoronary clot), thereby generating plasmin locally at that site, with less interference of fibrinogen in the general circulation. Nonetheless, bleeding remains the most important risk with all thrombolytic agents. Since rPA and TNK-tPA are mutants of tPA with longer half-lives, their major advantage is that they can be administered as boluses, which is more convenient and less prone to incorrect administration than the continuous intravenous infusions necessary for tPA and streptokinase.

Administration of thrombolytic agents in the early hours of an acute STEMI restores blood flow in the majority (70–80%) of coronary occlusions and significantly reduces the extent of tissue damage. Improved artery patency translates into substantially improved survival rates and fewer post-infarction complications. The rapid initiation of

thrombolytic therapy is crucial: patients who receive therapy within 2 hours of the onset of symptoms of STEMI have *half* the mortality rate of those who receive it after 6 hours of symptoms.

Successful reperfusion is marked by the relief of chest pain, return of the ST segments to baseline, and earlier-than-usual peaking of serum markers of necrosis, such as CK-MB and cardiac-specific troponins. During this phase, transient reperfusion arrhythmias are common and do not usually require treatment. To prevent immediate vessel reocclusion after successful thrombolysis, antithrombotic regimens are administered as described below.

Since the major risk of thrombolysis is bleeding, contraindications to such therapy include situations in which *necessary* fibrin clots within the circulation would be jeopardized (e.g., patients with active peptic ulcer disease or an underlying bleeding disorder, patients who have had a recent stroke or who are recovering from recent surgery). Consequently, approximately 30% of individuals may not be suitable candidates for thrombolysis.

Several large-scale comparisons of thrombolytic agents have been conducted. In 1993, the international GUSTO-1 trial found a small post-infarction survival advantage of t-PA compared with streptokinase, at the expense of a slightly increased risk of intracranial hemorrhage with tPA. More recent trials have compared tPA with the newer agents rPA and TNK-tPA and have found similar clinical efficacies of these three agents. The most important message from these trials is that early and sustained patency of the infarct-related coronary artery improves survival. No matter which thrombolytic is selected, it must be administered as soon as possible, ideally within 30 minutes of the patient's presentation to the hospital.

Primary Percutaneous Coronary Intervention

An alternative to thrombolytic therapy in acute MI is immediate cardiac catheterization and percutaneous coronary intervention (PCI) of the lesion responsible for the infarction (termed "primary PCI"). It is a particularly attractive option for patients with contraindications to thrombolytic drugs and offers the advantage of superior rates of coronary reperfusion. In clinical trials performed at highly experienced medical centers, primary PCI achieved optimal flow in the infarct-related artery in more than 95% of patients. When compared with thrombolytic therapy, primary PCI led to greater survival with a lower risk of serious bleeding complications. However, primary PCI is limited to centers that are very experienced in coronary angioplasty and are equipped to perform it on an emergency basis. Since the majority of hospitals in the United States do not meet those criteria, the administration of thrombolytic therapy remains the widespread standard.

Antithrombotic and Anti-Ischemic Medications in STEMI

Several additional therapies, many of which were described above for UA/NSTEMI, are also beneficial to patients with STEMI. These include antithrombotic drugs and other agents to 1) maintain patency of the coronary vessel in patients who receive thrombolysis, 2) restore balance between myocardial oxygen supply and demand, 3) relieve chest pain, and 4) prevent complications related to infarcted myocardium.

Antiplatelet therapy with **aspirin** decreases mortality rates and rates of reinfarction after STEMI. It should be administered immediately on presentation and continued daily thereafter. For aspirin-allergic patients, the thienopyridine clopidogrel is often substituted. The potent platelet GP IIb/IIIa antagonists are being tested in combination with thrombolytic agents in patients with STEMI, but as of this writing, mortality benefits have not been shown compared to thrombolytic therapy alone.

Intravenous unfractionated **heparin** is typically administered for 1–2 days to maintain patency of the coronary vessel after thrombolysis with tPA, rPA, or TNK-tPA (but is not required for the non–fibrin-specific agent streptokinase). Heparin should also be administered to prevent thromboembolism in MI patients with atrial fibrillation, LV thrombus, or a new anterior MI with a large wall motion abnormality (in which thrombus can form). All other patients can receive low-dose subcutaneous heparin while maintaining bedrest to prevent deep venous thrombosis in the lower extremities.

As is the case in UA/NSTEMI, several other therapies are beneficial in the management of STEMI. β-**Blockers** reduce myocardial oxygen demand and lower the risk of recurrent ischemia, arrhythmias, and reinfarction. In the absence of contraindications (e.g., asthma, hypotension, or significant bradycardia), a β-blocker should be administered, usually intravenously at first and then orally.

Nitrate therapy, usually intravenous nitroglycerin, is administered to help control ischemic pain and can also serve as a beneficial vasodilator in patients with heart failure or severe hypertension during acute infarction.

Adjunctive Therapies for both NSTEMI and STEMI

Angiotensin-converting enzyme (ACE) inhibitors limit adverse ventricular remodeling and reduce the incidence of heart failure, recurrent ischemic events, and mortality following an MI. Their benefit is additive to that of aspirin and β-blocker therapies, and they have shown the most favorable improvements in higher-risk patients—those with anterior wall infarctions or LV systolic dysfunction. As discussed in Chapter 6, ACE inhibition also reduces mortality rates in patients with chronic stable coronary artery disease. Thus, oral ACE inhibitors are frequently prescribed after an ACS and continued indefinitely.

Cholesterol-lowering **statins** (HMG CoA reductase inhibitors) reduce mortality rates of patients with coronary artery disease (see Chapter 5). Such therapy has typically been initiated sometime after hospitalization for patients with ACS. However, recent clinical trials have demonstrated that it is safe to begin statin therapy early during the course of an ACS and that doing so improves cardiac outcomes following hospitalization. The benefits of statin therapy may extend beyond lipid-lowering, as this group of drugs has attributes that can potentially improve endothelial dysfunction, inhibit platelet aggregation, and impair thrombus formation. Thus, the expanding trend is to start statin therapy early in the course of patients hospitalized for an acute coronary syndrome.

COMPLICATIONS

In UA, the potential complications include death (5–10%) or progression to MI (10–20%) over the ensuing days and weeks. Once infarction has transpired, complica-

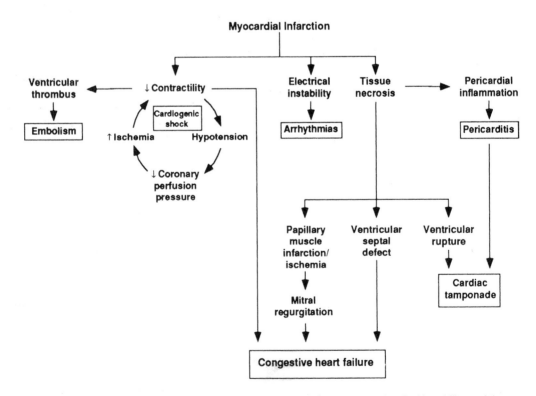

Figure 7.12. **Complications of MI.** Infarction results in decreased contractility, electrical instability, and tissue necrosis, which lead to these potential complications.

tions result from the inflammatory, mechanical, and electrical abnormalities induced by regions of necrosing myocardium (Fig. 7.12). Immediate complications result from myocardial necrosis itself. Those that develop several days to weeks later may be due to the inflammation and healing of necrotic tissue.

Recurrent Ischemia

Post-infarction angina has been reported to occur in 20–30% of patients following an MI. This rate has not been reduced by the use of thrombolytic therapy, but it is lower in those who have undergone percutaneous angioplasty or coronary stent implantation as part of early MI management. Indicative of inadequate residual coronary blood flow, it is a poor omen and correlates with an increased risk for reinfarction. Such patients usually require urgent cardiac catheterization, often followed by revascularization by angioplasty techniques or coronary artery bypass surgery.

Arrhythmias

Arrhythmias are extremely common during acute MI and are a major source of mortality before hospitalization. Modern coronary care units are highly attuned to the detection and treatment of rhythm disturbances, so that once a patient is hospitalized, arrhythmia-associated deaths are uncommon. Mechanisms that contribute to arrhythmogenesis after MI include the following (see Table 7.6):

1. Anatomic interruption of perfusion to structures of the conduction pathway (e.g., sinoatrial node, atrioventricular node, bundle branches); the normal perfusion of pertinent components of the conduction system is shown in Table 7.7.
2. Accumulation of toxic metabolic products (e.g., cellular acidosis) and abnormal transcellular ion concentrations due to membrane leaks.
3. Autonomic stimulation (sympathetic and parasympathetic).

4. Administration of potentially arrhythmogenic drugs (e.g., dopamine).

Ventricular Fibrillation

Ventricular fibrillation (rapid, disorganized electrical activity of the ventricles) is largely responsible for episodes of sudden cardiac death during the course of acute MI. Unfortunately, most fatal episodes oc-

TABLE 7.6. Arrhythmias in Acute Myocardial Infarction

Rhythm	Cause
Sinus bradycardia	• ↑Vagal tone • ↓SA nodal artery perfusion
Sinus tachycardia	• Pain and anxiety • CHF • Volume depletion • Pericarditis • Chronotropic drugs (e.g., dopamine)
APBs, atrial fibrillation	• CHF • Atrial ischemia
VPBs, VT, VF	• Ventricular ischemia • CHF
AV block (1°, 2°, 3°)	• IMI: ↑vagal tone and ↓AV nodal artery flow • AMI: extensive destruction of conduction tissue

SA, sinoatrial; *CHF*, congestive heart failure; *APBs*, atrial premature beats; *VPBs*, ventricular premature beats; *VT*, ventricular tachycardia; *VF*, ventricular fibrillation; *AV*, atrioventricular; *IMI*, inferior myocardial infarction; *AMI*, anterior myocardial infarction.

TABLE 7.7. Blood Supply of the Conduction System

Conduction Pathway	Primary Arterial Supply
SA node	• RCA (70% of patients)
AV node	• RCA (85% of patients)
Bundle of His	• LAD (septal branches)
RBB	• Proximal portion by LAD • Distal portion by RCA
LBB:	
Left anterior fascicle	• LAD
Left posterior fascicle	• LAD and PDA

SA, sinoatrial; *RCA*, right coronary artery; *AV*, atrioventricular; *LAD*, left anterior descending coronary artery; *RBB*, right bundle branch; *LBB*, left bundle branch; *PDA*, posterior descending artery.

cur before the arrival of medical assistance and hospitalization. Episodes of ventricular fibrillation that occur during the first 48 hours of MI are often related to transient electrical instability, and the long-term prognosis of survivors of such events is not affected. However, ventricular fibrillation occurring later than 48 hours after the acute MI usually reflects severe LV dysfunction and is associated with high subsequent mortality rates.

Ventricular ectopic beats, ventricular tachycardia, and ventricular fibrillation during an acute MI arise from either re-entrant circuits or enhanced automaticity of ventricular cells (see Chapter 11). Ventricular ectopy is common but usually not treated unless the abnormal beats become consecutive, multifocal, or frequent. Intravenous lidocaine (a class IB antiarrhythmic drug described in Chapter 17) is effective in preventing ventricular fibrillation in the ischemic setting, but is not indicated in the routine management of acute MI patients because of its potential side effects and because cardiac care unit personnel are proficient at arrhythmia detection and treatment should that complication occur.

Supraventricular Arrhythmias

Supraventricular arrhythmias are also common in acute MI. *Sinus bradycardia* results from either excessive vagal stimulation or sinoatrial nodal ischemia, usually in the setting of an inferior wall MI. *Sinus tachycardia* occurs frequently and may result from many causes, especially pain and anxiety, heart failure, drug administration (e.g., dopamine, nitrates), or intravascular volume depletion. Differentiating between heart failure and volume depletion may require the placement of a transvenous pulmonary artery catheter (described in Chapter 3): The pulmonary capillary wedge pressure is *low* in volume depletion, whereas it is *elevated* in heart failure. Because sinus tachycardia increases myocardial oxygen demand and could exacerbate ischemia, identifying and treating its cause are important. *Atrial premature beats* and

atrial fibrillation (see Chapter 12) may result from atrial ischemia or atrial distention secondary to LV failure.

Conduction Blocks

Conduction blocks (atrioventricular nodal block and bundle branch blocks) develop frequently in acute MI. They may result from ischemia or necrosis of conduction tracts (Table 7.7), or in the case of atrioventricular blocks, may develop transiently because of increased vagal tone. Vagal activity may be increased because of stimulation of afferent fibers by the inflamed myocardium or as a result of generalized autonomic activation in association with the pain of an acute MI.

Myocardial Dysfunction

Congestive Heart Failure

Acute cardiac ischemia results in impaired ventricular contractility (systolic dysfunction) and increased myocardial stiffness (diastolic dysfunction), both of which may lead to symptoms of heart failure. In addition, ventricular remodeling, arrhythmias, and acute mechanical complications of MI (described below) may culminate in heart failure. Signs and symptoms of such decompensation include dyspnea, pulmonary rales, and a third heart sound (S_3). Treatment consists of standard heart failure therapy (discussed in Chapter 9).

Cardiogenic Shock

Cardiogenic shock is a condition of severely decreased cardiac output and hypotension (systolic blood pressure < 90 mm Hg) with inadequate perfusion of peripheral tissues, which develops when more than 40% of the LV mass has infarcted. It may also follow certain severe mechanical complications of MI described below. Demise in cardiogenic shock is self-perpetuating because (see Fig. 7.12): 1) hypotension leads to decreased coronary perfusion, which exacerbates ischemic damage, and 2) decreased stroke volume increases LV size and therefore augments myocardial oxygen demand. Despite aggressive treatment, the mortality rate of patients in cardiogenic shock is greater than 70%.

Patients in cardiogenic shock require intravenous inotropic agents (e.g., dobutamine) to increase cardiac output and arterial vasodilators to reduce the resistance to LV contraction. Such patients are often stabilized by the placement of an **intra-aortic balloon pump.** This device is inserted into the aorta via a femoral artery and consists of an inflatable, flexible chamber that expands during diastole to increase intraaortic pressure, thus augmenting perfusion of the coronary arteries and the peripheral tissues. During systole it deflates to create a "vacuum" that serves to reduce the afterload of the left ventricle, thus aiding the ejection of blood into the aorta. Early cardiac catheterization and revascularization (angioplasty or CABG) has the potential to improve the long-term prognosis of patients in cardiogenic shock.

Right Ventricular Infarction

Approximately one-third of patients with infarction of the LV inferior wall also develop necrosis of portions of the right ventricle, because the same coronary artery (usually the right coronary) perfuses both regions in most individuals. The resulting abnormal contraction and decreased compliance of the right ventricle lead to signs of right-sided heart failure (e.g., jugular venous distention) out of proportion to signs of left-sided failure. In addition, profound hypotension may result because right ventricular dysfunction impairs blood flow through the lungs, so that the left ventricle becomes underfilled. In this setting, intravenous volume infusion often serves to correct hypotension, guided by hemodynamic measurements via a transvenous pulmonary artery catheter.

Mechanical Complications

Mechanical complications following MI result from tissue ischemia and necrosis.

Papillary Muscle Rupture

Ischemic necrosis and rupture of a LV papillary muscle may be rapidly fatal because of acute severe mitral regurgitation, as the valve leaflets lose their anchoring attachments. *Partial* rupture, with more moderate regurgitation, is not immediately lethal but may result in symptoms of heart failure or pulmonary edema. The posteromedial LV papillary muscle is more susceptible to infarction than the anterolateral one, because it has a more precarious blood supply; therefore, this complication is more common following an inferoposterior MI.

Ventricular Free Wall Rupture

An infrequent but deadly complication, rupture of the LV free wall through a tear in the necrotic myocardium, may occur within the first 2 weeks following MI. It is more common among women and individuals with a history of hypertension. Hemorrhage into the pericardial space owing to such rupture results in rapid cardiac tamponade, in which blood fills the pericardial space and severely restricts ventricular filling (see Chapter 14). Survival is rare.

On occasion, a **pseudoaneurysm** results if rupture of the free wall is incomplete and held in check by thrombus formation that "plugs" the hole in the myocardium. This situation is the cardiac equivalent of a time bomb, because subsequent complete rupture into the pericardium and tamponade could follow. If detected (usually by echocardiography), surgical correction may prevent an otherwise disastrous outcome.

Ventricular Septal Rupture

This complication is analogous to LV free wall rupture, but the abnormal flow of blood is not directed across the LV wall into the pericardium. Rather, blood is shunted across the ventricular septum from the left ventricle to the right ventricle, usually precipitating congestive heart failure because of subsequent volume overload of the pulmonary capillaries. A loud systolic murmur at the left sternal border, representing transseptal flow, is common in this situation. The murmur of ventricular septal rupture can be differentiated from that of acute mitral regurgitation by performing Doppler echocardiography or by measuring the O_2 saturation of blood in the right-sided heart chambers through a transvenous catheter. The O_2 content in the right ventricle is abnormally higher than that in the right atrium if there is shunting of oxygenated blood from the left ventricle across the septal defect.

True Ventricular Aneurysm

This is a late complication of MI, occurring weeks to months after the acute event. It develops as the ventricular wall is weakened, but not perforated, by the phagocytic clearance of necrotic tissue, and it results in a localized outward bulge (dyskinesia) when the residual viable heart muscle contracts. Unlike the pseudoaneurysm described above, there is no communication between the LV cavity and the pericardium, so that rupture and tamponade do not develop. Complications of LV aneurysm include 1) thrombus formation within this region of stagnant blood flow, serving as a potential source of emboli to peripheral organs; 2) ventricular arrhythmias associated with the stretched myofibers; and 3) heart failure due to reduced forward cardiac output, because some of the LV stroke volume is "wasted" by filling the aneurysm cavity during systole.

Clues to the presence of an LV aneurysm include persistent ST segment elevations on the ECG weeks after the acute ST-elevation MI and a bulge of the LV border on chest radiograph. The abnormality can usually be confirmed by echocardiography.

Pericarditis

Acute pericarditis may occur in the early (in-hospital) post-infarction period as necrosis and neutrophilic infiltrates extend from the myocardium to the adjacent pericardium. Sharp pain, fever, and a pericardial friction rub are often manifest in this situation and help distinguish pericarditis from the pain of recurrent myocardial ischemia.

Anticoagulants are relatively contraindicated in MI complicated by pericarditis to avoid hemorrhage from the inflamed pericardial lining. The frequency of MI-associated pericarditis has declined since the introduction of acute reperfusion strategies, because those approaches limit the extent of myocardial damage and inflammation.

Dressler Syndrome

Dressler syndrome is another uncommon form of pericarditis that can occur over the first several weeks following hospitalization for MI. The cause is unclear, but an immune process directed against damaged myocardial tissue is suspected to play a role. The syndrome is heralded by fever, malaise, and sharp, pleuritic chest pain typically accompanied by leukocytosis, an elevated erythrocyte sedimentation rate, and a pericardial effusion. Similar to other forms of acute pericarditis, Dressler syndrome generally responds to high-dose aspirin therapy.

Thromboembolism

Stasis of blood flow in regions of impaired LV contraction after an MI may incite intracavity thrombus formation, especially when the infarction involves the LV apex, or when a true aneurysm has formed. Subsequent thromboemboli can result in devastating infarction of peripheral organs (e.g., an embolism to the brain may cause a stroke).

POST-MI RISK STRATIFICATION AND MANAGEMENT

Most patients can be discharged safely from the hospital 5–6 days after an acute MI (sooner if aggressive reperfusion therapies were undertaken and complications had not occurred). The most important predictor of post-MI outcome is the *extent of LV dysfunction*. Other features that portend adverse outcomes include early recurrence of ischemia, a large volume of residual myocardium still at ischemic risk by coronary disease, and high-grade ventricular arrhythmias.

To identify patients at high risk for complications who may benefit from cardiac catheterization, exercise treadmill testing is performed (unless the patient has *already* undergone catheterization and corrective percutaneous revascularization for the presenting coronary syndrome). Typically a low-level exercise test is undertaken at the time of discharge with more rigorous testing 4–6 weeks later. Patients with significantly abnormal results, or those who demonstrate an early spontaneous recurrence of angina, are referred for cardiac catheterization to define their coronary anatomy.

Standard post-discharge therapy includes 1) aspirin, 2) a β-blocker, and 3) an ACE inhibitor (especially if LV dysfunction is demonstrated). Cholesterol-lowering therapy (usually an HMG CoA reductase inhibitor) is prescribed to achieve a long-term low-density lipoprotein value of <100 mg/dL. Rigorous attention to other cardiac risk factors, such as smoking, hypertension, and diabetes, is also mandatory, and a formal exercise rehabilitation program often speeds convalescence.

SUMMARY

1. ACS include UA, NSTEMI, and STEMI. Most ACS episodes are due to the formation of intracoronary thrombus at the site of atherosclerotic plaque. Plaque rupture is the usual trigger for thrombus formation through activation of platelets and the coagulation cascade. Atherosclerosis-induced endothelium dysfunction contributes to the process by producing decreased amounts of vasodilators and antithrombotic agents.
2. The classification of ACS is based on the severity of ischemia and whether necrosis results. ST-elevation MI generally results from an occlusive thrombus with severe ischemia and necrosis. Acute coronary conditions not associated with ST elevation (non-ST-elevation MI and UA) usually result from partially occlusive thrombi with less intense ischemia. Compared with UA, the insult in NSTEMI is of sufficient magnitude to cause some degree of myocardial necrosis.
3. ACS result in biochemical and mechanical changes that impair systolic contraction, decrease myocardial compliance (diastolic dysfunction), and predispose to dangerous arrhythmias. Infarction initiates an inflammatory response that clears necrotic tissue and leads to scar formation. Transient severe ischemia without infarction can cause "stunned" myocardium, a condition of contractile dysfunction that persists beyond the period of ischemia, with subsequent gradual recovery of function.
4. The diagnosis of, and distinction between, ACS relies on the patient's history, typical ECG abnormalities, and temporal evolution of specific serum biomarkers.
5. Acute treatment of UA/NSTEMI includes measures to restore balance between myocardial oxygen supply and demand (β-blockers, nitrates) and stabilization of the intracoronary thrombus (aspirin, heparin [unfractionated or low molecular weight], and sometimes additional antiplatelet therapies [e.g., thienopyridines, GP IIb/IIIa antagonists]). ACE inhibitor and statin therapies are often indicated. Early coronary angiography, with subsequent mechanical intervention, is beneficial in high-risk patients.
6. Acute treatment for STEMI includes early reperfusion strategies with thrombolytic drugs or PCI. Other important measures include aspirin, a β-blocker, and in appropriate circumstances, nitrate and heparin therapies. Similar to UA/STEMI, ACE inhibitor and statin therapies may be beneficial.
7. Potential complications of MI include arrhythmias such as ventricular tachycardia and fibrillation, atrioventricular blocks, bundle branch blocks, and supraventricular arrhythmias. Cardiogenic shock or congestive heart failure may develop because of ventricular dysfunction or mechanical complications including ventricular rupture, mitral regurgitation, and ventricular septal defect. In addition, wall motion abnor-

malities of the affected segment may predispose to thrombus formation.

8. Standard pharmacologic therapy following discharge from the hospital includes aspirin, a β-blocker, an ACE inhibitor (especially if LV dysfunction is present), and cholesterol-lowering therapy (usually a statin). Additional therapy may include a thienopyridine (clopidogrel) or systemic anticoagulation (if intraventricular thrombus or a large akinetic segment is present).

9. Post-ACS risk stratification seeks to identify patients at high risk of recurrent ischemia, reinfarction, or death. Impaired LV function, electrical instability (high-grade ventricular arrhythmias), and ischemic changes during exercise testing all portend unfavorable outcomes and warrant further investigations and treatment.

Acknowledgments   The authors thank Dr. Frederick Schoen for his helpful suggestions. Contributors to the previous editions of this chapter were J.G. Fletcher, MD; Marc S. Sabatine, MD; William Carlson, MD; Patrick T. O'Gara, MD; and Leonard S. Lilly, MD.

ADDITIONAL READING

Armstrong PW, Collen D. Fibrinolysis for acute myocardial infarction: current status and new horizons for pharmacological reperfusion. Circulation 2001;103:2862–2866.

Braunwald E, Antman EM, Beasley JW, et al. ACC/AHA guidelines for management of patients with unstable angina and non-ST-segment elevation myocardial infarction: a report of the American College of Cardiology/American Heart Association Task Force on Practice Guidelines (Committee on the Management of Unstable Angina). J Am Coll Cardiol 2000;36:970–1062.

Califf RM, Bengtson JR. Cardiogenic shock. N Engl J Med 1994;330:1724–1730.

Cannon CP, Weintraub WS, Demopoulos LA, et al. Comparison of early invasive and conservative strategies in patients with unstable coronary syndromes treated with the glycoprotein IIb/IIIa inhibitor tirofiban (TACTICS-TIMI 18). N Engl J Med 2001;344:1879–1887.

Clopidogrel in Unstable Angina to Prevent Recurrent Events (CURE) Trial Investigators. Effects of clopidogrel in addition to aspirin in patients with acute coronary syndromes without ST-segment elevation. N Engl J Med 2001;345:494–502.

Collins R, Peto R, Baigent C, et al. Aspirin, heparin, and fibrinolytic therapy in suspected acute myocardial infarction. N Engl J Med 1997;336:847–860.

Fibrinolytic Therapy Trialists (FTT) Collaborative Group. Indications for fibrinolytic therapy in suspected acute myocardial infarction: collaborative overview of early mortality and major morbidity results from all randomised trials of more than 1000 patients. Lancet 1994;343:311–322.

Fuster V, Badimon L, Badimon JJ, et al. The pathogenesis of coronary artery disease and the acute coronary syndromes. N Engl J Med 1992;326:242–250, 310–318.

Gavin BJ, Ridker PM. Novel clinical markers of vascular wall inflammation. Circulation Res 2001;89(9):763–771.

Grines CL, Browne KF, Marco J, et al. for the Primary Angioplasty in Myocardial Infarction Study Group. A comparison of immediate angioplasty with thrombolytic therapy for acute myocardial infarction. N Engl J Med 1993;328:673–679.

Kloner RA, Jennings RB. Consequences of brief ischemia: stunning, preconditioning, and their clinical implications: part 1. Circulation 2001;104(24):2981–2989.

Llevadot J, Giugliano RP, Antman EM. Bolus fibrinolytic therapy in acute myocardial infarction. JAMA 2001;286:442–449.

Miller WL, Reeder GS. Adjunctive therapies in the treatment of acute coronary syndromes. Mayo Clin Proc 2001;76:391–405.

Montalescot G, Barragan P, Wittenberg O, et al. for the ADMIRAL investigators. Platelet glycoprotein IIb/IIIa inhibition with coronary stenting for acute myocardial infarction. N Engl J Med 2001;344:1895–1903.

Pfeffer MA. ACE inhibition in acute myocardial infarction. Circulation 1998;97:2192–2194.

Puleo PR, Meyer D, Wathen C, et al. Use of a rapid assay of subforms of creatine kinase MB to diagnose or rule out acute myocardial infarction. N Engl J Med 1994;331:561–566.

Ryan TJ, Antman EM, Brooks NH, et al. 1999 update: ACC/AHA guidelines for the management of patients with acute myocardial infarction: executive summary and recommendations: a report of the American College of Cardiology/American Heart Association Task Force on Practice Guidelines (Committee on Management of Acute Myocardial Infarction). Circulation 1999;100:1016–1030.

Schwartz GG, Olsson AG, Ezekowitz MD, et al. for the Myocardial Ischemia Reduction with Aggressive Cholesterol Lowering Study Investigators. Effects of atorvastatin on early recurrent ischemic events in acute coronary syndromes: The MIRACL study: A randomized controlled trial. JAMA 2001;285:1711–1718.

Van de Werf F. Cardiac troponins in acute coronary syndromes. N Engl J Med 1996;335:1388–1389.

Yeghiazarians Y, Braunstein JB, Askari A, et al. Unstable angina pectoris. N Engl J Med. 2000;342:101–114.

Valvular Heart Disease

Patrick Yachimski and Leonard S. Lilly

Rheumatic Fever
Mitral Valve Disease
  Mitral Stenosis
  Mitral Regurgitation
  Mitral Valve Prolapse
Aortic Valve Disease
  Aortic Stenosis
  Aortic Regurgitation

Tricuspid Valve Disease
  Tricuspid Stenosis
  Tricuspid Regurgitation
Pulmonic Valve Disease
  Pulmonic Stenosis
  Pulmonic Regurgitation
Prosthetic Valves
Infective Endocarditis
  Pathogenesis
  Clinical Manifestations

This chapter reviews the pathophysiology and clinical assessment of patients with valvular heart disease. Each of the common valvular abnormalities is discussed separately, because unifying pathophysiologic principles do not govern the behavior of all stenotic or regurgitant valves.

The evaluation of valvular heart disease begins at the bedside with a careful history and physical examination, from which the trained clinician can usually identify the type of valvular abnormalities that are present. Accurate assessment of the severity of the valve lesion often requires additional information from the electrocardiogram, chest radiograph, and echocardiogram. In selected patients, further investigation by exercise testing or cardiac catheterization may be necessary to define fully the severity of the condition and guide therapy. Thus, effective management of patients with valvular disease requires accurate identification of the lesion, an evaluation of its severity, and a clear understanding of the pathophysiologic consequences and natural history of the condition.

RHEUMATIC FEVER

Acute rheumatic fever (ARF) was once among the most common causes of valvular heart disease, but its incidence has waned considerably in the past half-century in industrialized society. In the 1940s, the yearly incidence of ARF exceeded 200,000 cases in the United States, whereas the disease is now rare. The decline of this condition immediately preceded or coincided with the introduction of penicillin as well as with improvement of general health care and relief from overcrowding. Recent reports have identified occasional local outbreaks in the United States, but a major resurgence has not been seen. Nevertheless, in developing countries of the Middle East, Southeast Asia, and Indian subcontinent, ARF continues to be a scourge with fulminant consequences.

ARF is an inflammatory condition primarily involving the heart, skin, and connective tissues. It is a complication of upper respiratory tract infections caused by group A streptococci and mainly occurs in childhood and young adulthood. During epidemics, approximately 3% of patients with acute streptococcal pharyngitis develop ARF 2–3 weeks after the initial throat infection. The pathogenesis of ARF remains unknown but does not involve direct bacterial infection of the heart. Some proposed mechanisms include the elaboration of a toxin by the streptococci or autoimmune cross-reactivity between bacterial antigens and those on the endocardium. The most common presenting symptoms are chills, fever, migratory arthralgias, and fatigue. The cardinal symptoms and clinical manifestations of the disease that establish the diagnosis are known as the *Jones' criteria* (Table 8.1).

Pathologically, rheumatic carditis (i.e., cardiac inflammation) may affect all three layers of the heart (pericardium, myocardium, and endocardium). Histopathologic examination often demonstrates the "Aschoff body," an area of focal fibrinoid necrosis surrounded by inflammatory cells including lymphocytes, plasma cells, and macrophages that later resolve to form fibrous scar tissue. The most devastating sequelae result from inflammatory involvement of the valvular endocardium, which leads to chronic rheumatic heart disease, characterized by permanent deformity and impairment of one or more cardiac valves. Symptoms of valvular dysfunction, however, generally do not become manifest until *10–30 years* after ARF has subsided, although this latency period may be considerably shorter with more aggressive disease observed in developing countries.

During the acute episode, carditis may be associated with tachycardia, decreased left ventricular contractility, a pericardial friction rub, a transient murmur of mitral or aortic regurgitation, or a mid-diastolic murmur at the cardiac apex (termed the Carey-Coombs murmur). These transient murmurs may reflect turbulent flow across inflamed valve leaflets. Treatment of the acute episode of ARF includes the use of high-dose aspirin to reduce inflammation, penicillin to eliminate residual streptococcal infection, and therapy for complications such as congestive heart failure and pericarditis.

During the chronic phase, stenosis or regurgitation of cardiac valves is common, most often affecting the mitral valve. Forty percent of patients with rheumatic heart disease will develop mitral stenosis. An additional 25% will develop aortic regurgitation or stenosis in addition to the mitral abnormality. Infrequently, the tricuspid valve is affected as well.

ARF recurs in 10% of patients, and such recurrences can incite further cardiac damage. Therefore, patients who have experienced ARF should receive low-dose penicillin prophylaxis until young adulthood (i.e., approximately age 30), by which time exposure and susceptibility to the streptococcal infection have sufficiently diminished.

MITRAL VALVE DISEASE

Mitral Stenosis

Etiology

Mitral stenosis (MS) is almost always a sequela of rheumatic fever; therefore, virtually all adults with MS have typical rheumatic deformity of the valve on pathologic examination. Approximately 50% of patients with symptomatic MS provide a history of ARF that had occurred, on average, 20 years before presentation. Other rare causes of MS (less than 1%) include congenital stenosis of the mitral valve, prominent calcification extending from the mitral annulus in elderly patients, or endocarditis with very large vegetations that obstruct the valve orifice.

Pathology

Acute and recurrent inflammation produce the typical pathologic features of rheumatic MS. These include fibrous thickening and calcification of the valve leaflets, fusion of the commissures (the borders

---

TABLE 8.1. Jones' Criteria for Diagnosis of Rheumatic Fever[a]

Major criteria
  Carditis
  Polyarthritis
  Sydenham's chorea (involuntary movements)
  Erythema marginatum (skin rash with advancing
    edge and clearing center)
  Subcutaneous nodules

Minor criteria
  Migratory arthralgias
  Fever
  Increased acute phase reactants (ESR, leukocytosis)
  Prolonged PR interval on electrocardiogram

Evidence of streptococcal infection
  Antistreptolysin O antibodies
  Positive throat culture for Streptococci group A

[a]Diagnosis requires evidence of streptococcal infection and either: two major criteria, or one major plus two minor criteria.

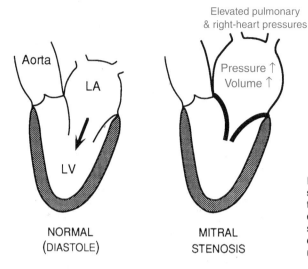

Figure 8.1. **Pathophysiology of mitral stenosis.** In the normal heart, blood flows freely from the left atrium (LA) into the left ventricle (LV) during diastole. In mitral stenosis, there is obstruction to LA emptying. Thus, LA pressure increases, which in turn elevates pulmonary and right-heart pressures.

where the leaflets meet), and thickening and shortening of the chordae tendineae.

Pathophysiology

In early diastole in the normal heart, the mitral valve opens and blood flows freely from the left atrium (LA) into the left ven-

tricle (LV), such that there is a negligible pressure difference between the two chambers. In MS, however, there is obstruction to blood flow across the valve such that emptying of the LA is impeded and there is an abnormal pressure gradient between the LA and LV (Figs 8.1 and 8.2). As a result, the left atrial pressure is higher than normal, a

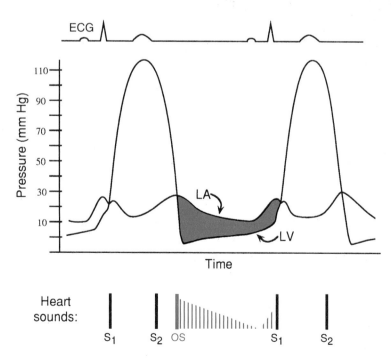

Figure 8.2. **Hemodynamic profile of mitral stenosis.** The left atrial (LA) pressure is elevated, and there is a pressure gradient (shaded area) between the LA and left ventricle (LV) during diastole. Compare with schematic of normal tracing (see Fig. 2.1). Abnormal heart sounds are present: there is a diastolic opening snap (OS) that corresponds to the opening of the mitral valve, followed by a decrescendo murmur. There is accentuation of the murmur just before S_1 due to the increased pressure gradient when the LA contracts.

necessary feature for blood to be propelled forward across the obstructed valve. The normal cross-sectional area of the mitral valve orifice is 4–6 cm^2. Hemodynamically significant MS becomes apparent when the valve area is reduced to less than 2 cm^2. Although left ventricular pressures are usually normal in MS, impaired filling of the chamber across the narrowed mitral valve may reduce LV stroke volume and cardiac output.

The high left atrial pressure in MS is passively transmitted to the pulmonary circulation, resulting in increased pulmonary venous and capillary pressures (see Fig. 8.1). This elevation of hydrostatic pressure in the pulmonary vasculature may cause transudation of plasma into the lung interstitium and alveoli. The patient may therefore experience dyspnea and other symptoms of congestive heart failure. In severe cases, significant elevation of pulmonary venous pressure leads to the opening of collateral channels between the pulmonary and bronchial veins. Subsequently, the high pulmonary vascular pressures may cause rupture of a bronchial vein into the lung parenchyma, resulting in hemoptysis (coughing blood).

The elevation of left atrial pressure in MS can result in two distinct forms of pulmonary hypertension: passive and reactive. Most patients with MS exhibit *passive* pulmonary hypertension, related to the backward transmission of the elevated LA pressure. This is actually an "obligatory" increase in pulmonary artery pressure that develops to preserve forward flow in the setting of increased left atrial and pulmonary venous pressures. Additionally, approximately 40% of patients with MS demonstrate *reactive* pulmonary hypertension with medial hypertrophy and intimal fibrosis of the pulmonary arterioles. On the one hand, reactive pulmonary hypertension is "beneficial" in that the increased arteriolar resistance impedes blood flow into the engorged pulmonary capillary bed and thereby reduces capillary hydrostatic pressure. Thus, reactive pulmonary hypertension "protects" the pulmonary capillaries from even higher pressures and lessens

pulmonary congestion. However, this benefit is at the cost of decreased blood flow through the pulmonary vasculature with resultant elevation of the *right*-sided heart pressures, as the right ventricle pumps against the increased resistance. Chronic elevation of the right ventricular pressure leads to hypertrophy of that chamber and ultimately to right-sided heart failure.

Chronic pressure overload of the left atrium in MS leads to left atrial enlargement. Left atrial dilatation stretches the atrial conduction fibers and may disrupt the integrity of the cardiac conduction system, resulting in *atrial fibrillation* (a rapid irregular heart rhythm described in Chapter 12). Atrial fibrillation causes the cardiac output to fall in MS because the increased heart rate shortens diastole. This reduces the time available for blood to flow across the obstructed mitral valve and results in markedly elevated left atrial pressure.

The relative stagnation of blood flow in the dilated left atrium in MS, especially when combined with the development of atrial fibrillation, predisposes to intra-atrial thrombus formation. Thromboemboli to peripheral organs may follow, leading to devastating complications such as cerebrovascular occlusion (stroke). The likelihood of developing systemic thromboembolic complications in a patient with MS correlates with the patient's age and the dimensions of the left atrial appendage (a portion of the left atrium); it correlates inversely with the patient's cardiac output. Patients at high risk require chronic anticoagulation therapy.

The turbulent blood flow across the obstructed mitral valve in MS predisposes to *infective endocarditis* (see below); however, that complication occurs less frequently in MS than in other forms of acquired valvular disease.

Clinical Manifestations and Evaluation

The natural history of MS without intervention leads to a significantly reduced lifespan with a median survival of 7 years after the onset of symptoms. Patients with even mild symptoms are likely to die

TABLE 8.2. Follow-up of Mitral Stenosis Patients Treated Without Surgery

	Status 10 years later (%)		
Status at Diagnosis	No change	Worse	Deceased
Asymptomatic	59	25	16
Mild symptoms	21	21	58
Moderate symptoms	4	11	85

Adapted from Rowe JC, Bland EF, Sprague HB, et al. The course of mitral stenosis without surgery. Ann Intern Med 1960;52:741.

within 10 years if the mitral valve is not repaired (Table 8.2).

The clinical presentation of MS depends in large part on the degree of reduction in valve area. The more severe the stenosis, the greater the symptoms related to elevation of left atrial and pulmonary venous pressures. The earliest manifestations are those of dyspnea and reduced exercise capacity. In mild MS, dyspnea may be absent at rest; however, it develops on exertion as LA pressure rises with the exercise-induced increase in blood flow through the heart and faster heart rate (i.e., decreased diastolic filling time). Other conditions and activities that increase heart rate and cardiac blood flow, and therefore exacerbate symptoms of MS, include fever, anemia, hyperthyroidism, pregnancy, rapid arrhythmias such as atrial fibrillation, exercise, emotional stress, and sexual intercourse.

With more severe MS (i.e., a smaller valve area) dyspnea occurs even at rest. Increasing fatigue and more severe signs of pulmonary congestion, such as orthopnea and paroxysmal nocturnal dyspnea, occur. With advanced MS and pulmonary hypertension, signs of right-sided heart failure ensue, including jugular venous distention, hepatomegaly, ascites, and peripheral edema. Compression of the recurrent laryngeal nerve by the enlarged pulmonary artery or left atrium may cause hoarseness.

Less often, the diagnosis of MS is heralded by one of its complications—atrial fibrillation, thromboembolism, infective endocarditis, or hemoptysis, as described in the pathophysiology section above.

On examination, there are several typical findings. Palpation of the precordium often reveals a right ventricular "tap" due to the increased right ventricular pressure. Auscultation discloses a loud S_1 (the heart sound associated with mitral valve closure) in almost all cases. This is so because the high atrial-ventricular pressure gradient keeps the mobile portions of the mitral valve leaflets widely separated throughout diastole; at the onset of systole, ventricular contraction abruptly slams the leaflets together from the relatively wide-open position, increasing the intensity of the valve closure sound (see Chapter 2).

A main feature of auscultation in MS is a high-pitched "opening snap" (OS) that follows S_2. The OS is thought to be due to the sudden tensing of the chordae tendineae and stenotic leaflets upon opening. The interval between S_2 and the OS relates inversely to the severity of MS. The more severe the MS, the higher the LA pressure, and the earlier the valve is forced open in diastole. The OS is followed by a low-frequency decrescendo murmur (termed a diastolic "rumble") due to turbulent flow across the stenotic valve during diastole (see Fig. 8.2 and page 40). The duration, but not the intensity, of the diastolic murmur relates to the severity of MS. The more severe the stenosis, the longer it takes for the LA to empty and for the gradient between the LA and LV to dissipate. Near the end of diastole, contraction of the LA causes the pressure gradient between the LA and LV to transiently rise (see Fig. 8.2); therefore, the murmur briefly becomes louder. This final accentuation of the murmur does not occur if atrial fibrillation has developed, as there is no effective atrial contraction in that situation.

Murmurs due to other valvular lesions are often found concurrently in patients with MS. For example, mitral regurgitation (see below) frequently coexists with MS. Additionally, right-sided heart failure caused by severe MS may induce tricuspid regurgitation. A diastolic decrescendo murmur along the left sternal border may be due to coexistent aortic regurgitation (because of rheumatic involvement of the aortic leaflets) or pulmonic regurgitation (because of MS-induced pulmonary hypertension).

The *electrocardiogram* in MS routinely shows left atrial enlargement and, if pulmonary hypertension has developed, right ventricular hypertrophy. Atrial fibrillation may be present. The *chest radiograph* reveals left atrial enlargement, pulmonary vascular redistribution, interstitial edema, and Kerley B lines due to edema within the pulmonary septae (see Chapter 3). With the development of pulmonary hypertension, right ventricular enlargement and prominence of the pulmonary arteries also appear.

Echocardiography is of major diagnostic value in MS. It reveals thickened mitral leaflets and abnormal fusion of their commissures with restricted separation during diastole. Left atrial enlargement can be assessed, and if present, intra-atrial thrombus may be visualized. The mitral valve area can be measured directly on cross-sectional views or calculated from Doppler-echocardiographic velocity measurements. Patients are stratified into groups of disease severity based in part on the mitral valve area. Recall from above that the normal mitral valve orifice measures between 4 and 6 cm^2. A reduced mitral valve area of $\leq$2 cm^2 correlates with mild MS, whereas a patient with a valve area $\leq$1 cm^2 typically falls into the category of *critical MS*.

Although *cardiac catheterization* is not necessary to confirm the diagnosis of MS, it is sometimes performed to accurately assess the valve area and to identify whether mitral regurgitation, pulmonary hypertension, or coronary artery disease is present.

Treatment

Therapy of MS includes prophylaxis against recurrent ARF in young individuals and against infective endocarditis in all patients (see below). Diuretics are used to treat symptoms of vascular congestion. Digoxin is useful only if MS is accompanied by impaired left ventricular contractile function or if atrial fibrillation has developed, in which case it can be used to slow the rapid ventricular rate (see Chapter 17). β-Blockers, or the calcium channel antago-

nists verapamil or diltiazem, may also be used to slow the heart rate. Anticoagulant therapy (to prevent thromboembolism) is recommended for patients with MS with atrial fibrillation or concurrent congestive heart failure, or if previous embolic episodes have occurred.

If symptoms of MS persist despite diuretic therapy and control of rapid heart rates, mechanical correction of the stenosis is warranted. *Percutaneous balloon mitral valvuloplasty* was first introduced in 1985 and is a "nonsurgical" approach performed via cardiac catheterization. During this procedure, a balloon catheter is advanced from the femoral vein into the right atrium, across the atrial septum (by creating a small hole there), and advanced through the narrowed mitral valve orifice. The balloon is then rapidly inflated, thereby "cracking" open the fused commissures. The procedure is most effective in the absence of complicating features, such as mitral regurgitation, extensive valve calcification, or atrial thrombus. The results of this procedure in randomized trials compare favorably with those of surgical treatment. Approximately 5% of patients undergoing balloon mitral valvuloplasty are left with residual atrial septal defects. Less frequent complications include cerebral emboli at the time of valvuloplasty, cardiac perforation, or the iatrogenic creation of mitral regurgitation requiring subsequent surgical repair.

Surgical options for correcting MS include *open mitral commissurotomy* (an operation in which the stenotic commissures are separated under direct visualization), and in severe disease, mitral valve replacement (MVR). Perioperative mortality for MVR is approximately 1–2%, and 10-year survival rates exceed 80%, a marked improvement over the natural history of this disease (see Table 8.2).

Mitral Regurgitation

Etiology

Normal closure of the mitral valve during systole requires the coordinated action of each component of the valve apparatus. Therefore, mitral regurgitation (MR) may

TABLE 8.3. Common Causes of Mitral Regurgitation

Myxomatous degeneration (e.g., mitral valve
  prolapse)
Ischemic heart disease with papillary muscle
  dysfunction
Infective endocarditis
Idiopathic ruptured chordae
Rheumatic deformity
Hypertrophic cardiomyopathy (see Chapter 10)
Significant left ventricular enlargement from any
  cause
Mitral annulus abnormalities (calcification or
  dilatation)

result from structural abnormalities of the mitral annulus, the valve leaflets, the chordae tendineae, or the papillary muscles (Table 8.3). Myxomatous degeneration of the valve (termed "mitral valve prolapse") causes MR because enlarged, redundant leaflets bow excessively into the LA during systole rather than opposing each other normally. Ischemic heart disease may scar or cause transient dysfunction of a papillary muscle, interfering with valve closure. Infective endocarditis can result in MR because of leaflet perforation or rupture of infected chordae. Primary (idiopathic) rupture of chordae tendineae is associated with acute, severe valvular incompetence. Rheumatic fever may lead to MS, as already discussed, or primarily MR if excessive shortening of the chordae tendineae and retraction of the leaflets occur. Hypertrophic cardiomyopathy (described in Chapter 10) is associated with abnormal systolic motion of the anterior mitral leaflet, which prevents normal valve closure, causing significant MR in 50% of patients. Marked left ventricular enlargement of any cause results in MR because of two mechanisms that interfere with mitral leaflet closure: 1) the spatial separation between the papillary muscles is augmented, and 2) the mitral annulus is stretched to an increased diameter. Calcification of the mitral annulus can occur with normal aging, but is more common among patients with hypertension or aortic stenosis. Such calcification immobilizes the basal portion of the valve leaflets, interfering with their excursion and systolic coaptation.

Pathophysiology

In MR, a portion of the left ventricular stroke volume is ejected backward into the low-pressure LA (Fig. 8.3). As a result, the forward cardiac output (into the aorta) is less than the left ventricle's total (forward flow + backward leak) output. Therefore, the direct consequences of MR include: 1) an elevation of the left atrial volume and pressure, 2) a reduction of forward cardiac output into the aorta, and 3) a volume-related stress on the LV when the regurgitated volume returns to the LV in diastole along with normal pulmonary venous return. To meet normal circulatory needs and to eject the additional volume, the LV stroke volume must increase. This is accomplished by the Frank-Starling mechanism (see Chapter 9) whereby the elevated LV diastolic volume causes increased myofiber stretch and an augmented stroke volume with each contraction. The subsequent hemodynamic consequences of MR vary depending on the severity of the regurgitation and how long it has been present.

The severity of MR and the ratio of forward cardiac output to backward flow are dictated by five factors: 1) the size of the mitral orifice during regurgitation, 2) the systolic pressure gradient between the LV and LA, 3) the systemic vascular resistance opposing forward LV blood flow, 4) the left atrial compliance, and 5) the duration of regurgitation with each systolic contraction.

The *regurgitant fraction* in MR is defined as:

$$\frac{\text{Volume of MR}}{\text{Total LV stroke volume}}$$

and this ratio rises whenever the resistance to aortic outflow is increased (i.e., the blood follows the path of least resistance). For example, high systemic blood pressure or the presence of aortic stenosis will increase the regurgitant fraction. The extent to which left atrial pressure rises in response to the regurgitated volume is determined by the left atrial compliance. (Compliance is a measure of the chamber's pressure-volume

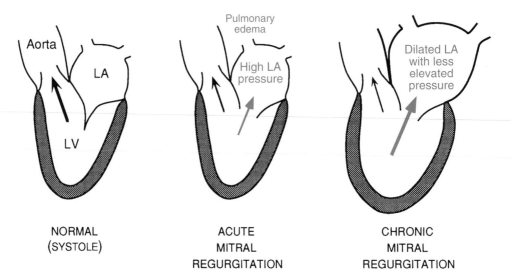

Figure 8.3. Pathophysiology of mitral regurgitation. In the normal heart, left ventricular (LV) contraction during systole forces blood exclusively through the aortic valve into the aorta; the closed mitral valve prevents regurgitation into the left atrium (LA). In mitral regurgitation (MR), a portion of LV output is forced backward into the LA, so that forward cardiac output into the aorta is reduced. In *acute* MR, the LA is of normal size and is relatively noncompliant, such that the LA pressure rises significantly and pulmonary edema may result. In *chronic* MR, the LA has enlarged and is more compliant, so that LA pressure is less elevated and pulmonary congestive symptoms are less common. There is LV enlargement and eccentric hypertrophy due to the chronically elevated volume load.

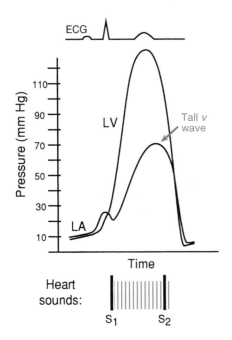

Figure 8.4. Hemodynamic profile of acute mitral regurgitation. A large systolic v wave is noted in the left atrial (LA) pressure tracing. A holosystolic murmur is present, beginning at the first heart sound (S_1) and continuing through the second heart sound (S_2). LV, left ventricle.

relationship, defined as the change in unit volume per change in unit pressure.)

In *acute MR* (e.g., due to sudden rupture of chordae tendineae), left atrial compliance undergoes little immediate change. This means that the left atrium is a relatively stiff chamber, and when it is suddenly exposed to the regurgitant flow, the elevated LA volume is accompanied by a large increase in LA pressure (see Fig. 8.3). This increased pressure helps to prevent further regurgitation; however, the high pressure is also transmitted to the pulmonary circulation. Therefore, acute MR can result in rapid pulmonary congestion and edema, a medical emergency.

In acute MR, measurements of the LA pressure, or the pulmonary capillary wedge pressure (an indirect measurement of LA pressure described in Chapter 3), demonstrate a prominent *v* wave (often referred to as a *"cv"* wave when it is so prominent that it merges with the preceding *c* wave), reflecting the increased LA filling during systole (Fig. 8.4). Additionally, as in MS, pulmonary artery and right heart pressures passively rise such that forward flow through the heart is maintained.

In acute MR, the LV accommodates the increased volume load from the LA according to the Frank-Starling relationship. Thus, the increased LV volume results in 1) an obligatory increase in LV diastolic pressure, and 2) a compensatory increase in the LV stroke volume, such that at the end of each systolic contraction, LV volume remains normal in the nonfailing heart. Systolic emptying of the ventricle is facilitated in MR by the fact that the total impedance to LV contraction is reduced (i.e., the afterload is lower than normal), since a portion of the LV output is directed into the relatively low-pressure left atrium, compared with normal outflow into the higher-pressure aorta.

In contrast to the acute situation, the more gradual development of *chronic* MR (e.g., due to rheumatic valve disease) permits the LA to undergo compensatory changes that lessen the effects of regurgitation on the pulmonary circulation (Fig. 8.3). In particular, the LA dilates and its compliance increases such that the chamber is able to accommodate larger volumes without a substantial increase in pressure. Left atrial dilatation is therefore adaptive in that it prevents significant increases in pulmonary vascular pressures. However, this adaptation occurs at the cost of inadequate forward cardiac output, because the compliant LA becomes a preferred low-pressure "sink" for left ventricular ejection, compared with the greater impedance of the aorta. Consequently, as progressively larger fractions of blood regurgitate into the LA, the main symptoms of chronic MR become those of low forward cardiac output (e.g., weakness and fatigue). In addition, chronic left atrial dilatation predisposes to the development of atrial fibrillation.

In *chronic MR,* the LV also undergoes gradual compensatory dilatation (eccentric hypertrophy, described in Chapter 9) in response to the volume load. Compared with acute MR, the increased ventricular compliance accommodates the augmented filling volume with relatively normal filling pressures. Forward output in chronic MR is pre-

served to near-normal levels by maintaining a high stroke volume via the Frank-Starling mechanism. Over time (usually several years), however, the chronic volume overload results in deterioration of left ventricular systolic function and leads to declining forward output and symptoms of heart failure.

In summary, the main differences between acute and chronic MR relate to left atrial size and compliance (see Fig. 8.3):

1. Acute MR: normal LA size and compliance → high LA pressure → high pulmonary venous pressure → pulmonary congestion.
2. Chronic MR: increased LA size and compliance → more normal LA and pulmonary venous pressures but low forward cardiac output.

Clinical Manifestations and Evaluation

As should be clear from the pathophysiology discussion above, patients with acute MR usually present with symptoms of pulmonary edema (Chapter 9). The symptoms of *chronic* MR are predominantly due to low cardiac output, especially during exertion, and consist of fatigue and weakness. Patients with severe MR or those who develop LV contractile dysfunction often complain of dyspnea and may describe orthopnea or paroxysmal nocturnal dyspnea. In severe chronic MR, symptoms of right heart failure (increased abdominal girth, peripheral edema) may develop as well.

The physical examination of a patient with MR reveals an apical holosystolic (also termed "pansystolic") murmur that radiates to the axilla (see Fig. 8.4). This description, accurate for rheumatic MR, has some exceptions. For example, when ischemic papillary muscle dysfunction interferes with normal mitral valve closure, the regurgitant jet may be directed toward the anterior left atrial wall immediately posterior to the aorta. In this setting, the murmur may be best heard in the "aortic" area (Chapter 2) and could be confused with the murmur of aortic stenosis (AS). Fortunately, the distinction between the systolic murmur of

MR and that of AS can be made by simple bedside maneuvers. If the patient is instructed to clench the fists, systemic vascular resistance will increase, and the severity of MR and its murmur will intensify, whereas the murmur of AS will not. Even more helpful in this distinction is to note the effect of varying cardiac cycle length (the time between consecutive heart beats) on the intensity of the systolic murmur. In a patient with atrial fibrillation or frequent premature beats, the LV fills to a degree that directly depends on the preceding cycle length (i.e., a longer cycle length permits greater left ventricular filling). The systolic murmur of AS becomes very loud after long cycle lengths because even small pressure gradients are amplified as more blood is ejected across the reduced aortic orifice. In MR, however, the murmur does not vary significantly because the change in the LV to LA pressure gradient is minimally affected by alterations in the cycle length.

In addition to the systolic murmur, a common finding in chronic MR is the presence of an S_3, which reflects increased volume returning to the LV in early diastole (see Chapter 2). In chronic MR, the palpated cardiac apical impulse is often laterally displaced toward the axilla, because of LV enlargement.

The *chest radiograph* in chronic MR demonstrates left ventricular and atrial enlargement. Calcification of the mitral annulus may be seen if that is the cause of the MR. The *electrocardiogram* typically demonstrates left atrial enlargement and signs of left ventricular hypertrophy. *Echocardiography* can often identify the structural cause of MR and grade its severity by color Doppler analysis. Left ventricular size and function (usually vigorous in the "compensated" heart because of the increased stroke volume) can be observed. *Cardiac catheterization* is useful for identifying a coronary ischemic cause (i.e., papillary muscle dysfunction) and for grading the severity of MR. The characteristic hemodynamic abnormality is a large v wave on the pulmonary capillary wedge pressure (reflecting LA pressure) tracing (see Fig. 8.4).

Natural History and Treatment

The natural history of chronic MR is related to its underlying cause. For example, in rheumatic heart disease, the course is one of very slow progression with a 15-year survival rate of 70%. On the other hand, abrupt worsening of chronic MR of any cause can occur with superimposed complications, such as rupture of chordae tendineae or endocarditis, and can result in an immediate life-threatening situation.

Medical therapy of MR involves augmenting forward cardiac output while reducing regurgitation into the LA and relieving pulmonary congestion. In acute MR with heart failure, treatment includes intravenous diuretics to relieve pulmonary edema and vasodilators (e.g., intravenous sodium nitroprusside) to reduce the resistance to forward flow and augment forward cardiac output. In chronic MR, improvement in forward flow can be accomplished by oral arteriolar vasodilators such as angiotensin enzyme-converting inhibitors or hydralazine.

Because chronic MR produces continuous left ventricular volume overload, it can slowly result in left ventricular contractile impairment and, ultimately, heart failure. Mitral valve surgery should be performed before such impairment occurs, but the operative mortality and the drawbacks associated with prosthetic valves are motivations for delaying surgery as long as possible. After more than 30 years' experience, the timing of surgery for a patient with chronic MR remains one of the most difficult decisions in the practice of cardiology. This is so because survival after *mitral valve replacement* is not clearly better than the natural history of the disease (because of potential complications of implanted artificial heart valves), even though symptomatic improvement is the rule. Fortunately, recent refinements in mitral valve surgery allow many patients to undergo *mitral valve repair* rather than replacement, eliminating many of the problems due to artificial valves. Mitral valve repair involves the surgical reconstruction of parts of the valve responsible for the regurgitation. For example, a perforated leaflet may be patched with transplanted autologous pericardium, or ruptured chordae may be reattached to a papillary muscle. In such patients, the postoperative survival rate appears to be better than the natural history of MR and has provided impetus toward earlier surgical intervention.

The operative mortality rate is approximately 2–4% for mitral valve repair and 8–10% for mitral replacement. The 10-year survival rate is about 80% for mitral repair and 50% for mitral replacement. In general, mitral valve repair is more often appropriate for younger patients with myxomatous involvement of the mitral valve, and mitral replacement is more often used in older patients with more extensive valve pathology.

Mitral Valve Prolapse

Mitral valve prolapse (MVP) is a common and usually asymptomatic billowing of the mitral leaflets into the LA during ventricular systole, sometimes accompanied by MR. Other names for this condition include "floppy" mitral valve, myxomatous mitral valve, or Barlow's syndrome. This condition may be inherited as a primary autosomal dominant disorder or may occur as a part of other connective tissue diseases such as the Marfan or Ehlers-Danlos syndromes. Pathologically, the valve leaflets, particularly the posterior leaflet, are enlarged, and the normal dense collagen and elastin matrix of the valvular fibrosa is fragmented and replaced with loose, "myxomatous" connective tissue. Additionally, in more severe lesions, elongated or ruptured chordae, annular enlargement, or thickened leaflets may be present. A recent rigorous echocardiographic study indicated that MVP occurs in about 2.4% of the population and is more common among women, especially those with a thin, lean body habitus.

Mitral prolapse is often asymptomatic, but affected individuals may describe chest pains or palpitations because of associated arrhythmias. Most often, it is found on routine physical examination, identified by the presence of a midsystolic "click" and late

systolic murmur heard best at the cardiac apex. The systolic click is thought to correspond to the sudden tensing of the involved mitral leaflet or chordae tendineae as the leaflet is forced back toward the left atrium; the murmur corresponds to regurgitant flow through the incompetent valve. The click and murmur are characteristically altered during dynamic auscultation at the bedside: maneuvers that increase the volume of the LV (e.g., sudden squatting) delay the occurrence of prolapse in systole and cause the click and murmur to occur later (i.e., further from S_1). Conversely, if the volume of blood in the LV is decreased (e.g., upon sudden standing), then prolapse occurs more readily and the click and murmur occur earlier in systole (closer to S_1).

Confirmation of the diagnosis is obtained by echocardiography, which demonstrates posterior displacement of one or both mitral leaflets into the left atrium during systole. The *electrocardiogram* and chest radiograph are usually normal unless chronic MR has resulted in left atrial and left ventricular enlargement.

The clinical course of mitral prolapse is most often benign. Treatment consists of reassurance about the usually good prognosis and antibiotic prophylaxis for endocarditis only if substantial valve thickening or MR are present. Of the potential complications, the most common is the development of gradually progressive MR. Occasionally, rupture of myxomatous chordae can cause sudden severe regurgitation and pulmonary edema. Other rare complications include infective endocarditis, peripheral emboli due to microthrombus formation behind the redundant valve tissue, and atrial or ventricular arrhythmias.

AORTIC VALVE DISEASE

Aortic Stenosis

Etiology

Aortic stenosis (AS) is often caused by age-related degenerative calcific changes of the valve, formerly termed "senile" AS. Calcific changes that progress to AS may also develop in patients with congenitally deformed aortic valves (about 1–2% of the population is born with an abnormal bicuspid aortic valve). Most patients who present with AS after the age of 65 have the age-related form, whereas the majority of younger patients have calcification of a congenitally bicuspid valve. AS may also result from chronic rheumatic valve disease, although the prevalence of this condition has decreased dramatically in recent decades in the United States. Approximately 95% of patients who are found to have rheumatic AS have coexisting rheumatic disease of the mitral valve.

Pathology

The pathologic appearance in AS is derived from its etiology. In age-related degenerative calcific AS, cumulative "wear-and-tear" leads to endothelial and fibrous damage, resulting in calcification of an otherwise normal trileaflet valve. In the case of a congenitally deformed valve, years of turbulent flow across the valve disrupt the endothelium and collagen matrix of the leaflets, resulting in gradual calcium deposition similar to that of the age-related degenerative form but appearing decades earlier. In rheumatic AS, endocardial inflammation leads to organization and fibrosis of the valve, resulting in fusion of the

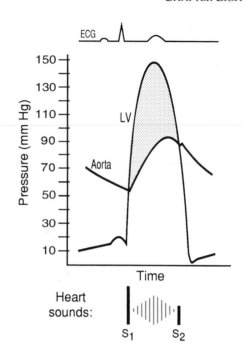

Figure 8.6. **Hemodynamic profile of aortic stenosis.** A systolic pressure gradient (shaded area) is present between the left ventricle (LV) and aorta. The second heart sound (S_2) is diminished in intensity, and there is a crescendo-decrescendo systolic murmur that does not extend beyond S_2.

commissures and the formation of calcified masses within the aortic cusps.

Regardless of the cause, the final pathologic findings in advanced AS are similar. Calcification is seen deep within the fibrosa of the valve cusps, extending toward the surface and resulting in heaped up or nodular deposition extending into the sinuses of Valsalva of the aortic root.

Pathophysiology

In AS, blood flow across the aortic valve is obstructed during systole (Fig. 8.5). When the valve orifice area is reduced by more than 50% of its normal size, significant elevation of left ventricular pressure is necessary to drive blood into the aorta (Fig. 8.6). In advanced AS, it is common to measure pressure gradients greater than 100 mm Hg between the LV and the aorta.

Since AS develops over a chronic course, the LV is able to compensate by undergoing concentric hypertrophy in response to the

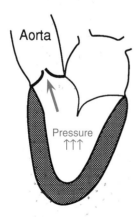

Figure 8.5. **Pathophysiology of aortic stenosis (AS).** Obstruction to systolic left ventricular (LV) outflow in AS results in elevation of intraventricular pressures and secondary LV hypertrophy.

high systolic pressure it must generate. Such hypertrophy serves an important role in reducing ventricular wall stress (remember from Chapter 6 that wall stress = P · r/2h); however, it also reduces the compliance of the ventricle. The resulting elevation in diastolic LV pressure also causes the LA to hypertrophy to fill the "stiff" LV. Whereas left atrial contraction contributes only a small portion of the left ventricular stroke volume in normal individuals, this LA "kick" may contribute more than 25% of the stroke volume to the stiffened LV in AS patients. Thus, left atrial hypertrophy is beneficial, and the loss of effective atrial contraction (e.g., the development of atrial fibrillation) can cause marked clinical deterioration.

Three major symptoms occur in patients with advanced AS: 1) angina, 2) syncope, and 3) congestive heart failure, all of which can be explained on the basis of the underlying pathophysiology. Each of these symptoms, in order, heralds an increasingly ominous prognosis (Table 8.4).

AS may result in *angina* because it creates a substantial imbalance between myocardial oxygen supply and demand. Myocardial oxygen *demand* is increased in two ways. First, the muscle mass of the hypertrophied LV is increased, requiring greater than normal perfusion. Second, wall stress is increased because of the elevated systolic ventricular pressure. In addition, AS reduces myocardial oxygen *supply* as the elevated left ventricular diastolic pressure reduces the coronary perfusion pressure gradient between the aorta and the myocardium.

AS may cause *syncope* during exertion. Although left ventricular hypertrophy allows the ventricle to generate a high pressure and maintain a normal cardiac output at rest, the ventricle cannot significantly increase its cardiac output during exercise because of the fixed stenotic aortic orifice. In addition, exercise leads to vasodilatation of the peripheral muscle beds. Thus, the combination of peripheral vasodilatation and the inability to augment cardiac output contribute to decreased cerebral perfusion pressure, and potentially, syncope upon exertion.

Finally, AS can result in symptoms of *congestive heart failure*. Early in the course of AS, the abnormal increase in left atrial pressure occurs mostly at the end of diastole, when the LA contracts into the thickened noncompliant LV. As a result, the mean left atrial pressure and the pulmonary venous pressure are not greatly affected early in the disease. However, with progression of the stenosis, the LV develops contractile dysfunction due to the insurmountably high afterload, leading to increased left ventricular end-diastolic volume and pressure. The accompanying marked elevation of LA and pulmonary venous pressures produces pulmonary alveolar congestion and the symptoms of congestive heart failure.

The normal aortic valve area is 3–4 cm². When the valve area is reduced to less than 2 cm², a significant pressure gradient between the LV and aorta first appears ("mild" AS). "Moderate" AS is characterized by a valve area of 1–1.5 cm². When the aortic valve area is reduced to less than 0.8 cm², critical valve obstruction is said to be present.

Clinical Manifestations and Evaluation

Angina, syncope, and congestive heart failure may appear after many asymptomatic years of slowly progressive valve stenosis. Once these symptoms develop, they confer a significantly decreased survival if surgical correction of AS is not undertaken (see Table 8.4).

Physical examination often permits accurate detection and estimation of the severity of AS. The key features of advanced AS include 1) a coarse late-peaking systolic ejection murmur (see Fig. 8.6 and

TABLE 8.4. Median Survival Time in Symptomatic Aortic Stenosis

Clinical Symptoms	Median Survival
Angina	5 years
Syncope	3 years
Congestive heart failure	2 years
Atrial fibrillation	6 months

Reprinted with permission from Ross J Jr, Braunwald E. Aortic stenosis. Circulation 1968; 38(Supplement v):61.

page 37), and 2) a weakened ("parvus") and delayed ("tardus") upstroke of the carotid artery pulsations due to the obstructed LV outflow. Other common findings on cardiac examination include the presence of an S_4 (because of atrial contraction into the "stiff" LV) and reduced intensity, or complete absence, of the aortic component of the second heart sound (see Fig. 8.6).

On the *electrocardiogram*, left ventricular hypertrophy is common in advanced AS, but *echocardiography* is a more sensitive technique to assess LV wall thickness. The transvalvular pressure gradient and aortic valve area can be calculated by Doppler echocardiography (see Chapter 3). *Cardiac catheterization* is sometimes used to confirm the severity of AS and also to define the coronary anatomy, because concurrent coronary artery bypass surgery is often necessary at the time of aortic valve replacement in patients with coexisting coronary disease.

Treatment

The natural history of severe, symptomatic, uncorrected AS is very poor. Data from the Mayo Clinic indicate that the 1-year survival rate is 57% for patients with severe AS who do not undergo surgery. The only effective treatment for advanced AS is surgical replacement of the valve.

Aortic valve replacement (AVR) is indicated for AS when patients with severe LV outflow obstruction develop symptoms, or when there is evidence of progressive LV dysfunction in the absence of symptoms. The left ventricular ejection fraction almost always increases after valve replacement, even in patients with impaired preoperative left ventricular function. The effect of AVR on the natural history of AS is dramatic, with the 10-year survival rate exceeding 75%.

Percutaneous valvuloplasty, unlike its role in the treatment of MS, has been disappointing in the treatment of AS. While balloon dilatation across the aortic valve orifice can fracture fused, calcified valve commissures leading to some immediate relief of outflow obstruction, up to 50% of patients experience valve restenosis within

6 months of the procedure. Valvuloplasty is occasionally a suitable option for patients who are poor surgical candidates or as a temporizing measure in patients too ill to proceed directly to valve replacement.

Mild, asymptomatic AS has a slow rate of progression such that over a 20-year period, only 20% of patients will progress to severe or symptomatic AS. Medical therapy for asymptomatic AS includes close clinical follow-up, endocarditis antibiotic prophylaxis, and avoidance of medications that could result in hypotension in this setting (e.g., vasodilators, diuretics, nitroglycerin).

Aortic Regurgitation

Etiology

Aortic regurgitation (AR), also termed aortic insufficiency, may result from 1) diseases of the aortic leaflets or 2) dilatation of the aortic root. The most common causes of AR are listed in Table 8.5.

Pathophysiology

In AR, abnormal regurgitation of blood from the aorta into the LV occurs during diastole. Therefore, with each contraction, the LV must pump the regurgitant volume *plus* the normal volume of blood returning from the LA. Hemodynamic compensation relies on the Frank-Starling mechanism to augment the LV stroke volume during systole. Factors influencing the severity of AR are analogous to those of MR: 1) the size of the regurgitant aortic orifice, 2) the pressure gradient across the aortic valve during diastole, and 3) the duration of diastole.

TABLE 8.5. Examples of Aortic Insufficiency

Abnormalities of valve leaflets
1. Rheumatic
2. Endocarditis
3. Congenital (bicuspid valve)

Dilatation of aortic root
1. Aortic aneurysm/dissection
2. Annulo-aortic ectasia
3. Marfan syndrome
4. Syphilis

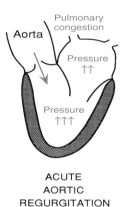

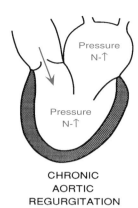

ACUTE
AORTIC
REGURGITATION

CHRONIC
AORTIC
REGURGITATION

Figure 8.7. Pathophysiology of acute and chronic aortic regurgitation (AR). Abnormal regurgitation of blood from the aorta into the left ventricle (LV) is shown in each schematic drawing (large arrows). In acute AR, the LV is of normal size and relatively low compliance, such that its diastolic pressure rises significantly; this is reflected back to the left atrium (LA) and pulmonary vasculature, resulting in pulmonary congestion or edema. In chronic AR, adaptive LV and LA enlargement have occurred, such that a greater volume of regurgitation can be accommodated with less of an increase in diastolic LV pressure, so that pulmonary congestion is less likely. N, normal.

As is the case with MR, the hemodynamic abnormalities and symptoms differ in acute and chronic AR (Fig. 8.7). In *acute* AR, the LV is of normal size and is relatively noncompliant. Thus, the volume load of regurgitation causes the LV diastolic pressure to rise substantially. The sudden high diastolic LV pressure is transmitted to the LA and pulmonary circulation, often producing dyspnea and pulmonary edema. Thus, acute severe AR is usually a surgical emergency, requiring immediate valve replacement.

In *chronic* AR, the LV undergoes compensatory adaptation in response to the long-standing regurgitation. AR subjects the LV primarily to volume overload, but also to excessive pressure; therefore, the ventricle compensates through dilatation and, to a lesser degree, hypertrophy. Over time, the dilatation increases the compliance of the LV and allows it to accommodate a large regurgitant volume with less of an increase in diastolic pressure, reducing the pressure transmitted into the LA and pulmonary circulation. However, by allowing the aorta to regurgitate a huge volume of blood during diastole, LV dilatation also causes the aortic (and therefore systemic arterial) diastolic pressure to drop substantially. The combination of a high LV stroke volume (and therefore high systolic arterial pressure) with a reduced aortic diastolic pressure produces a widened *pulse pressure* (the difference between arterial systolic and diastolic pressures), a hallmark of chronic AR (Fig. 8.8). As a result of the decreased aortic diastolic pressure, the coronary artery perfusion

pressure falls, potentially reducing myocardial oxygen supply. This, coupled with the increase in LV size (which causes increased wall stress and myocardial oxygen demand), can produce angina, even in the absence of atherosclerotic coronary disease.

Because left ventricular dilatation and hypertrophy are generally adequate to meet the demands of chronic AR, affected patients are usually asymptomatic for

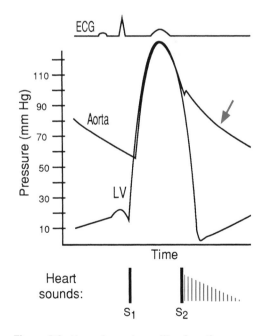

Figure 8.8. Hemodynamic profile of aortic regurgitation. During diastole, the aortic pressure falls rapidly (arrow), and left ventricular (LV) pressure rises as blood regurgitates from the aorta into the LV. A diastolic decrescendo murmur, beginning at the second heart sound (S₂), corresponds with the abnormal regurgitant flow.

many years. Gradually, however, progressive remodeling of the LV occurs, resulting in myocardial systolic dysfunction. This in turn results in decreased forward cardiac output as well as an increase in left atrial and pulmonary pressures. At that point, the patient develops symptoms of heart failure.

Clinical Manifestations and Assessment

Common symptoms of chronic AR include dyspnea on exertion, fatigue, decreased exercise tolerance, and the uncomfortable sensation of a forceful heartbeat associated with high pulse pressure. Physical examination may show bounding pulses and other stigmata of the widened pulse pressure (Table 8.6), in addition to a hyperdynamic LV impulse and the blowing murmur of AR in early diastole along the left sternal border (see Fig. 8.8). It is best heard with the patient leaning forward, after exhaling. In addition, a low-frequency mid-diastolic rumbling sound may be auscultated at the cardiac apex in some patients with severe AR. Known as the *Austin Flint* murmur, it is thought to reflect turbulent blood flow across the *mitral* valve during diastole due to downward displacement of the mitral anterior leaflet by the stream of AR. It can be distinguished from the murmur of MS by the absence of an opening snap or presystolic accentuation of the murmur.

In chronic AR, the *chest radiograph* shows an enlarged left ventricular silhouette. This is usually absent in acute AR, in which pulmonary vascular congestion is the more likely finding. *Doppler echocardiography* can identify and quantify the degree of AR and often can identify its cause. *Cardiac catheterization* with contrast angiography is useful for evaluation of left ventricular function, quantification of the degree of AR, and assessment of coexisting coronary artery disease.

Treatment

Data from the National Institutes of Health suggest that 60% of patients with asymptomatic chronic AR and normal LV contractile function will remain asymptomatic at 10-year follow-up. Therefore, asymptomatic patients simply need regular clinical evaluation, periodic assessment of LV function (usually by echocardiography), and endocarditis antibiotic prophylaxis. Symptomatic patients with preserved LV function may respond to therapy with diuretics and afterload reducing vasodilators (e.g., angiotensin-converting enzyme inhibitors). The calcium-channel blocker nifedipine has been shown to reduce LV enlargement, increase the LV ejection fraction, and delay the need for valve surgery in patients with severe AR who have normal LV contractile function.

The onset of symptoms in a patient with chronic AR usually heralds the development of LV contractile dysfunction, and the prognosis worsens once LV decompensation occurs. Symptomatic patients with severe chronic AR, or asymptomatic patients with impaired LV systolic function as a re-

TABLE 8.6. Physical Findings Associated with Widened Pulse Pressure in Chronic Aortic Regurgitation

Name	Description
Bisferiens pulse	Double systolic impulse in carotid or brachial artery
Corrigan's pulse	"Water-hammer" pulses with marked distention and collapse
de Musset's sign	Head-bobbing with each systole
Duroziez's sign	To-and-fro murmur heard over femoral artery with light compression
Hill's sign	Popliteal systolic pressure more than 60 mm Hg greater than brachial systolic pressure
Müller's sign	Systolic pulsations of the uvula
Quincke's sign	Capillary pulsations visible at lip or proximal nail beds
Traube's sign	"Pistol-shot" sound auscultated over the femoral artery

---

Box 8.1. Diet Drugs and Valvular Heart Disease

The role of diet drugs as causative factors in valvular heart disease has received considerable publicity over the past few years. Phentermine and fenfluramine, two well-known appetite suppressant drugs, had been in use for decades as weight-reduction agents. Phentermine is a noradrenergic central nervous system stimulant; fenfluramine promotes the release of serotonin and inhibits its uptake by neurons. During the 1990s, physicians began prescribing these two medications in combination, which became known as "fen-phen." When taken together, the two drugs were thought to be efficacious at lower doses than when either was used alone and with fewer side effects. It is estimated that in 1996, more than 18 million prescriptions were filled for phentermine and fenfluramine.

In August 1997, Connolly et al. published a report in the *New England Journal of Medicine* regarding new valvular disease associated with fen-phen use. The report described 24 women who had been taking fen-phen for weight reduction over 2–28 months. Twenty of the women presented with new cardiovascular symptoms, such as dyspnea or peripheral edema; the remaining 4 women presented with new cardiac murmurs.

All 24 women underwent echocardiography, which demonstrated mitral regurgitation and/or aortic regurgitation in each patient; half also had tricuspid valve involvement. None of the women were known to have had preexisting cardiovascular disease.

At the time of the report's publication, 5 of 24 patients had developed valvular dysfunction severe enough to warrant valve replacement. Postoperative examination of valve tissue from these individuals revealed histopathology similar to that of the carcinoid syndrome. (In carcinoid syndrome, high circulating levels of serotonin are thought to lead to fibroplastic changes of valvular endocardium.) This comparison led to speculation that fen-phen use led to excess serum serotonin levels, thereby causing the valvular lesions.

Following the initial report, subsequent analyses estimated that the prevalence of valvular heart disease in patients who had taken fen-phen was as high as 20–30%. Phentermine and fenfluramine were withdrawn from the market by their manufacturers in September 1997, one month after publication of the initial *New England Journal of Medicine* report.

Subsequent studies recruiting larger numbers of patients have confirmed increased rates of valvular disease in patients exposed to diet drugs (e.g., fenfluramine alone or in combination with phentermine), but with widely varying estimates of both prevalence and severity of the valvular lesions. The precise mechanism of valvular disease has still not been elucidated.

Fortunately, the most recent follow-up studies have shown no progression, and have even shown improvement, in valvular function once the drugs are discontinued.

REFERENCES

Connolly HM, Crary JL, McGoon MD, et al. Valvular heart disease associated with fenfluramine-phentermine. N Engl J Med 1997;337:581–588.

Gardin J, Weissman NJ, Leung C, et al. Clinical and echocardiographic follow-up of patients previously treated with dexfenfluramine or phentermine/fenfluramine. JAMA 2001;286:2011–2014.

Khan MA, Herzog CA, St. Peter JV, et al. The prevalence of cardiac valvular insufficiency assessed by transthoracic echocardiography in obese patients treated with appetite-suppressant drugs. N Engl J Med 1998;339:713–718.

sult of regurgitation, should undergo surgical valve replacement to prevent further deterioration of LV function.

TRICUSPID VALVE DISEASE

Tricuspid Stenosis

Tricuspid stenosis (TS) is rare and usually a consequence of rheumatic heart disease. The opening snap and diastolic murmur of TS are similar to those of MS, but the murmur is heard closer to the sternum and intensifies on inspiration because of increased right-heart blood flow. In TS, the neck veins are distended and show a large *a* wave due to right atrial contraction against the stenotic tricuspid valve orifice. Patients may develop abdominal distention and hepatomegaly due to passive venous congestion.

Symptoms of TS can be similar to those of MS, and the two conditions can coexist as sequelae of rheumatic heart disease. Surgical therapy is usually required (valvuloplasty or valve replacement).

Tricuspid Regurgitation

Tricuspid regurgitation (TR) is usually "functional" rather than structural; that is, it develops because of right ventricular enlargement (e.g., due to pressure or volume overload), rather than primary valve disease. In patients with rheumatic MS, 20% have significant TR (of whom 80% have "functional" TR because of pulmonary hypertension with right ventricular enlargement, and 20% have "organic" TR due to rheumatic involvement of the tricuspid valve). The most sensitive physical signs are prominent *v* waves in the jugular veins and a pulsatile liver because of regurgitation of right ventricular blood into the systemic veins. The systolic murmur of TR is heard at the lower left sternal border. It is often soft but becomes louder on inspiration. Doppler echocardiography is sensitive for the detection and quantification of TR. The primary therapy of functional TR is directed at the conditions responsible for the elevated right ventricular size or pressure

as well as diuretic therapy; surgical repair of the valve is indicated in severe cases.

PULMONIC VALVE DISEASE

Pulmonic Stenosis

Pulmonic stenosis (PS) is rare, and its cause is almost always congenital deformity of the valve. Severe cases are associated with a pressure gradient of greater than 80 mm Hg, moderate cases with a gradient of 40–80 mm Hg, and mild cases with a gradient of less than 40 mm Hg. Only those with moderate to severe gradients are symptomatic. Transcatheter balloon valvuloplasty is usually effective therapy for patients with severe or symptomatic PS.

Pulmonic Regurgitation

Pulmonic regurgitation most commonly develops in the setting of severe pulmonary hypertension and results from dilatation of the valve ring by the enlarged pulmonary artery. Auscultation reveals a high-pitched decrescendo murmur along the left sternal border that is often indistinguishable from AR (the two conditions are easily differentiated by Doppler echocardiography).

PROSTHETIC VALVES

The patient who undergoes valve replacement surgery often benefits dramatically from hemodynamic and symptomatic improvement, but also acquires a new set of potential complications related to the intracardiac prosthesis itself. Because all available valve substitutes have certain limitations, valve replacement surgery is not a true "cure."

Currently available valve substitutes are either mechanical or bioprosthetic (derived from animal or human tissue) in construction (Fig. 8.9). Older mechanical valves include a ball-in-cage design, the bulky shape of which often left a significant valvular gradient and occasionally produced intravascular hemolysis from mechanical red blood cell trauma. This valve, however, also has an impressive record for valve durabil-

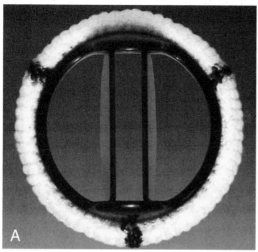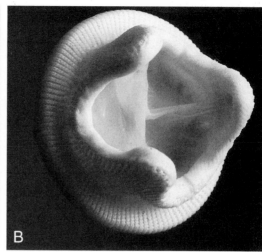

Figure 8.9. **Examples of prosthetic heart valves. A.** St. Jude mechanical bi-leaflet valve in the open position. (Courtesy of St. Jude Medical, Inc., St. Paul, MN.) **B.** A bioprosthetic aortic valve with leaflets in the closed position. (Courtesy of Medtronic, Inc., Minneapolis, MN.)

ity, with some models functioning well for more than 30 years. Newer mechanical valves, such as the St. Jude bileaflet prosthesis, provide a lower profile and superior hemodynamics without an apparent sacrifice of durability. It is an example of a hinged bi-leaflet valve consisting of two Pyrolyte carbon discs (see Fig. 8.9) that open opposite one another.

Mechanical valves, while extremely durable, present foreign thrombogenic surfaces to the circulating blood and require lifelong anticoagulation (usually with oral warfarin) to prevent thromboembolism.

The most commonly used bioprostheses (tissue valves) are made from glutaraldehyde-fixed porcine valves secured in a support frame. In recent years, bovine pericardium and human homograft (cryopreserved from human cadavers) prostheses have also been introduced. Bioprosthetic valves have limited durability compared with mechanical valves, and structural failure occurs in up to 50% of valves at 10 years, with failure rates accelerating thereafter. Structural failure rates vary greatly depending on the position of the valve. For example, bioprosthetic valves in the mitral position deteriorate more rapidly than those in the aortic position, probably because valve closure occurs during systolic

contraction in the mitral position and is therefore associated with higher leaflet stresses than those experienced by leaflets in the aortic position that close under lower diastolic pressures. The principal causes of bioprosthetic valve failure include leaflet tears and calcification. Despite their increased rate of deterioration, bioprosthetic valves have a very low rate of thromboembolism and do not require long-term anticoagulation therapy.

Common to all types of valve replacement is the risk of infective endocarditis, which occurs at an incidence of 1–2% per patient per year (see below). If endocarditis occurs in the first 60 days after surgery, the mortality rate is exceedingly high (50–80%). If endocarditis occurs later, mortality rates range from 20–50%. Reoperation is usually required if endocarditis involves a mechanical prosthesis, because an adjacent abscess is almost always present (the organism cannot infect the prosthetic material itself). Some cases of bioprosthetic valve endocarditis can be treated with antibiotic therapy alone.

Given their respective advantages and disadvantages, the mortality and complication rates of mechanical and bioprosthetic valves are similar for the first 10 years following replacement. Therefore, the decision about which type of prosthesis to use in an individual patient often centers on 1) the patient's expected lifespan in comparison to the functional lifespan of the valve, and 2) risk-versus-benefit considerations of chronic anticoagulation therapy. Mechanical valves are often recommended in younger patients and in those who will be tolerant of, and compliant with, anticoagulant therapy. Bioprosthetic valves are suitable choices in patients 65 years or older and in patients with contraindications to chronic anticoagulation therapy.

INFECTIVE ENDOCARDITIS

Infection of the endocardial surface of the heart, including the cardiac valves, by microbial organisms can lead to extensive tissue damage and is often fatal. Endocarditis carries a 10–30% mortality rate even with appropriate therapy and a 100% mortality rate if it is not recognized and treated correctly.

There are three clinically useful ways to classify infective endocarditis (IE): 1) by clinical course, 2) by host substrate, or 3) by the specific infecting microorganism. In the first classification scheme, IE is termed **acute bacterial endocarditis** (ABE) when the syndrome presents as an acute, fulminant infection, and a highly virulent and invasive organism such as *Staphylococcus aureus* is implicated. Because of the aggressiveness of the responsible microorganism, ABE may occur on previously healthy heart valves. When IE presents with a more insidious clinical course, it is termed **subacute bacterial endocarditis** (SBE), and less virulent organisms such as *Streptococcus viridans* are involved. SBE most frequently occurs in individuals with previous underlying valvular damage.

The second means of classification of IE is according to the host substrate: 1) native valve endocarditis (NVE), 2) prosthetic valve endocarditis (PVE), or 3) endocarditis in the setting of intravenous drug abuse (IVDA). Of these, NVE accounts for 60–80% of patients with endocarditis. Different microorganisms and clinical courses are associated with each of these categories. For example, the skin contaminant *Staphylococcus epidermidis*, is a common cause of prosthetic valve endocarditis, but that is rarely the case when endocarditis occurs on a native heart valve. Intravenous drug users are prone to *Staphylococcus aureus* and fungal endocarditis, particularly on right-sided heart valves.

The third classification of IE is according to the specific infecting microorganism (e.g., "*Staphylococcus aureus* endocarditis"). Although the remainder of this discussion focuses on the endocarditis syndromes based on clinical course, it is important to recognize that all three classifications of IE are used.

Pathogenesis

The pathogenesis of endocarditis requires several conditions: 1) endocardial surface injury, 2) thrombus formation at the site of injury, 3) bacterial entry into the circulation, and 4) bacterial adherence to the injured endocardial surface. The first two conditions provide an environment favorable to infection, whereas the latter two permit implantation of the organism on the endocardial surface. The most common cause of endothelial injury is turbulent blood flow resulting from underlying valvular disease; approximately 70% of patients with endocarditis have evidence of underlying structural or hemodynamic abnormalities (Table 8.7). Endothelial injury may also be incited by foreign material within the circulation, such as in-dwelling intravenous catheters or prosthetic heart valves.

Once an endocardial surface is injured, platelets adhere to the exposed subendocardial connective tissue and initiate the formation of a sterile thrombus (termed a "vegetation") through fibrin deposition. This process is referred to as nonbacterial thrombotic endocarditis (NBTE). NBTE makes the endocardium more hospitable to microbes in two ways. First, the fibrin-platelet deposits provide a surface for adherence by bacteria. Second, the fibrin covers adherent organisms and protects them from host defenses by inhibiting chemotaxis and migration of phagocytes.

When NBTE is present, the delivery of microorganisms in the bloodstream to the injured surface can lead to infective endocarditis. Three factors determine the ability

TABLE 8.7. Cardiac Lesions that Predispose to Endocarditis

- Rheumatic valvular disease
- Other acquired valvular lesions
    Calcific aortic stenosis
    Aortic regurgitation
    Mitral regurgitation
    Mitral valve prolapse (if murmur auscultated or detected by Doppler)
- Hypertrophic obstructive cardiomyopathy
- Congenital heart disease, including:
    Ventricular septal defect
    Patent ductus arteriosus
    Tetralogy of Fallot
    Aortic coarctation
    Bicuspid aortic valve
    Pulmonic stenosis
- Surgically implanted intravascular hardware, including:
    Prosthetic heart valves
    Pulmonary-systemic vascular shunts
    Ventriculo-atrial shunts for hydrocephalus
- Previous episode of endocarditis

of an organism to induce IE: 1) access to the bloodstream, 2) survival of the organism in the circulation, and 3) adherence of the bacteria to the endocardium. Bacteria can be introduced into the bloodstream whenever a mucosal or skin surface harboring an organism is traumatized, such as from the mouth during dental procedures or from the skin during intravenous drug use. However, while transient bacteremia is a relatively common event, only those microorganisms that are suited for survival in the circulation and are able to adhere to the vegetation will result in infective endocarditis. For example, gram-positive organisms account for approximately 90% of cases of endocarditis, in large part because of their resistance to destruction in the circulation by complement. Furthermore, the production by certain streptococcal species of dextran, a bacterial cell wall component that adheres to thrombus, correlates with their ability to incite endocarditis. Table 8.8 lists the infectious agents reported to be the most common causes of endocarditis and their relative frequencies of involvement. It should be noted, however, that recent trends show an increasing dominance of staphylococcal endocarditis in the tertiary-care hospital.

Once organisms adhere to the injured surface, they may be protected from phagocytic activity by the overlying fibrin. The organisms are then free to multiply, which further enlarges the infected vegetation. The latter provides a source for continuous bacteremia and can lead to several complications including 1) mechanical cardiac injury, 2) thrombotic or septic emboli, or 3) immune injury, mediated by antigen-antibody deposition. For example, local extension of the infection within the heart can result in progressive valvular damage (leading to heart failure), abscess formation, or erosion into the cardiac conduction system. Portions of a vegetation may embolize peripherally, often to the central nervous system, kidneys, or spleen, and incite infection or infarction of the target organs. Each of these is a potentially fatal complication. Additionally, immune complex deposition can result in glomerulonephritis, arthritis, or vasculitis.

Clinical Manifestations

A patient with *acute* IE is likely to report a history of an explosive and rapidly progressive illness with high fever and shaking chills. In contrast, *subacute* IE presents less dramatically with low-grade fever often accompanied by nonspecific constitutional symptoms such as fatigue, anorexia, weakness, myalgia, and night sweats. These symptoms are not specific for IE and could easily be mistaken for influenza or an up-

TABLE 8.8. Common Causes of Infective Endocarditis

Organism	Incidence (%)
Streptococci	70
Viridans	35
Enterococci	10
Other streptococci	25
Staphylococci	20
S. aureus	18
Coagulase-negative	2
Other organisms	10
(e.g., gram-negative, haemophilus, fungi)	

Reprinted with permission from Freeman R, Hall R. Infective endocarditis. In: Julian DG, et al. Diseases of the Heart. London: Bailliére Tindall, 1989:855.

per respiratory tract infection. Thus, the diagnosis of subacute IE requires a high index of suspicion. A history of a valvular lesion or other condition known to predispose to endocarditis is helpful. A thorough history should also inquire about intravenous drug use, recent dental procedures, or any other potential sources of bacteremia.

Cardiac examination may reveal a murmur representing the underlying valvular pathology that predisposed the patient to IE, or a *new* murmur of valvular insufficiency due to IE-induced damage. Right-sided valvular lesions, although rare in normal hosts, are particularly common in IVDA-associated endocarditis. Overall, murmurs are found more commonly in SBE than in ABE. However, serial examination in ABE may be especially useful as changes in a particular murmur (i.e., worsening regurgitation) over time may correspond with rapidly progressive valvular damage specific to ABE. During the course of endocarditis, severe valvular damage may result in congestive heart failure.

Other physical examination findings that may appear in IE are associated with septic embolism or immune complex deposition. Infected emboli may travel to any end-organ, including the skin, brain, kidney, viscera, or spleen. Central nervous system emboli are seen in up to 33% of patients, often resulting in new neurologic findings on physical examination. Injury to the kidneys, of embolic or immunologic origin, may manifest as flank pain, hematuria, or renal failure. Lung infarction (septic pulmonary embolism) or infection (pneumonia) are particularly common in right-sided endocarditis.

Embolic infarction and seeding of the vasa vasorum of arteries can cause localized aneurysm formation (termed a "mycotic aneurysm") that weakens the vessel wall and may rupture. Mycotic aneurysms may be found in the aorta, viscera, or peripheral organs but are particularly dangerous in cerebral vessels, as rupture can result in fatal intracranial hemorrhage.

Skin findings, due to septic embolism or immune complex vasculitis, are often collectively referred to as "peripheral stigmata of endocarditis." For example, petechiae may appear as tiny, circular, red-brown discolorations on mucosal surfaces or skin. "Splinter hemorrhages," the result of subungual microemboli, are small, longitudinal hemorrhages found beneath nails. Other peripheral stigmata of IE are rarely encountered today. They include painless, slightly nodular discolorations found on the palms and soles called "Janeway lesions." Tender, pea-sized, erythematous nodules found primarily in the pulp space of the fingers and toes are termed "Osler nodes." Emboli to the retina produce "Roth spots," microinfarctions that appear as white dots surrounded by hemorrhage.

The systemic inflammatory response produced by the infection is responsible for fever and splenomegaly as well as for a number of laboratory findings including an elevated white blood cell count with a leftward shift (increase in proportion of neutrophils and immature granulocytes), an elevated erythrocyte sedimentation rate, and in approximately 50% of cases, an elevated serum rheumatoid factor.

The *electrocardiogram* may help identify extension of the infection into the cardiac conduction system, manifest by various degrees of heart block or new arrhythmias. *Echocardiography* is used to visualize vegetations, valvular dysfunction, and associated abscess formation. Echocardiographic assessment can consist of transthoracic echocardiography (TTE) or transesophageal echocardiography (TEE) as described in Chapter 3. TTE is useful in detecting large vegetations and those involving right-sided heart valves. This technique has the advantage of being noninvasive and easy to obtain. However, while the estimated *specificity* of TTE for vegetations is high, the *sensitivity* for finding vegetations is less than 60%. TEE, on the other hand, is much more sensitive (>90%) for the detection of small vegetations and can be particularly useful for the evaluation of infection involving prosthetic valves. The absence of vegetations visualized by TTE or TEE does not exclude the diagnosis of IE.

Central to the diagnosis and appropriate treatment of endocarditis is the identification of the responsible microorganism by

TABLE 8.9. Duke Criteria for Diagnosis of Bacterial Endocarditis[a]

Major Criteria	Minor Criteria
A. Positive blood culture defined as: • Typical microorganism for IE from two separate blood cultures: Viridans streptococci, *S. bovis*, HACEK group; *or S. aureus* or *enterococci*, in the absence of a primary focus OR • Microorganisms consistent with IE from persistently positive blood cultures: • Blood cultures drawn > 12 hours apart, *or* • All of three, or a majority of four, separate cultures drawn at least 1 hour apart B. Evidence of endocardial involvement • Echocardiogram positive for endocarditis: • Oscillating intracardiac mass, *or* • Myocardial abscess, *or* • New partial detachment of prosthetic valve OR • New valvular regurgitation	Predisposing cardiac condition or intravenous drug use Fever (≥ 38.0° C) Vascular phenomena (septic arterial or pulmonary emboli, mycotic aneurysm, intracranial hemorrhage, conjunctival hemorrhage, Janeway lesions) Immunologic phenomena (glomerulonephritis, Osler's nodes, Roth spots, + rheumatoid factor) Positive blood cultures not meeting major criteria or serologic evidence of infection with organism consistent with IE Echocardiogram consistent with IE but not meeting major criteria

aDiagnosis of definitive endocarditis requires two major criteria, one major criteria plus three minor criteria, or five minor criteria.
IE, infective endocarditis; HACEK, *Haemophilus* spp., *Actinobacillus actinomycetemcomitans, Cardiobacterium hominis, Eikenella* spp. and *Kingella kingae.*
Modified from Durack DT, Lukes AS, Bright DK et al. New criteria for diagnosis of infective endocarditis: Utilization of specific echocardiographic findings. Am J Med 1994;96:200–209.

blood culture. Once positive culture results are obtained, treatment can be tailored to the causative organism according to its antibiotic sensitivities. A specific etiologic agent will be identified by culture approximately 95% of the time. Blood cultures may fail to grow the responsible organism if antibiotics have been recently administered or if the organism has unusual growth requirements.

Even after a careful history, examination, and evaluation of laboratory data, the diagnosis of IE can be elusive. In other cases, the finding of a positive blood culture can be misleading for this diagnosis. Attempts have therefore been made to standardize diagnostic criteria for endocarditis, resulting in the now widely used Duke criteria (Table 8.9). To confirm the diagnosis of endocarditis, either two major criteria, one major and three minor criteria, or five minor criteria must be met.

Treatment of endocarditis entails prolonged (4–6 weeks) high-dose intravenous antibiotic therapy. Although empiric broad-spectrum antibiotics may be used (after blood cultures are obtained!) in patients who are severely ill or hemodynamically unstable, specific, tailored therapy is prefer-

able once the causative microorganism has been identified. Surgical evaluation and intervention, usually with valve replacement, is indicated for patients with persistent bacteremia despite maximal antibiotic therapy, patients with severe valvular dysfunction leading to heart failure, and patients who develop myocardial abscesses or experience recurrent thromboembolic events.

Perhaps the most important aspect of therapy is prevention of endocarditis by administering specific antibiotics before procedures that result in bacteremia in susceptible individuals (i.e., those with underlying structural heart disease) (Table 8.10). Although randomized controlled trials have

TABLE 8.10. Procedures Warranting Endocarditis Prophylaxis

Dental manipulations that produce gingival bleeding
Rigid bronchoscopy and surgery of the upper respiratory tract
Genitourinary procedures, including:
  Indwelling bladder catheter
  Cystoscopy
  Prostatectomy
  Vaginal delivery (if peripartum infection present)
Gastrointestinal surgery, including cholecystectomy

TABLE 8.11. Summary of Major Valvular Lesions

Valve Lesion	Causes	Symptoms	Physical Findings	Compensatory Mechanisms
Mitral stenosis	Sequella of rheumatic fever	• Symptoms of left-sided (and later right-sided) heart failure[a]	• Loud S_1 • Opening snap • Diastolic rumble	• Pulmonary arteriolar constriction "protects" pulmonary vasculature
Mitral regurgitation	*Acute:* • Endocarditis • Ruptured chordae • Papillary muscle dysfunction *Chronic:* • Rheumatic • Mitral prolapse • Calcified annulus • LV dilatation	*Acute:* • Pulmonary edema *Chronic:* • Symptoms of left-sided heart failure[a] and low cardiac output (e.g., fatigue)	• Widely split S_2 • Holosystolic murmur at apex	*Acute:* • Frank-Starling mechanism increases stroke volume and maintains normal end-systolic volume *Chronic:* • Left atrial dilatation serves as volume "sink"
Aortic stenosis	• Congenital • Rheumatic • Senile calcific	• Chest pain • Syncope • Dyspnea on exertion	*Carotids:* delayed upstroke and decreased volume *Palpation:* suprasternal thrill *Auscultation:* • Soft A_2 • Late-peaking systolic ejection-type murmur	• Compensatory left ventricular hypertrophy
Aortic regurgitation	• Congenital (e.g., bicuspid valve) • Endocarditis • Rheumatic • Aortic root dilatation	• Dyspnea on exertion • Chest pain (sometimes)	• Wide pulse pressure • Bounding pulses • Early diastolic decrescendo murmur	• Frank-Starling mechanism increases stroke volume and maintains normal end-systolic volume • (Chronic) left ventricular hypertrophy

[a]Symptoms of left-sided heart failure include exertional dyspnea, orthopnea, paroxysmal nocturnal dyspnea; symptoms of right-sided heart failure include peripheral edema, abdominal bloating, and right upper quadrant tenderness (hepatic enlargement).

not been performed to demonstrate the efficacy of antibiotic prophylaxis against IE, such practice has become widespread.

SUMMARY

Valvular heart disease can be a significant source of disability and mortality. From simple bedside observations to complex physiologic measurements, much has been learned about the pathophysiology of these conditions. A summary of the important findings associated with major valve lesions is presented in Table 8.11.

Acknowledgments   Contributors to the previous editions of this chapter were Edward Chan, MD; Elia Duh, MD; Brian Stidham, MD; Stephen K. Frankel, MD; John A. Bittl, MD; and Leonard S. Lilly, MD.

ADDITIONAL READING

Bonow RO, Carabello B, de Leon AS Jr, et al. ACC/AHA guidelines for the management of patients with valvular heart disease: executive summary: a report of the American College of Cardiology/American Heart Association Task Force on Practice Guidelines. Circulation 1998;98:1949–1984.

Cabell CH, Jollis JG, Peterson GE, et al. Changing patient characteristics and the effect on mortality in endocarditis. Arch Intern Med 2002;162:90–94.

Carabello BA, Crawford FA. Valvular heart disease. N Engl J Med 1997;337:32–41.

Carroll JD, Feldman T. Percutaneous mitral balloon valvotomy and the new demographics of mitral stenosis. JAMA 1993;270:1731–1736.

Dajani AS, Ayoub E, Bierman FZ, et al. Guidelines for the diagnosis of rheumatic fever: Jones criteria, updated 1992. Circulation 1993;87:302–307.

Dajani AS, Taubert KA, Wilson W, et al. Prevention of bacterial endocarditis: recommendations by the American Heart Association. JAMA 1997;277:1794–1801.

Durack DT, Lukes AS, Bright DK. New criteria for diagnosis of infective endocarditis: utilization of specific echocardiographic findings: Duke Endocarditis Service. Am J Med 1994;96:211–219.

Freed LA, Levy D, Levine RA, et al. Prevalence and clinical outcome of mitral valve prolapse. N Engl J Med 1999;341:1–7.

Jamieson WRE, Edwards FH, Schwartz M, et al. Risk stratification for cardiac valve replacement. National cardiac surgery database. Ann Thorac Surg 1999;67:943–951.

Mylonakis E, Calderwood SB. Medical progress: infective endocarditis in adults. N Engl J Med 2001;345:1318–1330.

Pellikka PA, Nishimura RA, Bailey KR, et al. The natural history of adults with asymptomatic, hemodynamically significant aortic stenosis. J Am Coll Cardiol 1990;15:1012–1017.

Scognamiglio R, Rahimtoola SH, Fasoli G, et al. Nifedipine in asymptomatic patients with severe aortic regurgitation and normal left ventricular function. N Engl J Med 1994;331:689–694.

Vongpatanasin W, Hillis LD, Lange RA. Medical progress: prosthetic heart valves. N Engl J Med 1996;335:407–416.

Wisenbaugh T. Mitral valve disease. Curr Opin Cardiol 1994;9:146–151.

Heart Failure

George S.M. Dyer
and Michael A. Fifer

Physiology
 Determinants of Contractile Function in the Intact
  Heart
 Pressure-Volume Loops
Pathophysiology of Heart Failure
 Systolic Dysfunction
 Diastolic Dysfunction
 Right-Sided Heart Failure
Compensatory Mechanisms
 Frank-Starling Mechanism
 Neurohormonal Alterations
 Ventricular Hypertrophy and Remodeling
Myocyte Loss and Cellular Dysfunction
Precipitating Factors

Clinical Manifestations
 Symptoms
 Physical Signs
 Laboratory Tests
Prognosis
Treatment
 Diuretics
 Vasodilators
 Inotropic Drugs
 β-Blockers
 Additional Therapies
 Treatment of Diastolic Dysfunction
Acute Pulmonary Edema

The heart normally accepts blood at low filling pressures during diastole and then propels it forward at higher pressures in systole. Heart failure is defined as *the inability of the heart to pump blood forward at a sufficient rate to meet the metabolic demands of the body ("forward failure"), or the ability to do so only if the cardiac filling pressures are abnormally high ("backward failure"), or both.* Although conditions outside the heart may cause this definition to be met through inadequate tissue perfusion (e.g., severe hemorrhage) or increased metabolic demands (e.g., hyperthyroidism), in this chapter only *cardiac* causes of heart failure are considered.

Heart failure may be the final and most severe manifestation of nearly every form of cardiac disease, including coronary atherosclerosis, myocardial infarction, valvular diseases, hypertension, congenital heart disease, and the cardiomyopathies. More than 400,000 new cases of heart failure develop in the United States each year, and approximately 5 million people currently have this condition. It accounts for more than 12 million yearly medical office visits and is the most common diagnosis of hos-

pitalized patients age 65 and older. The incidence of heart failure is actually *increasing*, in part because the population is aging, and also because of interventions that prolong survival after acute cardiac insults such as myocardial infarction.

Heart failure most commonly results from conditions of impaired left ventricular function. Thus, this chapter begins by reviewing the physiology of normal myocardial contraction and relaxation.

PHYSIOLOGY

Experimental studies of isolated cardiac muscle segments have taught us several important physiologic principles that can be applied to the intact heart.

As an experimental muscle segment is stretched apart, the relation between its length and the tension it passively develops is curvilinear, reflecting its intrinsic elastic properties (Fig. 9.1A, lower curve). If the muscle is first passively stretched and then stimulated to contract while its ends are held at fixed positions (termed an "isometric" contraction), the total tension (active +

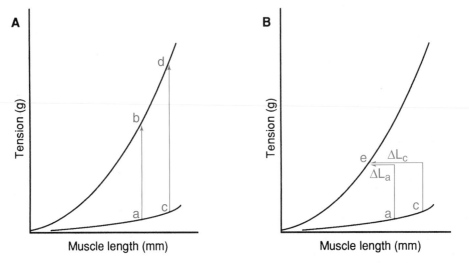

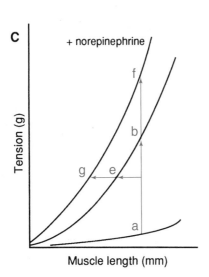

Figure 9.1. **A.** Passive (lower curve) and total (upper curve) length-tension relations for isolated cat papillary muscle. Lines ab and cd represent the force developed during isometric contractions. Initial passive muscle length c is longer (i.e., has been stretched more) than length a and therefore has a greater passive tension. When the muscle segments are stimulated to contract, the muscle with the longer initial length generates greater total tension (point d versus point b). **B.** If the muscle fiber preparation is allowed to shorten against a fixed load, the length at the end of the contraction is dependent on the load but not the initial fiber length; stimulation at point a or c results in the same final fiber length (e). Thus, the muscle that starts at length c shortens a greater distance (ΔL_c) than the muscle at length a (ΔL_a). **C.** The uppermost curve is the length-tension relation in the presence of the positive inotropic agent norepinephrine. For any given initial length, an isometric contraction in the presence of norepinephrine generates greater force (point f) than one in the absence of norepinephrine (point b). When contracting against a fixed load, the presence of norepinephrine causes greater muscle fiber shortening and a smaller final muscle length (point g) compared with contraction in the absence of the inotropic agent (point e). (Adapted from Downing SE, Sonnenblick EH. Cardiac muscle mechanics and ventricular performance: force and time parameters. Am J Physiol 1964;207:705–715.)

passive tension) generated by the fibers is proportional to the length of the muscle at the time of stimulation (see Fig. 9.1A, upper curve). That is, stretching the muscle before stimulation optimizes the overlap of myosin and actin filaments, increasing the number of cross bridges and the force of contraction. Stretching cardiac muscle fibers also increases the sensitivity of the myofilaments to calcium, which further augments force development.

The relationship between the initial fiber length and force development is of great importance in the intact heart: within a physiologic range, the larger the ventricular volume during diastole, the more the fibers are stretched before stimulation, and the greater will be the force of the next contraction. This is the basis of the Frank-Starling relationship, the observation that ventricular output increases in relation to the **preload** (the stretch on the myocardial fibers before contraction).

A second observation from the isolated muscle experiments arises when the fibers are not tethered at a fixed length but are allowed to *shorten* during stimulation against a fixed load (termed the **afterload**). In this situation (termed an "isotonic" contraction), the final length of the muscle at the end of contraction is directly related to the magnitude of the load, but is *independent* of the length of the muscle before stimulation (see Fig. 9.1B). That is, 1) the tension generated by the fiber is equal to the fixed load; 2) the greater the load opposing contraction, the less the muscle fiber can shorten; 3) if the fiber is stretched to a longer length before stimulation but the afterload is kept constant, the muscle shortens a greater distance and attains the same final length at the end of contraction; and 4) the maximum tension that a fiber can produce during isotonic contraction (i.e., such that the fiber is just unable to shorten) is the same as the force produced by an isometric contraction for the applied preload. The concept of afterload is also relevant to the intact heart: the pressure generated by the ventricle and the size of the chamber at the end of each contraction depend on the load against which the ventricle contracts (i.e., largely the arterial pressure), but are independent of the stretch on the myocardial fibers before contraction.

A third key experimental observation relates to myocardial **contractility** (also termed the **inotropic state**), which accounts for changes in the force of contraction independent of the initial fiber length and afterload. Contractility generally reflects chemical and hormonal influences on cardiac contraction, such as exposure to catecholamines. When contractility is enhanced pharmacologically (e.g., by a norepinephrine infusion), the relation between initial fiber length and force developed during contraction is shifted upward (see Fig. 9.1C) such that a greater total tension develops with isometric contraction at any given preload. Similarly, when contractility is augmented and the cardiac muscle is allowed to shorten against a fixed afterload, the fiber will contract to a greater extent and achieve

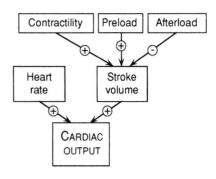

Figure 9.2. **Key mediators of cardiac output.** Determinants of the stroke volume include contractility, preload, and afterload. Cardiac output = heart rate × stroke volume.

a shorter final fiber length compared with the normal state. Enhanced contractility is likely induced by an increase in the cycling rate of actin-myosin cross-bridge formation.

Determinants of Contractile Function in the Intact Heart

In a healthy individual, the cardiac output is matched to the body's total metabolic need. Cardiac output (CO) is equal to the product of stroke volume (SV, the volume of blood ejected with each contraction) and the heart rate (HR):

$$CO = SV \times HR$$

The three major determinants of stroke volume are preload, afterload, and myocardial contractility, as shown in Figure 9.2.

Preload

The concept of preload (Table 9.1) in the intact heart was described by physiologists Frank and Starling a century ago. In experimental preparations, they showed that within physiologic limits, the more a normal ventricle is distended (i.e., filled with blood) during diastole, the greater the volume of blood ejected during the next systolic contraction. This relationship is illustrated graphically by the Frank-Starling curve, also known as the ventricular function curve (Fig. 9.3). The graph relates a measurement of cardiac performance (such

TABLE 9.1. Terms Related to Cardiac Performance

Term	Definition
Preload	The ventricular wall tension at the end of diastole. In clinical terms, it is the stretch on the ventricular fibers just before contraction, often approximated by the end-diastolic volume or end-diastolic pressure
Afterload	The ventricular wall tension during contraction; the resistance that must be overcome for the ventricle to eject its contents. It is often approximated by the systolic ventricular (or arterial) pressure
Contractility (inotropic state)	Property of heart muscle that accounts for changes in the strength of contraction, independent of the preload and afterload. Often reflects chemical or hormonal influences (e.g., catecholamines) on the force of contraction
Stroke volume	Volume of blood ejected from the ventricle during systole (= end-diastolic volume − end-systolic volume)
Ejection fraction (EF)	The fraction of end-diastolic volume ejected from the ventricle during each systolic contraction (normal range = 55–75%) $$EF = \frac{\text{stroke volume}}{\text{end-diastolic volume}}$$
Cardiac output	Volume of blood ejected from the ventricle per minute (= stroke volume × heart rate)
Compliance	Intrinsic property of a chamber that describes its pressure-volume relationship during filling. Reflects the ease or difficulty with which the chamber can be filled. Strictly defined, $$\text{Compliance} = \frac{\Delta \text{Volume}}{\Delta \text{Pressure}}$$

as cardiac output or stroke volume) on the vertical axis as a function of preload on the horizontal axis. As described above, the preload can be thought of as the amount of myocardial stretch at the end of diastole, just before contraction. Measurements that correlate with myocardial stretch, and that are often used to indicate the preload on the horizontal axis, are the ventricular end-diastolic volume (EDV) or end-diastolic pressure (EDP). Conditions that decrease intravascular volume, and thereby reduce ventricular preload (e.g., dehydration or severe hemorrhage), result in a smaller end-diastolic volume, and hence, a reduced stroke volume during contraction. Conversely, an increased volume within the left ventricle during diastole (e.g., a large intravenous infusion) results in a greater than normal stroke volume.

Afterload

Afterload (see Table 9.1) in the intact heart reflects the resistance that the ventricle must overcome to empty its contents. It is more formally defined as the ventricular wall stress that develops during systolic ejection. Wall stress (σ), like pressure, is expressed as force per unit area, and for the left ventricle, may be estimated from the LaPlace relation for a hollow sphere:

$$\sigma = \frac{P \cdot r}{2h}$$

in which P is ventricular pressure, r is ventricular chamber radius, and h is ventricular wall thickness. In general, a useful measurement to estimate the afterload is the arterial systolic pressure. Ventricular wall stress increases in response to a higher pressure load (e.g., hypertension) or an increased chamber size (e.g., a dilated left ventricle seen in many types of heart failure). Conversely, as discussed below, an increase in wall thickness serves a compensatory role in *reducing* wall stress, as the force is distributed over a greater mass per unit surface area of ventricular muscle.

Contractility

In the intact heart, as in the isolated muscle preparation, contractility accounts for

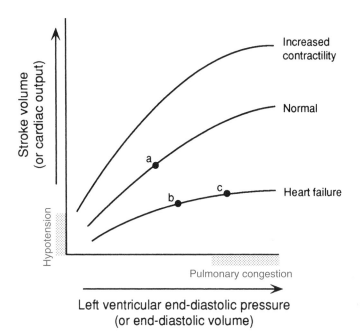

Figure 9.3. **Left ventricular (LV) performance (Frank-Starling) curves relate preload, measured as LV end-diastolic volume (EDV) or pressure (EDP), to cardiac performance, measured as ventricular stroke volume or cardiac output.** On the curve of a normal individual (middle line), cardiac performance continuously increases as a function of preload. States of increased contractility (e.g., norepinephrine infusion) are characterized by an augmented stroke volume at any level of preload (upper line). Conversely, decreased LV contractility (commonly associated with heart failure) is characterized by a curve that is shifted downward (lower line). Point a is an example of a normal individual at rest. Point b represents the same individual after developing systolic dysfunction and heart failure (e.g., after a large myocardial infarction): stroke volume has fallen, and the decreased LV emptying results in elevation of the EDV. Because point b is on the ascending portion of the curve, the elevated EDV serves a compensatory role because it results in an increase in subsequent stroke volume, albeit much less so than if operating on the normal curve. Further augmentation of LV filling (e.g., increased circulating volume) in the heart failure patient is represented by point c, which resides on the relatively flat part of the curve: stroke volume is only slightly augmented, but the significantly increased EDP results in pulmonary congestion.

changes in the force generated by the myocardium for a given set of preload and afterload conditions. By relating a measure of ventricular performance (stroke volume or cardiac output) to preload (left ventricular end-diastolic pressure or volume), each Frank-Starling curve is a reflection of the heart's current inotropic state (see Fig. 9.3). The effect on stroke volume by an alteration in preload is reflected by a change in position along a particular Frank-Starling curve. A change in contractility, on the other hand, actually shifts the entire curve in an upward or downward direction. Thus, when contractility is enhanced pharmacologically (e.g., by an infusion of norepinephrine), the ventricular performance curve is displaced upward such that at any

given preload, the stroke volume is increased. Conversely, when a drug that reduces contractility is administered, or the ventricle's contractile function is impaired (as in many types of heart failure), the curve shifts in a downward direction, so that at any given preload, the stroke volume and cardiac output are reduced.

Pressure-Volume Loops

Another useful graphic display to illustrate the determinants of cardiac function is the ventricular pressure-volume loop, which relates changes in ventricular volume to corresponding changes in pressure throughout the cardiac cycle (Fig. 9.4). In the left ventricle, filling of the chamber be-

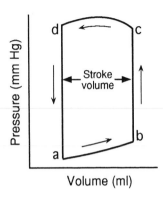

Figure 9.4. **Example of a normal left ventricular (LV) pressure-volume loop.** At point a the mitral valve opens. During diastolic filling of the LV (line ab), the volume increases in association with a gradual rise in pressure. When ventricular contraction commences and its pressure exceeds that of the left atrium, the mitral valve (MV) closes (point b) and iso-volumetric contraction of the LV ensues (the aortic valve is not yet open, and no blood leaves the chamber), as shown by line bc. When LV pressure rises to that in the aorta, the aortic valve (AV) opens (point c) and ejection begins. The volume within the LV declines during ejection (line cd), but LV pressure continues to rise until ventricular relaxation commences. At point d, the LV pressure during relaxation falls below that in the aorta, and the AV closes, leading to isovolumetric relaxation (line da). As the LV pressure falls further, the mitral valve reopens (point a). Point b represents the end-diastolic volume (EDV) and pressure, and point d is the end-systolic volume (ESV) and pressure. Stroke volume is the difference between the EDV and ESV.

gins after the mitral valve opens in early diastole (point a). The curve between points a and b represents diastolic filling. As the volume increases during diastole, it is associated with a small rise in pressure, in accordance with the passive length-tension properties or **compliance** (see Table 9.1) of the myocardium, analogous to the lower curve in Figure 9.1A for an isolated muscle preparation. Next, the onset of left ventricular systolic contraction causes the ventricular pressure to rise. When the LV pressure exceeds that of the left atrium (point b), the mitral valve is forced to close. As the pressure continues to increase, the ventricular volume does not immediately change, because the aortic valve has not yet opened; therefore, this phase is called **isovolumetric contraction.** When the ventricular pressure reaches the aortic diastolic pressure, the aortic valve is forced to open (point c), and

ejection of blood into the aorta commences. During ejection, the volume within the ventricle decreases, but its pressure continues to rise until ventricular relaxation begins. The pressure against which the ventricle ejects (afterload) is represented by the curve cd. Ejection ends during ventricular relaxation, when the pressure falls below that of the aorta and the aortic valve closes (point d). As the ventricle continues to relax, its pressure declines while its volume remains constant since the mitral valve has not yet opened (this phase is known as **isovolumetric relaxation**). When the ventricular pressure falls below that of the left atrium, the mitral valve opens again (point a), and the cycle repeats. Note that point b represents the pressure and volume at the end of diastole, whereas point d represents the pressure and volume at the end of systole. The difference between the end-diastolic and end-systolic volumes represents the quantity of blood ejected during contraction (i.e., the stroke volume).

Changes in any of the determinants of cardiac function are reflected by alterations in the pressure-volume loop. By analyzing the effects of a change in an individual parameter (preload, afterload, or contractility) on the pressure-volume relationship, the resulting alterations in ventricular pressure and stroke volume can be predicted (Fig. 9.5).

Alterations in Preload

If afterload and contractility are held constant, but preload is caused to increase (e.g., by administration of intravenous fluids), left ventricular end-diastolic volume will rise. This increase in preload augments the stroke volume via the Frank-Starling mechanism such that the end-systolic volume achieved is the same as it was before increasing the preload. This means that the normal LV is able to adjust its stroke volume and effectively empty its contents to match its diastolic filling volume, as long as contractility and afterload are kept constant.

Although end-diastolic volume and end-diastolic pressure are often used interchangeably as markers for preload, the relationship between filling volume and pressure known as ventricular compliance (see Table 9.1) largely governs the extent of ventricular filling. If ventricular compliance is reduced (e.g., in severe left ventricular hypertrophy), then the slope of the diastolic filling curve (see segment ab in Fig. 9.4) becomes steeper, as discussed below. A "stiff" or poorly compliant ventricle reduces the ability of the chamber to fill during diastole, resulting in a lower than normal ventricular end-diastolic volume. In this circumstance, if afterload and contractility remain unaltered, the *end-systolic* volume will remain unchanged, and therefore the stroke volume will be reduced.

Alterations in Afterload

If preload and contractility are held constant and afterload is augmented (e.g., in high-impedance states such as hyperten-

sion or aortic stenosis), then the pressure generated by the LV during ejection is caused to increase. In this situation, more ventricular work is expended in overcoming the resistance to ejection and less fiber shortening takes place. As shown in Figure 9-5B, an increase in afterload results in a higher ventricular systolic pressure and a higher than normal LV end-systolic volume. Thus, in the setting of increased afterload, the ventricular stroke volume (EDV–ESV) is reduced.

The dependence of the end-systolic volume on afterload is approximately linear: the greater the afterload, the higher the end-systolic volume. This relationship is depicted in Figure 9.5 as the end-systolic pressure volume relation (ESPVR) and is analogous to the total tension curve in the isolated muscle experiments described above.

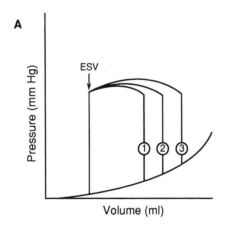

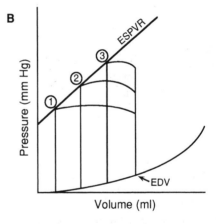

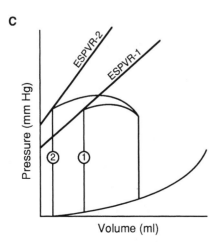

Figure 9.5. **The effect of varying preload, afterload, and contractility on the pressure-volume loop. A.** When arterial pressure (afterload) and contractility are held constant, sequential increases (lines 1, 2, 3) in preload (measured in this case as end-diastolic volume [EDV]) are associated with loops that have progressively higher stroke volumes but a constant end-systolic volume (ESV). **B.** When the preload (EDV) and contractility are held constant, sequential increases (points 1, 2, 3) in arterial pressure (afterload) are associated with loops that have progressively lower stroke volumes and higher end-systolic volumes. There is a nearly linear relationship between the afterload and ESV, termed the end-systolic pressure-volume relation (ESPVR). **C.** A positive inotropic intervention shifts the end-systolic pressure-volume relation upward and leftward from ESPVR-1 to ESPVR-2, resulting in loop 2, which has a larger stroke volume, and smaller end-systolic volume than the original loop 1.

Alterations in Contractility

The slope of the ESPVR line on the pressure-volume loop graph is a function of cardiac contractility. In conditions of increased contractility, the ESPVR slope becomes more steep; that is, it shifts upward and toward the left. Hence, at any given preload or afterload, the ventricle empties more completely (the stroke volume increases) and results in a smaller than normal end-systolic volume (see Fig. 9.5C). Conversely, in situations of reduced contractility, the ESPVR line shifts downward, consistent with a decline in stroke volume and a higher end-systolic volume. Thus, the end-systolic volume is *dependent* on the afterload against which the ventricle contracts and the inotropic state, but is *independent* of the end-diastolic volume before contraction.

In summary, the important physiologic concepts in this section are:

1. Ventricular stroke volume is a function of preload, afterload, and contractility. SV rises when there is an increase in preload, a decrease in afterload, or augmented contractility.
2. Ventricular end-diastolic volume (or end-diastolic pressure) is often used as a representation of preload. The end-diastolic volume is influenced by the chamber's compliance.
3. Ventricular end-systolic volume depends on the afterload and contractility but not the preload.

PATHOPHYSIOLOGY OF HEART FAILURE

Chronic heart failure may result from a wide variety of cardiovascular insults. The etiologies can be grouped into those that cause heart failure because of 1) impaired contractility, 2) increased afterload, or 3) impaired ventricular filling. Heart failure that results from an abnormality of ventricular emptying (due to impaired contractility or excessive afterload) is termed *systolic dysfunction*, whereas that due to abnormalities of diastolic relaxation or ventricular filling is termed *diastolic dysfunction*. Approximately two-thirds of patients with heart

failure have systolic dysfunction, and the remainder primarily have diastolic dysfunction. Figure 9.6 presents a general schema of cardiac conditions that may result in heart failure. Although this schema applies to chronic forms of heart failure, it should be recognized that a sudden overwhelming cardiac load (e.g., as may occur with an acute hypertensive crisis [Chapter 13], acute myocardial infarction [Chapter 7], or acute valvular insufficiency [Chapter 8]) can result in an acute form of heart failure (e.g., pulmonary edema), discussed later in this chapter.

Systolic Dysfunction

In systolic dysfunction, there is a diminished capacity of the affected ventricle to eject blood because of impaired myocardial contractility or pressure overload (i.e., excessive afterload). Loss of contractility may result from destruction of myocytes, abnormal myocyte function, or fibrosis. Pressure overload impairs ventricular ejection by significantly increasing resistance to flow. Figure 9.7A depicts the effects of systolic dysfunction due to impaired contractility on the pressure-volume loop. The ESPVR is shifted downward such that systolic emptying ceases at a higher end-systolic volume than normal. As a result, the stroke volume falls. When normal pulmonary venous return is added to the increased end-systolic volume that has remained in the ventricle because of incomplete emptying, the diastolic chamber volume increases, resulting in a higher than normal end-diastolic volume and pressure. While that increase in preload induces a compensatory rise in stroke volume (via the Frank-Starling mechanism), impaired contractility and the reduced ejection fraction cause the end-systolic volume to remain elevated.

During diastole, the persistently elevated left ventricular pressure is transmitted to the left atrium (through the open mitral valve) and to the pulmonary veins and capillaries. An elevated pulmonary capillary hydrostatic pressure, when sufficiently high (usually >20 mm Hg), results in the transudation of fluid into the pulmonary

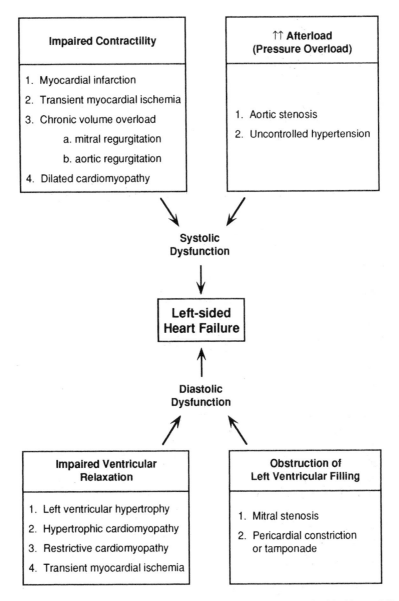

Figure 9.6. **Mechanisms and examples of conditions that cause left-sided heart failure.**

interstitium and symptoms of pulmonary congestion.

Diastolic Dysfunction

Approximately one-third of patients with clinical heart failure have normal ventricular contractile (systolic) function. Many of these individuals demonstrate abnormalities of *diastolic* function: either impaired early diastolic relaxation (an active, energy-dependent process), increased stiff-

ness of the ventricular wall (a passive property), or both. Acute myocardial ischemia is an example of a condition that *transiently* inhibits energy delivery and diastolic relaxation. Conversely, LV hypertrophy, fibrosis, or restrictive cardiomyopathy (see Chapter 10) causes the LV walls to become *chronically* stiffened. The effect of impaired diastolic function is reflected in the pressure-volume loop (see Fig. 9.7B): in diastole, filling of the ventricle occurs at higher than normal pressures because the lower part of

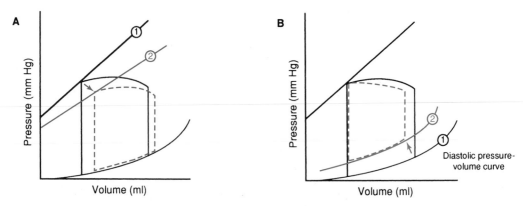

Figure 9.7. A. The normal pressure-volume loop (solid line) is compared with one demonstrating systolic dysfunction (dashed line). In systolic dysfunction due to decreased cardiac contractility, the end-systolic pressure-volume relation is shifted downward and rightward (from line 1 to line 2). As a result, the end-systolic volume (ESV) is increased (arrow). As normal venous return is added to the greater than normal ESV remaining in the ventricle, there is an obligatory increase in the end-diastolic volume (EDV) and pressure (preload), which serves a compensatory function by partially elevating stroke volume toward normal via the Frank-Starling mechanism. **B.** The pressure-volume loop of diastolic dysfunction due to increased stiffness (decreased compliance) of the ventricle (dashed line). The passive diastolic pressure-volume curve is shifted upward (from line 1 to line 2) such that at any diastolic volume, the ventricular pressure is greater than normal. The result is a decreased EDV (arrow) because of reduced filling of the stiffened ventricle at a higher than normal end-diastolic pressure.

the loop is shifted upward, due to the reduced chamber compliance. Patients with diastolic dysfunction often present with signs of vascular congestion because the elevated diastolic pressure is transmitted retrograde to the pulmonary and systemic veins.

Right-Sided Heart Failure

Whereas the above physiologic principles may be applied to right-sided and left-sided heart failure, there are distinct differences in function between the two ventricles. Compared with the left ventricle (LV), the right ventricle (RV) is a thin-walled, highly compliant chamber that accepts its blood volume at very low pressures and ejects against a low pulmonary vascular resistance. As a result of its high compliance, the RV has little difficulty accepting a wide range of filling volumes, without significant changes in its filling pressures. Conversely, the RV is quite susceptible to failure in situations that present a sudden increase in afterload, such as acute pulmonary embolism.

The most common cause of right-sided failure is actually left-sided heart failure (Table 9.2). In this situation, excessive after-

load confronts the right ventricle because of the elevated pulmonary vascular pressures that result from LV dysfunction. *Isolated* right heart failure is less common and usually reflects increased RV afterload due to diseases of the lung parenchyma or pulmonary vasculature. Right-sided heart disease that results from a primary pulmonary process is known as *cor pulmonale,* which often leads to right heart failure.

When the right ventricle fails, the elevated diastolic pressure is transmitted retrograde to the right atrium with subsequent congestion of the systemic veins, accompanied by signs of right-sided heart

---

TABLE 9.2. Examples of Conditions that Cause Right-Sided Heart Failure

Cardiac causes
  Left-sided heart failure
  Pulmonic valve stenosis
  Right ventricular infarction
Parenchymal pulmonary disease
  Chronic obstructive pulmonary disease
  Interstitial lung disease (e.g., sarcoidosis)
  Adult respiratory distress syndrome
  Chronic lung infection or bronchiectasis
Pulmonary vascular disease
  Pulmonary embolism
  Primary pulmonary hypertension

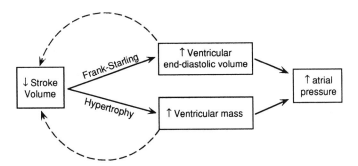

Figure 9.8. Compensatory mechanisms in heart failure. Both the Frank-Starling mechanism (which is invoked by the rise in ventricular end-diastolic volume) and myocardial hypertrophy (in response to pressure or volume overload) serve to maintain forward stroke volume (dashed lines). However, the chronic rise in EDV by the former, and increased ventricular stiffness by the latter, cause an increase in atrial pressure, which may result in manifestations of "backward" failure (e.g., pulmonary congestion in the case of left-sided heart failure).

failure (see below). Indirectly, isolated right heart failure may also influence left heart function: the decreased right ventricular output reduces blood return to the LV (↓ preload) and therefore left ventricular stroke volume may fall.

COMPENSATORY MECHANISMS

Several natural compensatory mechanisms are called into action in heart failure, which serve to buffer the fall in cardiac output and help to maintain sufficient blood pressure to perfuse the vital organs. These include 1) the Frank-Starling mechanism, 2) neurohormonal alterations, and 3) the development of myocardial hypertrophy and ventricular remodeling (Fig. 9.8).

Frank-Starling Mechanism

As shown in Figure 9.3, heart failure due to impaired left ventricular contractile function causes a downward shift of the ventricular performance curve. Therefore, at a given preload, stroke volume is decreased compared with normal. The reduced stroke volume results in incomplete chamber emptying; as a result, the volume of blood that accumulates in the ventricle during diastole is higher than normal (see Fig. 9.3, point b). This increased stretch on the myofibers acting via the Frank-Starling mechanism induces a greater stroke volume on subsequent contraction, which helps to empty the

enlarged LV and preserve forward cardiac output (see Fig 9.8). There are limits to this beneficial compensatory mechanism, however. In the case of severe heart failure and marked depression of contractility, the curve may be nearly flat at higher diastolic volumes, such that little augmentation of cardiac output is achieved by increased filling. Concurrently in such a circumstance, marked elevation of the end-diastolic volume and pressure (which is transmitted retrograde to the left atrium, pulmonary veins, and capillaries) may result in pulmonary congestion and edema (see Fig. 9.3, point c).

Neurohormonal Alterations

Neurohormonal activation encompasses a number of important compensatory mechanisms in heart failure that include 1) the adrenergic nervous system, 2) the renin-angiotensin system, and 3) increased production of antidiuretic hormone (ADH), all in response to decreased cardiac output (Fig. 9.9). In part, these mechanisms serve to increase systemic vascular resistance, which helps to maintain arterial perfusion to vital organs, even in the setting of a reduced cardiac output. That is, since blood pressure (BP) is equal to the product of cardiac output (CO) and total peripheral resistance (TPR):

$$BP = CO \times TPR$$

a rise in TPR induced by these compensatory mechanisms can nearly balance the

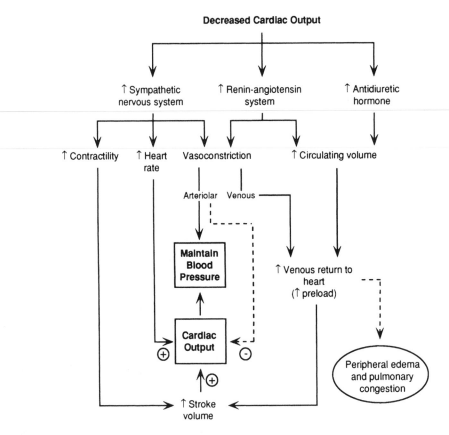

Figure 9.9. Compensatory neurohormonal stimulation develops in response to the reduced forward cardiac output and blood pressure of heart failure. Increased activity of the sympathetic nervous system, renin-angiotensin system, and antidiuretic hormone serve to support the cardiac output and blood pressure (boxes). However, adverse consequences of these activations (dashed lines) include an increase in afterload from excessive vasoconstriction (which may impede the cardiac output) and excess fluid retention, which contributes to peripheral edema and pulmonary congestion.

fall in CO, and in the early stages of heart failure maintain fairly normal BP. In addition, neurohormonal activation results in salt and water retention, which in turn increases intravascular volume and left ventricular preload, so as to maximize stroke volume via the Frank-Starling mechanism.

Although the acute effects of neurohormonal stimulation are compensatory and beneficial, chronic activation of these mechanisms often ultimately proves deleterious to the failing heart and contributes to a progressive downhill course, as described below.

Adrenergic Nervous System

The fall in cardiac output in heart failure is sensed as decreased perfusion pressure by baroreceptors in the carotid sinus and aortic arch. These receptors decrease their rate of firing in proportion to the fall in BP, and the signal is transmitted by the 9th and 10th cranial nerves to the cardiovascular control center in medulla. As a result, sympathetic outflow to the heart and peripheral circulation is increased, and parasympathetic tone is diminished. Three immediate consequences arise (see Fig. 9.9): 1) an increase in heart rate, 2) augmentation of ventricular contractility, and 3) vasoconstriction due to stimulation of α-receptors on the systemic veins and arteries.

The increased heart rate and ventricular contractility directly augment cardiac output (see Fig. 9.2). Vasoconstriction of the venous and arterial circulations is also *initially* beneficial. Venous constriction augments blood return to the heart, which increases preload and raises stroke volume through the Frank-Starling mechanism, if the ventricle is operating on the ascending portion of its ventricular performance curve (see Fig. 9.3). Arteriolar constriction increases the peripheral vascular resistance and therefore helps to maintain blood pressure (BP = CO × TPR). The regional distribution of α-receptors is such that during sympathetic stimulation, blood flow is redistributed to vital organs (e.g., heart and brain) at the expense of the skin, splanchnic viscera, and kidneys.

Renin-Angiotensin-Aldosterone System

This system is also activated early in patients with heart failure (see Fig. 9.9), mediated by increased renin release. The main stimuli for renin secretion from the juxtaglomerular cells of the kidney in heart failure patients include 1) decreased renal artery perfusion pressure secondary to low cardiac output, 2) decreased salt delivery to the macula densa of the kidney due to alterations in intrarenal hemodynamics, and 3) direct stimulation of juxtaglomerular β_2-receptors by the activated adrenergic nervous system.

Renin is an enzyme that cleaves circulating angiotensinogen to form angiotensin I, which is then rapidly cleaved by endothelial-cell bound angiotensin-converting enzyme (ACE) to form angiotensin II (AII), a potent vasoconstrictor (see Chapter 13). Increased AII constricts arterioles and raises total peripheral resistance, thereby helping to maintain systemic blood pressure. In addition, AII acts to increase intravascular volume by two mechanisms: 1) at the hypothalamus, it stimulates thirst and therefore water intake, and 2) it acts at the adrenal cortex to increase aldosterone secretion. The latter hormone promotes sodium reabsorption from the distal convoluted tubule of the kidney into the circulation (see Chapter 17), serving to augment intravascular volume. The rise in intravascular volume increases left ventricular preload and thereby augments cardiac output via the Frank-Starling mechanism in patients on the ascending portion of the ventricular performance curve (see Fig. 9.3).

Antidiuretic Hormone

Secretion of this hormone (also called arginine vasopressin) by the posterior pituitary is increased in many patients with heart failure, presumably mediated through left atrial and arterial baroreceptors, and by increased levels of AII. ADH contributes to increased intravascular volume because it promotes water retention in the distal nephron. The increased intravascular volume serves to augment left ventricular preload and cardiac output. ADH also appears to contribute to systemic vasoconstriction.

Although each of these neurohormonal activations in heart failure is initially beneficial, ultimately they prove harmful. For example, the increased circulating volume and augmented venous return to the heart may *worsen* engorgement of the lung vasculature, exacerbating congestive pulmonary symptoms. Furthermore, the elevated arteriolar resistance increases the afterload against which the failing left ventricle contracts and may *impair* stroke volume and reduce cardiac output (see Fig. 9.9). The increased heart rate augments metabolic demand and can therefore further reduce the performance of the failing heart. The continuous sympathetic activation results in downregulation of cardiac β-adrenergic receptors and upregulation of inhibitory G-proteins, contributing to a decrease in the myocardium's sensitivity to circulating catecholamines and a *reduced* inotropic response.

Chronically elevated levels of angiotensin II and aldosterone have additional detrimental effects. They provoke the production of cytokines (small proteins that mediate cell-cell communication and immune responses), activate macrophages, and stimulate fibroblasts, resulting in fibrosis and adverse remodeling of the failing heart.

Because the undesired consequences of chronic neurohormonal activation eventually outweigh their benefits, much of today's pharmacologic therapy of heart failure is designed to moderate these "compensatory" mechanisms, as will be examined below.

Conversely, the **natriuretic peptides** are natural "beneficial" hormones secreted in heart failure in response to increased intracardiac pressures. The best studied of these are atrial natriuretic peptide (ANP) and B-type natriuretic peptide (BNP). ANP is stored in atrial cells and is released in response to atrial distention. BNP is not detected in normal hearts but is produced when ventricular myocardium is subjected to hemodynamic stress (e.g., in heart failure or during myocardial infarction). Recent studies have shown a close relationship between serum BNP levels and the clinical severity of heart failure.

Actions of the natriuretic peptides are mediated via specific natriuretic receptors and are largely opposite to those of the other hormone systems activated in heart failure. They result in excretion of sodium and water, vasodilatation, inhibition of renin secretion, and antagonism of the effects of AII on aldosterone and vasopressin secretion. Whereas these effects are beneficial to patients with heart failure, they are usually not sufficient to fully counteract the vasoconstriction and volume-retaining effects of the other activated hormonal systems.

Another recently recognized substance that is released in heart failure is **endothelin,** a potent vasoconstrictor, derived from endothelial cells lining the vasculature (see Chapter 6). Drugs designed to inhibit endothelin receptors (and therefore blunt adverse vasoconstriction) improve LV function in heart failure, but long-term effects have not yet been studied.

Ventricular Hypertrophy and Remodeling

Ventricular hypertrophy and remodeling are important compensatory processes that develop over time in response to hemodynamic burdens. Wall stress (σ) is often increased in developing heart failure, because of either LV dilatation (increased chamber radius) or the need to generate high systolic pressures to overcome excessive afterload (e.g., in aortic stenosis or hypertension). A sustained increase in wall stress (along with neurohormonal and cytokine alterations)

stimulates the development of myocardial hypertrophy and deposition of extracellular matrix. This increased mass of muscle fibers serves as a compensatory mechanism that helps to maintain contractile force and *counteracts* the elevated ventricular wall stress (recall that wall thickness is in the denominator of the LaPlace wall stress formula). However, because of the increased stiffness of the hypertrophied wall, these benefits come at the expense of higher than normal diastolic ventricular pressures, which are transmitted to the left atrium and pulmonary vasculature (see Fig. 9.8).

The pattern of compensatory hypertrophy and remodeling that develops depends on whether the ventricle is subjected to chronic volume or pressure overload. Chronic chamber dilatation owing to *volume* overload (e.g., chronic mitral or aortic regurgitation) results in the synthesis of new sarcomeres in *series* with the old, causing the myocytes to elongate. The radius of the ventricular chamber therefore enlarges, doing so in proportion to the increase in wall thickness, and is termed *eccentric* hypertrophy. Chronic *pressure* overload (e.g., due to hypertension or aortic stenosis) results in the synthesis of sarcomeres in *parallel* with the old (i.e., the myocytes thicken), termed *concentric* hypertrophy. In this situation, the wall thickness increases without proportional chamber dilatation so that wall stress may be reduced substantially.

Such hypertrophy and remodeling help to reduce wall stress and maintain contractile force, but ultimately ventricular function deteriorates and causes the chamber to dilate out of proportion to wall thickness. When this occurs, the excessive hemodynamic burden on the contractile units produces a downward spiral of deterioration with progressive heart failure symptomatology.

MYOCYTE LOSS AND CELLULAR DYSFUNCTION

Impairment of ventricular function in heart failure may result from the actual loss of myocytes and/or impaired function of living myocytes. A loss of myocytes may be due to cellular *necrosis* (e.g., from myocardial infarction or exposure to cardiotoxic drugs such as doxorubicin) or *apoptosis* (programmed cell death). In apoptosis, genetic instructions activate intracellular pathways that cause the cell to fragment and undergo phagocytosis by other cells, without an inflammatory response. Factors implicated in triggering apoptosis in heart failure include elevated catecholamines, angiotensin II, inflammatory cytokines, and mechanical strain on the myocytes due to the augmented wall stress.

Even viable myocardium in heart failure is abnormal at the ultrastructural and molecular levels. Mechanical wall stress, neurohormonal activation, inflammatory cytokines (such as tumor necrosis factor-alpha [TNF-α]) are believed to activate changes in the genetic expression of contractile proteins, ion channels, catalytic enzymes, surface receptors, and secondary messengers in the myocyte. Recent experimental evidence has demonstrated such changes at the subcellular level that affect intracellular calcium handling by the sarcoplasmic reticulum, decrease the responsiveness of the myofilaments to calcium, impair excitation-contraction coupling, and alter cellular energy production. It is believed that the most important cellular factors contributing to dysfunction in heart failure are 1) a reduced cellular ability to maintain calcium homeostasis, and/or 2) changes in the production, availability, and utilization of high-energy phosphates. However, the exact subcellular alterations that result in heart failure have not yet been elucidated, and this remains one of the most active areas of cardiovascular research.

PRECIPITATING FACTORS

Many patients with heart failure remain asymptomatic for extended periods either because the impairment is mild or because cardiac dysfunction is balanced by the compensatory mechanisms described above. Often clinical manifestations occur only in the presence of precipitating factors that increase the cardiac workload and tip the balanced state into one of de-

compensation. Common precipitating factors are listed in Table 9.3. For example, conditions of increased metabolic demand such as fever or infection may not be matched by a sufficient increase in output by the failing heart, so that symptoms of cardiac insufficiency are precipitated. Tachyarrhythmias precipitate heart failure by decreasing diastolic ventricular filling time and by increasing myocardial oxygen demand. Excessively low heart rates directly cause a drop in cardiac output (remember, cardiac output = heart rate × stroke volume). An increase in salt ingestion, renal dysfunction, or failure to take prescribed diuretic medications may each increase the circulating volume, thus promoting systemic and pulmonary congestion. Uncontrolled hypertension depresses systolic function because of excessive afterload. A large pulmonary embolism results in both hypoxemia (and therefore decreased myocardial oxygen supply) and a substantial increase in right ventricular afterload. Ischemic insults (i.e., myocardial ischemia or infarction), ethanol ingestion, or negative inotropic medications (e.g., large doses of β-blockers and certain calcium channel blockers) can all depress myocardial contractility and precipitate

TABLE 9.3. Factors that may Precipitate Symptoms in Compensated Heart Failure

Increased metabolic demands
  Fever
  Infection
  Anemia
  Tachycardia
  Hyperthyroidism
  Pregnancy
Increased circulating volume (increased preload)
  Excessive sodium content in diet
  Excessive fluid administration
  Renal failure
Conditions that increase afterload
  Uncontrolled hypertension
  Pulmonary embolism (increased right ventricular afterload)
Conditions that impair contractility
  Negative inotropic medications
  Myocardial ischemia or infarction
  Ethanol ingestion
Failure to take prescribed heart failure medications
Excessively slow heart rate

symptoms in the otherwise compensated congestive heart failure patient.

CLINICAL MANIFESTATIONS

The clinical manifestations of heart failure result from impaired forward cardiac output and/or elevated venous pressures and relate to which of the ventricles has failed (Table 9.4). A patient may present with the chronic progressive symptoms of heart failure described here, or in certain cases with sudden decompensation of left-sided heart function (e.g., acute pulmonary edema, as described below).

Symptoms

The most prominent symptom of chronic left ventricular failure is *dyspnea* (breathlessness) on exertion. Controversy regarding the cause of this symptom has centered on whether it is primarily a manifestation of pulmonary venous congestion or decreased forward cardiac output. When the pulmonary venous pressure exceeds approximately 20 mm Hg, there is transudation of fluid into the pulmonary interstitium and congestion of the lung parenchyma. The resulting reduced pulmonary compliance increases the work of breathing to move the same volume of air. Moreover, the excess fluid in the interstitium compresses the walls of the bronchioles and alveoli, increasing the resistance to airflow and requiring greater effort of respiration. In addition, juxtacapillary receptors (J receptors) are stimulated which mediate rapid shallow breathing. The heart failure patient can also suffer from dyspnea even in the absence of pulmonary congestion, because reduced forward blood flow to the overworked respiratory muscles and accumulation of lactic acid may also contribute to that sensation. Heart failure may initially cause dyspnea only on exertion, but more severe dysfunction results in symptoms at rest as well.

Other manifestations of low forward output in heart failure may include a *dulled mental status* because of reduced cerebral perfusion and *impaired urine output* during the day because of decreased renal perfusion. The latter often gives way to increased urinary frequency at night *(nocturia)* when, while supine, blood flow is redistributed to the kidney, promoting renal perfusion and diuresis. Reduced skeletal muscle perfusion may result in *fatigue* and *weakness.*

Other congestive manifestations of heart failure include *orthopnea, paroxysmal nocturnal dyspnea (PND),* and *nocturnal cough.* Orthopnea is the sensation of labored breathing while lying flat and is relieved by sitting upright. It results from the redistribution of intravascular blood from the gravity-dependent portions of the body (abdomen and lower extremities) toward the lungs after lying down. The degree of orthopnea is generally assessed by the number of pillows on which the patient sleeps to avoid breathlessness. Sometimes, orthopnea is so significant that the patient may try to sleep upright in a chair.

TABLE 9.4. Most Common Symptoms and Physical Findings in Heart Failure

Symptoms	Physical Findings
Left-sided	
Dyspnea	Diaphoresis (sweating)
Orthopnea	Tachycardia, tachypnea
Paroxysmal nocturnal dyspnea	Pulmonary rales
Fatigue	Loud P_2
	S_3 gallop ($\pm$ S_4)
Right-sided	
Peripheral edema	Jugular venous distention
Right upper quadrant discomfort	Hepatomegaly
(due to hepatic enlargement)	Peripheral edema

TABLE 9.5. New York Heart Association Classification of Heart Failure

Class I	No limitation of physical activity
Class II	Slight limitation of activity. Dyspnea and fatigue with moderate physical activity (e.g., walking up stairs quickly)
Class III	Marked limitation of activity. Dyspnea with minimal activity (e.g., slowly walking up stairs)
Class IV	Severe limitation of activity. Symptoms are present even at rest

PND is severe breathlessness that awakens the patient from sleep 2–3 hours after retiring to bed. This frightening symptom results from the gradual reabsorption into the circulation of lower extremity interstitial edema after lying down, with subsequent expansion of intravascular volume and increased venous return to the heart and lungs. A nocturnal cough is another symptom of pulmonary congestion and is produced by a mechanism similar to orthopnea. Hemoptysis (coughing bright red blood) may result from rupture of engorged bronchial veins.

In right-sided heart failure, the elevated systemic venous pressures can result in *abdominal discomfort* because the liver becomes engorged and its capsule is stretched. Similarly, *anorexia* (decreased appetite) and nausea may result from edema within the gastrointestinal tract. *Peripheral edema*, especially in the ankles and feet, also reflects increased hydrostatic venous pressures. Because of the effects of gravity, it tends to worsen while the patient is upright during the day and is often improved by

morning after lying supine at night. Even before peripheral edema develops, the patient may note an unexpected *weight gain* due to the accumulation of interstitial fluid.

The symptoms of heart failure are commonly graded according to the New York Heart Association classification (Table 9.5). There is also a newer system that classifies patients according to their stage in the course of heart failure (Table 9.6).

Physical Signs

The physical signs of heart failure depend on the severity and chronicity of the condition and can be divided into those due to left or right cardiac dysfunction (see Table 9.4). Individuals with only mild impairment may appear well. However, the patient with chronic, severe heart failure may demonstrate *cachexia* (a frail, wasted appearance) due in part to poor appetite and to the metabolic demands of the increased effort of breathing. In decompensated left-sided heart failure, the patient may appear *dusky* (decreased cardiac output) and *diaphoretic* (sweating due to increased sympathetic nervous activity), and the extremities are cool because of peripheral arterial vasoconstriction. *Tachypnea* (rapid breathing) is common. The pattern of Cheyne-Stokes respiration may also be present in advanced heart failure, characterized by periods of hyperventilation separated by intervals of apnea (absent breathing). This pattern is related to the prolonged circulation time between the lungs and respiratory center of the brain in heart failure that interferes with the normal

TABLE 9.6 Stages of Heart Failure

Stage	Description
A	Patients at risk of developing heart failure who have not yet developed structural cardiac dysfunction (e.g., patients with coronary artery disease, hypertension, or family history of cardiomyopathy)
B	Patients with structural heart disease associated with heart failure but who have not yet developed symptoms
C	Patients with current or prior symptoms of heart failure associated with structural heart disease
D	Patients with structural heart disease and *marked* heart failure symptoms despite maximal medical therapy who require advanced interventions (e.g., cardiac transplantation)

Modified from Hunt SA, Baker DW, Chin MH, et al. ACC/AHA guidelines for the evaluation and management of chronic heart failure in the adult: executive summary. Circulation 2001;104:2996–3007.

feedback mechanism of systemic oxygenation. *Sinus tachycardia* (due to increased sympathetic nervous system activity) is also common. *Pulsus alternans* (alternating strong and weak contractions detected in the peripheral pulse) may be present as a sign of advanced ventricular dysfunction.

In left-sided heart failure, the auscultatory finding of *pulmonary rales* is created by the "popping open" of small airways that had been closed off by edema fluid before inspiration. This finding is initially apparent at the lung bases, where hydrostatic forces are greatest; however, more severe pulmonary congestion is associated with additional rales higher in the lung fields. Compression of conduction airways by pulmonary congestion may produce coarse rhonchi and wheezing; the latter finding in heart failure is termed "cardiac asthma."

Depending on the cause of heart failure, palpation of the heart may show that the left ventricular impulse is not focal but diffuse (in dilated cardiomyopathy), sustained (in pressure overload states such as aortic stenosis or hypertension), or lifting in quality (in volume overload states such as mitral regurgitation). Because elevated left heart filling pressures result in increased pulmonary vascular pressures, the pulmonic component of the second heart sound is often louder than normal. An early diastolic sound (S_3) is frequently heard in adults with systolic heart failure and is due to abnormal filling of the dilated chamber (see Chapter 2). A late diastolic sound (S_4) results from forceful atrial contraction into a stiffened ventricle and is common in states of decreased left ventricular compliance (diastolic dysfunction). The murmur of *mitral regurgitation* is sometimes auscultated in left-sided heart failure if the valve annulus is stretched and the papillary muscles are spread widely apart from one another because of left ventricular dilatation, thus preventing full closure of the mitral leaflets in systole.

In the presence of right-sided heart failure, different physical findings may be present. Cardiac examination may reveal a palpable parasternal *right ventricular heave*, representing right ventricular enlargement, or a right-sided S_3 or S_4 gallop. The murmur of *tricuspid regurgitation* may be auscultated and is due to right ventricular enlargement, analogous to mitral regurgitation that develops in left ventricular dilatation. The elevated systemic venous pressure produced by right heart failure is manifested by *distention of the jugular veins* as well as *hepatic enlargement* with abdominal right upper quadrant tenderness. *Edema* accumulates in the dependent portions of the body, beginning in the ankles and feet of ambulatory patients, and in the presacral regions of bedridden individuals.

Pleural effusions may develop in either left- or right-sided heart failure, because the pleural veins drain into both the systemic and pulmonary venous beds. The presence of pleural effusions is suggested on physical examination by dullness to percussion over the posterior lung bases.

Laboratory Tests

Normally the mean left atrial (LA) pressure is ≤10 mm Hg. If the LA pressure exceeds approximately 15 mm Hg, the chest radiograph shows upper zone vascular redistribution, such that the vessels supplying the upper lung lobes are larger than those supplying the lower lobes (see Fig. 3.5, page 49). This is explained as follows. When a patient is in the upright position, blood flow is normally greater to the lung bases than to the apices because of the effect of gravity. Redistribution of flow occurs when interstitial and perivascular edema develops, because such edema is most prominent at the lung bases, where the hydrostatic pressure is the highest, and compresses the blood vessels in that region, whereas flow into the upper lung zones is less affected. When the LA pressure surpasses 20 mm Hg, interstitial edema is usually manifested as indistinctness of the vessels and the presence of Kerley B lines (short linear markings at the periphery of the lower lung fields) indicating interlobular edema. If the LA pressure exceeds 25–30 mm Hg, alveolar pulmonary edema may develop, with opacification of the air spaces. The relationship between LA pressure and chest radiograph findings is modified in patients with chronic heart failure because of enhanced lymphatic drainage, such that higher pressures can be accommodated with fewer radiologic signs.

Depending on the cause of heart failure, the chest radiograph may show cardiomegaly, defined as a cardiothoracic ratio of greater than 0.5 on the posteroanterior film. A high right atrial pressure also causes enlargement of the azygous vein, a finding that can be visualized by chest radiography. Pleural effusions may be present.

The cause of heart failure in an individual is often evident from the history, such as a patient who has sustained a large myocardial infarction, or by physical examination, as in an individual with the murmur of mitral stenosis. In cases in which the cause is not clear from clinical evaluation, the first step is to determine whether systolic ventricular function is normal or depressed (see Fig. 9.6). Ventricular function can be assessed by a number of noninvasive tests, of which echocardiography is especially useful (described in Chapter 3). In a minority of cases, cardiac catheterization is necessary to determine the cause of heart failure, including valvular and ischemic etiologies.

PROGNOSIS

The prognosis of heart failure is dismal in the absence of a correctable underlying cause. Only 50% of patients remain alive 5 years after the diagnosis is made. Patients with severe symptoms (i.e., New York Heart Association Class III or IV) fare the least well, having a 1-year survival rate of only 40%. The greatest mortality is due to refractory heart failure, but a large number of patients die suddenly, presumably because of ventricular arrhythmias.

Ventricular dysfunction usually begins with an inciting insult but is a progressive process, contributed to by the maladaptive activation of neurohormones, cytokines, and continuous ventricular remodeling. Thus, it should not be surprising that measures of neurohormonal and cytokine stimulation predict survival in heart failure patients. For example, adverse prognosis correlates with the serum norepinephrine level (marker of sympathetic nervous system activity), serum sodium (reduced level reflects activation of renin-angiotensin system and alterations in intrarenal hemodynamics), endothelin, and cytokine TNF-α levels. Most recently, an assay for B-type natriuretic peptide has been shown to correlate very well with the degree of LV dysfunction and prognosis.

Despite the generally bleak prognosis, recent studies have demonstrated that survival in heart failure patients can be substantially prolonged by specific interventions, as discussed in the following section.

TREATMENT

There are five main goals of therapy in patients with chronic heart failure:

1. *Identification and correction of the underlying condition causing heart failure.* In some individuals, this may require surgical repair or replacement of dysfunctional cardiac valves, coronary artery bypass graft surgery, aggressive treatment of severe hypertension, or cessation of alcohol consumption.
2. *Elimination of the acute precipitating cause of symptoms* in the patient with heart failure who was previously in a compensated state. This may include, for example, treating acute infections or arrhythmias, removing sources of excessive salt intake, or eliminating drugs that can aggravate symptomatology (e.g., certain calcium channel blockers [negative inotropic effect] or nonsteroidal antiinflammatory drugs [which can contribute to volume retention]).
3. *Management of heart failure systems:*
    Treatment of pulmonary and systemic vascular congestion. This is most readily accomplished by dietary sodium restriction and diuretic medications.
    Increase of forward cardiac output and perfusion of vital organs through the use of vasodilators and positive inotropic drugs.

4. *Modulation of the neurohormonal response* to help prevent adverse ventricular remodeling in order to slow progression of LV dysfunction.

5. *Improvement in long-term survival.* There is now convincing evidence that longevity is enhanced by specific interventions, as described below.

Diuretics

The mechanism of action and pharmacology of diuretic drugs are summarized in Chapter 17. By promoting the elimination of sodium and water via the kidney, diuretics reduce intravascular volume and thus venous return to the heart. Therefore, the preload of the left ventricle is decreased, and its diastolic pressure falls out of the range that promotes pulmonary congestion (Fig. 9.10, point b). The judicious use of di-

uretics does not significantly reduce cardiac output in this setting, because the heart is operating on the "flat" portion of a depressed Frank-Starling curve. The intent is to reduce the end-diastolic pressure (and therefore hydrostatic forces contributing to pulmonary congestion) without a significant fall in stroke volume. However, overly vigorous diuresis *can* lower the left ventricular filling pressures into the steep portion of the ventricular performance curve, resulting in an undesired fall in cardiac output (see Fig. 9.10, point b'). Thus, diuretics should be used only if there is evidence of pulmonary congestion (rales) or peripheral interstitial fluid accumulation (edema).

Diuretics that act primarily at the renal loop of Henle (e.g., furosemide, torsemide, and bumetanide) are the most potent in heart failure. Thiazide diuretics (e.g., hydrochlorothiazide and metolazone) are also

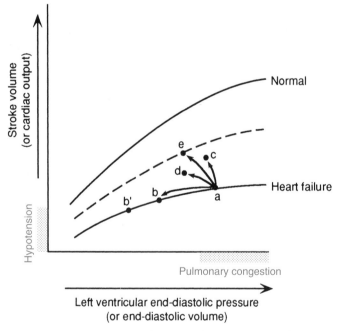

Figure 9.10. Examples of the effect of heart failure treatment on the left ventricular (LV) Frank-Starling curve. Point a represents the failing heart on a curve that is shifted downward compared with normal. The stroke volume is reduced (bordering on hypotension), and the end-diastolic pressure (LVEDP) is increased, resulting in symptoms of pulmonary congestion. Therapy with a diuretic or pure venous vasodilator (point b on the same Frank-Starling curve) reduces LV pressure without much change in stroke volume (SV). However, excessive diuresis or venous vasodilatation may result in an undesired fall in SV with hypotension (point b'). Inotropic drug therapy (point c) and arteriolar (or "balanced") vasodilator therapy (point d) augment SV, and because of improved LV emptying during contraction, the LVEDP becomes less. Point e represents the potential added benefit of combining an inotrope and vasodilator together. The dashed line shows one example of how the Frank-Starling curve shifts upward during inotropic/vasodilator therapy but does not achieve the level of a normal ventricle.

useful but are less effective in the setting of decreased renal perfusion, which is often present in this condition. The general side effects of diuretics are described in Chapter 17. The most important adverse effects with respect to heart failure include overdiuresis resulting in a fall in cardiac output and electrolyte disturbances (particularly hypokalemia and hypomagnesemia), which may contribute to dangerous arrhythmias. When diuretics are used in patients with pure diastolic left ventricular dysfunction to relieve congestive symptoms, one must be especially careful to avoid overdiuresis, as these patients *require* elevated diastolic filling pressures to adequately fill their stiffened left ventricles (see Fig. 9.7B). It is therefore often necessary to accept some degree of chronically elevated filling pressures in patients with diastolic ventricular dysfunction.

Vasodilators

One of the most important cardiac advances in the past quarter century was the introduction of vasodilator therapy for the treatment of heart failure, particularly the class of agents known as angiotensin-converting enzyme (ACE) inhibitors. As indicated above, neurohormonal compensatory mechanisms in heart failure often lead to excessive vasoconstriction, volume retention, and ventricular remodeling. Vasodilator drugs help to reverse these adverse consequences. Moreover, multiple studies have shown that certain vasodilator regimens significantly extend survival in patients with heart failure. The pharmacology of these drugs is described in Chapter 17.

Venous vasodilators (e.g., nitrates) increase venous capacitance, decrease venous return to the heart, and therefore reduce left ventricular preload. Consequently, left ventricular diastolic pressures fall and the pulmonary capillary hydrostatic pressure declines, similar to the hemodynamic effects of diuretic therapy. As a result, pulmonary congestion improves, and as long as the heart failure patient is on the relatively "flat" part of the depressed Frank-Starling curve (see Fig. 9.10), the cardiac output does not fall despite the reduction in ventricular filling pressure. However, venous vasodilatation in a patient who is operating on the steeper part of the curve may result in an undesired fall in stroke volume, cardiac output, and blood pressure.

Pure *arteriolar vasodilators* (e.g., hydralazine) reduce systemic vascular resistance and therefore LV afterload, which in turn permits increased ventricular muscle fiber shortening during systole (see Fig. 9.5B). This results in an augmented stroke volume and is represented on the Frank-Starling diagram as a shift in an upward direction (see Fig. 9.10). Although one might conclude that an arterial vasodilator would necessarily reduce blood pressure—an undesired effect in patients with heart failure who may already be hypotensive—this generally does not happen. As resistance is reduced by arteriolar vasodilatation, a concurrent *rise* in cardiac output usually occurs, such that blood pressure remains constant or decreases only mildly.

Some groups of drugs result in vasodilatation of both the venous and arteriolar circuits ("balanced" vasodilators). Of these, the most important are the *angiotensin-converting enzyme inhibitors*. These function as vasodilators by inhibiting the formation of the vasoconstrictor angiotensin II (AII), the production of which is stimulated in heart failure. In addition, because aldosterone levels fall in response to ACE inhibitor therapy, sodium elimination is facilitated, resulting in a reduction of intravascular volume and therefore improvement of systemic and pulmonary vascular congestion. ACE inhibitors also augment circulating levels of bradykinin (see Chapter 17), which is thought to play an important vasodilatory role in heart failure. Additionally, ACE inhibitors limit maladaptive ventricular remodeling in patients with heart failure and following acute myocardial infarction (see Chapter 7).

Supporting ACE inhibitors' beneficial hemodynamic and neurohormonal blocking effects, many recent large clinical trials have shown that such therapy reduces heart failure symptoms, improves stamina, reduces the need for hospitalization, and most importantly extends survival in patients with chronic heart failure. Thus, *ACE inhibitors are the standard first-line chronic therapy for patients with LV systolic dysfunction.*

The renin-angiotensin-aldosterone system can also be inhibited by the group of drugs known as *angiotensin II receptor blockers (ARBs)*, as will be described in Chapters 13 and 17. Since angiotensin II can be formed by pathways other than ACE, ARBs provide a more complete inhibition of the system through blockade of the actual AII receptor (see Fig. 17.6, p. 380). Conversely, ARBs do not stimulate the potentially beneficial rise in serum bradykinin. The net result is that the hemodynamic effects of ARBs in heart failure are similar to those of ACE inhibitors, and studies thus far have not shown any survival superiority of these agents over ACE inhibitors. Thus, they are prescribed to heart failure patients mainly when ACE inhibitors are not tolerated (e.g., because of the side effect of cough).

Chronic therapy using the combination of the venous dilator isosorbide dinitrate plus the arteriolar dilator hydralazine has also been shown to improve survival in patients with moderate symptoms of heart failure. However, when administration of the ACE inhibitor enalapril was compared with the hydralazine-isosorbide dinitrate (H-ISDN) combination, the ACE inhibitor was shown to produce the greater improvement in survival. Thus, H-ISDN is generally substituted only if a patient cannot tolerate ACE inhibitor therapy (e.g., because of renal insufficiency or hyperkalemia).

Nesiritide (human recombinant B-type natriuretic peptide) is a recent addition to the category of intravenous vasodilator drugs for hospitalized patients with decompensated heart failure. It causes rapid and potent vasodilatation, reduces elevated intracardiac pressures, augments forward cardiac output, and lessens the activation of the renin-angiotensin and sympathetic nervous systems. It promotes diuresis, reduces heart failure symptoms, has few side effects (mainly hypotension), and can be combined with diuretics and positive inotropic drugs. However, it is an expensive drug and its main use is for patients who have not responded to or cannot tolerate other intravenous vasodilators, such as intravenous nitroglycerin or nitroprusside (described in Chapter 17).

Inotropic Drugs

The inotropic drugs include β-adrenergic agonists, digitalis glycosides, and phosphodiesterase inhibitors (see Chapter 17). By increasing the availability of intracellular calcium, each of these groups of drugs increases the force of ventricular contraction and therefore shifts the Frank-Starling curve in an upward direction (see Fig. 9.10). As a result, stroke volume and cardiac output are augmented at any given ventricular end-diastolic volume. Therefore, these agents may be useful in the treatment of systolic ventricular dysfunction but not in patients with pure diastolic failure.

The *β-adrenergic agonists* (e.g., dobutamine and dopamine) are administered intravenously for temporary hemodynamic support in acutely ill, hospitalized patients. Their long-term use is limited by the lack of an oral form of administration and by the rapid development of drug tolerance. The latter refers to the progressive decline in effectiveness during continued administration of the drug, possibly due to downregulation of myocardial adrenergic receptors. The role of *phosphodiesterase inhibitors*, much like that of the β-adrenergic agonists, is limited to the intravenous treatment of congestive heart failure in acutely ill patients. Despite the initial promise of effective *oral* phosphodiesterase inhibitors, studies thus far have not demonstrated improved survival among patients so treated.

One of the oldest forms of inotropic therapy is *digitalis* (described in Chapter 17), which can be administered intravenously or orally. Digitalis preparations enhance contractility, reduce cardiac enlargement, improve symptoms, and augment cardiac output in patients with systolic heart failure. Digitalis also increases the sensitivity of the baroreceptors, so that the compensatory sympathetic drive in heart failure is blunted, a desired effect that reduces left ventricular afterload. Digitalis has an added benefit in patients with congestive heart failure and concurrent atrial fibrillation in helping to control the rate of ventricular contractions. Although digitalis can improve symptomatology in heart failure patients, it does not improve long-term survival. Its use is thus limited to patients who remain symptomatic despite other standard therapies, or to help slow the ventricular rate if atrial fibrillation is also present. Digitalis is *not* useful in the treatment of diastolic left ventricular dysfunction, because it does not improve ventricular relaxation properties.

β-Blockers

Historically, β-blockers have been contraindicated in patients with systolic dysfunction, as their negative inotropic effect would be expected to worsen symptomatology. Paradoxically, recent studies have actually shown that β-blockers have important *benefits* in heart failure, including augmented cardiac output, reduced hemodynamic deterioration, and improved survival. The explanation for this observation remains unclear but may relate to the reduction in heart rate, the blunting of chronic sympathetic activation, or the anti-ischemic properties of β-blocker drugs.

In clinical trials of patients with all classes of symptomatic heart failure, β-blockers have been well-tolerated in stable patients (i.e., those without recent deterioration of symptoms or active signs of volume overload) and have resulted in improved mortality rates and fewer hospitalizations compared with patients taking a placebo. Not all β-blockers have been tested in heart failure. Those that have and have been found to be successful include carvedilol (a nonselective β_1 and β_2 receptor blocker with weak α-blocking properties) and the β_1-selective metoprolol (in a sustained-release formulation). Nonetheless, β-blockers must be used cautiously in heart failure to prevent acute deterioration due to their negative inotropic effect. Regimens should be started at low dosages and augmented gradually.

Additional Therapies

Spironolactone is an aldosterone antagonist that has been used for decades as a potassium-sparing diuretic (see Chapter 17). There is growing evidence that chronic excess of aldosterone levels in heart failure may contribute to cardiac fibrosis and adverse ventricular remodeling. In a clinical trial of patients with advanced heart failure who were already taking an ACE inhibitor and diuretics, spironolactone substantially reduced mortality rates and improved heart failure symptoms. Although well-tolerated in this carefully controlled study, the serum potassium level needs to be closely monitored when prescribing spironolactone to heart failure patients (to prevent hyperkalemia), especially if there is renal impairment or concomitant ACE inhibitor therapy.

In summary, standard therapy of chronic congestive heart failure associated with left ventricular systolic dysfunction should include several drugs, the cornerstones of which are an ACE inhibitor and a beta-blocker. The general sequence of therapy is to start with an ACE inhibitor, as well as a diuretic if pulmonary or systemic congestive symptoms are present. If the patient is unable to tolerate the ACE inhibitor, then an ARB (or hydralazine plus isosorbide dinitrate) may be substituted. For patients without recent clinical deterioration or volume overload, a β-blocker should be added. For persistent symptoms, digoxin can also be prescribed. Those with advanced (NYHA class IV) heart failure may benefit from the addition of spironolactone.

Other therapies commonly administered to patients with systolic dysfunction include 1) anticoagulation to prevent intracardiac thrombus formation if left ventricular systolic function is significantly impaired (a controversial therapy because clear benefit has not yet been demonstrated by clinical trials), and 2) treatment of atrial and ventricular arrhythmias that frequently accompany chronic heart failure (see Chapter 12). For example, atrial fibrillation is very common among heart failure patients, and conversion back to sinus rhythm can substantially improve cardiac output. Ventricular arrhythmias are also frequently found. β-blockers may reduce the frequency of ventricular arrhythmias and are usually included in standard heart failure therapy as indicated above.

In terms of specific antiarrhythmic drugs, the most effective and least likely to *provoke* dangerous arrhythmias in heart failure patients is amiodarone. However, studies of amiodarone for asymptomatic ventricular arrhythmias in heart failure have not shown a consistent survival benefit. Heart failure patients with symptomatic or sustained ventricular arrhythmias (or those with inducible ventricular tachycardia during electrophysiologic testing) should receive an implantable defibrillator (see Chapter 11).

Resynchronization Therapy

Intraventricular conduction abnormalities with widened QRS complexes (such as left bundle branch block) are common in patients with advanced heart failure. These abnormalities can contribute to cardiac symptoms because of the uncoordinated right and left ventricular patterns of contraction. Special pacemakers have been devised that stimulate both ventricles simultaneously, thus resynchronizing the contractile effort. This technique of biventricular pacing has been studied in patients with reduced LV contractile function and QRS duration wider than 0.13 seconds (a little more than three small boxes on the ECG) and has been shown to improve exercise capacity and reduce heart failure exacerbations. Clinical trials are in progress to help determine which patients are most likely to benefit from this approach.

A patient with severe left ventricular dysfunction whose condition remains refractory to maximal medical management may be a candidate for cardiac transplantation. Because of a shortage of donor hearts, only approximately 2500 transplants are performed in the United States each year. Thus, alternative mechanical heart support therapies are undergoing intense development, including ventricular assist devices and totally implanted artificial hearts.

Treatment of Diastolic Dysfunction

Correctable causes of impaired diastolic function should be considered and addressed. For example, pericardiectomy would be undertaken for constrictive pericarditis (see Chapter 14), or therapy should be directed at coronary artery disease if transient ischemia is the mechanism of diastolic dysfunction. There is usually no role for inotropic drugs or vasodilators in the treatment of pure diastolic dysfunction. Diuretics may reduce pulmonary congestion and peripheral edema, but must be used cautiously to avoid decreased cardiac output or hypotension, as the stiffened left ventricle relies on higher filling pressures than normal to maintain its output. Calcium channel blockers are occasionally beneficial in diastolic dysfunction due to hypertension or hypertrophic cardiomyopathy (see Chapter 10) but have not been shown to be helpful when diastolic dysfunction is caused by other disorders.

ACUTE PULMONARY EDEMA

A severe, acute form of left-sided heart failure is cardiogenic pulmonary edema, in which elevated capillary hydrostatic pressure causes rapid accumulation of fluid within the interstitium and alveolar spaces of the lung. This condition is frequently accompanied by hypoxemia because of shunting of pulmonary blood flow through regions of hypoventilated alveoli. Pulmonary edema may appear suddenly in a previously asymptomatic individual in, for example, the setting of an acute myocardial infarction, or in patients with chronic compensated congestive heart failure following a precipitating event (see Table 9.3). Pulmonary edema is a horrifying experience for the patient, resulting in severe dyspnea and anxiety while struggling to breathe.

On examination, the patient is tachycardic and demonstrates cold, clammy skin due to peripheral vasoconstriction in response to the increased sympathetic outflow. Tachypnea and coughing of "frothy" sputum represent transudation of fluid into the alveoli. Rales are present initially at the bases and then throughout the lung fields, sometimes accompanied by wheezing because of edema fluid within the conductance airways.

In the presence of normal plasma oncotic pressure, pulmonary edema develops when the pulmonary capillary wedge pressure, which reflects LV diastolic pressure, exceeds approximately 25 mm Hg.

Pulmonary edema is a life-threatening emergency that requires immediate improvement of systemic oxygenation and elimination of the underlying cause. The patient should be seated upright to permit pooling of blood within the systemic veins of the lower body, so as to reduce venous return to the heart. Supplemental oxygen is provided by face mask. Morphine sulphate is administered intravenously to reduce anxiety and as a venous dilator to facilitate pooling of blood peripherally. A rapidly acting diuretic, such as intravenous furosemide, is administered in an attempt to further reduce left ventricular preload and pulmonary capillary hydrostatic pressure. Other means of reducing preload include administration of nitrates (often intravenously) or in extreme cases venous phlebotomy. Inotropic drugs (e.g., dopamine) can also be administered intravenously to augment forward cardiac output. During resolution of the pulmonary congestion and hypoxemia, attention should be directed at identifying and treating the underlying cause.

An easy to remember mnemonic for acute management of pulmonary edema is the alphabetic sequence: "LMNOP:"

Lasix (trade name for furosemide)
Morphine
Nitrates
Oxygen
Position (sit upright)

SUMMARY

1. Heart failure is present when cardiac output fails to meet the metabolic demands of the body or meets those demands only if the cardiac filling pressures are abnormally high. It most often results from impaired left ventricular systolic function, but may also arise from ventricular diastolic dysfunction and other cardiac abnormalities that interfere with ventricular filling or emptying.

2. Compensatory mechanisms in heart failure that help maintain circulatory function include 1) augmented stroke volume via the Frank-Starling mechanism, 2) activation of neurohormonal systems, and 3) ventricular hypertrophy. However, many of these compensations become maladaptive and contribute to adverse ventricular remodeling and progressive deterioration of ventricular function.

3. Symptoms of heart failure may be exacerbated by precipitating factors that increase metabolic demand, increase circulating volume, increase afterload, or decrease contractility (summarized in Table 9.3).

4. Successful treatment of heart failure requires identification of the underlying cause of the condition, elimination of precipitating factors, and modulation of neurohormonal activations. Standard medical treatment includes an ACE inhibitor, β-blocker and, as needed, diuretics and inotropic drugs (e.g., digoxin). For patients who do not tolerate an ACE inhibitor, an ARB or the combination of hydralazine plus nitrates can be substituted. Spironolactone should be considered for patients with advanced heart failure.

Acknowledgments   Contributors to the previous editions of this chapter were Arthur Coday, Jr, MD; Vikram Janakiraman, MD; Stephen K. Frankel, MD; and Michael A. Fifer, MD.

ADDITIONAL READING

Banerjee P, Banerjee T, Hkand A, et al. Diastolic heart failure: neglected or misdiagnosed? J Am Coll Cardiol 2002;39:138–141.

Colucci WS. Heart failure: cardiac function and dysfunction. In: Braunwald E, series ed. Atlas of Heart Disease. 2nd Ed. Philadelphia: Current Medicine, 1999.

Colucci WS. Nesiritide for the treatment of decompensated heart failure. J Cardiac Failure 2001;7:92–100.

Digitalis Investigation Group. The effect of digoxin on mortality and morbidity in patients with heart failure. N Engl J Med 1997;336:525–533.

Foody JM, Farrell MH, Krumholz HM. β-blocker therapy in heart failure: scientific review. JAMA 2002;287:883–889.

Garg R, Yusef S. Overview of randomized trials of angiotensin-converting enzyme inhibitors on mortality and morbidity in patients with heart failure. JAMA 1995;273:1450–1456.

Hunt SA, Baker DW, Chin MH, et al. ACC/AHA guidelines for the evaluation and management of chronic heart failure in the adult: executive summary. Circulation 2001;104:2996–3007.

Jong P, Demers C, McKelvie RS, et al. Angiotensin receptor blockers in heart failure: meta-analysis of randomized controlled trials. J Am Coll Cardiol 2002;39:463–470.

Katz AM. Heart Failure: Pathophysiology, Molecular Biology, Clinical Management. Philadelphia: Lippincott Williams & Wilkins, 2000.

Nohria A, Lewis E, Stevenson LW. Medical management of advanced heart failure. JAMA 2002; 287:628–640.

Towbin JA, Bowles NE. The failing heart. Nature 2002;415:227–233.

Weber KT. Aldosterone in congestive heart failure. N Engl J Med 2001;345:1689–1697.

Zile MR, Brutsaert DL. New concepts in diastolic dysfunction and diastolic heart failure. Circulation; 2002; 105:1387–1393.

The Cardiomyopathies

Yi-Bin Chen, G. William Dec, and Leonard S. Lilly

Chapter
10

Dilated Cardiomyopathy
  Etiology
  Pathology
  Pathophysiology
  Clinical Findings
  Physical Examination
  Diagnostic Studies
  Treatment
  Prognosis
Hypertrophic Cardiomyopathy
  Etiology
  Pathology

  Pathophysiology
  Clinical Findings
  Physical Examination
  Diagnostic Studies
  Treatment
  Prognosis
Restrictive Cardiomyopathy
  Pathophysiology
  Clinical Findings
  Physical Examination
  Diagnostic Studies
  Treatment

The cardiomyopathies are a group of heart disorders in which the major structural abnormality is limited to the myocardium. These conditions often result in symptoms of heart failure, and whereas the underlying cause of myocardial dysfunction can sometimes be identified, the etiology frequently remains unknown. Excluded from the definition of this group of diseases is heart muscle impairment due to other known cardiac conditions, such as hypertension, valvular disorders, or coronary artery disease.

Cardiomyopathies can be classified into three types by the anatomic appearance and abnormal physiology of the left ventricle (Fig. 10.1). **Dilated** cardiomyopathy is characterized by ventricular chamber enlargement with impaired *systolic* contractile function; **hypertrophic** cardiomyopathy by an abnormally thickened ventricular wall with abnormal *diastolic* relaxation but usually intact systolic function; and **restrictive** cardiomyopathy by an abnormally stiffened myocardium (because of fibrosis or an infiltrative process) such that diastolic relaxation is impaired, but systolic contractile function is normal or near-normal.

DILATED CARDIOMYOPATHY

Etiology

Cardiac enlargement in dilated cardiomyopathy (DCM) is due to ventricular dilatation with only minor hypertrophy. Myocyte damage leading to this condition results from a wide spectrum of genetic, toxic, metabolic, and infectious causes (Table 10.1). Although the majority of cases are idiopathic (i.e., the cause is undetermined), examples of conditions that *are* commonly recognized causes of DCM include viral myocarditis, alcohol toxicity, and gene mutations.

Acute viral myocarditis generally afflicts young, previously healthy individuals and is most often the result of Coxsackie group B or echovirus infection. It is usually a self-limited condition with full recovery, but for unclear reasons, some patients progress to DCM. It is hypothesized that myocardial destruction and fibrosis result from immune-mediated injury triggered by viral constituents. Nonetheless, immunosuppressive drugs have not been shown to improve the prognosis of this condition. Transvenous right ventricular biopsy during acute myocarditis may demonstrate active inflammation, and Coxsackie B RNA

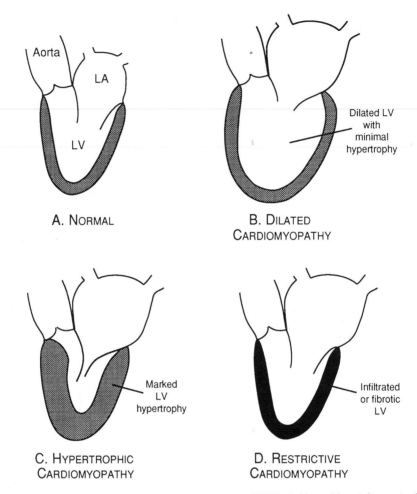

Figure 10.1. **Anatomic appearance of the cardiomyopathies (CMP). A.** Normal heart demonstrating left ventricle (LV) and left atrium (LA). **B.** Dilated CMP is characterized by ventricular dilatation with only mild hypertrophy. **C.** Hypertrophic CMP demonstrates significant ventricular hypertrophy, often predominantly involving the intraventricular septum. **D.** Restrictive CMP is due to infiltration or fibrosis of the ventricles, usually without enlargement of the cavities. Note that LA enlargement is common to all three types of CMP.

TABLE 10.1. Examples of Dilated Cardiomyopathies

Idiopathic
Familial (genetic)
Inflammatory
  Infectious (especially viral)
  Noninfectious
    Connective tissue diseases
    Peripartum cardiomyopathy
    Sarcoidosis
Toxic
  Chronic alcohol ingestion
  Chemotherapeutic agents (e.g., doxorubicin)
Metabolic
  Hypothyroidism
  Chronic hypocalcemia or hypophosphatemia
Neuromuscular
  Muscular or myotonic dystrophy

sequences have been demonstrated in some infected individuals.

Alcoholic cardiomyopathy develops in a small number of individuals who consume alcoholic beverages chronically. Although the pathophysiology is unknown, ethanol is thought to impair cellular function by inhibiting mitochondrial oxidative phosphorylation and fatty acid oxidation. Its clinical presentation and histologic features are similar to those of other dilated cardiomyopathies. Alcoholic cardiomyopathy is important to identify because it is one of the few reversible causes of DCM, in that cessation of alcohol consumption can result in dramatic improvement of ventricular function.

Recently, several familial forms of DCM have been identified and are believed to be responsible for 20–30% of what were once classified as idiopathic DCM. Autosomal dominant, autosomal recessive, X-linked, and mitochondrial patterns of inheritance have all been described, leading to defects in contractile force generation, force transmission, energy production, and myocyte viability. Genes identified thus far in this regard code for specific proteins, including troponin T, myosin, actin, and dystrophin (a myocyte cytoskeletal component). In certain families, associated phenotypical features have included auditory deficits, cardiac conduction system defects, and skeletal muscle abnormalities. Recognition of affected individuals and identification of their underlying genetic mutations can allow gene-based screening and diagnosis for family members and potentially earlier interventions to prevent the development of symptoms and complications.

Pathology

Marked enlargement of all four cardiac chambers is typical of DCM (Fig. 10.2), although sometimes the disease is limited to only the left or right side of the heart. The thickness of the ventricular walls may be increased, but chamber dilatation is out of proportion to any hypertrophy. Microscop-

ically, there is evidence of myocyte degeneration with irregular hypertrophy and atrophy of myofibers. Interstitial and perivascular fibrosis is often extensive.

Pathophysiology

The hallmark of DCM is ventricular dilatation with decreased contractile function (Fig. 10.3). Most often in DCM, both ventricles are impaired, but sometimes dysfunction is limited to the left ventricle (LV) and even less commonly to the right ventricle (RV).

As ventricular stroke volume and cardiac output decline because of impaired myocyte contractility, two compensatory effects are called into action: 1) the Frank-Starling mechanism, in which the elevated ventricular diastolic volume increases the stretch of the myofibers, thereby increasing the subsequent stroke volume, and 2) neurohormonal activation, initially mediated by the sympathetic nervous system (see Chapter 9). The latter contributes to an increased heart rate and contractility, which help to buffer the fall in cardiac output. These compensations may render the patient asymptomatic during the early stages of ventricular dysfunction; however, as progressive myocyte degeneration and volume overload ensue, clinical symptoms of heart failure develop.

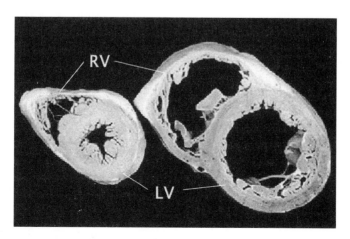

Figure 10.2. **Transverse sections of a normal heart (left) and a heart from a patient with dilated cardiomyopathy (DCM).** In the DCM specimen, there is biventricular dilatation without a proportional increase in wall thickness. RV, right ventricle; LV, left ventricle. (Modified from Emmanouilides GC (editor). Moss and Adams' Heart Disease in Infants, Children and Adolescents, 5/e. Baltimore: Lippincott Williams & Wilkins, 1995:86.)

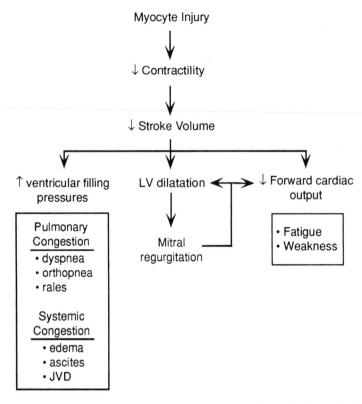

Figure 10.3. Pathophysiology of dilated cardiomyopathy. The reduced ventricular stroke volume results in decreased forward cardiac output and increased ventricular filling pressures. The listed clinical manifestations follow. JVD, jugular venous distention.

With a persistent reduction of cardiac output, the decline in renal blood flow prompts the kidneys to secrete increased amounts of renin. This activation of the renin-angiotensin-aldosterone axis increases peripheral vascular resistance (mediated through angiotensin II) and intravascular volume (because of increased aldosterone). As described in Chapter 9, these effects are also initially helpful in buffering the fall in cardiac output.

Ultimately, however, the "compensatory" effects of neurohormonal activation prove detrimental. Arteriolar vasoconstriction and increased systemic resistance render it more difficult for the LV to eject blood in the forward direction, and the rise in intravascular volume further burdens the ventricles, resulting in pulmonary and systemic congestion. In addition, chronically elevated circulating levels of angiotensin II and aldosterone contribute to increased myocardial and vascular remodeling with fibrosis.

As the cardiomyopathic process causes the ventricles to enlarge over time, the mitral and tricuspid valves may fail to coapt properly in systole, and valvular regurgitation ensues. Such regurgitation has three detrimental consequences: 1) excessive volume and pressure loads are placed on the atria, causing them to dilate, often leading to atrial fibrillation; 2) regurgitation of blood into the left atrium further decreases forward stroke volume into the aorta and systemic circulation; and 3) when the regurgitant volume returns to the LV during each diastole, there is an even greater volume load presented to the dilated LV.

Clinical Findings

The clinical manifestations of DCM are those of congestive heart failure. The most common symptoms of low forward cardiac output include fatigue, lightheadedness, and exertional dyspnea associated with decreased tissue perfusion. Pulmonary congestion results in dyspnea, orthopnea, and paroxysmal nocturnal dyspnea, whereas chronic systemic venous congestion causes ascites and peripheral edema. Because these symptoms may develop insidiously, the patient may complain only of recent weight gain (because of interstitial edema) and shortness of breath on exertion.

Physical Examination

Signs of decreased cardiac output are often present and include cool extremities (due to peripheral vasoconstriction), low arterial pressure, and tachycardia. Pulmonary venous congestion results in auscultatory crackles (rales), and basilar chest dullness on percussion may be present because of pleural effusions. Cardiac examination shows an enlarged heart with leftward displacement of a diffuse apical impulse. On auscultation, an S_3 is common as a sign of poor systolic function. The murmur of mitral valve regurgitation is common in association with significant left ventricular dilatation. If right ventricular heart failure has developed, signs of systemic venous congestion include jugular vein distention, hepatomegaly, ascites, and peripheral edema. Right ventricular enlargement and contractile dysfunction are often accompanied by the murmur of tricuspid valve regurgitation.

Diagnostic Studies

The *chest radiograph* shows an enlarged cardiac silhouette. If heart failure has developed, then pulmonary vascular redistribution, interstitial and alveolar edema, and pleural effusions are evident (see Fig. 3.5).

The *ECG* usually demonstrates atrial and ventricular enlargement. Patchy fibrosis of the myofibers results in a wide array of arrhythmias, most importantly atrial fibrillation and ventricular tachycardia. Conduction defects (left or right bundle branch block) occur in the majority of cases. Diffuse repolarization (ST and T wave) abnormalities are common. In addition, regions of dense myocardial fibrosis may produce

localized Q waves, resembling the pattern of previous myocardial infarction.

Echocardiography is valuable in the diagnosis of DCM. It demonstrates four-chamber cardiac enlargement with little hypertrophy and usually global reduction of systolic contractile function. Mitral and/or tricuspid regurgitation is also frequently visualized.

Cardiac catheterization is often performed to determine whether coexistent coronary artery disease is contributing to the impaired ventricular function. This procedure is most useful diagnostically in patients who describe episodes of angina pectoris or have evidence of previous myocardial infarction on the electrocardiogram. Typically, hemodynamic measurements show elevated right- and left-sided diastolic pressures and diminished cardiac output. While in the catheterization laboratory, a transvenous biopsy of the right ventricle is sometimes performed in an attempt to clarify the etiology of the cardiomyopathy. There is only a limited role for such a procedure, however, because it is rarely diagnostic in patients with DCM and only infrequently alters therapeutic decisions.

Treatment

The goal of therapy in DCM is to relieve symptoms, to prevent complications, and to improve long-term survival. Therefore, the therapeutic approach addresses the following: 1) treatment of the underlying cause if identified, 2) prevention of progressive ventricular dilatation, 3) relief of pulmonary and systemic congestion, 4) augmentation of low cardiac output, 5) prevention and treatment of arrhythmias, 6) prevention of thromboemboli, and 7) consideration of cardiac transplantation.

Approaches to the relief of vascular congestion and improvement in forward cardiac output are the same as standard therapies for heart failure as described in Chapter 9. Initial therapy of systemic or pulmonary congestion includes salt restriction and *diuretics*. One of the most important advances in the management of patients with heart failure in the past quarter century has been the introduction of vasodilator therapy. Improvement in hemodynamic measurements, quality of life, and survival times has been convincingly shown with the use of *angiotensin-converting enzyme (ACE) inhibitors,* and to a lesser extent with the combination of *hydralazine* (an arteriolar vasodilator) plus *isosorbide dinitrate* (a venous vasodilator). In addition, recent studies have shown that ACE inhibitor therapy can even benefit *asymptomatic* individuals with left ventricular dysfunction by slowing the progression to the symptomatic stages of heart failure. Thus, ACE inhibitors are first-line therapy for patients with DCM. *Angiotensin receptor blockers* (ARBs, described in Chapters 9 and 17) are appropriate substitutes for patients who cannot take an ACE inhibitor (e.g., because of ACE inhibitor-induced cough, a common side effect). If neither an ACE inhibitor nor ARB can be used (e.g., because of renal insufficiency or hyperkalemia), the combination of hydralazine plus isosorbide dinitrate is preferred.

As described in Chapter 9, *β-blockers* are now indicated for the majority of patients with stable heart failure associated with left ventricular contractile dysfunction. Although the use of such negative inotropic agents may seem counter-intuitive, multiple studies have shown improvement in symptoms, LV ejection fraction, exercise capacity, and survival in DCM with chronic β-blocker therapy. It is recommended that a β-blocker be prescribed for the majority of patients with stable symptoms of heart failure and continued indefinitely. Therapy must begin at low dosage and be augmented gradually so as not to *worsen* heart failure symptoms via the negative inotropic effect.

In patients with DCM, treatment with *digitalis* may further improve left ventricular function and reduce symptoms, but unlike ACE inhibitors and β-blockers, such therapy has not been shown to prolong survival. Finally, as discussed in Chapter 9, the potassium-sparing diuretic *spironolactone* reduces cardiac complications and mortality rates, when combined with a diuretic and ACE inhibitor, in patients with advanced (Class IV) symptoms of heart failure.

Atrial and ventricular arrhythmias are common in advanced DCM, and approximately 40% of deaths in this condition are due to ventricular tachycardia or fibrillation. It is important to maintain serum electrolytes (notably potassium and magnesium) within their normal ranges, especially during diuretic therapy, so as not to provoke serious arrhythmias. Unfortunately, studies to date have *not* shown that antiarrhythmic drugs prevent death related to ventricular arrhythmias in DCM. In fact, when used in patients with poor LV function, many antiarrhythmic drugs may *worsen* the rhythm disturbance. Amiodarone is the contemporary anti-arrhythmic studied most extensively in patients with DCM. Whereas there is no convincing evidence that it reduces mortality from ventricular arrhythmias in DCM, it is the safest antiarrhythmic for treating atrial fibrillation and other supraventricular arrhythmias in this population. In contrast to antiarrhythmic drugs, the placement of an implantable cardioverter-defibrillator (ICD) does reduce arrhythmic deaths in patients with DCM and severe ventricular rhythm disorders.

Patients with DCM are at increased risk for thromboembolic complications because of 1) stasis in the ventricles due to poor systolic function, 2) stasis in the atria due to chamber enlargement or atrial fibrillation, 3) an abnormally thrombogenic endocardial surface, and 4) venous stasis due to poor forward flow. Peripheral venous or right ventricular thrombus may lead to pulmonary emboli, whereas thromboemboli of left ventricular origin may lodge in any systemic artery, resulting in, for example, devastating cerebral, myocardial, or renal infarctions. Currently, the only *definite* indications for systemic anticoagulation in DCM patients are atrial fibrillation, a previous thromboembolic event, or an LV thrombus visualized by echocardiography. Chronic oral anticoagulation therapy (i.e., warfarin) is often also administered to DCM patients who have severe depression of ventricular function (e.g., LV ejection fraction <30%); however, prospective studies to evaluate the effectiveness of this therapy in patients with

DCM who are in sinus rhythm have not been performed.

Since many patients with DCM have ventricular conduction abnormalities, electronic pacemaker devices capable of stimulating both ventricles simultaneously have been devised to better synchronize systolic contraction as an adjunct to medical therapy. Short-term benefit with such therapy has been achieved in some patients, particularly those with left bundle branch block or other interventricular conduction abnormalities with a significantly prolonged QRS duration. Long-term benefits have not yet been demonstrated.

Finally, in suitable patients, cardiac transplantation offers a substantially better 5-year prognosis than the standard therapies for DCM described above. The current 5- and 10-year survival rates after transplantation are 74% and 55%, respectively. However, the scarcity of donor hearts greatly limits the availability of this technique. Fewer than 2500 transplants are performed in the United States per year, compared with approximately 20,000 patients who could potentially benefit from the procedure. As a result, other mechanical options have been explored and continue to undergo experimental refinements, including ventricular assist devices and completely implanted artificial hearts.

Prognosis

Despite advances in therapy, the prognosis for patients with DCM who do not undergo cardiac transplantation is poor—the average 5-year survival rate is less than 50%. Methods to reduce progressive LV dysfunction by early intervention in asymptomatic or minimally symptomatic patients and the prevention of sudden cardiac death remain major research goals in the treatment of this disorder.

HYPERTROPHIC CARDIOMYOPATHY

Hypertrophic cardiomyopathy (HCM) has received notoriety in the lay press because it is the most common cardiac abnormality found in young athletes who die suddenly during vigorous physical exertion. With an incidence of about 1/500 in the general population, HCM is characterized by septal or left ventricular hypertrophy that is not due to chronic pressure overload (i.e., *not* the result of systemic hypertension or aortic stenosis). Other terms frequently used to describe this disease are hypertrophic obstructive cardiomyopathy (HOCM) and idiopathic hypertrophic subaortic stenosis (IHSS). In this condition, systolic LV contractile function is vigorous but the thickened muscle is stiff, resulting in impaired ventricular relaxation and high diastolic pressures.

Etiology

HCM is a familial disease that can arise spontaneously as a new mutation, which is then passed on to subsequent generations. Inheritance follows an autosomal dominant pattern with variable penetrance, and a large variety of mutations in at least 10 different genes have been implicated in this condition. The proteins encoded by the responsible genes are all part of the sarcomere complex and include β-myosin heavy chain (β-MHC), cardiac troponin T, and myosin-binding protein C. The incorporation of these mutated peptides into the sarcomere is thought to cause impaired contractile function. The resultant increase in myocyte stress is then hypothesized to lead to compensatory hypertrophy and proliferation of fibroblasts.

The pathophysiology and natural history of familial HCM are quite variable and appear related to particular mutations within the disease-causing gene, rather than the actual gene involved. In fact, it has been shown that the precise genetic mutation determines the age of onset of hypertrophy, the extent and pattern of cardiac remodeling, and the individual's risk of developing symptomatic heart failure or sudden death. For example, more than 50 different mutations of the β-MHC gene have been identified, but some mutations (e.g., those that change the coded amino acid's charge) worsen prognosis more than others. It is hoped that better definition of the natural history of specific mutations will allow accurate risk stratification of patients and permit appropriate timing of therapeutic interventions.

Pathology

Although hypertrophy in HCM may involve any portion of the ventricles, asymmetric hypertrophy of the ventricular septum (Fig. 10.4) is most common (approximately 90% of cases). Less often, the hypertrophy involves the ventricular walls symmetrically or is localized to the apex or midregions of the LV.

Unlike ventricular hypertrophy due to hypertension, in which the myocytes enlarge uniformly and remain orderly, the histology of HCM is unusual. The myocardial fibers are in a pattern of extensive disarray (Fig. 10.5). Short, wide, hypertrophied fibers are oriented in chaotic directions and surrounded by numerous cardiac fibro-

blasts and extracellular matrix. This myocyte disarray and fibrosis are diagnostic of HCM and play a role in the abnormal diastolic stiffness and the arrhythmias that are so common in this disorder.

Pathophysiology

The predominant feature of HCM is significant ventricular hypertrophy that reduces the compliance and relaxation (*diastolic* function) of the chamber, such that filling becomes impaired (Fig. 10.6). Patients who have asymmetric hypertrophy of the upper interventricular septum may display additional findings due to transient obstruction of left ventricular outflow during *systole*. In that case, the mechanism of systolic obstruction is thought to involve abnormal motion of the anterior mitral valve leaflet toward the LV outflow tract where the thickened septum protrudes (Fig. 10.7). This process is explained as follows: 1) during ventricular contraction, ejection of blood past the upper septum is more rapid than usual, as it must flow through an outflow tract that is narrowed by the thickened septum; 2) this rapid flow creates Venturi forces that abnormally draw the anterior mitral leaflet toward the septum during contraction; 3) the anterior mitral leaflet approaches and transiently abuts the hypertrophied septum, causing brief obstruction of blood flow into the aorta.

It is useful to consider the pathophysiology of HCM based on whether transient systolic obstruction is present:

HCM Without Outflow Tract Obstruction

Although systolic contraction of the left ventricle is usually vigorous in HCM, the hypertrophied walls result in increased stiffness and impaired diastolic relaxation of the chamber. The reduced ventricular compliance alters the normal pressure-volume relationship, such that the passive diastolic filling curve shifts upward (Fig. 9.7B). The associated rise in diastolic LV pressure is transmitted backward, leading to elevated left atrial, pulmonary venous, and pulmonary capillary pressures. Dysp-

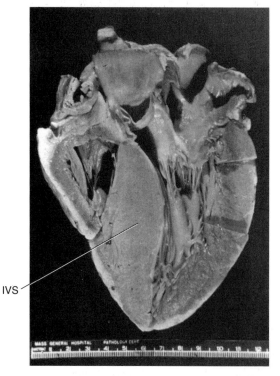

IVS

Figure 10.4. **Postmortem heart specimen from a patient with hypertrophic cardiomyopathy.** Significant left ventricular hypertrophy is seen, especially of the interventricular septum (IVS).

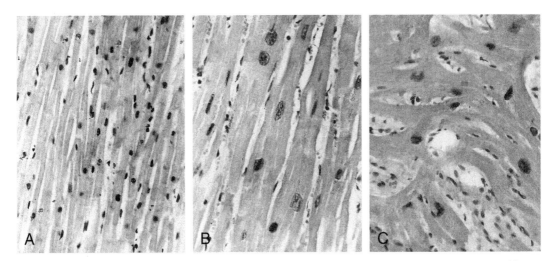

Figure 10.5. **Light microscopy of the hypertrophic myocardium. A.** Normal myocardium. **B.** Hypertrophic myocytes due to pressure overload in a patient with valvular heart disease. **C.** Disordered myocytes with fibrosis in a patient with hypertrophic cardiomyopathy. (Modified from Schoen FJ. Interventional and Surgical Cardiovascular Pathology: Clinical Correlations and Basic Principles. Philadelphia: WB Saunders, 1989:181.)

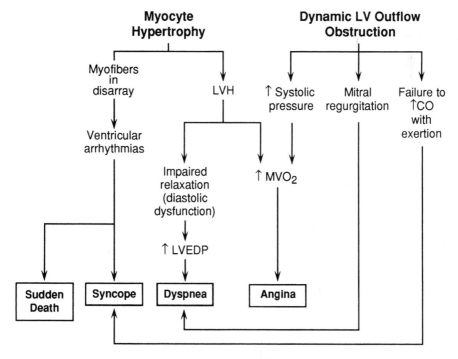

Figure 10.6. **Pathophysiology of hypertrophic cardiomyopathy.** The disarrayed and hypertrophied myocytes may lead to ventricular arrhythmias (which can cause syncope or sudden death) and impaired diastolic left ventricular (LV) relaxation (which causes elevated LV filling pressures and dyspnea). If dynamic left ventricular outflow obstruction is present, mitral regurgitation often accompanies it (which contributes to dyspnea), and the impaired ability to raise cardiac output with exertion can lead to exertional syncope. The thickened LV wall and systolic outflow tract obstruction both contribute to increased myocardial oxygen consumption (MVO_2) and can precipitate angina. LVH, LV hypertrophy; LVEDP, LV end-diastolic pressure; CO, cardiac output.

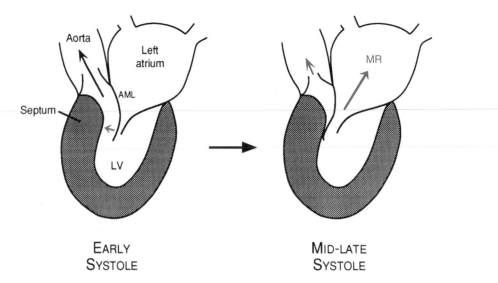

Figure 10.7. Pathophysiology of left ventricular (LV) outflow obstruction and mitral regurgitation in hypertrophic cardiomyopathy (HCM). Left panel. The LV outflow tract is abnormally narrowed between the hypertrophied interventricular septum and the anterior leaflet of the mitral valve (AML). It is thought that the rapid ejection velocity along the narrowed tract in early systole draws the AML toward the septum (small arrow). **Right panel.** As the mitral valve abnormally moves anteriorly and contacts the septum, outflow into the aorta is transiently obstructed. Because the mitral leaflets do not coapt normally in systole, mitral regurgitation (MR) also results.

nea, especially during exertion, is thus a common symptom in this disorder.

HCM with Outflow Obstruction

In patients with outflow obstruction, elevated left atrial and pulmonary capillary wedge pressures are due both to the decreased ventricular compliance and to the outflow obstruction during contraction. During systolic obstruction, a pressure gradient develops between the main body of the LV and the outflow tract distal to the obstruction (see Fig. 10.7). The elevated ventricular systolic pressure increases wall stress and myocardial oxygen consumption, which can result in anginal chest discomfort (see Fig. 10.6). In addition, because obstruction is due to abnormal motion of the anterior mitral leaflet toward the septum (and therefore *away* from the posterior mitral leaflet), the mitral valve does not close properly during systole, and mitral regurgitation may result. This further elevates left atrial and pulmonary venous pressures and may worsen symptoms of dyspnea as well as contribute to the development of atrial fibrillation.

The systolic pressure gradient observed in obstructive HCM is "dynamic" in that its magnitude varies during contraction and depends, at any given time, on the distance between the anterior leaflet of the mitral valve and the hypertrophied septum. Situations that *decrease* LV cavity size (e.g., reduced venous return because of intravascular volume depletion) bring the mitral leaflet and septum into closer proximity and *promote* obstruction. Conversely, conditions that *enlarge* the LV (e.g., augmented intravascular volume) increase the distance between the anterior mitral leaflet and septum and *reduce* the obstruction. Positive inotropic drugs (which augment the force of contraction) also force the mitral leaflet and septum into closer proximity and contribute to obstruction, whereas negative inotropic drugs (e.g., β-blockers, verapamil) have the opposite effect.

Although dynamic systolic outflow tract obstruction creates impressive murmurs and receives great attention, the symptoms of obstructive HCM appear to be primarily due to the increased LV stiffness and diastolic dysfunction that are also present in the nonobstructive form.

Clinical Findings

The symptoms of HCM vary widely, from the asymptomatic individual to those with significant physical limitations. The average age of presentation is in the mid-20s.

The most frequent symptom is *dyspnea* due to elevated diastolic LV (and therefore pulmonary capillary) pressures. This symptom is further exacerbated by the high systolic LV pressure and mitral regurgitation seen in individuals with outflow tract obstruction.

Angina is often described by patients with HCM, even in the absence of obstructive coronary artery disease. Myocardial ischemia may be contributed to by 1) the high oxygen demand of the increased muscle mass and 2) the narrowed small branches of the coronary arteries within the hypertrophied ventricular wall (i.e., decreased vasodilator reserve, hence reduced myocardial oxygen supply). If outflow tract obstruction is present, the high systolic ventricular pressure also increases myocardial oxygen demand, because of the increased wall stress.

Syncope in HCM may result from cardiac arrhythmias that develop because of the structurally abnormal myofibers (see below). In patients with outflow tract obstruction, syncope may also be induced by exertion, when the pressure gradient is made worse by the increased force of contraction, thereby causing a transient fall in cardiac output. Orthostatic lightheadedness is also common in patients with outflow tract obstruction. This occurs because venous return to the heart is reduced upon standing by the gravitational pooling of blood in the lower extremities. The LV thereby decreases in size, and outflow tract obstruction intensifies, transiently reducing cardiac output and cerebral perfusion.

When arrhythmias occur, symptoms of HCM may be exacerbated. For example, atrial fibrillation is not well tolerated, as the loss of the normal "atrial kick" further impairs diastolic filling and can worsen symptoms of pulmonary congestion. Of greatest concern, the first clinical manifestation of HCM may be ventricular fibrillation, resulting in *sudden cardiac death,* particularly in young adults with HCM during strenuous physical exertion. Risk factors for sudden death among patients with known HCM include a history of syncope, a family history of sudden death, certain high-risk mutations, and extreme hypertrophy of the LV wall (>30 mm in thickness).

Physical Examination

Patients with mild forms of HCM are often asymptomatic, and the findings of the physical examination may be entirely normal. A common finding is the presence of a fourth heart sound (S_4). It is generated by left atrial contraction into the stiffened LV (see Chapter 2). The forceful atrial contraction may also result in a palpable presystolic impulse over the cardiac apex (creating what is known as a "double" apical impulse).

Other findings are common in patients with systolic outflow obstruction. The carotid pulse rises briskly in early systole but then quickly declines as obstruction to cardiac outflow appears. The characteristic systolic murmur of LV outflow obstruction is rough and crescendo-decrescendo in shape, heard best at the left lower sternal border (due to turbulent flow through the narrowed outflow tract). In addition, as the stethoscope is moved toward the apex, the holosystolic blowing murmur of mitral regurgitation may be auscultated. Although the LV outflow obstruction murmur may be soft at rest, bedside maneuvers that alter preload and afterload can dramatically increase its intensity and help differentiate this murmur from other conditions, such as aortic stenosis (Table 10.2).

A commonly used technique in this regard is the Valsalva maneuver, produced by

TABLE 10.2. Effect of Maneuvers on Murmurs of Aortic Stenosis (AS) and Hypertrophic Cardiomyopathy (HCM)

	Valsalva	Squatting	Standing
Preload	↓	↑	↓
Afterload	↓	↑	↓
HCM murmur	↑	↓	↑
AS murmur	↓	↑ (usually)	↓

asking the patient to "bear down" (technically defined as forceful exhalation with the nose, mouth, and glottis closed). The Valsalva maneuver increases intrathoracic pressure, which decreases venous return to the heart and transiently reduces LV size. This action brings the hypertrophied septum and anterior leaflet of the mitral valve into closer proximity, creating greater obstruction to forward flow. Thus, during Valsalva, the murmur of HCM will *increase* in intensity. In contrast, the murmur of aortic stenosis decreases in intensity during Valsalva, because of the reduced flow across the stenotic valve.

Diagnostic Studies

The *ECG* typically shows left ventricular hypertrophy and left atrial enlargement. Prominent Q waves are common in the inferior and lateral leads, representing forces of initial depolarization of the hypertrophied septum. In some patients, diffuse T wave inversions are present, which can predate clinical, echocardiographic, or other electrocardiographic manifestations of HCM. Atrial and ventricular arrhythmias are frequent, especially atrial fibrillation. Ventricular arrhythmias are particularly ominous because they may herald ventricular fibrillation and sudden death, even in previously asymptomatic patients.

Echocardiography is most helpful in the evaluation of HCM. The degree of LV hypertrophy can be measured and regions of asymmetrical wall thickness readily identified. Signs of left ventricular outflow obstruction may also be demonstrated and include abnormal anterior motion of the mitral valve as it is drawn toward the hypertrophied septum during systole, and partial closure of the aortic valve in midsystole as flow across it is transiently obstructed. Doppler recordings during echocardiography accurately measure the outflow pressure gradient and quantify any associated mitral regurgitation. Children and adolescents with apparently mild HCM should undergo serial echocardiographic assessment over time, as the degree of hypertrophy may increase during puberty and early adulthood.

Cardiac catheterization is reserved for patients for whom the diagnosis is uncertain or if cardiac surgery is planned. The major feature, in patients with obstruction, is the finding of a pressure gradient within the outflow portion of the left ventricle, either at rest or during maneuvers that transiently reduce LV size and promote outflow tract obstruction. Myocardial biopsy at the time of catheterization is not necessary, because histologic findings do not predict disease severity or long-term prognosis.

Although genetic testing for HCM is not currently feasible on a wide-scale basis, future genotyping may provide a noninvasive technique for definitive diagnosis and risk stratification.

Treatment

β-Blockers are the standard therapy for HCM because they 1) reduce myocardial oxygen demand by slowing the heart rate and the force of contraction (and therefore diminish angina and dyspnea), 2) lessen the LV outflow gradient during exercise by reducing the force of contraction (allowing the chamber size to increase, thus separating the anterior leaflet of the mitral valve from the ventricular septum), 3) increase passive diastolic ventricular filling time due to the decreased heart rate, and 4) decrease the frequency of ventricular ectopic beats. Despite the antiarrhythmic effect, β-blockers have not been shown to prevent sudden arrhythmic death in this condition.

Calcium channel antagonists can reduce ventricular stiffness and are sometimes useful in improving exercise capacity in patients whose conditions fail to respond to β-blockers. Patients who develop pulmonary congestion may benefit from mild diuretic therapy, but such drugs must be administered cautiously to avoid volume depletion; reduced intravascular volume decreases LV size and could exacerbate outflow tract obstruction. Vasodilators (including nitrates) similarly reduce LV size and should also be avoided.

Because atrial fibrillation is poorly tolerated in HCM, it should be controlled aggressively, most commonly with *antiar-*

rhythmic drugs. Effective antiarrhythmics for atrial fibrillation in HCM include amiodarone and disopyramide (a type IA antiarrhythmic drug, described in Chapter 17, that also possesses negative inotropic properties that may help reduce LV outflow tract obstruction). Digitalis should be avoided in HCM as its *positive* inotropic effect increases the force of contraction and could worsen LV outflow tract obstruction.

Because sudden cardiac death has a propensity to occur in association with physical exertion, strenuous exercise and competitive sports should be avoided. Sudden death in this syndrome is almost always due to ventricular tachycardia/fibrillation. Although amiodarone may reduce the frequency of ventricular arrhythmias, HCM patients who have survived a cardiac arrest, or those who display high-risk ventricular arrhythmias, should receive an implantable cardioverter defibrillator.

Infective endocarditis can develop in patients with obstructive HCM because of turbulent blood flow through the narrowed LV outflow tract and in association with the accompanying mitral regurgitation. *Antibiotic prophylaxis* (see Chapter 8) is therefore indicated to prevent endocardial infection during surgical procedures that result in bacteremia.

Some studies have shown clinical improvement when patients with obstructive HCM are treated with a dual-chamber permanent pacemaker, the electrodes of which are placed in the right atrium and right ventricle. The LV outflow gradient may become reduced by this procedure, possibly by altering the normal sequence of ventricular contraction, such that septal-mitral valve apposition becomes less prominent. This technique seems to be useful for only a small percentage of patients.

Surgical therapy (*myomectomy*) is considered for patients whose conditions do not respond to pharmacologic therapy. This procedure involves excision of portions of the hypertrophied muscle mass and usually results in improved symptomatology. A less invasive experimental alternative is transcatheter septal ablation, in which ethanol is injected directly into the first major septal coronary artery (a branch of the left anterior descending artery) causing a small, controlled infarction. This results in reduced septal thickness and can lessen outflow tract obstruction.

Finally, genetic counseling should be provided to all patients with HCM. As this is an autosomal dominant disease, children of affected individuals have a 50% chance of inheriting the abnormal gene. In addition, first-degree relatives of patients with HCM should be screened for the condition by physical examination, electrocardiography, and echocardiography. Even if affected individuals are asymptomatic, they are at increased risk of complications, including sudden death, and must be monitored closely.

Prognosis

The incidence of sudden death is 2–4% per year in adults and 4–6% in children and adolescents. It has become clear that different mutations have vastly different phenotypes. Some cause extreme hypertrophy in childhood without any clinical symptoms until the occurrence of sudden death; others manifest later in life with heart failure symptoms. The majority produce only mild hypertrophy and are associated with a normal life expectancy. As the clinical outcomes of specific mutations are better defined, the use and timing of specific therapeutic interventions will likely be clarified.

RESTRICTIVE CARDIOMYOPATHY

The restrictive cardiomyopathies are less common than DCM and HCM. They are characterized by abnormally rigid (but not necessarily thickened) ventricles with impaired diastolic filling but usually normal, or near-normal, systolic function. This condition results from either 1) fibrosis or scarring of the endomyocardium or 2) infiltration of the myocardium by an abnormal substance, such as amyloid (Table 10.3). The pathologic appearance is varied depending on etiology.

TABLE 10.3. Examples of Restrictive Cardiomyopathy

Myocardial	Endomyocardial
Noninfiltrative	Endomyocardial fibrosis
Idiopathic	Hypereosinophilic syndrome
Scleroderma	Metastatic tumors
Infiltrative	Radiation therapy
Amyloidosis	
Sarcoidosis	
Storage diseases	
Hemochromatosis	
Glycogen storage	
diseases	

Pathophysiology

Reduced compliance of the ventricles due to fibrosis or infiltration results in an upward shift of the passive ventricular filling curve (see Fig. 9.7B) such that intraventricular pressure is abnormally high throughout diastole. There are two major consequences: 1) elevated systemic and pulmonary venous pressures, with signs of right- and left-sided vascular congestion, and 2) reduced ventricular cavity size with decreased stroke volume and cardiac output.

Clinical Findings

It follows from the underlying pathophysiology that signs of left- and right-sided heart failure are expected (Fig. 10.8). Decreased cardiac output is manifested by fatigue and decreased exercise tolerance. Systemic congestion (often more prominent than pulmonary congestion in this syndrome) leads to jugular venous distention, peripheral edema, and ascites with a large, tender liver. Arrhythmias such as atrial fibrillation are common. Infiltrative etiologies

that involve the cardiac conduction system can cause various types of heart block.

Physical Examination

Signs of congestive heart failure are often present including pulmonary rales, distended neck veins, ascites, and peripheral edema. Similar to constrictive pericarditis (see Chapter 14), jugular venous distention may paradoxically worsen with inspiration (**Kussmaul's sign**) as the right ventricle is not able to accommodate the increased venous return.

Diagnostic Studies

The chest radiograph usually shows a normal-sized heart with signs of pulmonary congestion. The ECG often displays nonspecific ST- and T-wave abnormalities; conduction disturbances such as atrioventricular block or a bundle branch block may be present.

As described in Chapter 14, the restrictive cardiomyopathies share nearly identical symptoms, physical signs, and hemodynamic profiles with constrictive pericarditis. However, it is important to distinguish between these two entities, because constrictive pericarditis is a treatable condition, whereas the restrictive cardiomyopathies generally are not treatable.

The most useful diagnostic tools to differentiate restrictive cardiomyopathy from constrictive pericarditis are transvenous endomyocardial biopsy, computed tomography (CT), and magnetic resonance imaging (MRI). For example, in restrictive cardiomyopathy, a transvenous endomyocardial

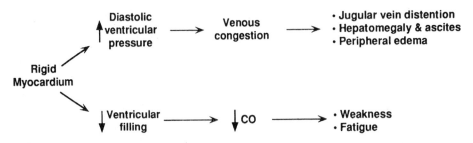

Figure 10.8. **Pathophysiology of restrictive cardiomyopathy.** The rigid myocardium results in elevated ventricular diastolic pressures and decreased ventricular filling. The resultant symptoms can be predicted from these abnormalities. CO, cardiac output.

biopsy may demonstrate the presence of infiltrative matter such as amyloid, iron deposits (hemochromatosis), or metastatic tumors. Conversely, CT or MRI scans are useful to identify the thickened pericardium of constrictive pericarditis, a finding that is not expected in restrictive cardiomyopathy.

Treatment

Restrictive cardiomyopathy typically has a very poor prognosis, except when treatment can be targeted at an underlying cause. For example, phlebotomy and iron chelation therapy may be helpful in the early form of hemochromatosis. Symptomatic therapy for all etiologies includes salt restriction and cautious use of diuretics to improve symptoms of systemic and pulmonary congestion. Unlike the dilated cardiomyopathies, digitalis and vasodilators are not helpful because systolic function is usually preserved. Maintenance of sinus rhythm is important to maximize diastolic filling and forward cardiac output. Some restrictive cardiomyopathies are prone to intraventricular thrombus formation, in which case chronic oral anticoagulant therapy is warranted.

SUMMARY

1. The cardiomyopathies are diseases of heart muscle that are classified by their pathophysiologic presentation into dilated, hypertrophic, or restrictive types (Table 10.4).

TABLE 10.4. Summary of the Cardiomyopathies

	Dilated Cardiomyopathy	Hypertrophic Cardiomyopathy	Restrictive Cardiomyopathy
Ventricular morphology	Dilated LV with little hypertrophy	Marked hypertrophy, often asymmetric	Fibrotic or infiltrated myocardium
Symptoms	Fatigue, weakness, dyspnea, orthopnea, PND (symptoms of congestive heart failure)	Dyspnea, angina, syncope	Dyspnea, fatigue
Physical exam	Pulmonary rales, S3; If RVfailure present: JVD, hepatomegaly, peripheral edema	S4; If outflow obstruction present: systolic murmur loudest at left sternal border, accompanied by mitral regurgitation	Signs of RV failure: JVD, hepatomegaly, peripheral edema
Pathophysiology	Impaired systolic contraction	Impaired diastolic relaxation; LV systolic function vigorous, often with dynamic obstruction	"Stiff" LV with impaired diastolic relaxation but normal systolic function
Cardiac size on chest radiograph	Dilated	Normal or dilated	Usually normal
Echocardiogram	Dilated, poorly contractile LV	LV hypertrophy, often more pronounced in septum; systolic anterior movement of MV with mitral regurgitation	Usually normal systolic contraction; "speckled" appearance in infiltrative disorders

LV, left ventricle; PND, paroxysmal nocturnal dyspnea; RV, right ventricle; JVD, jugular venous distension; MV, mitral valve.

2. Dilated cardiomyopathies are characterized by ventricular dilatation with impaired systolic function. Progressive left ventricular enlargement often leads to symptomatic heart failure, ventricular arrhythmias, and/or embolic complications.

3. HCM is characterized by a significantly thickened left ventricle with impaired diastolic relaxation. Dynamic LV outflow tract obstruction during systole may be present. The most common symptoms are dyspnea and exertional angina. Ventricular arrhythmias may lead to sudden cardiac death.

4. The restrictive cardiomyopathies are uncommon and are characterized by impairment of diastolic ventricular relaxation due to an infiltrated or fibrotic myocardium. Symptoms of heart failure are typical.

Acknowledgments   The authors thank Dr. Christine Seidman for reviewing the manuscript and Dr. Frederick Schoen for providing pathology specimens. Contributors to the previous editions of this chapter were Kay Fang, MD; David Grayzel, MD; G. William Dec, MD; and Leonard S. Lilly, MD.

ADDITIONAL READING

Costanzo NW, Augustine S, Bourge R, et al. Selection and treatment of candidates for heart transplantation. A statement for health professionals from the Committee on Heart Failure and Cardiac Transplantation of the Council of Clinical Cardiology, American Heart Association. Circulation 1995;92: 3593–3612.

Dec GW, Fuster VF. Idiopathic dilated cardiomyopathy. N Engl J Med 1994;331:1564–1575.

Kushwaha SS, Fallon JT, Fuster V. Medical progress: restrictive cardiomyopathy. N Engl J Med 1997;336:267–276.

Marian AJ, Roberts R. The molecular genetic basis for hypertrophic cardiomyopathy. J Mol Cell Cardiol 2001;33:655–670.

Maron BJ. Hypertrophic cardiomyopathy: a systemic review. JAMA 2002;287:1308–1320.

Maron BJ, Shen WK, Link MS, et al. Efficacy of implantable cardioverter-defibrillators for the prevention of sudden death in patients with hypertrophic cardiomyopathy. N Engl J Med 2000;342:365–373.

Richardson P, McKenna W, Bristow M, et al. Report of the 1995 World Health Organization/International Society and Federation of Cardiology Task Force on the Definition and Classification of Cardiomyopathies. Circulation 1996;93:841–842.

Roberts R, Sigwart U. New concepts in hypertrophic cardiomyopathies, part I. Circulation 2001;104: 2113–2116.

Schonberger J, Seidman C. Many roads lead to a broken heart: the genetics of dilated cardiomyopathy. Am J Hum Genet 2001;69:249–260.

Seidman JG, Seidman C. The genetic basis for cardiomyopathy: from mutation identification to mechanistic paradigms. Cell 2001;104:557–567.

Mechanisms of Cardiac Arrhythmias

Jennifer E. Ho, William G. Stevenson,
Gary R. Strichartz, and Leonard S. Lilly

Normal Impulse Formation
  Ionic Basis of Automaticity
  Native and Latent Pacemakers
  Overdrive Suppression
  Electrotonic Interactions
Altered Impulse Formation
  Alterations in Sinus Node Automaticity
  Escape Rhythms

Enhanced Automaticity of Latent Pacemakers
Abnormal Automaticity
Triggered Activity
Altered Impulse Conduction
  Conduction Block
  Unidirectional Block and Reentry
Approach to Antiarrhythmic Treatment
  Bradyarrhythmias
  Tachyarrhythmias

Normal cardiac function relies on the flow of electrical impulses through the heart in an exquisitely coordinated fashion. Abnormalities of the electrical rhythm are known as *arrhythmias* (also termed *dysrhythmias*) and are among the most common clinical problems encountered. Their presentations range from benign palpitations to severe symptoms of low cardiac output and death, so that a thorough understanding of these disorders is important to the daily practice of medicine.

This chapter describes the mechanisms by which arrhythmias develop, followed by a general description of treatment. Chapter 12 summarizes specific rhythm disorders and how to recognize and treat them.

Disorders of heart rhythm result from alterations of **impulse formation,** of **impulse conduction,** or both. This chapter first addresses how alterations of impulse formation and conduction occur and under what circumstances they cause arrhythmias. Figure 11.1 provides an organizational schema for this discussion.

NORMAL IMPULSE FORMATION

As presented in Chapter 1, electrical impulse formation in the heart arises from the intrinsic automaticity of specialized cardiac cells. **Automaticity** refers to a cell's ability to depolarize itself to a threshold voltage in a rhythmic, repeated fashion, such that *spontaneous* action potentials are generated. Although atrial and ventricular myocytes do not have this property under normal conditions, the cells of the specialized conducting system do possess natural automaticity and are therefore termed **pacemaker cells.** The specialized conducting system includes the sinoatrial (SA) node, the atrioventricular (AV) nodal region, and the ventricular conducting system. The latter is composed of the bundle of His, the bundle branches, and the Purkinje fibers. In *pathologic situations*, myocardial cells outside the conducting system may also acquire the property of automaticity.

Ionic Basis of Automaticity

Cells with natural automaticity do not have a static resting potential. Rather, they display a gradual depolarization during phase 4 of the action potential (Fig. 11.2) If this spontaneous diastolic depolarization reaches the threshold voltage, an action potential is generated. An important ionic flow largely responsible for phase 4 sponta-

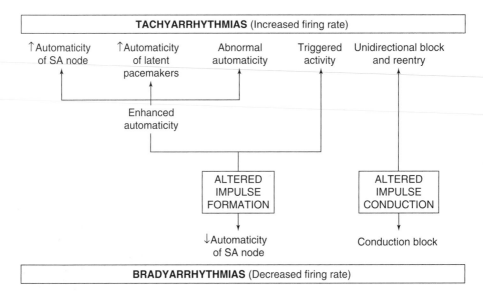

Figure 11.1. Arrhythmias result from alterations in impulse formation and/or impulse conduction. Tachy-arrhythmias result from enhanced automaticity, triggered activity, and unidirectional block with reentry. Brady-arrhythmias result from decreased automaticity or conduction block.

neous depolarization is known as the **pacemaker current (I_f).** This current is activated by hyperpolarization (increasingly negative voltages) and is carried mainly by sodium ions. The channels that carry I_f open when the membrane voltage becomes more negative than approximately -50 mV, and are *different* from the fast sodium channels responsible for rapid phase 0 depolarization in nonpacemaker cells. The inward

flow of Na^+ through these slow channels, driven by its concentration gradient and the negative intracellular charge, forces the membrane potential to depolarize toward the threshold voltage.

In the pacemaker cells of the sinoatrial node, alterations in two other ionic currents also contribute to phase 4 depolarization: 1) a slow inward calcium current, the channels of which become activated at voltages

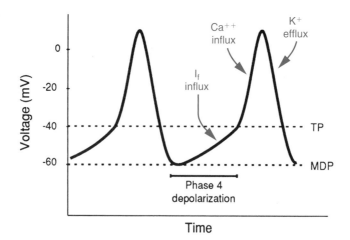

Figure 11.2. The action potential (AP) of a pacemaker cell. Note the slow phase 4 depolarization, largely caused by the I_f (pacemaker) current through slow Na^+ channels, which drives the cell to threshold potential (approximately -40mV). The upstroke of the AP is due to the slow inward current of Ca^+ ions. Inactivation of the calcium channels and K^+ efflux through potassium channels are responsible for repolarization. MDP, maximum negative diastolic potential; TP, threshold potential.

reached near the end of phase 4, and 2) a progressive decline of an *outward* potassium current. The latter current is responsible for cellular repolarization during phase 3 of the action potential, and it progressively diminishes during phase 4. The combination of the inward I_f, inward Ca^{++}, and reduced outward K^+ currents acts to gradually depolarize the SA nodal cells to the threshold potential.

When the membrane potential of the pacemaker cell reaches the threshold value, the upstroke of the action potential is generated. In distinction to the phase 0 upstroke of cells in the Purkinje system, that of cells in the sinus and AV nodes is much slower (see Fig. 11.2; compare with Fig. 1.14, page 18). This is so because the number of available (or resting-state) fast sodium channels responsible for the rapid upstroke of the action potential increases as the resting membrane potential becomes more negative. Because sinus and AV nodal cells have *less negative* maximum diastolic membrane voltages (typically -50 to -60 mV) as compared to Purkinje cells (typically -90 mV), a greater proportion of the fast sodium channels is chronically inactivated in the pacemaker cells. Thus, the action potential upstroke relies on *calcium* ion inflow (through the relatively slower opening Ca^{++} channels) and is less steep in these cells.

The repolarization phase of pacemaker cells depends on inactivation of the calcium channels and the opening of K^+ specific voltage-gated potassium channels that permit efflux of potassium from the cells.

Native and Latent Pacemakers

The different populations of automatic cells in the specialized conduction pathway have distinct intrinsic rates of firing. These rates are determined by three variables that influence how fast the membrane potential reaches threshold: 1) the rate (i.e., the slope) of phase 4 spontaneous depolarization, 2) the maximum negative diastolic potential, and 3) the threshold potential. A more negative maximum diastolic potential, or a less negative threshold potential, slows the rate

of impulse initiation because it takes longer to reach that threshold value (Fig. 11.3). Conversely, the greater the I_f, the steeper the slope of phase 4, and the faster the cell depolarizes. The rate of I_f depends on the number and kinetics of the individual pacemaker channels through which this current flows.

Because all the healthy myocardial cells are electrically connected by gap junctions, an action potential generated in one part of the myocardium will ultimately spread to all other regions. When an impulse arrives at a cell that is not yet close to threshold, current from the depolarized cell will bring the adjacent cell membrane potential to the threshold level so that it will fire (regardless of how close its intrinsic I_f has brought it to threshold). Thus, the pacemaker cells with the fastest rate of depolarization set the heart rate. In the normal heart, the dominant pacemaker is the *sinoatrial node*, which at rest initiates impulses at a rate of 60–100 bpm. Because the sinus node rate is faster than that of the other tissues that possess automaticity, its repeated discharges prevent spontaneous firing of other potential pacemaker sites.

Because the SA node normally sets the heart rate, it is known as the **native pacemaker.** Other cells within the specialized conduction system harbor the potential to act as pacemakers when called on to do so and are therefore called **latent pacemakers** (also termed **ectopic pacemakers**). In contrast to the SA node, the AV node and the bundle of His have intrinsic firing rates of 50–60 bpm, and cells of the Purkinje system have rates of approximately 30–40 bpm. These latent sites may initiate impulses and take over the pacemaking function if the faster pacemakers (i.e., cells of the SA node) fail or if conduction abnormalities block the normal wave of depolarization from reaching them.

Overdrive Suppression

Not only does the cell population with the fastest intrinsic rhythm preempt all other automatic cells from spontaneously firing, it also directly *suppresses* their auto-

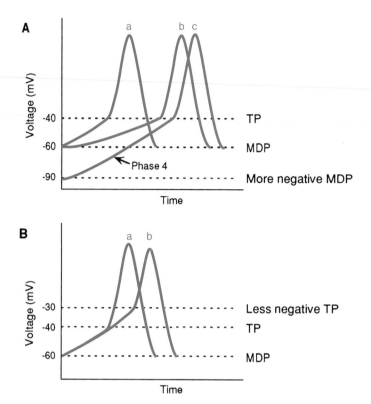

Figure 11.3. **A.** Alterations in the pacemaker current (I_f) and in the magnitude of the maximum diastolic potential (MDP) alter the cell firing rate. (a) The normal action potential (AP) of a pacemaker cell. (b) Reduced I_f renders the slope of phase 4 less steep; thus, the time required to reach threshold potential (TP) is increased. (c) The MDP is more negative; therefore, the time required to reach TP is increased. **B.** Alterations in TP change the firing rate of the cell. Compared with the normal TP (a), the TP in b is less negative; thus, the duration of time to achieve threshold is increased, and the firing rate decreases.

maticity. This phenomenon is called over-drive suppression. Cells maintain their trans-sarcolemmal ion distributions because of the continuously active Na$^+$/K$^+$-ATPase pump that extrudes three Na$^+$ ions

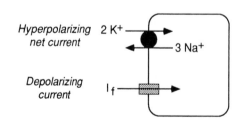

Figure 11.4. Competition between the depolarizing pacemaker current (I_f) and the Na$^+$/K$^+$ pump, which produces a hyperpolarizing current. The Na$^+$/K$^+$ pump transports three positive charges outside the cell for every two it pumps in. The hyperpolarizing current acts to suppress automaticity by antagonizing I_f, and contributes to overdrive suppression in cells that are stimulated more rapidly than their intrinsic firing rate.

from the cell in exchange for two K$^+$ ions transported in (Fig. 11.4). Because its net transport effect is one positive charge in the outward direction, the Na$^+$/K$^+$ pump creates a *hyperpolarizing* current (i.e., it tends to make the inside of the cell *more negative*). As the cell potential becomes increasingly negative, additional time is required for spontaneous phase 4 depolarization to reach the threshold voltage (see Fig. 11.3A), and therefore the rate of spontaneous firing is decreased. Although the hyperpolarizing current antagonizes I_f, pacemaker cells firing at their own intrinsic rate have an I_f current sufficiently large to overcome this hyperpolarizing influence (see Fig. 11.4).

The hyperpolarizing current *increases* when a cell is forced to fire faster than its intrinsic pacemaker rate. The more frequently the cell is depolarized, the greater the quantity of Na$^+$ ions that enter the cell per unit time. As a result, the Na^+/K^+ pump becomes more active, so as to restore the normal transmembrane Na^+ gradient. This increased pump activity provides a larger hyperpolarizing current, opposing the depolarizing current I_f, and further decreases rates of spontaneous depolarization. In this fashion, overdrive suppression decreases a cell's automaticity when that cell is forced to fire faster than its intrinsic discharge rate.

Electrotonic Interactions

In addition to overdrive suppression, *anatomic connections* between pacemaker and non-pacemaker cells are important in suppressing latent pacemaker foci. Myocardial cells that are not part of the specialized conducting system repolarize to a resting potential of −90 mV, whereas pacemaker cells repolarize to a maximum diastolic potential of about −60 mV. When these two cell types are adjacent to one another, *electrical coupling* occurs through gap junctions in their intercalated discs. This coupling results in an equilibration of electrical potentials, causing relative *hyperpolarization* of the pacemaker cell, and relative *depolarization* of the non-pacemaker cell (Fig. 11.5). The hyperpolarizing current in the coupled pacemaker cell competes with I_f and causes the slope of phase 4 diastolic depolarization to be less steep, thereby reducing the cell's automaticity. This mechanism may be particularly important in suppressing automaticity in the AV node (via connections between atrial myocytes and AV nodal cells) and in the distal Purkinje fibers (which are anatomically adjacent to nonautomatic ventricular myocardial cells). In contrast, cells of the SA node are less tightly coupled to atrial myocytes; thus, their automaticity is less subject to electrotonic interactions.

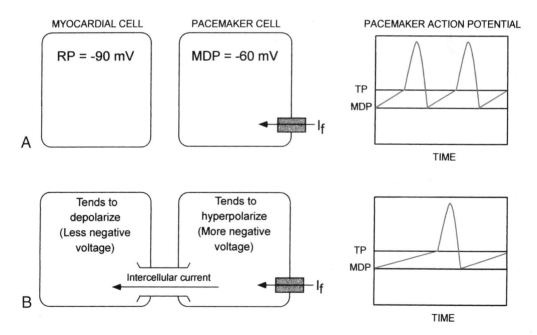

Figure 11.5. Electrotonic interaction between pacemaker (e.g., AV nodal) and non-pacemaker (myocardial) cells. A. When pacemaker cells are not coupled to myocardial cells (as in the SA node), they have a maximum negative potential (MDP) of approximately −60 mV, whereas myocardial cells have a resting potential (RP) of approximately −90 mV. **B.** When pacemaker cells and myocytes neighbor one another, they may be connected electrically by gap junctions in their intercalated discs (e.g., in the AV node). In this situation, a positive electrical current flows from the pacemaker cell toward the myocardial cell, tending to equilibrate voltages and hyperpolarize the former and depolarize the latter. This action opposes I_f of the pacemaker cell, the slope of phase 4 depolarization is less steep, and therefore cellular automaticity is suppressed. If a disease state causes the loss of the intercellular connection, then the pacemaker cell is no longer hyperpolarized by the neighboring cell and thus depolarizes to threshold more readily, much like SA nodal cells. TP, threshold potential.

Decoupling of normally suppressed cells, such as those in the AV node (e.g., by ischemic damage), may reduce the inhibitory electrotonic influence and *enhance* automaticity, producing ectopic rhythms by the latent pacemaker tissue.

ALTERED IMPULSE FORMATION

Arrhythmias may arise from altered impulse formation at the SA node or from other sites, including the specialized conduction pathways or from regions of cardiac muscle. The main abnormalities of impulse initiation that lead to arrhythmias are 1) **altered automaticity** (of the sinus node, of latent pacemakers within the specialized conduction pathway, or abnormal automaticity in atrial or ventricular myocytes) and 2) **triggered activity.**

Alterations in Sinus Node Automaticity

The rate of impulse initiation by the sinus node, as well as by the latent pacemakers of the specialized conducting system, is regulated primarily by neurohumoral factors.

Increased Sinus Node Automaticity

The most important modulator of normal sinus node automaticity is the autonomic nervous system. Sympathetic stimulation, acting through β_1-adrenergic receptors, increases the probability of the pacemaker channels being open (Fig. 11.6), through which I_f can flow. The increase in I_f leads to a steeper slope of phase 4 depolarization, such that the SA node reaches threshold and fires earlier than normal, and the heart rate increases.

In addition, sympathetic stimulation shifts the action potential threshold to more negative voltages by increasing the probability that voltage-sensitive Ca^{++} channels are open (recall that calcium carries the current of phase 0 depolarization in pacemaker cells). Therefore, diastolic depolarization reaches the threshold potential earlier. Thus, sympathetic activity increases sinus node automaticity both by causing the ac-

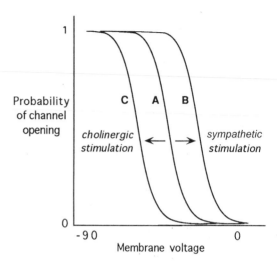

Figure 11.6. **The channels through which the pacemaker current (I_f) flows are voltage-gated, opening at more negative membrane potentials.** At any given voltage, there exists a probability between 0 and 1 that a specific channel will be open. Compared with normal baseline behavior (curve A), sympathetic stimulation (curve B) or treatment with anticholinergic drugs shifts this probability to a higher value for any given level of membrane voltage, thus increasing the number of open channels and the rate at which the cell will fire. Curve C shows that parasympathetic stimulation (or treatment with β-blockers) has the opposite effect, decreasing the probability of a channel being open, and therefore inhibiting depolarization.

tion potential threshold to become more negative and by increasing the rate of pacemaker depolarization via I_f. Examples of this normal physiologic effect occur during exercise or emotional stress, when sympathetic stimulation appropriately increases the heart rate.

Decreased Sinus Node Automaticity

Normal decreases in SA node automaticity are mediated by reduced sympathetic stimulation and by increased activity of the parasympathetic nervous system. Whereas the sympathetic nervous system exerts a dominant effect on the heart rate during times of stress, the parasympathetic nervous system is the major mediator of the heart rate at rest.

Cholinergic (i.e., parasympathetic) stimulation via the vagus nerve acts at the SA node to reduce the probability of pacemaker channels being open (see Fig. 11.6). Thus, I_f and the slope of phase 4 depolarization are reduced, and the intrinsic firing rate of the cell is slowed. In addition, the probability of the Ca^+ channels being open is decreased; thus, the action potential threshold increases to a more positive potential. Furthermore, cholinergic stimulation increases the probability of certain K^+ channels being open at rest. Because positively charged K^+ ions exit through these channels, the cell becomes hyperpolarized, and the maximum diastolic potential becomes more negative. The overall effect of reduced I_f, more negative maximum diastolic potential, and a less negative threshold level is a slowing of the intrinsic firing rate and therefore a reduced heart rate.

It follows that the use of pharmacologic agents that modify the effects of the autonomic nervous system will also affect the firing rate of the SA node. For example, β-blocking drugs antagonize the β-adrenergic sympathetic effect; therefore, they *decrease* the rate of phase 4 depolarization of the SA node and slow the heart rate. Conversely, atropine, an anticholinergic (antimuscarinic) drug has the opposite effect—by blocking the parasympathetic response, the rate of phase 4 depolarization *increases*, and the heart rate accelerates.

Escape Rhythms

If the sinus node becomes suppressed and fires less frequently than normal, the site of impulse formation usually shifts to a latent pacemaker within the specialized conduction pathway. When a latent pacemaker initiates an impulse because the SA node rate has slowed, it is called an **escape beat.** Persistent impairment of the SA node will allow a continued series of escape beats, termed an **escape rhythm.** Escape rhythms are protective in that they prevent the heart rate from becoming too slow when SA node firing is impaired.

As discussed in the previous section, suppression of sinus node activity may occur because of increased parasympathetic tone. Different regions of the heart vary in their sensitivity to parasympathetic (vagal) stimulation. The SA node and the AV node are most sensitive to such an influence, followed by atrial tissue. The ventricular conducting system is the least sensitive. Therefore, moderate parasympathetic stimulation slows the sinus rate and allows the pacemaker to shift to another atrial site. However, very strong parasympathetic stimulation suppresses excitability at both the SA node and atrial tissue, can cause conduction block at the AV node, and may therefore result in the emergence of a ventricular escape pacemaker.

Enhanced Automaticity of Latent Pacemakers

Another means by which a latent pacemaker can assume control of impulse formation is if it develops an intrinsic rate of depolarization *faster* than that of the sinus node. Termed an **ectopic beat,** the impulse is *premature* relative to the normal rhythm, whereas an escape beat is *late* and terminates a pause caused by a slowed sinus rhythm. A sequence of similar ectopic beats is called an **ectopic rhythm.**

Ectopic beats may arise in several circumstances. For example, high catecholamine concentrations can enhance the automaticity of latent pacemakers, and if the resulting rate of depolarization exceeds that of the sinus node, then an ectopic rhythm will develop. Ectopic beats are also commonly induced during periods of hypoxemia, ischemia, electrolyte disturbances, and because of certain drug toxicities (such as digitalis, as described in Chapter 17).

Abnormal Automaticity

Cardiac tissue injury may lead to pathologic changes in impulse formation whereby myocardial cells *outside* the specialized conduction system acquire automaticity and spontaneously depolarize. Although such activity may appear similar to impulses originating from latent pacemakers within the specialized conduction pathways, these ectopic beats arise from cells that do not usually possess automaticity. If the rate of depolarization of such cells ex-

Figure 11.7. **Triggered activity.** An early afterdepolarization (arrow) occurs before the triggering action potential (AP) has fully repolarized. Repetitive afterdepolarizations (dashed curve) may produce a rapid sequence of triggered action potentials and hence a tachyarrhythmia.

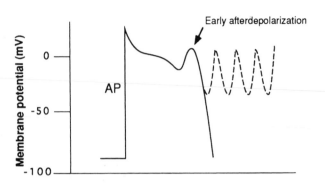

ceeds that of the sinus node, they transiently take over the pacemaker function and become the source of an abnormal ectopic rhythm.

Because these myocardial cells have few or no activated pacemaker channels, they do not normally carry I_f. How injury allows such cells to spontaneously depolarize has not been fully elucidated. However, when myocytes become injured, their membranes become "leaky." As such, they are unable to maintain the concentration gradients of ions, and the resting potential becomes less negative (i.e., the cell partially depolarizes). When a cell's membrane potential is reduced to a value less negative than −60 mV, gradual phase 4 depolarization can be demonstrated even among non-pacemaker cells. This slow spontaneous depolarization is probably related to a slow calcium current and by closure of a subset of K^+ channels that normally help repolarize the cell.

Triggered Activity

Under certain conditions, an action potential can "trigger" abnormal depolariza-

tions that result in extra heart beats or rapid arrhythmias. This process may occur when the first action potential leads to oscillations of the membrane voltage known as *afterdepolarizations*. Unlike the *spontaneous* activity seen when enhanced automaticity occurs, this type of automaticity is *stimulated* by a preceding action potential. As illustrated in Figures 11.7 and 11.8, there are two types of afterdepolarizations depending on their timing after the inciting action potential: *early* afterdepolarizations occur during the repolarization phase of the inciting beat, whereas *delayed* afterdepolarizations occur shortly after repolarization has been completed. In either case, abnormal action potentials are triggered if the afterdepolarization reaches a threshold voltage.

Early afterdepolarizations are changes of the membrane potential in the positive direction that interrupt normal repolarization (see Fig 11.7). They can occur either during the plateau of the action potential (phase 2) or during rapid repolarization (phase 3). Early afterdepolarizations are more likely to develop in conditions that prolong the action potential duration (and

Figure 11.8. **Triggered activity.** A delayed afterdepolarization (arrow) arises after the triggering action potential (AP) has fully repolarized. If the delayed afterdepolarization reaches the threshold voltage, a propagated action potential is fired (dashed curve).

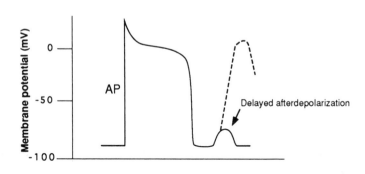

therefore the electrocardiographic QT interval), as may occur during therapy with certain drugs (as described in Chapter 17) and in the inherited long QT syndromes.

The ionic current responsible for an early afterdepolarization depends on the membrane voltage at which the triggered event occurs. If the early afterdepolarization occurs during phase 2 of the action potential, when most of the Na^+ channels are in an inactivated state, the upstroke of the triggered beat relies on an inward Ca^{++} current. If, however, it occurs during phase 3 (when the membrane voltage is more negative), there is partial recovery of the fast Na^+ channels, which are then available to contribute to the current.

An early afterdepolarization-triggered action potential can be self-perpetuating and lead to a series of depolarizations (see Fig. 11.7). Long sequences of these appear to be the mechanism responsible for the arrhythmia "torsades de pointes" discussed in the next chapter.

When **delayed afterdepolarizations** occur, they appear shortly after repolarization is complete (see Fig. 11.8). They most commonly develop in states of *high intracellular calcium*, as may be present with digitalis intoxication (see Chapter 17), or during marked catecholamine stimulation. It is thought that intracellular Ca^{++} accumulation causes the activation of chloride currents or of the Na^+/Ca^{++} exchanger that results in brief inward currents which generate the delayed afterdepolarization.

As with early afterdepolarizations, if the amplitude of the delayed afterdepolarization reaches a threshold voltage, an action potential will be generated. Such action potentials can be self-perpetuating and lead to tachyarrhythmias. For example, many arrhythmias associated with digitalis toxicity are thought to be the result of delayed afterdepolarizations, as described in Chapter 17.

ALTERED IMPULSE CONDUCTION

Alterations in impulse conduction, primarily conduction blocks, also may lead to arrhythmias. Conduction blocks generally lead to slowed heart rates (bradyarrhyth-mias); however, under certain circumstances, reentry (described below) can ensue and produce faster rhythms (tachyarrhythmias).

Conduction Block

A propagating impulse is blocked when it encounters a region of the heart that is electrically unexcitable. Conduction block can be either transient or permanent and may be unidirectional (i.e., conduction proceeds when the involved region is stimulated from one direction, but not when stimulated from the opposite direction) or bidirectional (conduction is blocked in both directions). A variety of conditions may cause conduction block, including ischemia, fibrosis, and trauma. It may also be precipitated temporarily by certain drugs. Most commonly, conduction block occurs because a propagating impulse encounters either cardiac cells that are still refractory (from a previous depolarization) or tissue that is intrinsically unable to conduct because of fibrosis or scarring.

Impulse blockade within the specialized conducting system prevents normal propagation from the sinus node to more distal sites, so it removes the normal overdrive suppression that keeps latent pacemakers in check. Thus, conduction block anywhere along the specialized conduction pathway can result in escape beats or escape rhythms, as the more distal sites assume the pacemaker function.

Conduction blocks between the atria and ventricles (termed AV blocks) are particularly common, and the major types of these are presented in Chapter 12.

Unidirectional Block and Reentry

A common mechanism by which altered stimulus conduction leads to tachyarrhythmias is termed **reentry.** A reentrant rhythm represents a self-sustaining electrical circuit that repeatedly depolarizes a region of cardiac tissue.

During normal cardiac conduction, each electrical impulse that originates in the SA node travels in an orderly, sequential fashion through the rest of the heart, depolarizing all the myocardial fibers. Because cellular refractoriness prevents reactivation of tissue that was just stimulated, the impulse then stops. However, if not all of the myocardium was depolarized (as occurs in conduction blocks), the original impulse can continue to propagate.

Figure 11.9 illustrates the conditions that set the stage for reentry to occur. The figure depicts electrical activity as it flows through a branch point anywhere within the conduction pathways. Panel A shows propagation of a normal action potential. At point x, the impulse reaches two parallel pathways (α and β) and travels down each into the more distal conduction tissue. Since the α and β pathways have identical conduction velocities and refractory periods, impulse wavefronts along these respective pathways will collide in the distal conduction tissue and extinguish each other.

Panel B shows what happens if conduction is blocked in one limb of the pathway. In this example, the action potential is blocked when it encounters the β pathway from above and therefore propagates only down the α tract into the distal tissue. As the impulse continues to spread, it will encounter the distal end of the β pathway (at point y). If the tissue in the distal β tract is also unable to conduct, then the impulse will simply continue to propagate into the deeper tissues, and reentry will not occur. However, if the impulse at point y *is* able to propagate retrogradely (backward) into pathway β, one of the necessary conditions for reentry will be met.

When an action potential is able to pass retrogradely in a conduction pathway, whereas it had been prevented from doing so in the forward direction, **unidirectional block** is said to be present. Unidirectional block may occur in states of cellular dysfunction, in tissues with pathologic differences in the refractory periods of neighboring cells, and in contiguous fibers with functionally different electrophysiologic properties.

As shown in Panel C of Figure 11.9, if the impulse is able to propagate retrogradely up the β pathway, it will again arrive at point x. If at that time the α pathway has not yet repolarized from the previous action potential that had occurred moments earlier, then that limb will be refractory to repeat stimulation, and the returning impulse will die out at that point.

However, in Panel D, consider what happens if the velocity of retrograde conduction in the diseased β path is not normal but *slower than normal*. In that case, sufficient time may have elapsed for the α pathway to repolarize before the returning impulse reaches point x from the β limb. Then, the impulse is free to stimulate the α pathway once again, and the cycle repeats itself. This circular action can continue indefinitely, and each pass of the impulse through the loop excites cells of the distal conduction tissue, which propagates to the rest of the myocardium, resulting in various tachyarrhythmias.

For the mechanism of reentry to occur, the propagating impulse must continuously encounter excitable tissue. Thus, the time it takes for the impulse to travel around the reentrant loop must be greater than the refractory period of the tissue to be restimulated. If the loop conduction time is shorter, the impulse will encounter refractory tissue and stop. Since normal conduction velocity is approximately 50 cm/sec, and the average effective refractory period is about 200 msec, the circuit would need to be at least 10 cm long for reentry to occur. Most clinical cases of reentry occur within much smaller regions of tissue. Therefore, slowing of the conduction velocity within the reentrant loop, as described in this example, is usually necessary to sustain a reentrant rhythm.

In practice, a region of cardiac tissue may develop reentry if two main conditions are met: 1) unidirectional block, and 2) slowed conduction through the loop of tissue. These conditions may exist if neighboring cells display different conduction velocities and refractory periods. In some cases reentry occurs over an anatomically fixed circuit or path, such as AV reentry using an accessory pathway (see below). Reentry around distinct anatomic pathways usually appears as a "monomorphic" tachycardia on

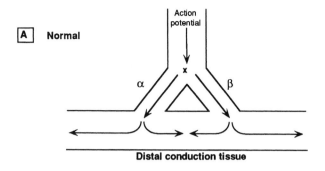

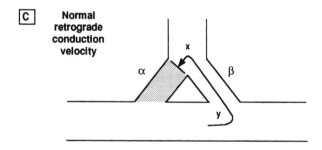

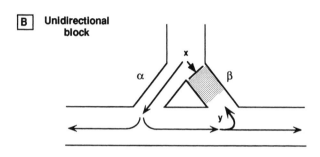

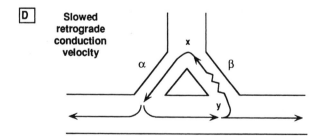

Figure 11.9. **Mechanism of reentry. A.** Normal conduction. When an action potential (AP) reaches a division in the conduction pathway (point x), the impulse travels down both fibers (α and β) to excite distal conduction tissue. **B.** Unidirectional block. Forward passage of the impulse is blocked in the β pathway but proceeds normally down the α pathway. When the impulse reaches point y, if retrograde conduction of the β pathway is intact, the AP can enter β from below and conduct in a retrograde fashion. **C.** When point x is reached, if the α pathway has not had sufficient time to repolarize, then the impulse stops. **D.** However, if conduction through the retrograde pathway is abnormally slow (jagged line), it reaches point x after the α pathway has completed repolarization. Thus, the impulse is free to excite pathway α again, and a reentrant loop is formed.

the ECG (i.e., in the case of ventricular tachycardia, all the QRS complexes have the same appearance). Other types of reentry can occur in electrophysiologically heterogeneous myocardium in which a wave of reentrant excitation spirals through the tissue, continually changing its path. For example, ischemic myocardium provides a setting for reentry because such tissue is a mosaic of nonexcitable and partially excitable zones with reduced conduction velocities. When reentry through an area of ischemia causes ventricular tachycardia, the reentry circuit is continually changing and the QRS complexes vary from beat to beat causing a "polymorphic" ventricular tachycardia pattern on the ECG.

Bypass Tracts

In the normal heart, the impulse generated by the SA node propagates through atrial tissue to the AV node, where there is a short delay before continuing on to the ventricles. In some individuals, there is an additional "accessory" pathway between atrium and ventricle that bypasses the AV node (hence the term "bypass tract"). The most common accessory pathway is called a bundle of Kent, which consists of a band of myocardium that connects atrial to ventricular tissue by spanning the AV groove,

as shown in Figure 11.10. Because accessory pathway tissue conducts impulses rapidly, the conduction delay that normally occurs at the AV node does not take place, stimulation of the ventricles occurs earlier than normal, and therefore the PR interval of the ECG is *shortened* (usually to less than 0.12 sec [i.e., < 3 small boxes]). Furthermore, ventricular depolarization in such individuals represents the combination of electrical activity over the accessory tract *plus* that over the normal conducting system. This results in a *wider than normal* QRS complex on the ECG, with an *earlier than normal* upstroke, known as the "delta wave" (Fig. 11.10).

In the presence of a bypass tract, a large anatomic loop may be created, with the accessory pathway serving as one limb and the normal conduction pathway through the AV node as the other. Because the conduction velocity and refractory period of the accessory pathway are usually different from those of the normal conduction pathway, an appropriately timed stimulus can initiate a reentrant tachycardia, as described in Chapter 12.

The mechanisms of altered impulse formation and conduction are the basis of all common arrhythmias, which can be divided into two groups: abnormally slow rhythms (bradyarrhythmias) and abnormally fast

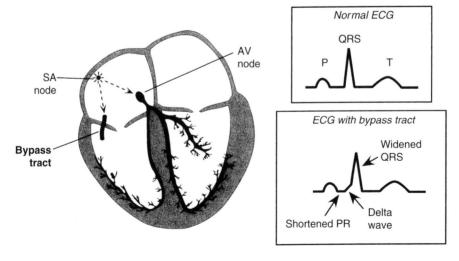

Figure 11.10. Bypass tract. Example of an atrioventricular bypass tract (Kent bundle), shown schematically, which can conduct impulses from the atrium directly to the ventricles, bypassing the AV node. The ECG demonstrates a shortened PR interval and delta wave, due to early excitation of the ventricles via the bypass tract.

rhythms (tachyarrhythmias). Table 11.1 lists the underlying mechanisms and examples of their commonly associated arrhythmias.

APPROACH TO ANTIARRHYTHMIC TREATMENT

The treatment of arrhythmias is aimed at correcting the basic mechanisms of abnormal impulse formation and conduction, altering conduction and refractoriness to prevent reentry, and protecting the patient from the consequences of the arrhythmia. This section summarizes the common therapeutic modalities, and Chapter 12 describes how these are used to treat specific rhythm disorders.

Bradyarrhythmias

Not all slow heart rhythms require specific treatment. When they do, pharmacologic therapy can be used to increase the heart rate acutely. Electronic pacemakers are used for a more sustained effect.

Pharmacologic Therapy

Pharmacologic therapies of bradyarrhythmias modify the autonomic input to the heart in one of two ways:

1. *Anticholinergic drugs.* Vagal stimulation reduces the heart rate and decreases conduction through the AV node through the release of acetylcholine onto muscarinic receptors. Anticholinergic drugs (i.e., anti-muscarinic agents directed to M_2 receptors), such as atropine, block the vagal effect and thus increase the heart rate and enhance AV nodal conduction.
2. *β_1-receptor agonists* (e.g., isoproterenol) mimic the effect of endogenous catecholamines, which increase heart rate and speed AV nodal conduction.

Atropine and isoproterenol are administered intravenously. Although these drugs are useful in treating certain slow heart rhythms acutely, it is not practical to continue these over the long term for persistent bradyarrhythmias.

TABLE 11.1. Mechanisms of Arrhythmia Development

Abnormality	Mechanism	Examples
Bradyarrhythmias		
Altered impulse formation		
• Decreased automaticity	Decreased phase 4 depolarization (e.g., parasympathetic stimulation)	Sinus bradycardia
Altered impulse conduction		
• Conduction blocks	Ischemic, anatomic, or drug-induced impaired conduction	First-, second-, and third-degree AV blocks
Tachyarrhythmias		
Altered impulse formation		
• Enhanced automaticity		
Sinus node	Increased phase 4 depolarization (e.g., sympathetic stimulation)	Sinus tachycardia
Ectopic focus	Acquires phase 4 depolarization	Ectopic atrial tachycardia
• Triggered activity		
Early afterdepolarization	Prolonged action potential duration	Torsades de pointes
Delayed afterdepolarization	Intracellular calcium overload (e.g., digitalis toxicity)	APBs, VPBs, digitalis-induced arrhythmias
Altered impulse conduction		
• Reentry	Unidirectional block plus slowed conduction	
Anatomical		Atrial flutter, AV nodal reentrant tachycardia
Functional		Atrial fibrillation, ventricular fibrillation

AV, atrioventricular; *APB,* atrial premature beat; *VPB,* ventricular premature beat.

Electronic Pacemakers

Electronic pacemakers apply repeated electrical stimulation to the heart to initiate depolarizations at a desired rate, thereby assuming control of the rhythm. Pacemakers may be installed on a temporary or a permanent basis. Temporary units are used to stabilize patients who are awaiting implantation of a permanent pacemaker or to treat transient bradyarrhythmias. For example, a bradyarrhythmia brought on by drug toxicity requires pacing only until the drug effect resolves.

There are two types of temporary pacemakers. The first uses **transthoracic** stimulation. An electrical current is applied to the patient's chest through large adhesive electrodes on the skin. Application of sufficient current initiates a cardiac depolarization. As one might imagine, this technique can be quite uncomfortable, as it also causes contraction of the thoracic muscles and stimulates nerves. Nonetheless, in an emergency, this form of pacing may be applied rapidly and can be life-saving.

The other option for temporary pacing is a **transvenous** device, in which an electrode-tipped catheter is passed into the heart through a peripheral or central vein and connected to an external power source, referred to as a pulse generator. Electrical pulses are applied directly to the heart via the electrode catheter placed in the right ventricle or right atrium to achieve the desired heart rate. This type of pacemaker is effective for a few days, but thereafter the risk of infection and thrombosis increases.

Permanent pacemakers are more sophisticated than the temporary variety. Different configurations can sense and capture the electrical activity of the atria and/or ventricles. One or more wires (known as leads) are generally passed through a subclavian vein into the right ventricle, right atrium, or through the coronary sinus (for the purpose of stimulating the left ventricle). The pulse generator, not much larger than three silver dollars stacked on top of one another, is connected to the leads and implanted under the skin. The pacemaker battery typi-

cally lasts 10–12 years. Permanent pacemakers are programmable, in that their modes of action can be altered noninvasively by transcutaneous radio signals.

Although the most common indications for permanent pacemakers are bradyarrhythmias, some special devices are used to improve hemodynamic performance in patients with severe heart failure (see Chapter 9).

Tachyarrhythmias

The treatment of tachyarrhythmias is directed at 1) the specific mechanism responsible for the abnormal rhythm, and 2) protection of the patient from consequences of the arrhythmia. Pharmacologic agents and cardioversion/defibrillation are commonly used therapies, but innovative electrical devices and transvenous catheter-based techniques have revolutionized treatment of these disorders.

Pharmacologic Therapy

Pharmacologic management of tachyarrhythmias is directed against the underlying mechanism (abnormal automaticity, reentrant circuits, or triggered activity). Many antiarrhythmic drugs are available, the pharmacology and actions of which are addressed in Chapter 17. The choice of drug relies on an understanding of the cause of the specific arrhythmia. From the mechanisms presented in this chapter, the following strategies emerge:

To eliminate rhythms due to *increased automaticity,* desired drug effects are:

1. To reduce the slope of phase 4 spontaneous depolarization of the automatic cells.
2. To make the diastolic potential more negative.
3. To make the threshold potential less negative.

By altering the diastolic and/or threshold potentials, or slowing the rate of spontaneous diastolic depolarization, the firing rate of ectopic pacemakers can be inhibited.

To interrupt *reentrant circuits,* desired antiarrhythmic effects are:

1. To decrease cellular conduction velocity, such that impulse propagation within the slowly conducting limb of the circuit becomes even slower and eventually stops.
2. To increase the refractory period within the reentrant circuit so that a propagating impulse finds tissue within the loop unexcitable, and the impulse stops.

To eliminate *triggered activity,* desired antiarrhythmic drug effects are:

1. To shorten the action potential duration (to prevent early afterdepolarizations).
2. To correct conditions of calcium overload (to prevent delayed afterdepolarizations).

For each of the tachyarrhythmia mechanisms, the treatment goals can be achieved by drugs that modulate the action potential through interactions with ion channels, surface receptors, and transport pumps. The reader should look through the antiarrhythmic drug section of Chapter 17 at this time to become familiar with the general mechanisms of action and names of antiarrhythmic drugs.

It is extremely important to recognize that in addition to suppressing an arrhythmia, antiarrhythmic drugs also have the potential to *aggravate* or provoke arrhythmias. Furthermore, all drugs have potentially toxic systemic side effects. Such problems with antiarrhythmic drug therapy have led to a decrease in their chronic use and increased reliance on nonpharmacologic treatment options discussed below.

Vagotonic Maneuvers

A useful bedside technique frequently used to arrest certain reentrant tachyarrhythmias is **carotid sinus massage.** Located at the bifurcation of the internal and external carotid arteries on either side of the neck, the carotid sinuses respond to stimulation (such as rubbing one of them firmly in a circular fashion for 3–5 sec) by enhancing central nervous system parasympathetic outflow and inhibiting sympathetic

activity. The result is a decrease in the sinus node rate of discharge and slowing of AV nodal conduction. The latter may interrupt supraventricular tachycardias in which the AV node is a part of a reentrant circuit.

Electrical Cardioversion and Defibrillation

Cardioversion and defibrillation are similar techniques used to treat certain tachycardias, in which an electrical current is momentarily discharged across the chest. This action simultaneously depolarizes the bulk of the excitable myocardial tissue, interrupts reentrant circuits, establishes electrical homogeneity, and allows the sinus node (the site of fastest spontaneous discharge) to regain pacemaker control. Tachyarrhythmias that are due to reentry usually terminate by this procedure, whereas those associated with enhanced automaticity may not be stopped, if the responsible ectopic focus continues to discharge at a rate faster than the SA node.

Cardioversion is performed by briefly sedating the patient and then placing two electrode paddles against the chest on either side of the heart. The electrical discharge is electronically *synchronized* to fire at the time of a QRS complex (i.e., when ventricular depolarization occurs). This prevents the possibility of discharge during the relative refractory period of the ventricle (see Fig. 1.16, p. 21), which could induce ventricular fibrillation.

Defibrillation is performed (with the same equipment as that used for cardioversion) in emergency situations for ventricular fibrillation. Unlike cardioversion, in this technique the electrical discharge is *not synchronized* to the QRS complex, because the latter is not discernible in ventricular fibrillation (see Chapter 12).

Implantable Cardioverter Defibrillators

Individuals at high risk for sudden cardiac death, such as patients with sustained ventricular tachycardia or survivors of cardiac arrest, are often treated with the permanent implantation of a small defibrillator into the body (known as an implantable cardioverter-defibrillator [ICD]). These devices appear similar to permanent pacemakers but are capable of delivering a high-voltage shock through leads placed in the heart to convert ventricular fibrillation or tachycardia back to a normal rhythm. The device continuously monitors for these dangerous rhythms and automatically delivers appropriate electrical therapy as needed.

For more stable tachycardias, ICDs can be programmed to perform antitachycardia pacing (also termed "burst" pacing). The idea of this mode is to artificially depolarize a portion of a reentrant circuit, rendering it refractory to further immediate stimulation. Consequently, when a reentrant impulse returns to the zone already depolarized by the device, it encounters unexcitable tissue, cannot propagate further, and the circuit is broken.

Catheter Ablation

For patients with recurrent symptomatic supraventricular arrhythmias involving distinct anatomical circuits or automatic foci, electrophysiologic mapping techniques may be used to localize the region of myocardium or conduction tissue responsible for the disturbance. It is then often possible to ablate the site via a catheter that applies radiofrequency current to heat and destroy the tissue. Such procedures have revolutionized the management of patients with many types of supraventricular tachycardias, as they often offer a permanent therapeutic solution that spares individuals the need for chronic antiarrhythmic drugs.

SUMMARY

1. Arrhythmias result from disorders of impulse formation, impulse conduction, or both.
2. Bradyarrhythmias develop because of decreased impulse formation (e.g., sinus bradycardia) or decreased impulse conduction (e.g., AV nodal conduction blocks).
3. Tachyarrhythmias result from 1) increased automaticity (of the SA node, latent pacemakers, or abnormal myocardial sites), 2) triggered activity, or 3) unidirectional block and reentry.
4. Bradyarrhythmias are usually treated with drugs that accelerate the rate of sinus node discharge and enhance AV nodal conduction (atropine, isoproterenol) or electronic pacemakers.
5. Tachyarrhythmias respond to pharmacologic therapy directed at the mechanism of arrhythmia formation. For refractory tachyarrhythmias, or in emergency situations, electrical cardioversion/defibrillation is used. Catheter-based ablative techniques are a popular method for long-term control of certain tachyarrhythmias.

Chapter 12 summarizes the diagnosis and treatment of the most common arrhythmias. Additional reading suggestions are listed at the end of that chapter. Chapter 17 describes currently available antiarrhythmic drugs.

Acknowledgment   Contributors to the previous editions of this chapter were Wendy Armstrong, MD; Nicholas Boulis, MD; Mark S. Sabatine, MD; Elliott M. Antman, MD; Leonard I. Ganz, MD; Gary R. Strichartz, PhD; and Leonard S. Lilly, MD.

Clinical Aspects of Cardiac Arrhythmias

Jennifer E. Ho, William G. Stevenson, and Leonard S. Lilly

Bradyarrhythmias
  Sinoatrial Node
  Escape Rhythms
  Atrioventricular Conduction System

Tachyarrhythmias
  Supraventricular Arrhythmias
  Ventricular Arrhythmias
  Differentiation of Wide Complex Tachycardias

Arrhythmias appear frequently in patients with heart disease and can occur in healthy individuals as well. Chapter 11 presented the mechanisms by which abnormal heart rhythms develop. This chapter describes how to recognize and treat specific common arrhythmias. Table 12.1 categorizes the disorders considered in this chapter.

There are five basic questions to consider when confronted with a patient with an abnormal heart rhythm, as detailed in the sections that follow:

1. Definition: What is the arrhythmia?
2. Pathogenesis: What is the underlying mechanism?
3. Precipitating factors: What conditions provoke it?
4. Clinical presentation: What symptoms and signs accompany the arrhythmia?
5. Treatment: What to do about it?

BRADYARRHYTHMIAS

Bradyarrhythmias are rhythms in which the heart rate is <60 bpm. They arise from disorders of impulse formation or impaired impulse conduction.

Sinoatrial Node

Sinus Bradycardia

Sinus bradycardia (Fig. 12.1) is simply a slowing of the normal heart rhythm, as a result of decreased firing of the sinoatrial (SA) node, to a rate <60 bpm. Trained athletes and normal elderly individuals at rest may have perfectly benign sinus bradycardia. It is incumbent on the physician to decide whether sinus bradycardia in a particular patient is appropriate or pathologic, and whether treatment is required. This decision can be made on the basis of a patient's age, underlying heart disease, level of physical activity, symptoms, and whether the heart rate increases appropriately with exercise.

Sinus bradycardia can result from either intrinsic SA node disease or extrinsic factors that affect the node. Depressed intrinsic automaticity can be due to aging or can result from underlying conditions such as ischemic heart disease or cardiomyopathy. Extrinsic factors that can suppress the SA node include medications (e.g., β-blockers, certain calcium channel blockers) and metabolic causes (e.g., hypothyroidism). Highly trained athletes often have elevated vagal tone, which results in *physiologic* (i.e., appropriate) sinus bradycardia. However, transient periods of high vagal tone can also occur in any individual experiencing pain or illness, resulting in *inappropriate* sinus bradycardia.

Sinus bradycardia is usually asymptomatic and does not require treatment. However, a pronounced reduction of the heart rate can lead to fatigue, lightheadedness, or syncope. In such cases, any extrinsic provocative factors should be corrected, and specific therapy instituted, as described in the next section.

TABLE 12.1. Common Arrhythmias

Location	Bradyarrhythmias	Tachyarrhythmias
SA node	Sinus bradycardia Sick sinus syndrome	Sinus tachycardia
Atria		Atrial premature beats Atrial flutter Atrial fibrillation Paroxysmal supraventricular tachycardias Ectopic atrial tachycardia Multifocal atrial tachycardia
AV node	Conduction blocks Junctional escape rhythm	Paroxysmal reentrant tachycardias (AV or AV nodal)
Ventricles	Ventricular escape rhythm	Ventricular premature beats Ventricular tachycardia Torsades de pointes Ventricular fibrillation

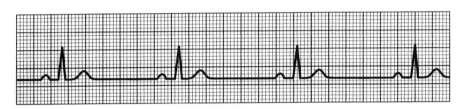

Figure 12.1. **Sinus bradycardia.** The P wave and QRS complexes are normal but the rate is <60 bpm.

Sick Sinus Syndrome

Intrinsic SA node dysfunction that causes periods of inappropriate bradycardia is known as sick sinus syndrome (SSS). This condition often leads to intermittent reductions of cardiac output and hypotension, which can cause dizziness, confusion, or syncope.

Patients with acute symptoms of SSS (or any other cause of symptomatic sinus bradycardia) can be treated with intravenous anticholinergic drugs (e.g., atropine) or β-adrenergic agents (e.g., isoproterenol), which transiently speed the heart rate. Permanent pacemaker placement is required for chronic symptomatic bradycardia.

SSS often coexists with periods of inappropriate, rapid supraventricular tachyarrhythmias (e.g., atrial fibrillation and atrial flutter), a combination known as the *bradycardia-tachycardia syndrome* (Fig. 12.2). This condition is thought to result from atrial fibrosis that impairs function of the SA node and also predisposes to atrial fibrillation and flutter. During tachyarrhythmia, overdrive suppression of the SA node occurs; when tachycardia terminates, profound periods of sinus bradycardia ensue.

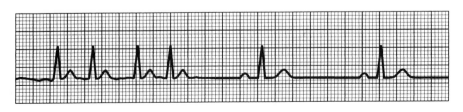

Figure 12.2. **Bradycardia-tachycardia syndrome.** A brief irregular tachycardia is followed by slow sinus node discharge.

Treatment generally requires the combination of antiarrhythmic drug therapy to suppress the tachyarrhythmias plus a permanent pacemaker to prevent bradycardia.

Escape Rhythms

Cells in the atrioventricular (AV) node and His-Purkinje system are capable of automaticity, but typically have slower firing rates than the sinus node and are therefore suppressed during normal sinus rhythm. However, if SA node activity becomes impaired or if there is conduction block of the impulse from the SA node, escape rhythms can emerge from the more distal latent pacemakers (Fig. 12.3).

Junctional escape beats arise from the AV node or proximal bundle of His. They are characterized by a normal, narrow QRS complex, and when they occur in sequence (termed a **junctional escape rhythm**), appear at a rate of 40–60 bpm. The QRS complexes are not preceded by normal P waves because the impulse originates below the atria. However, *retrograde* P waves may be observed as an impulse propagates from the more distal pacemaker backward to the atrium. Retrograde P waves typically *follow* the QRS complex and are *inverted* (negative deflection on the ECG) in limb leads II, III, and aVF, indicating activation of the atria from the inferior direction.

Ventricular escape rhythms are characterized by even slower rates (30–40 bpm) and *widened* QRS complexes. The complexes are wide because the ventricles are not depolarized by the normal rapid simultaneous conduction over the right and left bundle branches, but rather from a more distal point in the conduction system. Depending on the site of origin of the escape rhythm, the QRS may show different morphologies. For example, an escape rhythm originating from the left bundle branch will cause a right bundle branch block QRS pattern, because the impulse depolarizes the left ventricle first and then spreads more slowly through the right ventricle. Conversely, an escape rhythm originating in the right bundle branch would cause the QRS to appear with a left bundle branch block configuration. Escape rhythms that originate more distally, in the ventricular myocardium itself, are characterized by even wider QRS complexes because such impulses are conducted outside the rapidly propagating Purkinje fibers.

Junctional and ventricular escape rhythms are protective back-up mechanisms that maintain a heart rate and cardiac output when the sinus node or normal AV conduction fail. The clinical findings and treatment of bradycardia associated with escape rhythms are identical to those of SSS described earlier.

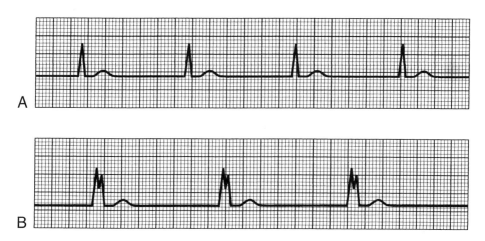

Figure 12.3. **Escape rhythms.** No P waves are evident. **A.** Junctional escape rhythm with normal-width QRS complexes. **B.** Wide QRS complexes typical of a ventricular escape rhythm.

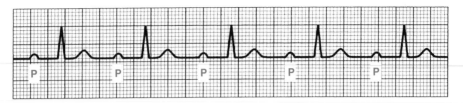

Figure 12.4. **First-degree AV block.** The PR interval is prolonged.

Atrioventricular Conduction System

The AV conduction system includes the AV node, bundle of His, and the left and right bundle branches. Impaired conduction through these structures can cause three "degrees" (types) of AV conduction block.

First-Degree AV Block

First-degree AV block, shown in Figure 12.4, indicates prolongation of the normal delay between atrial and ventricular depolarization, such that the PR interval is lengthened (>0.2 sec, which is >5 small boxes on the ECG). However, the 1:1 relationship between P waves and QRS complexes is preserved. The impairment of conduction is usually within the AV node itself and can be due to a transient influence or a structural defect. *Reversible* causes include heightened vagal tone, transient AV nodal ischemia, and drugs that depress conduction through the AV node including digitalis glycosides, β-blockers, and certain Ca^{++} channel antagonists. *Structural* causes of first-degree AV block include myocardial infarction and chronic degenerative diseases of the conduction system, which commonly occur with aging.

Generally, first-degree AV block is a benign, asymptomatic condition that does not require treatment. However, it can increase susceptibility to higher degrees of AV block if drugs are administered that further impair AV conduction.

Second-Degree AV Block

Second-degree AV block is characterized by *intermittent failure* of AV conduction, such that some P waves are not followed by a QRS complex (i.e., intermittent failure of 1:1 atrioventricular conduction). There are two forms of second-degree AV block: in **Möbitz type I** block (also termed **Wenckebach** block) shown in Figure 12.5, the degree of AV delay gradually increases with each beat until an impulse is completely blocked, such that ventricular stimulation does not follow a P wave for a single beat. Therefore, the ECG shows a progressive increase in the PR interval from one beat to the next until a single QRS complex is absent, after which the PR interval resets to the initial length, and the cycle starts anew. Möbitz type I block is almost always due to impaired conduction in the AV node (rather than more distally in the conduction system). It is usually benign and may be seen in children, trained athletes, and individuals with increased vagal tone, particularly during sleep. It may also occur during an acute inferior wall infarc-

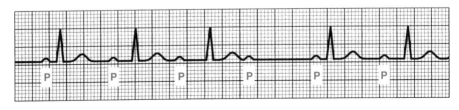

Figure 12.5. **Second-degree AV block: Möbitz I (Wenckebach).** The P wave rate is constant, but the PR interval progressively lengthens until a QRS is completely blocked (after fourth P wave).

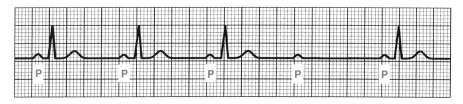

Figure 12.6. **Second-degree AV block: Möbitz II.** A QRS complex is blocked (after the fourth P wave) without gradual lengthening of the preceding PR intervals.

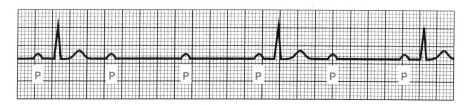

Figure 12.7. **High-grade AV block.** Sequential QRS complexes are blocked (after the second and third P waves).

tion due to increased vagal stimulation or ischemia of the AV node, but is usually transient. Treatment is typically not necessary, but in symptomatic cases, this rhythm usually responds to intravenous atropine or isoproterenol. Placement of a permanent pacemaker is required for symptomatic block that does not resolve spontaneously or persists despite the correction of aggravating factors.

Möbitz type II second-degree AV block is more dangerous and is characterized by the sudden and unpredictable loss of AV conduction, without preceding gradual lengthening of the PR interval (Fig. 12.6). The block may persist for two or more beats (i.e., two sequential P waves not followed by QRS complexes), in which case it is known as **high-grade** AV block (Fig. 12.7). Möbitz type II second-degree block is usually due to conduction block beyond the AV

node (in the bundle of His or more distally in the Purkinje system). Therefore, the QRS complexes are often wide and in the pattern of right or left bundle branch block. This type of block may arise from extensive myocardial infarction involving the septum or chronic degeneration of the His-Purkinje system. The rhythm may progress to third-degree block without warning; therefore, treatment with a pacemaker is usually warranted, even in asymptomatic patients.

Third-Degree AV Block

Third-degree AV block, also termed "complete" heart block (Fig. 12.8), is present when there is complete failure of conduction between the atria and ventricles. In adults, the most common causes are acute myocardial infarction, drug toxicity (especially digitalis), and chronic degeneration

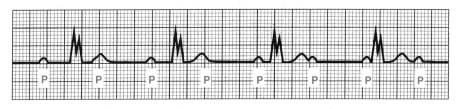

Figure 12.8. **Third-degree AV block.** The P wave and QRS rhythms are independent of one another. The QRS complexes are widened as they originate within the distal ventricular conduction system, not at the bundle of His. The second and fourth P waves are superimposed on normal T waves.

of the conduction pathways. Third-degree AV block divides the heart into two unconnected zones: there is no relationship between the P waves and QRS complexes, as the atria depolarize in response to SA node activity, while a more distal escape rhythm drives the ventricles independently. Thus, the P waves "march out" at a rate that is not related to the intervals at which QRS complexes appear. Depending on the site of the escape rhythm, the QRS complexes may be of normal width and occur at 40–60 bpm (originating from the AV node) or may be widened and occur at slower rates (originating from the His-Purkinje system). As a result of the slow rate, lightheadedness or syncope may occur. Permanent pacemaker therapy is almost always necessary.

The term **atrioventricular dissociation (AV dissociation)** is a general description that refers to any situation in which the atria and ventricles beat independently, without any direct relationship between P waves and QRS complexes. Third-degree AV block is an example of AV dissociation.

TACHYARRHYTHMIAS

Whenever the heart rate is >100 bpm for three beats or more, a tachyarrhythmia is said to be present. Tachyarrhythmias result from one of three mechanisms (see previous chapter): 1) enhanced cellular automaticity, 2) triggered activity, or 3) unidirectional block and reentry. Tachyarrhythmias are categorized into those that arise *above* (supraventricular) and those that arise *within* the ventricles, and can usually be differentiated by the width of the QRS complex, the morphology and rate of the P waves, the relationship between the P waves and the QRS complexes, and the response of the rhythm to vagal maneuvers such as carotid sinus massage (Fig. 12.9).

Supraventricular Arrhythmias

Sinus Tachycardia

Sinus tachycardia (ST) is characterized by an SA node discharge rate of 100–180 bpm and normal P waves and QRS complexes (Fig. 12.10). This rhythm most often arises because of increased sympathetic and/or decreased vagal influences on the SA node, with acceleration of the normal discharge rate. ST is an appropriate physiologic response to exercise. However, it may also result from sympathetic stimulation in pathologic conditions, including fever, hypovolemia, and hypoxemia. Because the increased rate is usually a response to stimuli external to the heart, the treatment of ST is directed at the underlying cause.

Atrial Premature Beats

Atrial premature beats (APBs) are common in healthy and diseased hearts (Fig. 12.11). They originate from automaticity or reentry in an atrial focus outside the SA node and are often exacerbated by sympathetic stimulation. APBs are usually asymptomatic but may cause palpitations. On ECG, an APB appears as an earlier-than-expected P wave with an *abnormal shape* (the impulse does not arise from the SA node, such that conduction through the atria is abnormal). The QRS complex that follows the P wave is usually normal, resembling the QRS during sinus rhythm, because ventricular conduction is not impaired. However, if the abnormal atrial focus fires very soon after the previous beat, the impulse may encounter an AV node that is refractory to excitation, such that the impulse is blocked and does not conduct to the ventricles. The premature P wave is then *not* followed by a QRS complex and is termed a "blocked" APB. Similarly, if the ectopic focus fires just a bit later in diastole, it may conduct through the AV node, but encounter portions of the His-Purkinje system that are still refractory. As a result, the impulse is conducted through those territories and to the ventricular myocytes in a slower-than-normal fashion, resulting in QRS complexes that are abnormally wide.

APBs require treatment only if they are symptomatic. Because caffeine ingestion, alcohol, and adrenergic stimulation (e.g., emotional stress) can all predispose to APBs, it is important to address these exposures. β-blockers are the initial preferred pharmacologic treatment if needed.

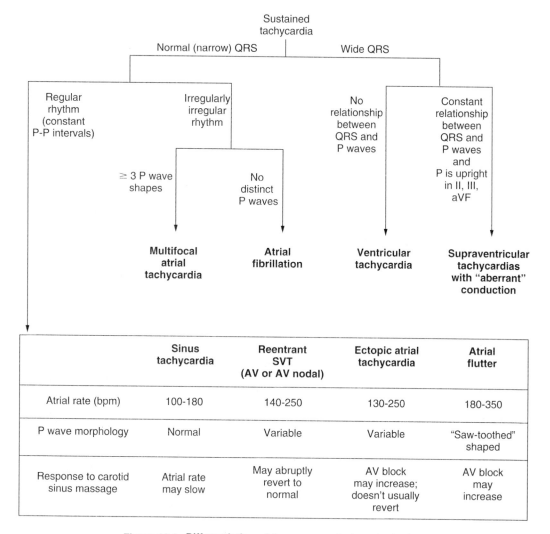

Figure 12.9. Differentiation of the common tachyarrhythmias.

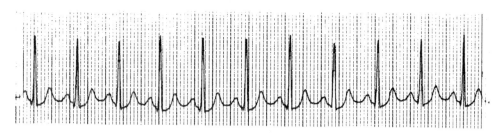

Figure 12.10. Sinus tachycardia. The P wave and QRS complexes are normal but the rate is >100 bpm.

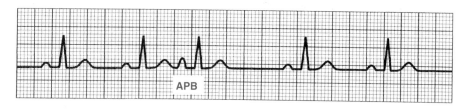

Figure 12.11. Atrial premature beat (APB). The P wave occurs earlier than expected, and its shape is abnormal.

Atrial Flutter

Atrial flutter is characterized by rapid, regular atrial activity at a rate of 180–350 bpm (Fig. 12.12). Many of these fast impulses reach the AV node during its refractory period and do not conduct to the ventricles, so that the ventricular rate is slower, often at an even fraction of the atrial rate. Thus, if the atrial rate is 300 bpm, and 2:1 block occurs at the AV node (i.e., every other atrial impulse finds the AV node refractory), then the ventricular rate would be 150 bpm. Because vagal maneuvers (e.g., carotid sinus massage) decrease AV nodal conduction, they increase the degree of block, temporarily slowing the ventricular rate and allowing better visualization of the underlying atrial activity. In general, atrial flutter is caused by reentry over a large anatomically fixed circuit. In the common form of atrial flutter, this circuit involves a specific pathway that runs through the interatrial septum and the roof and free wall of the right atrium. Because large parts of the atrium are depolarized throughout the cycle, P waves often have a sinusoidal or "sawtooth" appearance. Large flutter circuits can occur in other parts of the right or left atrium as well.

Atrial flutter generally occurs in individuals with preexisting heart disease. It may be paroxysmal and transient, persistent (lasting for days or weeks), or permanent. Frequently, it degenerates into atrial fibrillation. Symptoms of atrial flutter depend on the accompanying ventricular rate. If the rate is <100 bpm, the patient may be asymptomatic. Conversely, faster rates often cause palpitations, dyspnea, or weakness. Atrial flutter may paradoxically become more dangerous if the atrial rate *slows* somewhat, either spontaneously or due to pharmacologic intervention, to a rate that allows the AV node more time to recover between impulses. In that situation, the AV node may begin to conduct in a 1:1 fashion, producing very rapid ventricular rates. For example, consider a patient with atrial flutter at an atrial rate of 280 bpm with 2:1 conduction block at the AV node. The ventricular rate in that circumstance would be 140 bpm. If the atrial rate then slows to 220 bpm, the AV node may be able to recover sufficiently between depolarizations to conduct every atrial impulse (i.e., 1:1 conduction), such that the ventricular rate *accelerates* to 220 bpm. In individuals with limited cardiac reserve, this acceleration may result in a profound reduction of cardiac output and hypotension.

There are several approaches to the treatment of atrial flutter:

1. For symptomatic patients with recent-onset atrial flutter, the most expeditious therapy is electrical cardioversion to restore sinus rhythm. This technique is also used to revert chronic atrial flutter that has not responded to other approaches.
2. Flutter can be terminated by rapid atrial stimulation (burst pacing) using a temporary or permanent pacemaker (see Chapter 11). This procedure can be used when temporary atrial pacing wires are already present, such as in the postoperative period after cardiac surgery. In ad-

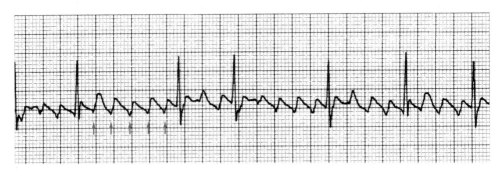

Figure 12.12. **Atrial flutter is typified by rapid "saw-toothed" atrial activity (arrows).**

dition, certain types of permanent pacemakers and implanted defibrillators can be programmed to perform burst pacing automatically when atrial flutter occurs.

3. For patients without the immediate need for cardioversion, pharmacologic therapy is begun. First, the ventricular rate is slowed by drugs that increase AV block (β-blockers, calcium channel blockers [e.g., verapamil, diltiazem], or digoxin). Once the rate is effectively slowed, attempts are made to restore sinus rhythm using antiarrhythmic drugs that slow conduction or prolong the refractory period of the atrial myocardium (Class IA, IC, or III agents, described in Chapter 17). Should such drugs fail to convert the rhythm, elective electrical cardioversion can then be undertaken. Once sinus rhythm has been restored, class IA, IC, or III antiarrhythmic drugs may be administered chronically to prevent recurrences.

4. Radiofrequency catheter ablation of atrial flutter is often a better alternative than chronic drug therapy. An electrode catheter is inserted into the femoral vein, passed via the inferior vena cava to the right atrium, and used to localize and cauterize ("ablate") part of the reentrant loop to permanently interrupt the flutter circuit.

Atrial Fibrillation

Atrial fibrillation (AF) is a chaotic rhythm with an atrial rate so fast (350–600 discharges/min) that discrete P waves are not discernible on the ECG (Fig. 12.13). Like atrial flutter, many of the atrial impulses encounter refractory tissue at the AV node, so that only some of the depolarizations are conducted to the ventricles, in a very irregular fashion. The average ventricular rate in untreated AF is approximately 160 bpm. Because discrete P waves are not visible on the ECG, the baseline shows low amplitude undulations punctuated by QRS complexes and T waves.

In most cases, the mechanism of AF appears to involve multiple "wandering" reentrant circuits within the atria, and in some patients, the rhythm repetitively shifts between fibrillation and atrial flutter. For the arrhythmia to sustain itself, a minimum number of reentrant circuits is needed and an enlarged atrium increases the potential for this to occur. Thus, AF is often associated with right or left atrial enlargement. A second mechanism by which AF can develop involves a rapidly firing atrial ectopic focus that drives the atria into fibrillation.

AF is common in patients with hypertension, coronary artery disease, alcohol intoxication, thyrotoxicosis, pulmonary disease, and following cardiothoracic surgery. It is a potentially dangerous arrhythmia for two reasons: 1) rapid ventricular rates may compromise cardiac output, resulting in hypotension and pulmonary congestion (especially in individuals with a hypertrophied or "stiff" left ventricle in whom the loss of normal atrial contraction can significantly compromise left ventricular filling and stroke volume), and 2) the absence of organized atrial contraction promotes blood stasis in the atria, which increases the risk of thrombus formation, particularly in the left atrial appendage. Embolization of left atrial thrombi is an important cause of stroke. Treatment of AF therefore focuses

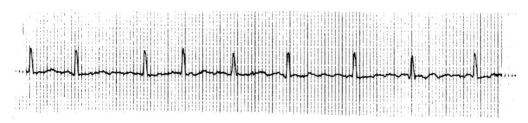

Figure 12.13. **Atrial fibrillation is characterized by chaotic atrial activity without organized P waves, and irregularity of the ventricular (QRS) rate.**

on three aspects of the arrhythmia: 1) ventricular rate control, 2) attempts to restore sinus rhythm, and 3) assessment of the need for anticoagulation to prevent thromboembolism.

Antiarrhythmic drug treatment of AF is similar to that of atrial flutter. β-blockers or certain Ca^{++} channel antagonists (diltiazem, verapamil) are administered to promote block at the AV node and to reduce the ventricular rate. Digitalis is less effective for this purpose, although it may be useful in patients with accompanying impairment of ventricular contractile function. For those who remain symptomatic despite adequate rate control, conversion back to sinus rhythm is usually attempted. If AF has been present for more than 48 hours, there is a risk that intraatrial thrombus has formed, and systemic anticoagulation (for at least 3 weeks) is usually warranted to reduce the risk of thromboembolism. In urgent situations, a transesophageal echocardiogram can be performed to evaluate for thrombus; if no thrombus is found, cardioversion can proceed expeditiously. Otherwise, it should be deferred until a course of anticoagulation has been completed so that thromboembolism does not occur when cardioversion restores organized atrial contraction.

Cardioversion back to sinus rhythm can be attempted chemically by administration of class IA, IC, or III antiarrhythmic drugs (see Chapter 17). If such drugs do not restore sinus rhythm, electrical cardioversion can be undertaken. Once successfully converted to sinus rhythm, antiarrhythmic drugs are often continued to prevent recurrences. Although antiarrhythmic drugs do not always maintain sinus rhythm during long-term follow-up, they can reduce the number of AF episodes. However, these drugs can also cause serious, sometimes lethal, side effects (as described in Chapter 17). Thus, in patients with *asymptomatic* AF, it is often safer to simply continue chronic anticoagulation therapy and to control the ventricular rate with β-blockers, calcium channel blockers, or digoxin.

There are other more permanent, nonpharmacologic options for management of AF, but these are not widely available. The surgical "maze procedure" places multiple incisions in the left and right atria such that the formation of reentry circuits is prevented. More recently, catheter ablation of rapidly firing atrial foci, typically localized near the insertion of the pulmonary veins, has been shown to be effective at suppressing AF in some patients. When sinus rhythm cannot be maintained and the heart rate cannot be controlled adequately with medications, catheter ablation of the AV junction can be undertaken to intentionally create complete heart block, as a means to permanently slow the ventricular rate. Such a procedure usually requires the simultaneous placement of a permanent pacemaker to ensure an adequate ventricular heart rate.

Paroxysmal Supraventricular Tachycardias

Paroxysmal supraventricular tachycardias (PSVTs) (Fig. 12.14) are manifest by: 1) sudden onset and termination, 2) atrial rates between 140–250 bpm, and 3) narrow (normal) QRS complexes, unless "aberrant conduction" is present, as described below. The mechanism of PSVT is most often reen-

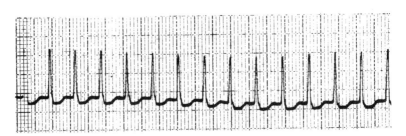

Figure 12.14. **Paroxysmal supraventricular tachycardia due to AV nodal reentry.** Retrograde P waves in this example occur simultaneously with, and are "hidden" in, the QRS complexes.

try involving the AV node, SA node, atrium, or accessory pathways between an atrium and ventricle. Enhanced automaticity and triggered activity are less common causes.

AV Nodal Reentrant Tachycardia

AV nodal reentrant tachycardia (AVNRT) is the most common form of PSVT in adults. In most individuals, the AV node is a lobulated structure that consists of a compact portion and several atrial extensions. The latter constitute two (or more) potential pathways for conduction through the AV node (Fig. 12.15). In some people, these extensions conduct at different velocities, providing both slow-conducting and fast-conducting pathways. The fast pathway is characterized by a rapid conduction velocity but a relatively long refractory period, whereas the slow pathway demonstrates a less rapid conduction velocity and a shorter refractory period. Thus, although the fast pathway conducts rapidly, it takes longer to recover between impulses compared with the slow pathway.

Normally, a stimulus arriving at the AV node travels down both pathways, but the impulse traveling down the fast pathway reaches the bundle of His first. By the time the impulse traversing the slow pathway reaches the bundle of His, it encounters refractory tissue and is extinguished. Thus, under normal conditions, only the fast pathway impulse makes its way forward to the ventricles (see Fig 12.15A).

However, consider what happens when an APB spontaneously occurs. Because the refractory period of the fast pathway is relatively long, an APB would find that pathway unexcitable and unable to conduct the impulse. However, the impulse *is* able to conduct over the slow pathway (which *is* excitable because it has a shorter refractory period than the fast pathway and has already repolarized when the APB arrives). By the time this impulse travels down the slowly conducting pathway and reaches the compact portion of the AV node, the distal end of the fast pathway may have had time to repolarize, and the impulse is able to propagate both distally (to the bundle of His and ventricles) *and* backward to the atria, up the fast pathway in a retrograde direction. Upon reaching the atria, the impulse can then circulate back down the slow pathway, completing the reentrant loop and initiating tachycardia as this sequence repeats. Thus, the fundamental conditions for reentry in AVNRT are transient unidirectional block in the fast pathway (e.g., an APB encountering refractory tissue) and relatively slow conduction through the other pathway (see Fig 12.15B).

The ECG in AVNRT shows a regular tachycardia with normal-width QRS complexes. P waves may not be apparent, because retrograde atrial depolarization typically occurs simultaneously with ventricular depolarization. Thus, the retrograde P wave and QRS are inscribed at the same time and the P is typically "hidden" in the QRS complex. In cases in which P waves *are* visualized, they are superimposed on the terminal portion of the QRS complex and are inverted (negative deflection) in limb leads II, III, and aVF because of the caudocranial direction of atrial activation.

Rarely, the reentrant loop revolves in the reverse direction, with anterograde conduction down the fast pathway, and retrograde conduction up the slow pathway. This is known as "uncommon AVNRT" and, unlike the more common rhythm, results in clearly visible retrograde P waves following the QRS complex on ECG.

AVNRT often presents in teenagers or young adults. It is usually well-tolerated but causes palpitations that many patients find frightening, and rapid tachycardias can cause lightheadedness or shortness of breath. In elderly patients or those with underlying heart disease, more severe symptoms may result, such as syncope, angina, or pulmonary edema.

Treatment of AVNRT is aimed at preventing reentry by purposefully impairing conduction in the AV node. Vagal maneuvers such as carotid sinus massage transiently increase parasympathetic input to the AV node, slowing (and in some cases blocking) AV conduction, thereby breaking the reentrant circuit and termi-

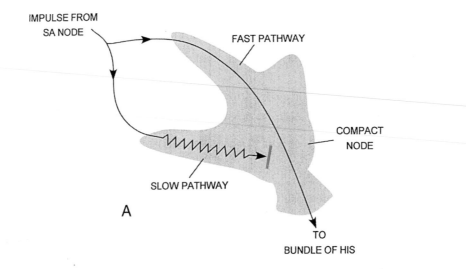

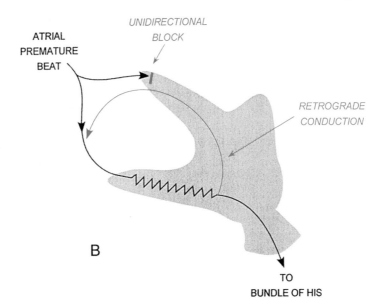

Figure 12.15. **Common mechanism of AV nodal reentry.** In most patients, the AV node (gray-colored region in the drawing) is a lobulated structure consisting proximally of several atrial extensions and distally of a compact node portion. **A.** In patients with AV nodal reentry, two functionally distinct tracts exist within the AV node (termed the slow and fast pathways). The slow pathway conducts slowly and has a short refractory period, whereas the fast pathway conducts more rapidly but has a long refractory period. Impulses from above conduct down both pathways; because the fast pathway impulse reaches the distal common pathway first, it continues to the bundle of His. Conversely, the slow pathway impulse arrives later and encounters refractory tissue. **B.** An atrial premature beat arrives at the entrance of the two pathways. The fast pathway is still refractory from the preceding beat and the impulse is blocked, but the slow pathway has repolarized and is able to conduct. When the impulse reaches the distal portion of the fast pathway after traveling down the slower pathway, the fast pathway has repolarized and is able to conduct the impulse in a retrograde direction (exemplifying unidirectional block). The impulse can then travel through the atrium and back to the slow pathway, and a reentrant loop is initiated.

nating the tachycardia. The most rapidly effective pharmacologic treatment is intravenous adenosine, which impairs AV nodal conduction and often aborts the reentrant rhythm (see Chapter 17). Other drug options include intravenous calcium channel antagonists (verapamil and diltiazem) or β-blockers. Digitalis also slows conduction through the AV node but is less useful in treating an acute episode of

AVNRT because of its slow onset of action.

Most patients with AVNRT have infrequent episodes that terminate with vagal maneuvers and do not require other specific interventions. Frequent symptomatic episodes, particularly when requiring visits to the emergency department for treatment, warrant preventive therapy—oral β-blocker, Ca^{++} channel blockers, or digoxin are often successful for this purpose. If ineffective, the circuit can be permanently interrupted with radiofrequency catheter ablation of the slow pathway. Chronic class IA or IC antiarrhythmic drugs are also effective but are less desirable because of associated risks and side effects.

Atrioventricular Reentrant Tachycardias

Atrioventricular reentrant tachycardias (AVRTs) are similar to AVNRTs except that in the former, one limb of the reentrant loop is constituted by an accessory pathway ("bypass tract"), rather than by separate fast and slow pathways within the AV node itself. As described in Chapter 11, an accessory pathway is an abnormal band of myocytes that spans the AV groove and connects atrial to ventricular tissue separately from the normal conduction system. Approximately 1 in 1500 people have such a pathway.

Several different types of bypass tracts have been described, of which the bundle of Kent is the most common (see Fig. 11.10). Such accessory connections can allow an impulse to abnormally conduct from atrium to ventricle (anterograde conduction), from ventricle to atrium (retrograde conduction), or in both directions. Depending on the direction of conduction, two characteristic entities can result: 1) the ventricular preexcitation syndrome or 2) a concealed bypass tract.

VENTRICULAR PREEXCITATION SYNDROME

In patients with ventricular preexcitation, atrial impulses can pass in an anterograde direction to the ventricles through both the AV node *and* the accessory pathway. Because conduction through the accessory pathway is usually faster than via the AV node, the ventricles are stimulated *earlier* (preexcited) than by the normal impulse. An example of ventricular preexcitation is **Wolff-Parkinson-White (WPW) syndrome,** in which the baseline ECG shows three characteristic abnormalities (Figs. 12.16 and 12.17): 1) the PR interval is shortened, because ventricular stimulation begins earlier than normal via the accessory pathway; 2) a slurred rather than sharp upstroke of the QRS (the "delta wave") is apparent due to initial ventricular activation by the accessory pathway; and 3) the QRS complex is abnormally widened, because it represents fusion of two excitation wavefronts through the ventricles, one from the accessory pathway and one from the normal His-Purkinje system.

Patients with WPW syndrome are predisposed to PSVTs since the accessory pathway provides a potential limb of a reentrant loop. The most common form of PSVT in patients with this syndrome is *orthodromic* atrioventricular reentrant tachycardia (orthodromic AVRT). During this tachycardia, an impulse travels *antegradely* down the AV

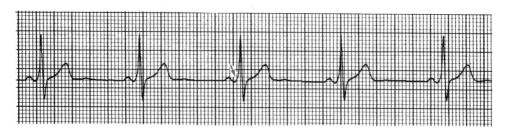

Figure 12.16. Wolff-Parkinson-White syndrome. The delta wave (arrow) indicates preexcitation of the ventricles. (Courtesy of Dr. Eric Isselbacher, Massachusetts General Hospital, Boston, MA.)

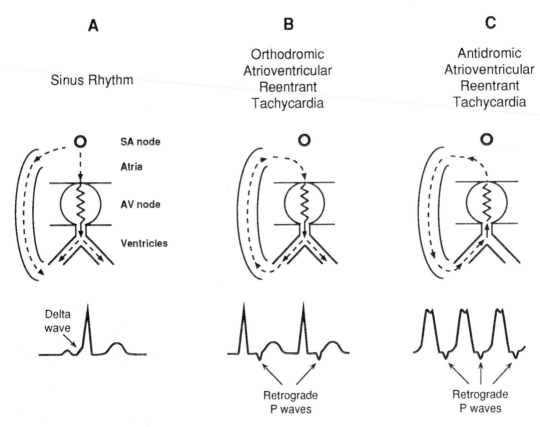

Figure 12.17. Wolff-Parkinson-White syndrome. A. During normal sinus rhythm, the shortened PR interval, delta wave, and widened QRS complex indicate fusion of ventricular activation via the AV node and accessory pathway. **B.** An atrial premature beat can trigger an orthodromic atrioventricular reentrant tachycardia, in which impulses are conducted antegradely down the AV node and retrogradely up the accessory pathway. Retrograde P waves are visible immediately after the QRS complex. There is no delta wave because antegrade ventricular stimulation passes exclusively through the AV node. **C.** Antidromic atrioventricular reentrant tachycardia in which impulses are conducted antegradely down the accessory tract and retrogradely up the AV node. The QRS complex is very widened because the ventricles are stimulated by abnormal conduction through the accessory pathway.

node to the ventricles, then *retrogradely* up the accessory tract back to the atria (Fig. 12.17B). Because the ventricles in this situation are depolarized during each cycle via the normal conduction system (through the AV node and bundle of His), there is no delta wave during the tachycardia and the width of the QRS is usually normal. Retrograde P waves are often visible soon after each QRS complex, as the atria are stimulated from below, via retrograde conduction through the bypass tract.

In fewer than 10% of patients with AVRT involving an accessory pathway, the reentrant arrhythmia travels in the opposite direction. Impulses conduct *antegradely* down the accessory pathway and *retrogradely* up

the AV node (Fig. 12.17C). Termed *antidromic* AVRT, its ECG pattern is characterized by a *widened* QRS complex, because the ventricles are activated entirely from antegrade conduction over the accessory pathway (thus representing an exaggerated form of the delta wave).

A third type of arrhythmia encountered in patients with WPW syndrome is antegrade conduction over the accessory pathway when atrial fibrillation or flutter is present. Since accessory pathways typically have short refractory periods, they allow very rapid rates of ventricular stimulation, unlike the AV node which has a longer refractory period. Thus, during AF or atrial flutter, ventricular rates as fast as 300 bpm may result. Such rates are poorly tolerated and can lead to ventricular fibrillation and cardiac arrest, even in a young, otherwise healthy patient.

Pharmacologic management of arrhythmias in patients with the WPW syndrome requires greater caution than in AVNRT. Although digitalis, β-blockers, and certain Ca^{++} channel blockers are effective at blocking conduction through the AV node during AF, they do *not* slow conduction over most accessory pathways. Sometimes, these drugs can actually *shorten* the refractory period of the accessory pathway, thus *speeding* conduction. Therefore, they could precipitate even faster ventricular rates (and hemodynamic collapse) when administered to patients with WPW syndrome who develop atrial fibrillation or flutter. In contrast, Na^+ channel blockers (specifically, class IA and IC antiarrhythmics) and some class III antiarrhythmics slow conduction and prolong the refractory period of accessory pathways as well as the AV node; therefore, these are the preferred treatments of this condition.

When a patient with WPW presents with a wide QRS tachycardia, first-line treatment options include administration of intravenous procainamide (a class IA agent that slows conduction in both the AV node and the accessory pathway) or electrical cardioversion if the patient's condition is unstable. Chronic oral therapy should include one of the drugs that slows accessory pathway conduction (class IA, IC, and III agents), rather than an agent that only impairs AV node conduction. Tachycardias due to this condition can be prevented altogether by performing percutaneous radiofrequency catheter ablation of the accessory pathway.

Another type of ventricular preexcitation is the **Lown-Ganong-Levine syndrome,** an uncommon entity also characterized by a short PR interval but a normal, narrow QRS complex (i.e., no delta wave) during sinus rhythm. Although it has been suggested that a short accessory pathway connects the atria directly to the His-Purkinje system in this condition, most patients just have enhanced conduction through the normal AV node, thus shortening the PR interval.

CONCEALED BYPASS TRACTS

Accessory pathways do not always result in ECG findings of ventricular preexcitation (i.e., short PR, delta wave). Approximately 25% of accessory pathways are capable of only *retrograde* conduction. In that case, during sinus rhythm the ventricles are depolarized normally through the AV node alone (i.e., the accessory pathway is *concealed*). However, because the abnormal pathway *is* capable of retrograde conduction, it can form a limb of a reentrant circuit and participate in orthodromic AVRT.

Management of patients with tachycardia involving a concealed accessory pathway is the same as for patients with AVNRT. Because the reentrant circuit travels antegradely down the AV node, vagal maneuvers and drugs that interrupt conduction over the AV node (e.g., adenosine, verapamil, diltiazem, and β-blockers) can abort the tachycardia. Another option in patients with recurrent episodes is catheter

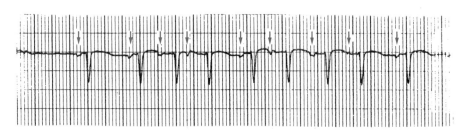

Figure 12.18. Multifocal atrial tachycardia. Each QRS is preceded by a P wave (arrows) of varying morphology. (Courtesy of Dr. Eric Isselbacher, Massachusetts General Hospital, Boston, MA.)

ablation of the accessory pathway, which permanently prevents recurrences in most patients.

Ectopic Atrial Tachycardia

Ectopic atrial tachycardia results from automaticity of an atrial focus and less commonly on the basis of reentry. The ECG has the appearance of sinus tachycardia, with a P wave before each QRS complex, but the P wave morphology is different from that of sinus rhythm, indicating depolarization of the atrium from an abnormal site. The arrhythmia can be paroxysmal and of limited duration, or it can persist. Short, asymptomatic bursts of atrial tachycardia are commonly observed on 24-hour ECG recordings, even in otherwise healthy people.

Atrial tachycardia can be caused by digitalis toxicity and is also aggravated by elevated sympathetic tone (e.g., during exertion or periods of illness). Initial treatment includes correction of any aggravating factors. Unlike reentrant supraventricular tachycardias, vagal maneuvers (such as carotid sinus massage) usually have no effect on atrial discharges from the ectopic pacemaker focus. However, β-blockers, calcium channel blockers, and Class IA, IC, and III antiarrhythmic drugs can be effective. Catheter ablation is also an option for symptomatic patients.

Multifocal Atrial Tachycardia

In multifocal atrial tachycardia (MAT) the ECG shows an irregular rhythm with multiple (at least three) P wave morphologies, and the average atrial rate is >100 bpm. An isoelectric (i.e., "flat") baseline between P waves distinguishes MAT from the chaotic baseline of AF. This rhythm is probably due to triggered automaticity of several foci within the atria (Fig. 12.18) and most often occurs in the setting of severe pulmonary disease and hypoxemia. Because individuals with this rhythm are usually critically ill from the underlying disease, the mortality rate is high, and treatment is aimed at resolving the causative disorder. The Ca^{++} channel blocker verapamil is often effective at slowing the ventricular rate as a temporizing measure.

Ventricular Arrhythmias

The common ventricular arrhythmias are 1) ventricular premature beats, 2) ventricular tachycardia, and 3) ventricular fibrillation. Ventricular arrhythmias are usually more dangerous than supraventricular rhythm disorders and are responsible for the majority of sudden cardiac deaths.

Ventricular Premature Beats

Similar to APBs, ventricular premature beats (VPBs) are common even among healthy individuals and are often asymptomatic and benign (Fig. 12.19). A VPB arises when an ectopic ventricular focus fires an action potential. On the ECG, a VPB appears as a *widened* QRS complex, because the impulse travels from its ectopic site through the ventricles via slow cell-to-cell connections rather than through the normal rapid conduction system pathway. Furthermore, the ectopic beat is not related to a preceding P wave.

VPBs are not dangerous by themselves. In individuals without heart disease, they

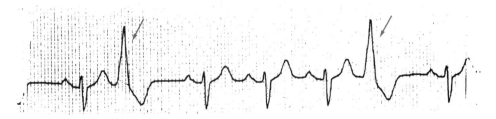

Figure 12.19. **Ventricular premature beats (arrows).**

confer no added risk of sudden cardiac death. However, they take on added significance in patients who have structural heart disease, as they may infer an increased risk of ventricular tachycardia or fibrillation. For example, they are common following an acute myocardial infarction. When VPBs occur frequently in that setting (more than 10/hour) or appear in **couplets** (two in a row) or **triplets** (three in a row), they are markers of increased mortality.

VPBs can also occur in a grouped pattern in which a fixed number of normal beats are followed by a VPB, then the series repeats. When every alternate beat is a VPB, the rhythm is termed **bigeminy.** When two normal beats precede every VPB, **trigeminy** is said to be present. Three preceding normal beats are referred to as quadrigeminy, and so on.

In healthy individuals, treatment of VPBs mainly involves reassurance and, if needed, symptomatic control using β-blockers.

Ventricular Tachycardia

Ventricular tachycardia (VT) is a series of three or more VPBs in a row (Fig. 12.20). VT is divided arbitrarily into two categories. If it persists for more than 30 seconds or requires termination because of severe symptoms, it is called **sustained VT;** otherwise, it is termed **nonsustained VT.** Both forms are found most commonly in patients with structural heart disease.

The QRS complexes of VT are typically wide (>0.12 sec) and occur at a rate of 100–200 bpm. VT is further categorized according to its QRS morphology. When every

QRS complex appears the same and the rate is regular, it is referred to as **monomorphic** VT (see Fig. 12.20). In this case, there is usually a structural abnormality supporting a reentry circuit, most commonly a region of old infarction. Occasionally, monomorphic VT occurs as a result of an ectopic ventricular focus in an otherwise healthy individual.

When the QRS complexes continually change in shape and the rate varies from beat to beat, the VT is referred to as **polymorphic.** Multiple ectopic foci or a continually changing reentry circuit is the cause. Torsades de pointes (see below) and acute myocardial ischemia or infarction are the most common causes of polymorphic VT.

The symptoms of VT vary depending on the duration of the tachycardia, the rate, and the underlying condition of the heart. When VT provokes symptoms, the major manifestations are hypotension and loss of consciousness due to low cardiac output.

Other arrhythmias may mimic VT, including supraventricular tachycardias that conduct to the ventricles with bundle branch block morphology. Differentiation of these from VT relies heavily on the relationship between the P waves and QRS complexes, since AV dissociation (no relationship between the P waves and QRS complexes) confirms the presence of VT (as described below).

Symptomatic or sustained episodes of VT are dangerous because they can deteriorate into ventricular fibrillation, which is fatal if not quickly corrected. Acute treatment usually consists of electrical cardioversion, followed by antiarrhythmic drugs for chronic suppression. Patients at high risk for VT receive an implanted cardioverter

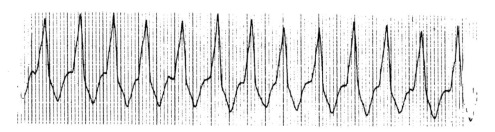

Figure 12.20. **Monomorphic ventricular tachycardia.**

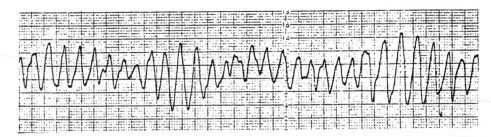

Figure 12.21. **Torsades de pointes.** The widened polymorphic QRS complexes demonstrate a waxing and waning pattern; the QT interval was prolonged before the onset of the arrhythmia (not shown).

defibrillator (ICD) to automatically and promptly terminate future episodes.

Asymptomatic nonsustained VT and simple ventricular ectopic beats usually do not warrant specific antiarrhythmic drugs, because such therapy has not been shown to improve survival and has the potential to *aggravate* dangerous arrhythmias. Rather, β-blockers are often the first-line agents to reduce symptoms of ventricular arrhythmias that are not life-threatening.

Torsades de Pointes

Torsades de pointes ("twisting of the points") is a form of polymorphic VT presenting as varying amplitudes of the QRS, as if the complexes are "twisting" about the baseline (Fig. 12.21). It can be produced by early afterdepolarizations (triggered activity), particularly in patients who have a *prolonged QT interval*. QT prolongation (which indicates a lengthened action potential duration) can result from electrolyte disturbances (especially hypokalemia or hypomagnesemia) and certain drugs, including many *anti*arrhythmic agents (particularly Class III agents sotalol, ibutilide, and dofetilide; and some Class I drugs, including quinidine, procainamide, and disopyramide). Other medications that can prolong the QT interval and predispose to torsades de pointes are erythromycin and phenothiazines. A rare group of hereditary ion channel abnormalities can produce *congenital* QT prolongation, which places the patient at continuous risk for torsades de pointes.

Torsades de pointes is usually symptomatic but frequently self-limited. Its danger results from syncope during the rhythm or its degeneration into ventricular fibrilla-

tion. When it is drug- or electrolyte-induced, correcting the underlying cause abolishes the arrhythmia. Administration of intravenous magnesium often suppresses recurrent episodes. Other preventive strategies are aimed at shortening the QT interval by increasing the underlying heart rate. Such strategies include administering intravenous β-adrenergic *stimulating* agents (e.g., isoproterenol) and accelerating the heart rate via an artificial pacemaker. Paradoxically, when torsades de pointes appears in patients with congenital prolongation of the QT interval, β-*blocking* drugs are the treatment of choice, because sympathetic stimulation actually aggravates the arrhythmia in such individuals. An implantable defibrillator is often used for these patients.

Ventricular Fibrillation

Ventricular fibrillation (VF) is the most life-threatening arrhythmia (Fig. 12.22). It results in disordered rapid stimulation of the ventricles, preventing them from contracting in a coordinated fashion. The result is a severe drop in cardiac output and death if not quickly reversed. This rhythm most often occurs in individuals with severe heart disease and is the major cause of mortality in acute myocardial infarction.

VT usually precedes VF. It is thought that degeneration of VT results in multiple small wavelets of reentry that constitute the VF rhythm. On the ECG, VF is characterized by a chaotic irregular appearance with complexes of varying amplitude and morphology, without discrete QRS waveforms.

Untreated, VF rapidly leads to death. The only effective therapy is prompt electri-

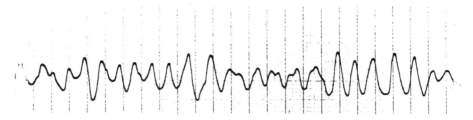

Figure 12.22. **Ventricular fibrillation.**

cal defibrillation. As soon as the heart has been converted to a safe rhythm, the underlying cause of the arrhythmia (e.g., electrolyte imbalances, hypoxemia, or acidosis) should be sought and corrected to prevent further episodes. Intravenous antiarrhythmic drug therapy may be administered to prevent recurrences. If no reversible inciting cause is found, survivors of VF usually receive an ICD.

Differentiation of Wide Complex Tachycardias

VT can usually be distinguished from supraventricular tachycardia (SVT) by the width of the QRS complex. It is routinely wide in the former and narrow (i.e., normal) in the latter, as illustrated in Figure 12.9. However, under certain circumstances, arrhythmias that arise from sites above the ventricles *can* result in wide QRS complexes. This may occur because either 1) the patient has an underlying conduction abnormality (e.g., a bundle branch block), such that the QRS is abnormally wide even when in normal sinus rhythm, or 2) repetitive rapid stimulation of the ventricles during SVT finds portions of the ventricular conduction system refractory, because of insufficient time to recover from the previous depolarization. As a result, the impulse propagating through the ventricles is partially blocked, causing the QRS to become distorted and widened (termed "SVT with aberrant conduction").

Certain clinical and electrocardiographic features help to distinguish wide QRS complexes of VT from those of supraventricular rhythms with aberrant conduction. In patients with a history of prior myocardial infarction, congestive heart failure, or left ventricular dysfunction, a wide complex tachycardia is more likely to be VT rather than SVT with aberrancy. At the bedside, SVT is more probable if vagal maneuvers (such as carotid sinus massage) affect the rhythm, as indicated in Figure 12.9.

Electrocardiographically, a *supraventricular* tachyarrhythmia is more likely if the morphology of the QRS at the rapid rate is similar to that on the patient's ECG tracing obtained while in sinus rhythm (i.e., the complex is widened because of an underlying bundle branch block). Conversely, *ventricular* tachycardia is more likely if 1) there is no relationship between the QRS complexes and any observed P waves (atrioventricular dissociation), and 2) the QRS complexes in each of the chest leads (V_1 through V_6) are oriented in the same direction [i.e., they are all either positive or negative ("concordance" of the precordial QRS complexes)]. These features are summarized in Table 12.2. Other morphologic ECG features have been used to distinguish VT from SVT with aberrancy, but the distinction is often difficult. Most patients

TABLE 12.2. **Differentiation of Wide Complex Tachycardias**

Supports SVT with "Aberrant" Conduction	Supports Ventricular Tachycardia
• QRS morphology same as when in sinus rhythm • Rhythm responds to vagal maneuvers (see Fig. 12.9)	• No relationship between P wave and QRS complexes • Concordance of QRS complexes in the chest leads (V_1–V_6)

SVT, supraventricular tachycardia.

with wide QRS tachycardia should be
managed as though they have VT until
proven otherwise.

SUMMARY

1. Disorders of impulse formation and
   conduction result in bradyarrhythmias
   and tachyarrhythmias, the most common of which are presented in this
   chapter. Through careful analysis of the
   ECG, it is usually possible to distinguish between the array of rhythm disorders so that appropriate therapy can
   be administered.
2. When evaluating a patient with a slow
   heart rhythm (Figs. 12.1–12.8), the key
   questions to address are:
   • Are P waves present?
   • What is the relationship between the
     P waves and the QRS complexes?
3. Differentiation of tachyarrhythmias requires assessment of:
   • The width of the QRS complex (nor-
     mal or wide)
   • The morphology and rate of the P
     waves
   • The relationship between the P waves
     and the QRS complexes
   • The response to vagal maneuvers (see
     Fig. 12.9).

Each of the ECG texts listed at the end of
Chapter 4 provides additional examples of
the rhythm disorders presented in this
chapter.

*Acknowledgment   Contributors to the previous
editions of this chapter were Wendy Armstrong, MD;
Nicholas Boulis, MD; Marc S. Sabatine, MD;
Leonard I. Ganz, MD; Elliott M. Antman, MD; and
Leonard S. Lilly, MD.*

ADDITIONAL READING

Cannom DS, Prystowsky EN. Management of ventricular arrhythmias: detection, drugs, and devices.
JAMA 1999;281:172–179.

Falk RH. Atrial fibrillation. N Engl J Med. 2001;344:
1067–1078.

Ganz LI, Friedman PL. Supraventricular tachycardia.
N Engl J Med 1995;332:162–173.

Glikson M, Friedman PA. The implantable cardioverter defibrillator. Lancet 2001;357:1107–1117.

Gollob MH, Green MS, Tang AS, et al. Identification of
a gene responsible for familial Wolff-Parkinson-
White syndrome. N Engl J Med 2001;344:1823–1831.

Gregoratos G, Cheitlin MD, Conill A, et al. ACC/AHA
guidelines for implantation of cardiac pacemakers
and antiarrhythmia devices: a report of the American College of Cardiology/American Heart Association Task Force on Practice Guidelines (Committee on Pacemaker Implantation). J Am Coll Cardiol
1998;31:1175–1209.

Huikuri HV, Castellanos A, Myerburg RJ. Sudden
death due to cardiac arrhythmias. N Engl J Med
2001;345:1473–1482.

Kusumoto FM, Goldschlager N. Cardiac pacing. N
Engl J Med 1996;334:89–97.

Kusumoto FM, Goldschlager H. Device therapy for
cardiac arrhthmias. JAMA 2002;287:1848–1852.

Mangrum JM, DiMarco JP. The evaluation and management of bradycardia. N Engl J Med 2000;342:
703–709.

Morady F. Radio-frequency ablation as treatment for
cardiac arrhythmias. N Engl J Med 1999;340:
534–544.

Viskin S. Long QT syndromes and torsade de pointes.
Lancet 1999;354:1625–1633.

Zipes D, Jalife J. Cardiac Electrophysiology: From Cell
to Bedside. 3rd Ed. Philadelphia: WB Saunders,
2000.

Hypertension

Rajeev Malhotra, Gordon H. Williams, and Leonard S. Lilly

What Is Hypertension?
How Is Blood Pressure Regulated?
Blood Pressure Reflexes
Essential Hypertension
Severity
Epidemiology
Experimental Findings
Natural History
Secondary Hypertension
Exogenous Causes
Renal Causes

Mechanical Causes
Endocrine Causes
Consequences of Hypertension
Clinical Signs and Symptoms
Organ Damage due to Hypertension
Hypertensive Crises
Treatment of Hypertension
Nonpharmacologic Treatment
Pharmacologic Treatment

More than 50 million Americans have hypertension—blood pressure high enough to be a danger to their well-being. Hypertension can be implicated in as many as 800,000 deaths per year as well as nonlethal myocardial infarctions, strokes, and permanent damage to the retina and kidney. Nonetheless, nearly one-third of hypertensive individuals are unaware that they have this condition. Because elevated blood pressure is usually asymptomatic until an acute cardiovascular event strikes, screening for hypertension is a critical aspect of preventive medicine.

Hypertension is also a scientific problem of unexpected complexity. In almost 95% of affected patients, the cause of the blood pressure elevation is unknown, a condition termed primary or **essential hypertension (EH).** Evidence suggests that there are multiple, diverse causes for EH, and considerable insight into these factors can be achieved by studying the normal physiology of blood pressure control, as will be examined.

High blood pressure attributed to a *definable* cause is termed **secondary hypertension.** Although far less common than EH, conditions that cause secondary hypertension are very important because

they are often amenable to permanent cure. Following the discussions of essential and secondary hypertension, this chapter considers the clinical consequences of elevated blood pressure and approaches to treatment.

WHAT IS HYPERTENSION?

Blood pressure values vary widely in the population. Diastolic pressures follow the smooth bell-shaped distribution shown in Figure 13.1, and both systolic and diastolic pressures rise with increasing age, as illustrated in Figure 13.2. The risk of complications of elevated pressure increases progressively with higher values, so that the exact cutoff point for the definition of hypertension is somewhat arbitrary; nevertheless, the currently established criteria are listed in Table 13.1. By these criteria, a diastolic pressure consistently at or above 90 mm Hg or a systolic pressure at or above 140 mm Hg establishes the diagnosis of hypertension. Those with "high normal" blood pressure have an increased risk of developing definite hypertension and therefore need to be monitored closely. The definitions in Table 13.1 are based on studies that examined

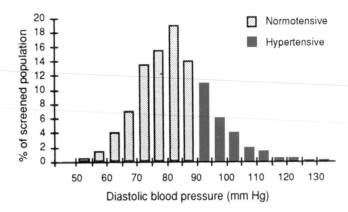

Figure 13.1. **Distribution of diastolic blood pressure values in the 30- to 69-year age group (n = 158,906).** Hypertension is arbitrarily defined as diastolic blood pressure ≥ 90 mm Hg. (Modified from Hypertension Detection and Follow-up Program. A progress report. Circ Res 1977;40(Suppl1):106.)

the incidence of cardiovascular complications related to blood pressure values. Although the emphasis has historically been on the level of *diastolic* pressure, recent evidence implicates *systolic* pressure as equally or more important in predicting hypertensive complications.

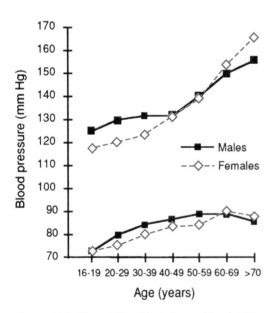

Figure 13.2. **The relationship between blood pressure and age (n = 1029). Systolic (upper curves) and diastolic (lower curves) values are shown.** Note that by age 60, the average systolic pressure of women exceeds that of men. (Modified from Kotchen JM, McKean HE, Kotchen TA. Blood pressure trends with aging. Hypertension 1982;4(Suppl 3):111–129.)

HOW IS BLOOD PRESSURE REGULATED?

Blood pressure (BP) is the product of cardiac output (CO) and total peripheral resistance (TPR):

$$BP = CO \times TPR$$

In turn, CO is the product of cardiac stroke volume (SV) and heart rate (HR):

$$CO = SV \times HR$$

in which the stroke volume is largely determined by cardiac contractility and by the amount of venous return to the heart (i.e., the preload, as described in Chapter 9).

It follows that at least three systems are directly responsible for blood pressure regulation: the *heart*, which supplies the pumping pressure; *blood vessel tone*, which largely determines systemic resistance; and the *kidney*, which regulates intravascular volume. Figure 13.3 shows how these three systems contribute to the CO and TPR.

The renal component of blood pressure regulation deserves special mention, in light of the temptation to view hypertension as a "cardiovascular problem." No matter how high the CO and how constricted the blood vessels, renal excretion has the capacity to completely return blood pressure to normal levels by reducing intravascular volume. Therefore, the maintenance of chronic hypertension requires renal participation, even though the factors

TABLE 13.1. Classification of Blood Pressure in Adults

Category	Systolic Pressure (mm Hg)		Diastolic Pressure (mm Hg)
Optimal	<120	and	<80
Normal	<130	and	<85
High-Normal	130–139	or	85–89
Hypertension			
Stage 1	140–159	or	90–99
Stage 2	160–179	or	100–109
Stage 3	≥ 180	or	≥ 110

Modified from The sixth report of the Joint National Committee on Prevention, Detection, Evaluation, and Treatment of High Blood Pressure. Arch Intern Med 1997;157:2413–2446.

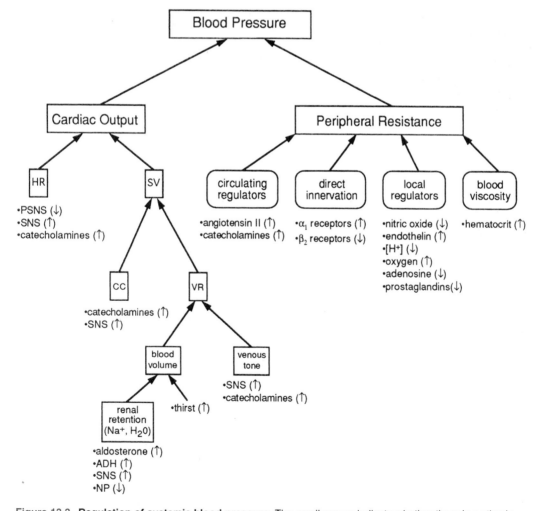

Figure 13.3. Regulation of systemic blood pressure. The small arrows indicate whether there is a stimulatory (↑) or inhibitory (↓) effect on the boxed parameters. HR, heart rate; SV, stroke volume; PSNS, parasympathetic nervous system; SNS, sympathetic nervous system; CC, cardiac contractility; VR, venous return; ADH, antidiuretic hormone; NP, natriuretic peptides.

responsible may lie outside of the renal parenchyma. Examples of such factors include reduced blood perfusion to the kidney because of restricted flow through the renal artery, or aberrant secretion of circulating hormones that enhance renal sodium retention, as described below.

Blood Pressure Reflexes

The cardiovascular system is endowed with feedback mechanisms that continuously monitor arterial pressure—they sense when the pressure becomes excessively high or low and then respond rapidly to these changes. One such mechanism is the **baroreceptor reflex,** which is mediated by receptors in the walls of the aortic arch and the carotid sinuses. These baroreceptors monitor changes in pressure by sensing the stretch and deformation of the arteries. If the arterial pressure rises, the baroreceptors are stimulated, increasing their transmission of impulses to the central nervous system (i.e., the medulla). Negative feedback signals are then sent back to the circulation via the autonomic nervous system, causing the blood pressure to fall back to its baseline level.

The higher the blood pressure rises, the more the baroreceptors are stretched and the greater the impulse transmission rate to the medulla. Such signals from the carotid sinus receptors are carried by the glossopharyngeal nerve (cranial nerve IX), whereas the signals from the aortic arch receptors are carried by the vagus nerve (cranial nerve X). These nerve fibers converge at the tractus solitarius in the medulla, where the baroreceptor impulses *inhibit* sympathetic nervous system outflow and *excite* parasympathetic effects. The net result is: 1) a decline in peripheral vascular resistance (i.e., vasodilation), and 2) a reduction in CO (due to a lower heart rate and reduced force of cardiac contraction). Each of these effects tends to lower arterial pressure back toward its baseline. On the other hand, when a fall in systemic pressure is sensed by the baroreceptors, fewer impulses are transmitted to the medulla and there is a reflex *increase* in blood pressure back to its baseline.

The main effect of the baroreceptors is to reduce moment-by-moment variations in systemic blood pressure. However, the baroreceptor reflex is not involved in the long-term regulation of mean blood pressure and does not prevent the development of chronic hypertension. This is so because the baroreceptors constantly reset themselves. After a day or two of exposure to higher-than-baseline pressures, the baroreceptor firing rate slows back to its control value.

ESSENTIAL HYPERTENSION

Almost 95% of hypertensive patients have blood pressures that are elevated for no readily definable reason; they are therefore said to suffer from essential hypertension (EH). The diagnosis of EH is one of exclusion; it is the option left to the clinician after ruling out all the causes of secondary hypertension described later in this chapter.

EH is more a description than a diagnosis, indicating only that a patient manifests a specific physical finding (high blood pressure) for which no cause has been found. In all likelihood, different underlying defects are responsible for the elevated pressure in different subpopulations of patients. Because the exact nature of these defects is unknown, to understand EH is to understand the possibilities—what could go wrong with normal physiology to produce chronically elevated blood pressure?

This discussion of EH therefore reflects what is currently known about its severity, epidemiology and genetics, experimental findings, and natural history. The picture that will emerge is that EH likely results from the synergy of multiple defects of blood pressure regulation that interact with environmental stressors. The regulatory defects may be acquired or genetically determined and may be independent of each other. As a result, EH patients exhibit varied combinations of regulatory defects and therefore have different physiologic bases for their elevated blood pressures.

Severity

Approximately 80% of EH patients have stage 1 hypertension; only 10% have either moderate or severe degrees. Although the cardiovascular danger of high blood pressure is greater for those with higher pressures, it is the stage 1 and 2 hypertensive patients who, because of their sheer numbers, account for the vast morbidity and mortality attributable to EH.

Epidemiology and Genetics

Heredity appears to play an important role in EH, but definite genetic markers have not yet been identified. There is clearly a higher rate of elevated blood pressures among first-degree relatives of hypertensives than in the general population. Concordance between identical twins is not complete, but is high and significantly greater than that for dizygotic twins. Hypothesized genetic abnormalities include defects in the renal excretion of sodium, abnormal sodium transport across cell membranes, and an abnormally high autonomic nervous system response to exogenous stress. Of note, normotensive relatives of EH patients can often be shown to exhibit physiologic abnormalities of a type that, in conjunction with other regulatory defects, could lead to an elevated pressure (e.g., abnormalities of renal blood flow regulation).

A genetic component to EH is also suggested by the uneven distribution of hypertension among racial groups. For example, in most age distributions, blacks are significantly more likely to be hypertensive than are individuals of other races. Environmental differences may also contribute to this disparity, as suggested by the concordance of blood pressures among spouses. In addition, populations of lower educational backgrounds and socioeconomic status suffer from higher levels of blood pressure. Finally, age is an important factor, as there is an increased prevalence of hypertensives among older individuals.

Experimental Findings

Multiple defects of blood pressure regulation have been found in essential hypertensives and their relatives. By themselves, or in conjunction with one another, these abnormalities might contribute to chronic blood pressure elevation.

The *heart* can contribute to a high CO-based hypertension due to abnormal neural or catecholamine stimulation. For example, when tested under psychologically stressful conditions, hypertensive patients (and their first-degree relatives) often develop excessive heart rate acceleration compared with control subjects, suggesting an excessive sympathetic response.

The *blood vessels* can contribute to peripheral vascular resistance-based hypertension by constricting in response to 1) malregulation of the sympathetic nervous system; 2) abnormal regulation of vascular tone by local factors, including nitric oxide, endothelin, and natriuretic factors; or 3) ion channel defects in contractile vascular smooth muscle.

The *kidney* can induce volume-based hypertension by retaining excessive sodium and water due to 1) failure to regulate renal blood flow appropriately, 2) ion channel defects (e.g., reduced basolateral Na^+/K^+-ATPase) directly causing sodium retention, or 3) inappropriate hormonal regulation. For example, the renin-angiotensin-aldosterone axis is an important hormonal regulator of peripheral vascular resistance. Renin levels in EH patients (relative to normotensives) are subnormal in 30%, normal in 60%, and high in 10%. Since renin secretion should be *suppressed* by high blood pressure, even "normal" levels of renin secretion are inappropriate in hypertensive patients. Thus, abnormalities of renin regulation may play a role in some individuals with EH.

Figure 13.4 highlights these and other potential mechanisms of EH. Note that although the heart, blood vessels, and kidneys are the organs ultimately responsible for producing the pressure, primary defects may be located elsewhere as well (e.g., the central nervous system, arterial barorecep-

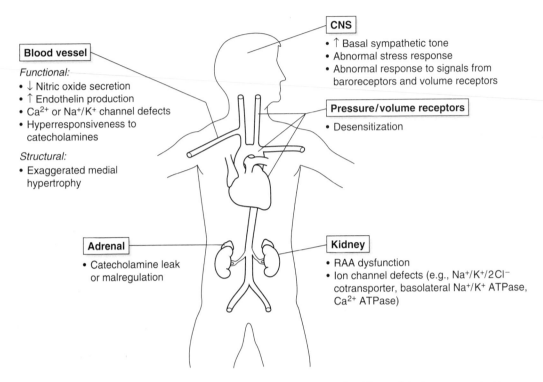

Blood vessel

Functional:
- ↓ Nitric oxide secretion
- ↑ Endothelin production
- Ca^{2+} or Na^{+}/K^{+} channel defects
- Hyperresponsiveness to catecholamines

Structural:
- Exaggerated medial hypertrophy

CNS
- ↑ Basal sympathetic tone
- Abnormal stress response
- Abnormal response to signals from baroreceptors and volume receptors

Pressure/volume receptors
- Desensitization

Adrenal
- Catecholamine leak or malregulation

Kidney
- RAA dysfunction
- Ion channel defects (e.g., $Na^{+}/K^{+}/2Cl^{-}$ cotransporter, basolateral Na^{+}/K^{+} ATPase, Ca^{2+} ATPase)

Figure 13.4. **Potential primary abnormalities in essential hypertension.** These defects are supported by experimental evidence, but their specific contributions to essential hypertension remain unclear. CNS, central nervous system; RAA, renin-angiotensin-aldosterone system.

tors, and adrenal gland hormone secretion). Although abnormal regulation at these sites can contribute to elevated blood pressure, it is important to remember that without renal complicity, malfunction of other systems would not produce sustained hypertension, because the normal kidney is capable of eliminating sufficient volume to return the blood pressure to normal.

Recent research has shown that another potentially important factor in the development of EH relates to the hormone insulin. In many patients with hypertension, especially those who are obese or have type II diabetes mellitus, there is impaired insulin-dependent transport of glucose into the peripheral tissues (termed *insulin resistance*). As a result, serum glucose levels rise, stimulating the pancreas to release greater amounts of insulin. Such hyperinsulinemia can theoretically raise arterial pressure by at least four mechanisms: 1) insulin stimulates renal sodium reabsorption, thereby increasing intravascular volume; 2) insulin increases sympathetic nervous system ac-

tivity and raises the concentration of circulating catecholamines; 3) insulin is a mitogen that stimulates arterial vascular smooth muscle hypertrophy; and 4) insulin alters cell membrane ion transport which can lead to increased intracellular calcium and heightened vascular tone.

Obesity itself has been directly associated with hypertension. One theory proposes that excessive leptin release by adipose tissue may contribute to elevated blood pressure. Leptin is a protein synthesized by fat tissue that is thought to promote appetite suppression but also to stimulate sympathetic nervous system activity. Whether hyperinsulinemia and obesity truly play important roles in the genesis of EH is unknown and remains a subject of ongoing investigation.

Natural History

EH characteristically arises after young adulthood. Its prevalence increases with age; more than 60% of Americans older than 60 years of age have a diastolic pressure greater than 90 mm Hg, and an additional number have isolated elevation of systolic pressure.

In addition, the hemodynamic characteristics of blood pressure elevation in EH tend to change over time (Fig. 13.5). In hypertensive patients younger than age 40, blood pressure tends to be driven by high CO in the setting of normal TPR, termed the "hyperkinetic" phase of EH. Eventually, however, the contribution by CO tends to decline, while TPR increases as the heart and vessels adapt to the prolonged stress. For example, the development of left ventricular hypertrophy in chronic hypertension compromises diastolic filling (which in turn reduces stroke volume and CO), whereas medial hypertrophy of the arterioles reduces the lumen diameter and increases the resistance to forward blood flow. Thus, older hypertensive patients tend to have elevated TPR as the principal abnormality, with a normal or reduced CO. This progression from "high CO, normal TPR" to "normal CO, high TPR" occurs independent of whether the mean arterial pressure rises over time or remains unchanged.

Thus, EH is a syndrome that may arise from many potential abnormalities, but it exhibits a characteristic hemodynamic profile and natural history. It is likely that multiple defects, separately inherited or acquired, acting together chronically raise blood pressure in affected individuals. Although we may not understand the precise underlying mechanism in any individual hypertensive patient, we can at least describe what kind of pathophysiology might be at fault. EH, although idiopathic, is not entirely a "black box."

SECONDARY HYPERTENSION

Although EH dominates the clinical picture, in 5% of patients with hypertension, there is a defined structural or hormonal cause. Although cases of such secondary hypertension are relatively uncommon, their identification is important, because these conditions are often curable and may require therapy different from that administered for EH. Moreover, if left uncontrolled, adaptive cardiovascular changes may develop analogous to those of longstanding EH, which could cause the elevated pressures to persist even after the underlying cause is corrected.

Although secondary forms should be considered in the workup of all patients with hypertension, there are clinical clues that a given patient may have one of the correctable conditions (Table 13.2):

1. **Age.** If a patient develops hypertension before age 20 or after age 50 (outside the usual range of EH), secondary hypertension is more likely.
2. **Severity.** Secondary hypertension often causes blood pressure to rise into the

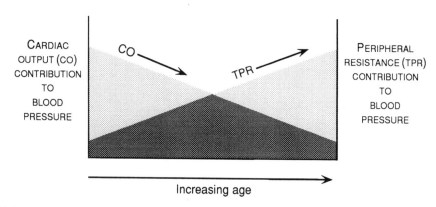

Figure 13.5. Hemodynamic progression of essential hypertension. Schematic representation of the changing contribution of cardiac output and total peripheral resistance as age increases in many patients with essential hypertension.

TABLE 13.2. Causes of Hypertension

Type	Percent of Hypertensive Patients	Clinical Clues
Essential	95%	• Age of onset: 20–50 years • Family history of hypertension • Normal serum [K$^+$], urinalysis
Chronic renal disease	2–4%	• $\uparrow$ [Creatinine], abnormal urinalysis
Renovascular	1%	• Abdominal bruit • Sudden onset (especially if age > 50 or < 20) • $\downarrow$ Serum [K$^+$]
Pheochromocytoma	0.2%	• Paroxysms of palpitations, diaphoresis, and anxiety • Episodic hypertension in one-third of patients
Coarctation of the aorta	0.1%	• Blood pressure in arms > legs, or right arm > left arm • Midsystolic murmur between scapulae • CXR: aortic indentation, rib-notching due to collaterals
Primary aldosteronism	0.1%	• $\downarrow$ Serum [K$^+$]
Cushing's syndrome	0.1%	• "Cushingoid" appearance (e.g., central obesity, hirsutism)

stage 3 (severe) category, whereas most EH patients have stage 1 to 2 (mild to moderate) hypertension.

3. **Onset.** Secondary forms of hypertension often present abruptly in a patient who was previously normotensive, rather than gradually progressing over years as is the usual case in EH.

4. **Associated signs and symptoms.** The process that induces hypertension may give rise to other characteristic abnormalities, identified by the history and physical examination. For example, a renal artery "bruit" (swishing sound due to turbulent blood flow through a stenotic artery) may be heard on abdominal examination in a patient with renal artery stenosis.

5. **Family history.** EH patients often have hypertensive first-degree relatives, whereas secondary hypertension more commonly occurs sporadically.

The usual clinical evaluation of a patient with recently diagnosed hypertension begins with a careful history and physical examination, including a search for clues to the secondary forms. For example, repeated urinary tract infections may suggest the presence of chronic pyelonephritis with renal damage as the cause of hypertension. Excessive weight loss may be an indicator of pheochromocytoma, whereas weight

gain may point to the presence of Cushing's syndrome. A history of certain drug use (e.g., glucocorticoids or estrogen) may clarify the underlying cause of hypertension.

Certain laboratory tests are commonly assessed in the evaluation of a hypertensive patient. Typical screening studies include the following: 1) urinalysis and serum concentration of creatinine and blood urea nitrogen to evaluate for renal abnormalities; 2) serum potassium level (abnormally low in renovascular hypertension or primary aldosteronism); 3) blood glucose level (abnormally high in diabetes, which is strongly associated with hypertension and renal vascular disease); 4) serum cholesterol, high-density lipoprotein (HDL) cholesterol, and triglyceride levels (abnormal levels may identify a predisposition for arteriosclerosis); and 5) chest radiograph (e.g., abnormal in aortic coarctation). If no abnormalities are found, the patient is presumed to have EH and treated accordingly. If, however, the patient's blood pressure is refractory to usual therapy, then more detailed diagnostic testing is performed to search for other specific forms of secondary hypertension.

Exogenous Causes

A number of medications can elevate blood pressure. For example, oral contraceptives may cause secondary hypertension in some women. The mechanism is likely related to increased activity of the renin-angiotensin system. Estrogens increase the hepatic synthesis of angiotensinogen, leading to greater production of angiotensin II (Fig. 13.6). Angiotensin II raises blood pressure by several mechanisms, most notably by direct vasoconstriction and by stimulating the adrenal release of aldosterone. The latter hormone causes renal sodium retention and therefore increased intravascular volume.

Other medications that can raise blood pressure include glucocorticoids, cyclosporine A (an antirejection drug used in patients with organ transplants), erythropoietin (a hormone that increases bone marrow red blood cell formation; elevation of BP is due to increased blood viscosity and reversal of local hypoxic vasodilatation), and sympathomimetic drugs (which are common in over-the-counter cold remedies).

Two other substances that may contribute to hypertension are cocaine and chronic excessive ethanol consumption. Both of these are associated with increased sympathetic nervous system activity.

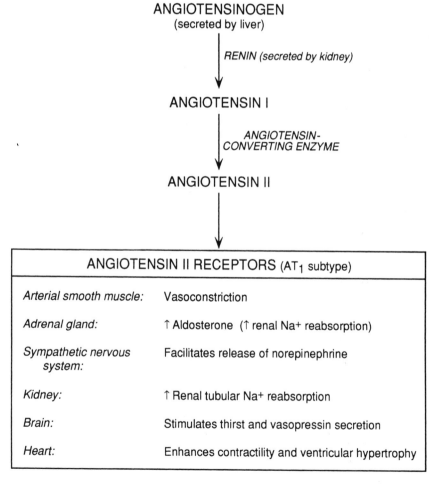

Figure 13.6. **The renin-angiotensin-aldosterone system.** Liver-derived angiotensinogen is cleaved in the circulation by renin (of kidney origin) to form angiotensin I (AI). AI is rapidly cleaved in the circulation to the potent vasoconstrictor angiotensin II (AII) by angiotensin-converting enzyme. AII also modulates the release of aldosterone from the adrenal cortex. Aldosterone in turn acts to reabsorb Na^+ from the distal nephron, resulting in increased intravascular volume. The other listed effects of AII receptor stimulation may also contribute to the development and maintenance of hypertension.

Renal Causes

Given the crucial role of the kidney in the control of blood pressure, it is not surprising that renal dysfunction can lead to hypertension. In fact, renal disease contributes to the two leading endogenous causes of secondary hypertension: renal parenchymal disease, accounting for 2–4% of hypertensive patients, and renal arterial stenosis, which accounts for approximately 1%.

Renal Parenchymal Disease

Parenchymal damage to the kidney can result from diverse pathologic processes. The major mechanism by which injury leads to elevated blood pressure is through increased intravascular volume. Damaged nephrons are unable to excrete normal amounts of sodium and water, leading to a rise in volume, elevated CO, and hence increased blood pressure.

If renal function is only mildly impaired, then the blood pressure may stabilize at a level at which the higher systemic pressure (and therefore renal perfusion pressure) enables sodium excretion to balance sodium intake. Conversely, if a patient has end-stage renal failure, the glomerular filtration rate is so greatly decreased that the kidney simply cannot excrete sufficient volume, and malignant-range blood pressures may follow.

Renal parenchymal disease may contribute to hypertension even if the glomerular filtration rate is not greatly reduced, through the excessive elaboration of renin.

Renovascular Hypertension

Stenosis of one or both renal arteries leads to hypertension. Although emboli, vasculitis, and external compression of the renal arteries can be responsible, the two most common causes of renovascular hypertension (RH) are atherosclerosis and fibromuscular dysplasia. *Atherosclerotic* lesions arise from extensive plaque formation either within the renal artery or in the aorta at the origin of the renal artery. This form accounts for about two-thirds of cases of RH and occurs most commonly in elderly men.

Fibromuscular lesions, in contrast, consist of discrete regions of fibrous or muscular proliferation, generally within the arterial media. Fibromuscular dysplasia accounts for one-third of cases of RH and characteristically occurs in young women.

The elevated blood pressure in RH arises from reduced renal blood flow to the affected kidney, which responds to the lower perfusion pressure by secreting renin. The latter raises the blood pressure through the subsequent actions of angiotensin II (vasoconstriction) and aldosterone (sodium retention), shown in Figure 13.6.

The diagnosis of RH is suggested by an abdominal bruit, which can be identified in 40–60% of patients, or by the presence of unexplained hypokalemia (owing to excessive renal excretion of potassium because of the elevated aldosterone levels). RH is a correctable form of hypertension that is often successfully treated by percutaneous catheter interventions or surgical reconstruction of the stenosed vessel. Medical therapy, particularly with angiotensin-converting enzyme (ACE) inhibitors, can also be effective initial therapy in patients with unilateral renal artery disease. ACE inhibitors negate the effect of elevated circulating renin in this situation by impeding the formation of angiotensin II (see Chapter 17).

Mechanical Causes

Coarctation of the Aorta

Coarctation is an infrequent congenital narrowing of the aorta typically located just distal to the origin of the left subclavian artery (see Chapter 16). As a result of the relative obstruction to flow, the blood pressure in the aortic arch, head, and arms is higher than that in the descending aorta and its branches and in the lower extremities. Sometimes the coarctation involves the origin of the left subclavian artery, so that the pressure of the left arm may be lower than that of the right.

Hypertension in this condition arises by two mechanisms. First, reduced blood flow to the kidneys stimulates the renin-angiotensin system, resulting in vasoconstriction (via angiotensin II). Second, high pressures proximal to the coarctation stiffen the aortic arch through medial hyperplasia and accelerated atherosclerosis, blunting the normal baroreceptor response to elevated intravascular pressure.

Clinical clues to the presence of coarctation include symptoms of inadequate blood flow to the legs or left arm, such as claudication or fatigue, or the finding of weakened or absent femoral pulses. A midsystolic murmur associated with the stenotic segment of the aorta may be auscultated, especially over the back, between the scapulae. The chest radiograph may show indentation of the aorta at the level of the coarctation. It may also demonstrate a notched appearance of the ribs secondary to the enlargement of collateral intercostal arteries, which shunt blood around the aortic narrowing. Treatment options include angioplasty or surgery to correct the stenosis. However, the hypertension may not abate completely after mechanical correction, possibly because of persistent desensitization of the arterial baroreceptors.

Endocrine Causes

Circulating hormones play an important role in the control of normal blood pressure, so that it is not surprising that endocrine diseases may cause hypertension. When suspected, the presence of such endocrine conditions is evaluated in four ways:

1. History of characteristic signs and symptoms
2. Measurement of hormone levels
3. Assessment of hormone secretion in response to stimulation or inhibition
4. Imaging studies to identify tumors secreting the excessive hormone

Pheochromocytoma

Pheochromocytomas are catecholamine-secreting tumors of neuroendocrine cells (usually in the adrenal medulla) that cause approximately 0.2% of cases of hypertension. The release of epinephrine and norepinephrine by the tumor results in intermittent or chronic vasoconstriction, tachycardia, and other sympathetic-mediated effects. A char-

acteristic presentation consists of paroxysmal rises in blood pressure accompanied by "autonomic attacks" due to the increased catecholamine levels: severe throbbing headaches, profuse sweating, palpitations, and tachycardia. Although some patients are actually normotensive between attacks, most have sustained hypertension. Ten percent of pheochromocytomas are malignant.

Determination of plasma catecholamine levels, or urine catecholamines and their metabolites (e.g., vanillylmandelic acid and metanephrine), obtained under controlled circumstances, are used to identify this condition. Because some pheochromocytomas secrete only episodically, diagnosis may require measurement of catecholamines immediately following an attack.

Pharmacologic therapy of pheochromocytomas includes the combination of an α-receptor blocker (e.g., phenoxybenzamine) combined with a β-blocker. However, once the tumor is localized by computed tomography (CT), magnetic resonance imaging (MRI), or by angiography, the definitive therapy is surgical resection. For patients with inoperable disease, treatment consists of α and β blockade as well as drugs that inhibit catecholamine biosynthesis (e.g., α-methyltyrosine).

Adrenocortical Hormone Excess

Among the hormones produced by the adrenal cortex are mineralocorticoids and glucocorticoids. Excess of either of these can result in hypertension.

Mineralocorticoids, primarily aldosterone, increase blood volume by stimulating reabsorption of sodium into the circulation by the distal portions of the nephron. This occurs in exchange for potassium excretion into the urine, and the resulting hypokalemia is an important diagnostic marker of mineralocorticoid excess. *Primary aldosteronism,* found in approximately 0.1% of hypertensive patients, is generally the result of an adrenal adenoma (termed Conn's syndrome), but may also result from bilateral hyperplasia of the adrenal glands. Clinically, the disease may be asymptomatic, so diagnosis relies on detection of hypokalemia, and is confirmed by measurement of excessive aldosterone secretion and suppressed plasma renin levels. Therapy includes either surgical removal of the adenoma or medical management with aldosterone receptor antagonists (e.g., spironolactone). *Secondary aldosteronism* can result from increased angiotensin II (AII) production stimulated by the very rare renin-secreting tumor.

Much more commonly, angiotensin II levels may be elevated in women taking oral contraceptives (which stimulate hepatic production of angiotensinogen, as indicated above) or because of decreased AII degradation in chronic liver diseases.

Glucocorticoids, such as cortisol, also elevate blood pressure when present in excess amounts, likely via blood volume expansion and increased renin synthesis. Recent evidence indicates that cortisol also inhibits normal cholinergic vasodilation. Nearly 80% of patients with Cushing's syndrome, a disorder of glucocorticoid excess, have some degree of hypertension. These patients often present with classic "cushingoid" features: a characteristic rounded facial appearance, central obesity, proximal muscle weakness, and hirsutism. The primary lesion may be either a pituitary adrenocorticotropic hormone (ACTH)-secreting adenoma, a peripheral ACTH-secreting tumor (either of which causes adrenal cortical hyperplasia), or an adrenal cortisol-secreting adenoma. The diagnosis of Cushing's syndrome is evaluated by a 24-hour urine collection for the measurement of cortisol, or by a dexamethasone test, which evaluates whether it can suppress cortisol secretion.

Thyroid Hormone Abnormalities

Approximately one-third of *hyperthyroid* and one-fourth of *hypothyroid* patients have significant hypertension. Thyroid hormones exert their cardiovascular effects by 1) inducing sodium-potassium ATPases in the heart and vessels, 2) increasing blood volume, and 3) stimulating tissue metabolism and oxygen demand, with secondary accumulation of metabolites that modulate local vascular tone.

Hyperthyroid patients develop hypertension through cardiac hyperactivity and an increase in blood volume. Hypothyroid patients likely become hypertensive via a mechanism mediated through local control: as basal metabolic rate falls, so does the accumulation of local vasodilating metabolites, such that relative vasoconstriction develops.

CONSEQUENCES OF HYPERTENSION

Whatever the cause of blood pressure elevation, the ultimate consequences are similar. High blood pressure itself is generally asymptomatic but can result in devastating effects on many organs, especially the blood vessels, heart, kidney, and retina.

Clinical Signs and Symptoms

In the past, "classic" symptoms of hypertension were considered to include headache, epistaxis (nose bleeds), and dizziness. The usefulness of these symptoms has been called into question, however, by studies that indicate that they are found no more frequently among hypertensive patients than in the general population. Other symptoms, such as flushing, sweating, and blurred vision, do seem more common in the hypertensive population. In general, however, the majority of hypertensive patients are asymptomatic and are diagnosed simply by blood pressure measurement during routine physical examinations.

Several physical signs of hypertension discussed in the following section directly result from elevated pressure, including left ventricular hypertrophy and retinopathy. In addition, hypertension complicated by atherosclerosis can manifest by arterial bruits, particularly in the carotid and femoral arteries.

Organ Damage due to Hypertension

Target organ complications of hypertension reflect the degree of chronic blood pressure elevation. Such organ damage can be attributed to 1) the increased workload of

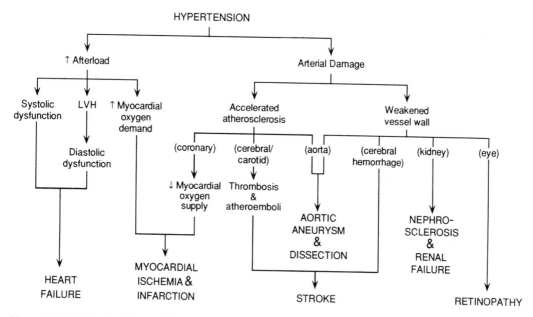

Figure 13.7. **Pathophysiology of the major consequences of hypertension.** LVH, left ventricular hypertrophy.

the heart, and 2) arterial damage due to the combined effects of the elevated pressure itself (weakened vessel walls) and accelerated atherosclerosis (Fig. 13.7). Abnormalities of the vasculature that result from elevated pressure include smooth muscle hypertrophy, endothelial cell dysfunction, and fatigue of elastic fibers. Chronic hypertensive trauma to the endothelium promotes atherosclerosis possibly by disrupting normal protective mechanisms such as the secretion of nitric oxide and by initiating smooth muscle cell hypertrophy. Arteries lined by atherosclerotic plaque may throm-

bose or may serve as a source of cholesterol emboli that occlude distal vessels, causing organ infarction (such as cerebrovascular occlusion, resulting in a stroke). In addition, atherosclerosis of large arteries hinders their elasticity, resulting in systolic pressure spikes that can further traumatize endothelium or provoke events such as aneurysm rupture.

The major target organs for the destructive complications of chronic hypertension are the heart, the cerebrovascular system, the aorta and peripheral vascular system, the kidney, and the retina (Table 13.3). Left

TABLE 13.3. Target Organ Damage in Hypertension

Organ System	Manifestations
Heart	• Left ventricular hypertrophy • Heart failure • Myocardial ischemia and infarction
Cerebrovascular	• Stroke
Aorta and peripheral vascular	• Aortic aneurysm and/or dissection • Arteriosclerosis
Kidney	• Nephrosclerosis • Renal failure
Retina	• Arterial narrowing • Hemorrhages, exudates, papilledema

untreated, approximately 50% of hypertensive patients die of coronary artery disease or congestive heart failure, about 33% from stroke, and 10–15% from renal failure.

Heart

The major cardiac effects of hypertension relate to the increased afterload against which the heart must contract and accelerated atherosclerosis within the coronary arteries.

Left Ventricular Hypertrophy and Diastolic Dysfunction

The high arterial pressure (heightened afterload) increases the wall tension of the left ventricle, which compensates through hypertrophy. *Concentric hypertrophy* (without dilatation) is the normal pattern of compensation, although conditions that elevate blood pressure by virtue of increased circulating volume (e.g., primary aldosteronism) may instead cause *eccentric* hypertrophy with chamber dilatation (see Chapter 9). Left ventricular hypertrophy (LVH) results in increased stiffness of the left ventricle with diastolic dysfunction, manifest by an elevation of LV filling pressure that can result in pulmonary congestion.

Physical findings of LVH may include a heaving LV impulse on chest palpation, indicative of the increased muscle mass. It is frequently accompanied by a fourth heart sound, as the left atrium contracts into the stiffened left ventricle (see Chapter 2).

LVH is one of the strongest predictors of cardiac morbidity in hypertensive patients. The degree of hypertrophy correlates with the development of congestive heart failure, angina, arrhythmias, myocardial infarction, and sudden cardiac death.

Systolic Dysfunction

Although LVH initially serves a compensatory role, later in the course of systemic hypertension, the increased LV mass may be insufficient to balance the high wall tension caused by the elevated pressure. As LV contractile capacity deteriorates, findings of systolic dysfunction become evident (reduced CO and pulmonary congestion). Systolic dysfunction is also provoked by the accelerated development of coronary artery disease with resultant periods of myocardial ischemia.

Coronary Artery Disease

Chronic hypertension is a major contributor to the development of myocardial ischemia and infarction. These complications reflect the combination of accelerated coronary atherosclerosis (decreased myocardial oxygen supply) and the high systolic workload (increased oxygen demand). Not only is acute myocardial infarction more common among hypertensives than among normotensives, but the former also have a higher incidence of post-myocardial infarction complications such as rupture of the ventricular wall, LV aneurysm formation, and congestive heart failure. In fact, 60% of patients who die of transmural myocardial infarctions have a history of hypertension.

Cerebrovascular System

Hypertension is the major modifiable risk factor for strokes (cerebrovascular accidents [CVAs]). Although diastolic pressure is important, it is the magnitude of the systolic pressure that has been most closely linked to CVAs. The presence of isolated systolic hypertension more than doubles an individual's chance of this complication.

Hypertension-induced strokes can be hemorrhagic or, more commonly, atherothrombotic. *Hemorrhagic* CVAs result from rupture of microaneurysms induced in cerebral parenchymal vessels by longstanding hypertension. *Atherothrombotic,* or thromboembolic, CVAs arise when portions of atherosclerotic plaque within the carotids or major cerebral arteries, or thrombi that form on those plaques, break off and embolize to smaller distal vessels. Additionally, intracerebral vessels may directly occlude by local atherosclerotic plaque rupture and thrombosis.

Occlusion of small penetrating arteries can result in multiple tiny infarcts. As these lesions soften and are absorbed by phago-cytic cells, small (≤3 mm diameter) cavities form, termed *lacunae*. Such lacunar infarc-tions are seen almost exclusively in patients with long-standing hypertension and are usually localized to the penetrating branches of the middle and posterior circulation of the brain.

The generalized arterial narrowing found in hypertensive patients reduces col-lateral flow to ischemic tissues and also im-poses structural requirements for higher perfusion pressure to maintain adequate tissue flow. This leaves the hypertensive pa-tient vulnerable to cerebral infarcts in areas supplied by the distal ends of arterial branches ("watershed" infarcts) if blood pressure should fall suddenly.

Effective treatment of hypertension di-minishes the risk of stroke and has con-tributed to a 50% reduction in deaths attrib-uted to cerebrovascular events over the past quarter century.

Aorta and Peripheral Vasculature

The accelerated atherosclerosis associ-ated with hypertension may result in plaque formation and narrowing throughout the arterial vasculature. In addition to the coro-nary arteries, lesions most commonly ap-pear within the aorta and the major arteries to the lower extremities, neck, and brain.

Chronic hypertension may lead to the development of aortic aneurysms, particu-larly of the abdominal aorta (see Chapter 15). An **abdominal aortic aneurysm** (AAA) is a dilatation of the aorta, usually located below the level of the renal arteries, caused by the mechanical stress of the high pres-sure on an arterial wall already weakened by medial damage and atherosclerosis. Aneurysms greater than 6 cm in diameter have a very high likelihood of rupture within 2 years if not surgically corrected.

Another life-threatening vascular conse-quence of high blood pressure is **aortic dis-section** (see Chapter 15). Elevated blood pressure, especially in the highest ranges, accelerates degenerative changes in the me-dia of the aorta. When the weakened wall is further exposed to high pressure, the intima

may tear, allowing blood to dissect into the aortic media and propagate in either direc-tion within the vessel wall, "clipping off" and obstructing major branch vessels along the way (e.g., coronary or carotid arteries). The mortality rate of aortic dissection is greater than 90% unless treated emergently, usually by surgical repair if the proximal aorta is involved. Rigorous control of hy-pertension is essential.

Kidney

Hypertension-induced kidney disease (nephrosclerosis) is a leading cause of renal failure that results from damage to the renal vasculature. Histologically, the vessel walls become thickened with a hyaline infiltrate, known as hyaline arteriolosclerosis (Fig. 13.8). Higher levels of hypertension can in-duce smooth muscle hypertrophy and even necrosis of capillary walls, termed fibrinoid necrosis. These changes result in reduced vascular supply and subsequent ischemic atrophy of tubules and, to a lesser extent, glomeruli. Because intact nephrons can usually compensate for those damaged by patchy ischemia, mild hypertension rarely leads to renal insufficiency in the absence of other insults to the kidney. However, ma-lignant levels of hypertension can inflict permanent damage to the point that dialy-sis becomes necessary.

One of the consequences of hypertensive renal failure is perpetuation of elevated blood pressure. For example, progressive renal failure compromises the ability of the kidney to regulate blood volume, which further contributes to chronic hypertension.

Retina

The retina is the only location where sys-temic arteries can be directly visualized by physical examination. High blood pressure induces abnormalities that are collectively termed **hypertensive retinopathy.** Al-though vision may be compromised when the damage is extensive, more commonly the changes serve as an asymptomatic clin-ical marker for the severity of hypertension and its duration.

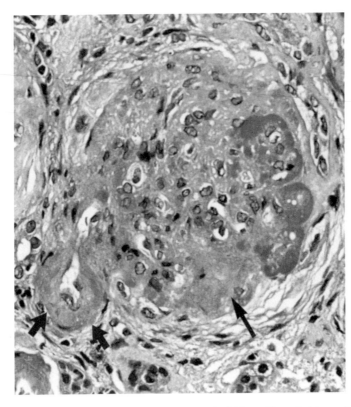

Figure 13.8. **Histologic effects of chronic hypertension on the kidney.** The arteriolar walls are thickened by hyaline infiltrate (short arrows). The glomeruli (long arrow) appear partially sclerosed because of reduced vascular supply. (Courtesy of Dr. Helmut G. Rennke, Brigham and Women's Hospital, Boston, MA.)

Severe hypertension that is *acute in onset* (e.g., uncontrolled and/or malignant hypertension) may burst small retinal vessels, causing *hemorrhages, exudation of plasma lipids,* and areas of *local infarction.* If ischemia of the optic nerve develops, patients may describe generalized blurred vision. Retinal ischemia caused by hemorrhage leads to more patchy loss of vision. **Papilledema,** or swelling of the optic disc with blurring of its margins, may arise from high intracranial pressure when the blood pressure reaches malignant levels and cerebrovascular autoregulation begins to fail.

Chronically elevated blood pressure results in a different set of retinal findings. Papilledema is absent, but vasoconstriction results in arterial narrowing, and medial hypertrophy thickens the vessel wall, which "nicks" (indents) crossing veins. With more severe chronic hypertension, arterial sclerosis is evident as an increased reflection of light through the ophthalmoscope (termed "copper" or "silver" wiring). Although these changes are not in themselves of major functional import, they indicate that the patient has had long-standing, poorly controlled hypertension.

HYPERTENSIVE CRISES

Hypertensive crises are medical emergencies characterized by a severe elevation of blood pressure. In the past, such elevations were usually a consequence of inadequate blood pressure treatment. Now, hypertensive crises are more often due to acute hemodynamic insults (e.g., acute renal disease) superimposed on a chronic hypertensive state. As a result of rapid pathologic changes (fibrinoid necrosis) within the blood vessels and kidney, a spiraling increase in blood pressure evolves. Further volume expansion and vasoconstriction occur as renal perfusion drops and serum renin and angiotensin levels rise.

Severe BP elevation results in increased intracranial pressure, and patients may present with *hypertensive encephalopathy* manifested by headache, blurred vision, confusion, somnolence, and sometimes coma. When hypertension results in acute damage to retinal vessels, *accelerated-malignant hypertension* is said to be present. Funduscopic examination shows the effects of the rapid pressure rise as hemorrhages, exudates, and sometimes papilledema. The increased load on the left ventricle during hypertensive crises may precipitate angina (because of increased myocardial oxygen demand) or pulmonary edema.

Hypertensive crises require rapid therapy to reduce blood pressure to prevent permanent vascular complications. Correction of blood pressure is generally followed by reversal of the acute pathologic changes, including papilledema and retinal exudation, although renal damage often persists.

TREATMENT OF HYPERTENSION

The therapeutic approach to the hypertensive patient should be tempered by two considerations. First, a single elevated blood pressure measurement does not establish the diagnosis of hypertension, because blood pressure varies considerably from day to day. Moreover, blood pressure measurement in the hospital or doctor's office may be affected by the "white coat" effect resulting from patient anxiety. The average of multiple readings taken at two or three separate office visits and/or in the home environment provides a more reliable basis for labeling a patient as hypertensive.

Second, although mild hypertension is a major public health problem because so many people suffer from it, for the individual with stage 1 hypertension, the risks are small. For example, the additional risk of a stroke is approximately 1 in 850 per year. Hence, observation for a few months to see whether the low-level hypertension is persistent, or whether lifestyle changes can reduce the pressure, is a recommended alternative to immediate drug therapy. This is especially true in the absence of other cardiovascular risk fac-

tors such as smoking or high serum cholesterol.

In the majority of hypertensive patients, drug therapy is ultimately the most effective way to prevent future complications, but that should not deter consideration of other beneficial lifestyle changes.

Nonpharmacologic Treatment

Weight Reduction

Studies have consistently found obesity and hypertension to be highly correlated with each other, as described above, especially when the obesity is of a central (abdominal) distribution. Blood pressure reduction follows weight loss in a large portion of hypertensives who are more than 10% over their ideal weights.

Exercise

Sedentary normotensive people have a 20–50% higher risk of developing hypertension than their more active peers. Regular aerobic exercise, such as walking, jogging or bicycling, has been shown to contribute to blood pressure reduction over and above any resulting weight loss. A hypertensive patient who becomes physically conditioned manifests a lower resting heart rate and reduced levels of circulating catecholamines than before training, suggesting a fall in sympathetic tone.

Diet

In addition to caloric restriction for weight loss, changes in the composition of a patient's diet may be important for blood pressure reduction. For example, a diet high in fruits, vegetables, and low-fat dairy products has been shown to reduce blood pressure.

Sodium

Salt restriction for people with high blood pressure is a controversial issue, but there are several epidemiologic and clinical trials that support the benefit of moderating sodium intake. In normotensive individuals, excess salt ingestion is simply excreted by the kidneys, but approximately 50% of essential hypertensives are found to have blood pressures that vary with sodium intake, suggesting a defect in natriuresis. Sensitivity to sodium levels is more common in black and elderly hypertensive patients. Because low-salt diets tend to increase the effectiveness of antihypertensive medications in general, the current recommendation is to limit salt intake to <6 g sodium chloride (<2.3 g sodium) per day , which is one-third less than the average U.S. consumption.

Potassium

Total body potassium content tends to be decreased by a diet low in fruits and vegetables or in individuals who take potassium-wasting diuretics. Potassium deficiency has several theoretical effects that may raise blood pressure, and dietary supplements to replete low potassium levels are routinely recommended. Thus far, however, there is no solid evidence that adding potassium supplements to the diet of a normokalemic hypertensive will lower blood pressure.

Alcohol

The chronic intake of alcoholic beverages correlates with high blood pressure and resistance to antihypertensive medications. Moreover, experimental evidence shows that blood pressure (especially systolic) may rise acutely following alcohol consumption. The reason for this link remains incompletely understood, but decreases in chronic alcohol intake have been shown to lower blood pressure.

Other

Low calcium intake and magnesium depletion have been associated with elevated blood pressure, but the responsible mechanisms and the implications for therapy are unclear. Caffeine ingestion transiently increases blood pressure (as much as 5–15 mm Hg after two cups of coffee), but routine use does not seem to produce chronic pressure elevation.

Smoking

Cigarette smoking transiently increases blood pressure, probably via a nicotine effect on autonomic ganglia, and is a risk factor for the development of sustained hypertension. In addition, the atherogenic effect of smoking may contribute to the development of RH. Cigarette usage is associated with many other health hazards, and all patients should be discouraged from smoking.

Relaxation Therapy

Blood pressure frequently rises under conditions of stress. In addition, essential hypertensive patients and their relatives often show higher than normal basal sympathetic tone and exaggerated autonomic responses to mental stress. Hence, relaxation techniques have been advocated as a method to control hypertension. Available methods include biofeedback and meditation. The effectiveness of such therapy has not been consistently demonstrated in clinical trials and seems to depend on the patient's attitude and long-term compliance.

In summary, nonpharmacologic therapy offers a wide range of options that do not have the expense and potential side effects of prescribed drug use. The effectiveness of these therapies should come as no surprise, given the extent to which environmental factors play a role in hypertension. Therefore, such behavior-based interventions are recommended as first-line therapy in individuals whose hypertension is not an immediate danger to life and well-being.

Pharmacologic Treatment

Antihypertensive medications are the standard means to lower chronically elevated blood pressure and are indicated if nonpharmacologic treatment proves inadequate. More than 100 drug preparations are available to treat hypertension, but fortunately the most commonly used medications fall into four classes: diuretics, sympatholytics, vasodilators, and drugs that interfere with the renin-angiotensin system (Table 13.4). The individual actions of these groups on the physiologic abnormalities in hypertension are shown in Figure 13.9. The pharmacology and use of the antihypertensive drugs are described in greater detail in Chapter 17.

Diuretics have been used for many years as a treatment of hypertension. They reduce circulatory volume, CO, and mean arterial pressure and are most effective in patients with mild to moderate hypertension who have normal renal function. They are especially effective in black and in elderly individuals, who tend to be salt-sensitive. In clinical trials, diuretics have reduced the

TABLE 13.4. Classes of Antihypertensive Medications

Drug Class	Types (see Chapter 17)
Diuretics	Thiazides Aldosterone-antagonists
Sympatholytics	β-blockers Combined α-β-blockers Central α_2-agonists Peripheral α_1-blockers
Vasodilators	Calcium channel blockers Direct vasodilators (e.g., hydralazine, minoxidil)
Renin-angiotensin system antagonists	Converting-enzyme inhibitors Angiotensin II receptor blockers

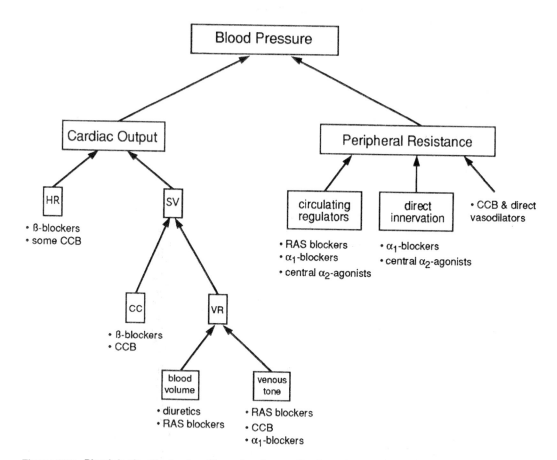

Figure 13.9. Physiologic effects of antihypertensive medications. Note that some antihypertensive medications work at multiple sites. HR, heart rate; SV, stroke volume; CC, cardiac contractility; VR, venous return; RAS blockers, renin-angiotensin system blockers (i.e., angiotensin-converting enzyme inhibitors and angiotensin II receptor blockers); CCB, Ca^{++} channel blockers.

risk of strokes and cardiovascular events in hypertensives and are inexpensive compared with other agents. Thiazide diuretics (e.g., hydrochlorothiazide) and potassium-sparing diuretics (e.g., spironolactone) promote Na^+ and Cl^- excretion in the nephron. Loop diuretics (e.g., furosemide) are generally too potent and their actions too short-lived for use as antihypertensive agents. However, they *are* useful in lowering blood pressure in patients with renal insufficiency, who often do not respond to other diuretics.

Diuretics may result in adverse metabolic side effects, including elevation of serum glucose, cholesterol, and triglyceride levels. In addition, hypokalemia, hyperuricemia, and decreased sexual function are common side effects. However, when diuretics are prescribed in low dosages, it is often possible to accrue the desired antihypertensive effect while minimizing adverse complications.

Sympatholytic agents include 1) β-blockers, 2) central α-adrenergic *agonists*, and 3) systemic α-adrenergic blocking drugs. **β-blockers,** such as propranolol, are believed to lower blood pressure by 1) reducing CO through a decrease in heart rate and mild decrease in contractility, and 2) decreasing the secretion of renin (and therefore levels of angiotensin II), causing a decrease in TPR. β-blockers are less effective than diuretics in hypertensives who are elderly or African American. Adverse effects of β-blockers include bronchospasm (because of bronchiolar β_2 receptor blockade), fatigue, impotence, and hyperglycemia. They may also adversely alter lipid metabolism. Most β-blockers cause an increase in serum triglyceride levels and a decrease in "good" HDL cholesterol levels. However, β-blockers with intrinsic sympathomimetic activity (see Chapter 17) or those with combined α-blocking properties (such as labetalol) do not adversely affect HDL levels.

Centrally acting α_2 adrenergic agonists, such as methyldopa and clonidine, reduce sympathetic outflow to the heart, blood vessels, and kidneys. These are rarely used today, owing to their high frequency of side effects (e.g., dry mouth, sedation). **Systemic α_1**

antagonists, such as prazosin, terazosin, and doxazosin, cause a decrease in TPR through relaxation of vascular smooth muscle. They may be beneficial for hypertension in some older men, as they also improve symptoms of prostatic enlargement. However, they are otherwise not often recommended, because a recent hypertension study showed that an α-blocker was associated with a greater number of adverse cardiovascular events compared with a diuretic.

Peripheral **vasodilators** include Ca^{++} channel blockers, hydralazine, and minoxidil. Ca^{++} **channel blockers** reduce the influx of calcium responsible for cardiac and vascular smooth muscle contraction, thus reducing cardiac contractility and TPR (see Chapter 17). Long-acting (i.e., sustained-release drugs taken once a day) Ca^{++} channel blockers are frequently used to treat hypertension. The shorter acting Ca^{++} channel blocker preparations are no longer used for this purpose. They are less convenient and have been associated with adverse cardiovascular outcomes (see Chapter 6). **Hydralazine** and **minoxidil** lower blood pressure by directly relaxing vascular smooth muscle of precapillary resistance vessels. However, this action can result in a reflex increase in heart rate, so that combined β-blocker therapy is frequently recommended. The use of these direct vasodilators in treating hypertension has waned with the advent of newer agents with fewer side effects.

Drugs that interfere with the renin-angiotensin system include ACE inhibitors and angiotensin II receptor blockers. **ACE inhibitors** decrease blood pressure by blocking the conversion of angiotensin I to angiotensin II (see Fig. 17.6, p. 380), thereby reducing the vasopressor activity of AII and also the secretion of aldosterone. Thus, there is a reduction in TPR and sodium retention by the kidney. An additional antihypertensive effect of ACE inhibitors is to increase the concentration of the circulating vasodilator bradykinin (see Fig. 17.6). ACE inhibitors are important drugs that have been shown to reduce mortality rates in patients following an acute myocardial infarction, in individuals with chronic symptomatic systolic heart failure (see Chapter 9), and even in people at high risk of developing cardiovascular disease. They also slow the deterioration of renal function in patients with diabetic nephropathy. The most common side effect of ACE inhibitors is the development of a reversible dry cough (likely related to the increased bradykinin effect); hyperkalemia and azotemia may also occur, as described in Chapter 17.

Angiotensin II receptor blockers (ARBs) are the newest class of antihypertensive agents. The action of this group is to block the binding of angiotensin II to its receptors (i.e., subtype AT_1 receptors) in blood vessels and other targets (see Fig. 17.6). By inhibiting the effects of angiotensin II (and thereby causing vasodilatation and reduced secretion of aldosterone), blood pressure falls. In clinical trials, the antihypertensive efficacy of this group is similar to that of ACE inhibitors. However, they are very well tolerated, and unlike with the use of ACE inhibitors, cough is not a common side effect. In a recent study of patients with hypertension and LVH, an ARB was superior to a β-blocker in preventing cardiovascular complications, especially strokes.

Given the large number of antihypertensive drugs available, the choice of which drug to use as initial therapy in an individual patient can seem daunting. The first-line drugs for uncomplicated hypertension recommended by the Joint National Committee on Detection, Evaluation, and Treatment of High Blood Pressure are diuretics and β-blockers because of their proven long-term benefits at reducing morbidity and mortality as well as their low cost. In certain circumstances, or if initial therapy with one drug is not sufficient, ACE inhibitors, angiotensin receptor blockers, Ca^{++} channel antagonists, or α_1-receptor blockers are added or substituted. For example, an ACE inhibitor should be given prime consideration in patients with concurrent heart failure, diabetes, or LV dysfunction following myocardial infarction.

There are some other guiding principles. First, the chosen drug regimen should conform to the patient's specific needs. For example, an anxious young patient in the throes of the "hyperkinetic" phase of EH might be best treated with a β-blocker, whereas a more effective choice for the same patient many years later, after the pressure becomes more dependent on peripheral vascular resistance, could be a vasodilator (e.g., long-acting Ca^{++} channel blocker). Because therapy is likely to continue for many years, consideration of adverse effects and impact of drug therapy on the patient's quality of life are very important.

Another helpful principle of antihypertensive drug therapy concerns the use of multiple agents. The effects of one drug, acting at one physiologic control point, can be defeated by natural compensatory mechanisms. For example, the drop in renal perfusion by a direct vasodilator can activate the renin-angiotensin system, prompting the kidney to retain more volume, thereby blunting the antihypertensive benefit. Combination drug therapy is aimed at preventing such an action by utilizing agents acting at different complementary sites. In this example, a direct vasodilator is often paired with a low-dose diuretic to avoid the undesired volume expansion effect.

In conclusion, hypertension emerges as a fascinating clinical problem, important because of its prevalence and devastating consequences, and interesting because of its usually obscure cause(s). The workup and treatment of a patient with hypertension require methodical consideration of the ways in which normal cardiovascular physiology can go astray. Because most patients still fall unsatisfyingly into the idiopathic category of EH, there is still much room for creative thought and research in this area.

SUMMARY

1. Hypertension is defined as a chronic diastolic blood pressure $\geq$ 90 mm Hg or systolic blood pressure $\geq$ 140 mm Hg.
2. Hypertension is of unknown cause in 95% of patients (EH). Secondary hypertension may arise from many causes, including 1) renal parenchymal disease, 2) renovascular hypertension, 3) pheochromocytoma, 4) coarctation of the aorta, and 5) primary aldosteronism.

3. Most hypertensive patients remain asymptomatic until complications arise. Complications include 1) stroke, 2) myocardial infarction, 3) heart failure, 4) aortic aneurysms and dissection, 5) renal damage, and 6) retinopathy.

4. Treatment of hypertension includes lifestyle and dietary changes, followed by pharmacologic therapy. Commonly used antihypertensive drugs include diuretics, β-blockers, ACE inhibitors, angiotensin receptor blockers, long-acting Ca^{++} channel antagonists, and α_1-receptor blockers.

Acknowledgment   Contributors to the previous editions of this chapter were Rajesh S. Magrulkar, MD; Peter A. Nigrovic, MD; Rahul Deshmukh, MD; Allison McDonough, MD; Thomas J. Moore, MD; and Leonard S. Lilly, MD.

ADDITIONAL READING

Alderman M. Dietary sodium and blood pressure. N Engl J Med 2001;344:1716–1719.

Benetos A, Thomas F, Bean K, et al. Prognostic value of systolic and diastolic blood pressure in treated hypertensive men. 2002;162:577–581.

Dahlöf B, Devereux RB, Kjeldsen SE, et al. Cardiovascular morbidity and mortality in the Losartan Intervention For Endpoint reduction in hypertension study (LIFE): a randomised trial against atenolol. Lancet 2002;359:995–1003.

Furberg CD, Psaty BM, Pahor M, et al. Clinical implications of recent findings from the Antihypertensive and Lipid-Lowering Treatment to Prevent Heart Attack Trial (ALLHAT) and other studies of hypertension. Ann Intern Med 2001;135:1074–1078.

Goodfriend TL, Elliott ME, Catt KJ. Angiotensin receptors and their antagonists. N Engl J Med 1996; 334:1649–1654.

Hollenberg NK. Hypertension: mechanisms and therapy. In: Braunwald E, ed. Atlas of Heart Diseases. St. Louis: CV Mosby, 1995.

Johnson RJ, Herrera-Acosta J, Schreiner GF, et al. Subtle acquired renal injury as a mechanism of salt-sensitive hypertension. N Engl J Med 2002;346: 913–923.

Kannel WB. Blood pressure as a cardiovascular risk factor. JAMA 1996;275:1571–1576.

Sixth report of the Joint National Committee on Prevention, Detection, Evaluation, and Treatment of High Blood Pressure. Arch Intern Med 1997;157: 2413–2446.

Stevens VJ, Obarzanek E, Cook NR, et al. Long-term weight loss and changes in blood pressure: results of the Trials of Hypertension Prevention, phase II. Ann Intern Med 2001;134:1–11.

Vollmer WM, Sacks FM, Ard J, et al. Effects of diet and sodium intake on blood pressure: subgroup analysis of the DASH-Sodium Trial. Ann Intern Med 2001;135:1019–1028.

Weber MA, ed. Hypertension Medicine. Totowa, NJ: Humana Press, 2001.

Williams GH. Hypertensive vascular disease. In: Braunwald E, Fauci AS, Kasper DL, et al., eds. Harrison's Principles of Internal Medicine. 15th Ed. New York: McGraw-Hill, 2001:1414–1430.

Diseases of the Pericardium

Leonard S. Lilly

Anatomy and Function
Acute Pericarditis
  Etiology
  Pathogenesis
  Pathology
  Clinical Features
  Diagnostic Approach
  Treatment
Pericardial Effusion
  Etiology
  Pathophysiology
  Clinical Features
  Diagnostic Studies
  Treatment

Cardiac Tamponade
  Etiology
  Pathophysiology
  Clinical Features
  Diagnostic Approach
  Treatment
Constrictive Pericarditis
  Etiology and Pathogenesis
  Pathology
  Pathophysiology
  Clinical Features
  Diagnostic Approach
  Treatment

Diseases of the pericardium form a spectrum that ranges from benign, self-limited pericarditis to life-threatening cardiac tamponade. The clinical manifestations of these disorders and the approaches to their management can be predicted from an understanding of pericardial anatomy and pathophysiology, as presented in this chapter.

ANATOMY AND FUNCTION

The pericardium is a two-layered sac that encircles the heart. The inner serosal layer (*visceral pericardium*) adheres to the outer wall of the heart and is reflected back on itself, at the level of the great vessels, to line the tough fibrous outer layer (*parietal pericardium*). A thin film of pericardial fluid slightly separates the two layers and decreases the friction between them.

The pericardium appears to serve three functions: 1) it fixes the heart within the mediastinum and limits its motion, 2) it prevents extreme dilatation of the heart during sudden rises of intracardiac volume, and 3) it may function as a barrier to limit the spread of infection from the adjacent lungs. However, patients with complete absence of the pericardium (either congenitally or after surgical removal) are generally asymptomatic, casting doubt on its actual importance in normal physiology. Yet like the unnecessary appendix, the pericardium can become diseased and cause great harm.

In the healthy heart, intrapericardial pressure varies during the respiratory cycle from −5 mm Hg (during inspiration) to +5 mm Hg (during expiration) and nearly equals the pressure within the pleural space. However, pathologic changes in pericardial stiffness, or the accumulation of fluid within the pericardial sac, may profoundly increase this pressure.

ACUTE PERICARDITIS

The most common affliction of the pericardium is acute pericarditis, which refers to inflammation of its layers. Many disease states and etiologic agents can produce this syndrome (Table 14.1), the most common of which are described here.

TABLE 14.1. Most Common Causes of Acute Pericarditis

Infectious
  Viral
  Tuberculosis
  Pyogenic bacteria

Noninfectious
  Postmyocardial infarction
  Uremia
  Neoplastic disease
  Radiation-induced
  Connective tissue diseases
  Drug-induced

Etiology

Infectious

Idiopathic and Viral Pericarditis

Acute pericarditis is most often of idiopathic origin, meaning that the actual cause is unknown. However, serologic studies have demonstrated that many such episodes are actually caused by viral infection, especially by echovirus or Coxsackie virus group B. Although a viral origin could be confirmed in infected patients by comparing antiviral titers of acute and convalescent serum, this is rarely done in the clinical setting because the patient has usually recovered by the time those results would be available. Thus, idiopathic and viral pericarditis are considered similar clinical entities, and the terms are used interchangeably.

Other viruses known to cause pericarditis include those responsible for influenza, varicella, mumps, hepatitis B, and infectious mononucleosis. Pericarditis has been found with increased frequency among patients with acquired immune deficiency syndrome (AIDS), possibly related to human immunodeficiency virus (HIV) itself, but often due to superimposed tuberculous or other bacterial infections in this immunocompromised population.

Tuberculous Pericarditis

Although tuberculosis remains a worldwide problem, its incidence in the United States is low. It is, however, an important cause of pericarditis in immunosuppressed individuals, such as those with AIDS. Tuberculous pericarditis arises from reactivation of the organism in mediastinal lymph nodes, with spread into the pericardium. It can also extend directly from a site of tuberculosis within the lungs, or the organism can arrive at the pericardium by hematogenous dissemination.

Nontuberculous Bacterial Pericarditis (Purulent Pericarditis)

Bacterial pericarditis has become rare since the advent of antibiotics. Pneumococcus and staphylococci are responsible most frequently, whereas gram-negative infection occurs less often. Common mechanisms by which bacterial invasion of the pericardium develops include 1) perforating trauma to the chest (e.g., stab wound), 2) contamination during chest surgery, 3) extension of an intracardiac infection (i.e., infective endocarditis), 4) extension of pneumonia or a subdiaphragmatic infection, and 5) hematogenous spread from a remote infection. Bacterial pericarditis is a fulminant illness but is rare in otherwise healthy individuals; it is most likely to occur in immunocompromised persons, including those with severe burns and malignancies.

Noninfectious

Pericarditis Following Myocardial Infarction

There are two forms of pericarditis associated with acute myocardial infarction (MI). The early form occurs within the first few days after an MI. It likely results from inflammation extending from the epicardial surface of the injured myocardium to the adjacent pericardium; therefore, it is most common in patients with transmural (as opposed to subendocardial) infarctions. The prognosis following acute MI is not affected by the presence of pericarditis; its major importance is in distinguishing it from the pain of recurrent myocardial ischemia. This form of pericarditis occurs in fewer than 5% of patients with acute MI who are treated acutely with thrombolytic agents, but it is more common in those who do not receive reperfusion therapy and who therefore sustain larger infarctions.

The second form of post-MI pericarditis is known as *Dressler's syndrome,* which develops 2 weeks to several months following an acute infarction. Its cause is unknown, but it is thought to be of autoimmune origin, possibly directed against antigens released from necrotic myocardial cells. A clinically similar form of pericarditis may occur weeks to months following heart surgery (termed *postpericardiotomy pericarditis*).

Uremic Pericarditis

Pericarditis is a serious complication of chronic renal failure, but its pathogenesis is unknown. Studies have shown no correlation between the plasma level of nitrogen waste products and the incidence of pericarditis, and it may even develop in patients during the first few months of dialysis therapy.

Neoplastic Pericarditis

Tumor within the pericardium most commonly results from metastatic spread or local invasion by cancer of the lung, breast, or lymphoma. Primary tumors of the pericardium are rare. Neoplastic effusions are usually large and hemorrhagic and frequently lead to cardiac tamponade, a severe complication described below.

Radiation-Induced Pericarditis

Pericarditis may complicate previous radiation therapy to the thorax (e.g., administered for the treatment of certain tumors), especially if the cumulative dose has exceeded 4000 rads (40 Gy). Radiation-induced damage causes a local inflammatory response that can result in pericardial effusions and fibrosis. Cytologic examination of the pericardial fluid helps to distinguish radiation-induced pericardial damage from that of tumor invasion.

Pericarditis Associated with Connective Tissue Diseases

Pericardial involvement is common in many connective tissue diseases, including systemic lupus erythematosus (SLE), rheumatoid arthritis, and progressive systemic sclerosis. For example, 20–40% of patients with SLE experience clinically detectable pericarditis during the course of their disease. Customary treatment of the underlying connective tissue disease usually ameliorates the pericarditis as well.

Drug-Induced Pericarditis

Many pharmaceutical agents can result in pericarditis, often by inducing a systemic lupus-like syndrome (Table 14.2). Drugs that most commonly induce this syndrome include the antiarrhythmic *procainamide* and the vasodilator *hydralazine.* Drug-induced pericarditis usually abates when the causative drug is discontinued.

Pathogenesis

Similar to other inflammatory processes, pericarditis is characterized by three stages: 1) local *vasodilation* with transudation of protein-poor, cell-free fluid into the pericardial space; 2) *increased vascular permeability,* with leak of protein into the pericardial space; and 3) *leukocyte exudation,* initially by neutrophils, followed later by mononuclear cells.

TABLE 14.2. Examples of Drug-Induced Pericarditis

Due to drug-induced lupus syndrome
　Procainamide
　Hydralazine
　Methyldopa
　Isoniazid
　Phenytoin

Not related to drug-induced lupus
　Anthracycline antineoplastic agents (doxorubicin, daunorubicin)
　Minoxidil

The leukocytes are of critical importance because they help contain or eliminate the offending infectious or autoimmune agent. However, metabolic products released by these cells may prolong inflammation, cause pain and local cellular damage, and mediate somatic symptoms such as fever. Therefore, the immune response to pericardial injury may significantly contribute to tissue damage and symptomatology.

Pathology

The pathologic appearance of the pericardium depends on the underlying cause and severity of inflammation. **Serous pericarditis** is characterized by scant polymorphonuclear leukocytes, lymphocytes, and histiocytes. The exudate is a thin fluid secreted by the mesothelial cells lining the serosal surface of the pericardium. This likely represents the early inflammatory response common to all types of acute pericarditis.

Serofibrinous pericarditis is the most commonly observed morphologic pattern in patients with pericarditis. The pericardial exudate contains plasma proteins, including fibrinogen, yielding a grossly rough and shaggy appearance (termed "bread and butter" pericarditis). Portions of the visceral and parietal pericardium may become thickened and fused. Occasionally, this process leads to a dense scar that restricts movement and diastolic filling of the cardiac chambers, as described below.

Suppurative (or purulent) pericarditis is an intense inflammatory response associated most commonly with bacterial infection. The serosal surfaces are erythematous and coated with purulent exudate.

Hemorrhagic pericarditis refers to a grossly bloody form of pericardial inflammation and is most often due to tuberculosis or malignancy.

Clinical Features

History

The most frequent symptoms of acute pericarditis are *chest pain* and *fever* (Table 14.3). The pain may be severe and most often localizes to the retrosternal area and left

TABLE 14.3. Clinical Features of Acute Pericarditis

Pleuritic chest pain
Fever
Pericardial friction rub
ECG abnormalities

precordium; it may also radiate to the back and ridge of the left trapezius muscle. What differentiates it from myocardial ischemia or infarction is that the pain of pericarditis is typically sharp and *pleuritic* (it is aggravated by inspiration and coughing) and *positional* (e.g., sitting and leaning forward often lessen the discomfort). *Dyspnea* is common during acute pericarditis, but is not exertional and probably results from a reluctance of the patient to breathe deeply because of pleuritic pain.

Patients with idiopathic or viral pericarditis are typically young and previously healthy. Pericarditis of other causes should be suspected in individuals with the underlying diseases in Table 14.1 who develop the typical sharp, pleuritic chest pains and fever.

Physical Examination

A scratchy pericardial *friction rub* is common in acute pericarditis and is produced by the movement of the inflamed pericardial layers against one another. Auscultation of the rub is best heard using the diaphragm of the stethoscope with the patient leaning forward while exhaling (which brings the pericardium closer to the chest wall and stethoscope). In its full form, the rub consists of three components, corresponding to the phases of greatest cardiac movement: ventricular contraction, ventricular relaxation, and atrial contraction. Characteristically, the pericardial rub is evanescent, so that it may come and go from one examination to the next.

Diagnostic Approach

The presence of pleuritic, positional chest pain and the characteristic pericardial friction rub implicate the presence of acute pericarditis. However, certain laboratory studies are helpful to confirm the diagnosis and to assess any impending complications.

The *electrocardiogram (ECG)* is abnormal in 90% of patients with acute pericarditis and helps to distinguish it from other forms of cardiac disease, such as an acute MI. The most important ECG pattern, which reflects inflammation of the adjacent myocardium, consists of *diffuse ST segment elevation* in most of the ECG leads, usually with the exception of aV$_R$ and V$_1$ (Fig. 14.1). In addition, *PR segment depression* is often evident, reflecting abnormal atrial repolarization related to atrial epicardial inflammation. These abnormalities are in contrast to the ECG of acute MI, in which the ST segments are elevated only in the leads overlying the region of infarction, and PR depression is not expected.

Further testing in acute pericarditis often includes *echocardiography* to evaluate for the presence and hemodynamic significance of a pericardial effusion. Additional studies that may be useful in individual cases to define the cause of pericarditis include: 1) purified protein derivative (PPD) skin test for tuberculosis, 2) serologic tests (Antinu-

clear antibodies and rheumatoid factor) to screen for connective tissue diseases, and 3) a careful search for malignancy, especially of the lung and breast (physical examination supplemented by chest radiograph and mammogram). The yield of diagnostic pericardiocentesis (removal of pericardial fluid through a needle) in uncomplicated acute pericarditis is low and should be reserved for patients with very large effusions or evidence of cardiac chamber compression, as discussed below.

Treatment

Idiopathic or viral pericarditis is a self-limited disease that usually runs its course in 1–3 weeks. Management consists of *rest*, to reduce the interaction of the inflamed pericardial layers, and *pain relief* by analgesic and anti-inflammatory drugs (aspirin and other nonsteroidal anti-inflammatory agents). Oral corticosteroids are often effective for severe or recurrent pericardial pain but should *not* be used in uncomplicated cases, because of potentially severe side effects and because even gradual withdrawal of this form of therapy often leads to recurrent symptoms of pericarditis.

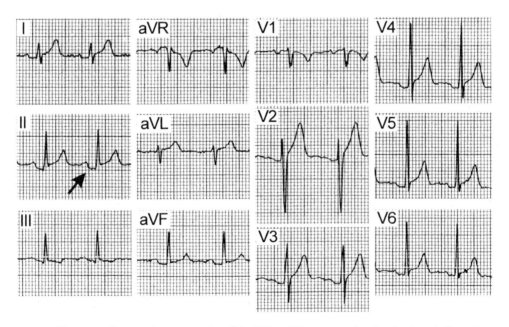

Figure 14.1. **Electrocardiogram in acute pericarditis.** Diffuse ST segment elevation is present. Also note depression of the PR segment (arrow).

The forms of pericarditis that follow MI are treated in a similar fashion, with rest and aspirin. Other nonsteroidal anti-inflammatory agents are often avoided in this form of pericarditis because of experimental evidence linking them to delayed healing of the infarction.

Purulent pericarditis requires more aggressive treatment, including catheter drainage of the pericardium and intensive antibiotic therapy. Nevertheless, even with such therapy, the mortality rate is very high. Tuberculous pericarditis requires prolonged multidrug antituberculous therapy. Pericarditis in the setting of uremia often resolves following intensive dialysis. Neoplastic pericardial disease usually indicates widely metastatic cancer, and therapy is unfortunately only palliative, often using radiation or chemotherapy.

PERICARDIAL EFFUSION

Etiology

The normal pericardial space contains 15–50 ml of pericardial fluid, a plasma ultrafiltrate secreted by the mesothelial cells that line the serosal layer. However, a larger volume of fluid may accumulate in association with any of the forms of acute pericarditis discussed above.

In addition, noninflammatory serous effusions may result from conditions of 1) increased capillary permeability (e.g., severe hypothyroidism), 2) increased capillary hydrostatic pressure (e.g., congestive heart failure), or 3) decreased plasma oncotic pressure (e.g., cirrhosis or the nephrotic syndrome). Chylous effusions may occur in the presence of lymphatic obstruction of pericardial drainage, due most commonly to neoplasms and tuberculosis.

Pathophysiology

Because the pericardium is a relatively stiff structure, the relationship between its internal volume and pressure is not linear (Fig. 14.2, curve A). Note that the initial portion of this curve is nearly flat, indicating that at the low volumes normally present within the pericardium, a small increase in volume leads to only a small rise in pressure. However, when the intrapericardial volume expands beyond a critical level (arrow in Fig. 14.2), a dramatic increase in pressure is incited by the nondistensible sac. At that point, even a minor increase in volume can translate into an enormous compressive force on the heart.

Three factors determine whether a pericardial effusion remains clinically silent or whether symptoms of cardiac compression

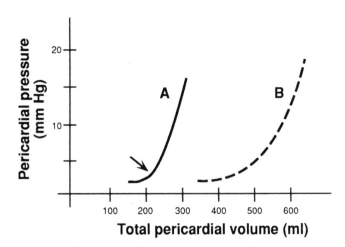

Figure 14.2. Schematic representation of the volume-pressure relationship of the normal pericardium. A. At the very lowest levels, a small rise in volume results in a small rise in pressure. However, when the limits of pericardial stretch are reached (arrow), the curve becomes very steep, and a further small rise in intrapericardial volume results in significantly increased pressure. **B.** Chronic slow accumulation of volume allows the pericardium to gradually stretch over time, so that the curve shifts to the right and much larger volumes are accommodated at lower pressures. (Modified from Freeman GL, LeWinter MM. Pericardial adaptations during chronic dilation in dogs. Circ Res 1984;54:294.)

ensue: 1) the *volume* of fluid, 2) the *rate* at which the fluid accumulates, and 3) the *compliance* characteristics of the pericardium.

A *sudden* increase of pericardial volume, as may occur in chest trauma with intrapericardial hemorrhage, results in significant elevation of pericardial pressure (Fig. 14.2, steep portion of curve A) and the potential for severe cardiac chamber compression. Even lesser amounts of fluid may cause significant elevation of pressure if the pericardium is pathologically noncompliant and stiff, as may occur in the presence of tumor or fibrosis of the sac. In contrast, if the pericardial effusion accumulates *slowly*, over weeks to months, the pericardium gradually stretches, such that the volume-pressure relationship curve shifts toward the right (see Fig. 14.2, curve B). With this adaptation, the pericardium can accommodate larger volumes (e.g., 1–2 *liters*) without marked elevation of intrapericardial pressure.

Clinical Features

There is a spectrum of possible symptoms associated with pericardial effusions. For example, the patient with a large effusion may be asymptomatic, may complain of a dull constant ache in the left side of the chest, or may present with symptoms of cardiac tamponade, as described below. In addition, the effusion may cause symptoms due to compression of adjacent structures, such as dysphagia (difficult swallowing because of esophageal compression), dyspnea (shortness of breath resulting from lung compression), hoarseness (due to recurrent laryngeal nerve compression), or hiccups (because of phrenic nerve stimulation).

On examination (Table 14.4), a large pericardial fluid "insulates" the heart from the chest wall, and the heart sounds may be muffled. In fact, a friction rub that had been present during the acute phase of pericarditis may disappear if a large effusion develops and separates the inflamed layers from one another. Dullness to percussion of the left lung over the angle of the scapula may be present (this is known as Ewart's sign) owing to compressive atelectasis by the enlarged pericardial sac.

TABLE 14.4. Clinical Features of Large Pericardial Effusion

Soft heart sounds
Reduced intensity of friction rub
Ewart's sign (dullness over posterior left lung)

Diagnostic Studies

The *chest radiograph* may be normal if only a small pericardial effusion is present. However, if more than approximately 250 ml has accumulated, the cardiac silhouette enlarges in a globular, symmetric fashion. In large effusions, the *electrocardiogram* may demonstrate reduced voltage of the complexes. In the presence of extremely large effusions, the height of the QRS complex may vary from beat to beat (*electrical alternans*); this results from a constantly changing electrical axis as the heart swings from side-to-side within the large pericardial volume.

One of the most useful laboratory tests in the evaluation of an effusion is *echocardiography* (Fig. 14.3), which can identify pericardial collections as small as 20 ml. This noninvasive technique can quantify the volume of pericardial fluid, determine whether ventricular filling is compromised and, when necessary, help direct the placement of a pericardiocentesis needle.

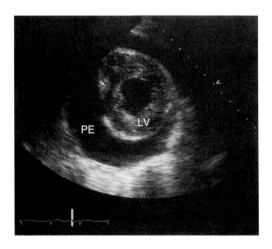

Figure 14.3. **Two-dimensional echocardiogram (parasternal short-axis view) of a pericardial effusion (PE) surrounding the heart.** LV, left ventricle.

Treatment

If the cause of the effusion is known, then therapy is directed toward the underlying disorder (e.g., intensive dialysis for uremic effusion). If the cause is not evident, the clinical state of the patient determines whether pericardiocentesis (removal of pericardial fluid) should be undertaken. An asymptomatic effusion, even of large volume, can be observed for months or years, without specific intervention. However, if serial examination demonstrates a precipitous rise in pericardial volume, or hemodynamic compression of the cardiac chambers becomes evident, then pericardiocentesis should be performed for therapeutic drainage and for analysis of the fluid.

CARDIAC TAMPONADE

At the opposite end of the spectrum from the asymptomatic pericardial effusion is cardiac tamponade. In this condition, pericardial fluid accumulates under high pressure, compresses the cardiac chambers, and severely limits filling of the heart. As a result, ventricular stroke volume and cardiac output decline, potentially leading to hypotensive shock and death.

Etiology

Any etiology of acute pericarditis (see Table 14.1) can progress to cardiac tamponade, but the most common causes are neoplastic, postviral, and uremic pericarditis. Acute hemorrhage into the pericardium is also an important cause of tamponade, which can result from 1) blunt or penetrating chest trauma, 2) rupture of the left ventricular (LV) free wall following MI (see Chapter 7), or 3) as a complication of a dissecting aortic aneurysm (see Chapter 15).

Pathophysiology

As a result of the surrounding tense pericardial fluid, the heart is compressed, and *the diastolic pressure within each chamber becomes elevated and equal to the pericardial pressure.* The pathophysiologic consequences of

this are illustrated in Figure 14.4. Because normal venous return to the heart cannot be accommodated by the compromised cardiac chambers, the systemic and pulmonary venous pressures rise. The increase of systemic venous pressure results in signs of right-sided heart failure (e.g., jugular venous distention), whereas elevated pulmonary venous pressure leads to pulmonary congestion. In addition, reduced filling of the ventricles during diastole decreases the systolic stroke volume, and the cardiac output declines.

These derangements trigger compensatory mechanisms aimed at maintaining tissue perfusion, initially through activation of the sympathetic nervous system. Nonetheless, failure to evacuate the effusion leads to inadequate perfusion of vital organs, shock, and ultimately death.

Clinical Features

Cardiac tamponade should be suspected in any patient with known pericarditis, pericardial effusion, or chest trauma who develops signs and symptoms of systemic vascular congestion and decreased cardiac output (Table 14.5). The key physical findings include 1) jugular venous distention, 2) systemic hypotension, and 3) a "small, quiet heart" on physical examination, due to the insulating effects of the effusion. Other signs include sinus tachycardia and pulsus paradoxus (described below). Dyspnea and tachypnea reflect pulmonary congestion and decreased oxygen delivery to peripheral tissues.

If tamponade develops suddenly, symptoms of profound hypotension are evident, including confusion and agitation. However, if the effusion develops more slowly, over a period of weeks, then fatigue (due to low cardiac output) and peripheral edema (owing to right-sided heart failure) may be the presenting complaints.

Pulsus paradoxus is an important physical sign in cardiac tamponade that can be recognized at the bedside using a blood pressure cuff. It refers to a cyclical *decrease of systolic blood pressure (more than 10 mm Hg) during normal inspiration.*

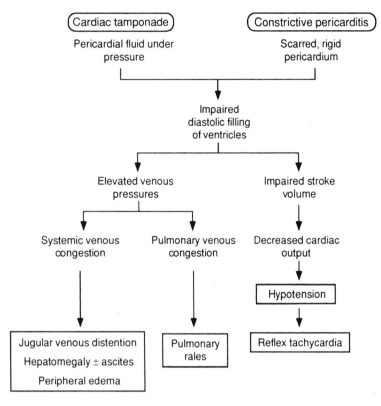

Figure 14.4. Pathophysiology of cardiac tamponade and constrictive pericarditis. The symptoms and signs (boxes) arise from impaired diastolic filling of the ventricles in both conditions.

Pulsus paradoxus is not really "paradoxical"; it is just an exaggeration of appropriate cardiac physiology. Normally, expansion of the thorax during inspiration causes the intrathoracic pressure to become more negative compared with the expiratory phase. This facilitates systemic venous return to the chest and augments filling of the right ventricle (RV). The transient increase in RV size shifts the interventricular septum toward the left, which slightly diminishes *LV* filling. As a result, in normal individuals, LV stroke volume and systolic blood pressure decline slightly following inspiration.

In cardiac tamponade, this situation is exaggerated as both ventricles share a reduced, fixed volume due to external compression by the tense pericardial fluid. In this case, the inspiratory increase of right ventricular volume and bulging of the interventricular septum toward the left have a proportionally greater effect on the limitation of LV filling. Thus, in tamponade there is a more substantial reduction of LV stroke

volume (and therefore systolic blood pressure) following inspiration.

Pulsus paradoxus may also be manifest by other conditions in which inspiration is exaggerated, including severe asthma and chronic obstructive airways disease.

Diagnostic Approach

Echocardiography is the most useful noninvasive technique to evaluate whether pericardial effusion has led to cardiac tamponade physiology. An important indicator of high-pressure pericardial fluid is compression of the RV and right atrium during

TABLE 14.5. Clinical Features of Cardiac Tamponade

Jugular venous distention
Hypotension with pulsus paradoxus
Quiet precordium on palpation
Sinus tachycardia

diastole (see Fig. 3.12). In addition, echocardiography can differentiate between cardiac tamponade and other causes of low cardiac output, such as ventricular contractile dysfunction.

The definitive diagnostic procedure for cardiac tamponade is cardiac catheterization with measurement of intracardiac and intrapericardial pressures, usually combined with therapeutic pericardiocentesis, as described in the next section.

Treatment

Removal of the high-pressure pericardial fluid is the only intervention that reverses the life-threatening physiology of this condition. Pericardiocentesis is best performed in the cardiac catheterization laboratory, where the hemodynamic effect of fluid removal can be assessed. The patient is positioned head up at a 45° angle to promote pooling of the effusion, and a needle is inserted into the pericardial space through the skin, just below the xiphoid process (which is the safest location to avoid piercing a coronary artery). A catheter is then threaded into the pericardial space and connected to a transducer for pressure measurement. Another catheter is threaded through a systemic vein into the right side of the heart, and simultaneous recordings of intracardiac and intrapericardial pressures are compared. In tamponade, the pericardial pressure is elevated and *equal* to the diastolic pressures within the cardiac chambers; all of the latter are elevated to the same degree because of the surrounding compressive force of the effusion.

In addition, the right atrial pressure tracing, which is equivalent to the jugular venous pulsations observed on physical examination, displays a characteristic abnormality (Fig. 14.5). During early diastole in a normal individual, as the right ventricular pressure falls and the tricuspid valve opens, blood quickly flows from the right atrium into the RV, such that there is a rapid decline in the right atrial (RA) pressure tracing (y descent). In tamponade, however, the pericardial fluid compresses the right ventricle and prevents its rapid expansion. Thus, the RA cannot empty quickly, and *the y descent is blunted.*

Following successful pericardiocentesis, the pericardial pressure falls to normal and is no longer equal to the pressures within the heart chambers, which also decline to their normal levels. After initial aspiration of fluid, the pericardial catheter may be left in place for a day or two to allow more complete drainage.

When pericardial fluid is obtained for diagnostic purposes, it should be stained and cultured for bacteria, fungi, and acid-fast bacilli (tuberculosis), and cytologic examination should be performed to evaluate for malignancy. Other common measurements of pericardial fluid include cell counts (e.g., white cell count is elevated in bacterial infections and other inflammatory conditions) and protein and lactate dehydrogenase (LDH) levels. If the concentration ratio of pericardial protein to serum protein is >0.5, or of pericardial LDH to serum LDH is >0.6, then the fluid is consistent with an exudate; otherwise, it is more likely a transudate. When tuberculosis is suspected, it is also useful to measure the level of adenosine deaminase in the pericardial fluid. Some studies have indicated that an elevated level is highly sensitive and specific for tuberculosis.

If cardiac tamponade recurs following pericardiocentesis, the procedure can be repeated. In some cases, a more definitive surgical undertaking (removal of part or all of the pericardium) is required to prevent recurrent collections of effusion.

CONSTRICTIVE PERICARDITIS

The other major potential complication of pericardial diseases is constrictive pericarditis. This is a condition not often encountered but important to understand, because it can masquerade as other, more common disorders. In addition, it is an affliction that may cause profound symptoms, yet is fully correctable if recognized.

Etiology and Pathogenesis

In the early part of the 20th century, tuberculosis was the major cause of constrictive pericarditis, but that is much less common today in industrialized societies. The

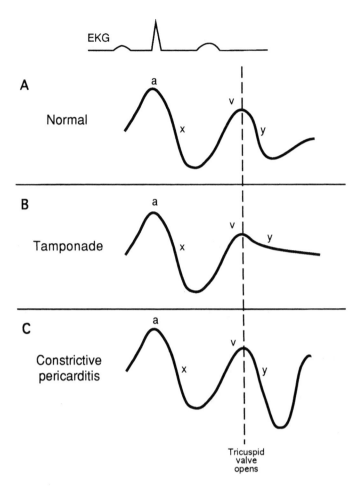

Figure 14.5. **Schematic diagrams of right atrial (or jugular venous) pressure recordings. A.** Normal. The initial *a* wave represents atrial contraction. The *v* wave reflects passive filling of the atria during systole, when the tricuspid and mitral valves are closed. After the tricuspid valve opens, the right atrial pressure falls (*y* descent) as blood empties into the right ventricle. **B.** Cardiac tamponade. High-pressure pericardial fluid compresses the heart, impairing right ventricular filling, so that the *y* descent is blunted. **C.** Constrictive pericarditis. The *earliest* phase of diastolic filling is not impaired so that the *y* descent is not blunted. The y descent appears accentuated because it descends from a higher than normal right atrial pressure. The right atrial *c* wave (described in Chapter 2) is not shown.

most frequent cause now is "idiopathic" (i.e., months to years following presumed idiopathic/viral acute pericarditis). However, any cause of pericarditis (see Table 14.1) can lead to this complication.

Pathology

Following an episode of acute pericarditis, any pericardial effusion that has accumulated usually undergoes gradual resorption. However, in patients who later develop constrictive pericarditis, the fluid undergoes organization, with subsequent fusion of the pericardial layers, followed by fibrous scar formation. In some patients, calcification of the adherent layers ensues, further stiffening the pericardium.

Pathophysiology

The pathophysiologic abnormalities in constrictive pericarditis occur during diastole; systolic contraction of the ventricles is usually normal. In this condition, a rigid, scarred pericardium encircles the heart and *inhibits normal filling of the cardiac chambers.* In diastole, as blood passes from the right atrium into the right ventricle, the RV size expands and quickly reaches the limit imposed by the constricting pericardium. At that point, further filling is suddenly arrested, and venous return to the right heart ceases. Thus, systemic venous pressure rises, and signs of right-sided heart failure ensue. In addition, the impaired filling of the left ventricle causes a reduction in stroke volume, cardiac output, and therefore blood pressure.

Clinical Features

The symptoms and signs of constrictive pericarditis usually develop over months to years. They result from 1) reduced cardiac output (fatigue, hypotension, reflex tachycardia) and 2) elevated systemic venous pressures (jugular venous distention, hepatomegaly with ascites, and peripheral edema). Because the most impressive physical findings are often the insidious development of hepatomegaly and ascites, such patients are often mistakenly thought to have hepatic cirrhosis or an intra-abdominal tumor. It is only after careful inspection of the jugular veins that a cardiac source of the problem is identified, and the correct diagnosis of constrictive pericarditis ultimately made.

On cardiac examination, an early diastolic "knock" may follow S_2 (see Chapter 2) in patients with severe calcific constriction. It represents the sudden cessation of ventricular diastolic filling imposed by the rigid pericardial sac.

Unlike cardiac tamponade, pericardial constriction does not usually result in pulsus paradoxus. Recall that in tamponade, this finding reflects inspiratory augmentation of right ventricular filling, at the expense of LV filling. However, in constrictive pericarditis, the negative intrathoracic pressure generated by inspiration is not transmitted through the rigid pericardial shell to the right-sided heart chambers; therefore, inspiratory augmentation of right ventricular filling does not occur. Rather, when a patient with severe pericardial constriction inhales, the negative intrathoracic pressure draws blood toward the thorax, where it cannot be accommodated by the constricted right-sided cardiac chambers. Thus,

the increased venous return accumulates in the intrathoracic systemic veins, causing the jugular veins to become more distended during inspiration (**Kussmaul's sign**). This is the opposite of normal physiology, in which inspiration results in a *decline* in jugular venous pressure, as venous return is drawn into the heart. The usual effect of respiration in pericardial disease is summarized as follows:

	Constrictive pericarditis	Cardiac tamponade
Pulsus paradoxus	−	+
Kussmaul's sign	+	−

Diagnostic Approach

The *chest radiograph* in constrictive pericarditis shows a normal or mildly enlarged cardiac silhouette. Historically, calcification of the pericardium has been detected in up to 50% of affected patients. The *ECG* generally shows only nonspecific ST and T wave abnormalities, although atrial arrhythmias are common.

Echocardiographic evidence of constriction is subtle. The pericardium, if well-imaged, is thickened; the ventricular cavities are small and contract vigorously, and diastolic ventricular filling terminates abruptly in early diastole, as the chambers reach the limit imposed by the surrounding rigid shell.

Computed tomography or *magnetic resonance imaging* is superior to echocardiography in the assessment of pericardial anatomy and thickness. The presence of normal pericardial thickness (<2 mm) by these modalities is generally a reliable indication that constrictive pericarditis is *not* present.

The diagnosis of constrictive pericarditis can be confirmed by *cardiac catheterization*. There are three key features: 1) elevation and equalization of the diastolic pressures in each of the cardiac chambers; 2) the right and left ventricular tracings show an early diastolic "dip and plateau" configuration (Fig. 14.6)— this pattern reflects blood flow into the ventricles at the very onset of diastole, just after the tricuspid and mitral valves open, followed by sudden cessation

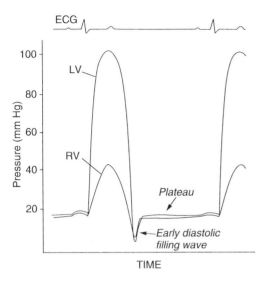

Figure 14.6. Schematic tracings of left ventricular (LV) and right ventricular (RV) pressures in constrictive pericarditis. Early diastolic ventricular filling abruptly halts as the volume in each ventricle quickly reaches the limit imposed by the constricting pericardium. Throughout most of diastole, the LV and RV pressures are abnormally elevated and equal.

of filling as further expansion of the ventricles is arrested by the surrounding rigid pericardium; and 3) the right atrial pressure tracing shows a *prominent y* descent (see Fig. 14.5). After the tricuspid valve opens, the right atrium quickly empties into the RV during the very brief period before filling is arrested. This is in contrast to cardiac tamponade, in which the external compressive force throughout the cardiac cycle *prevents* rapid ventricular filling, even in early diastole, such that the *y* descent is blunted.

The clinical and hemodynamic findings of constrictive pericarditis are often similar to those of restrictive cardiomyopathy (see Chapter 10), another uncommon condition. Distinguishing between these two syndromes is important, however, because pericardial constriction is correctable, whereas most cases of restrictive cardiomyopathy are not correctable. An endomyocardial biopsy is sometimes necessary to distinguish between these (biopsy results are normal in constriction but usually abnormal in restrictive cardiomyopathy; see Chapter 10).

Treatment

The only effective treatment of severe constrictive pericarditis is surgical removal of the pericardium. Symptoms and signs of constriction may not resolve immediately because of the associated stiffness of the neighboring outer walls of the heart, but eventual symptomatic improvement is expected in the majority of patients who undergo this procedure.

SUMMARY

1. Acute pericarditis is most often of idiopathic/viral cause and is usually a self-limited illness. More serious forms of pericarditis arise from the conditions listed in Table 14.1.
2. Common findings in acute pericarditis include 1) pleuritic chest pain, 2) fever, 3) pericardial friction rub, and 4) diffuse ST segment elevation on the ECG, often accompanied by PR segment depression.
3. Complications of pericarditis include cardiac tamponade (accumulation of pericardial fluid under high pressure, which compresses the cardiac chambers) and constrictive pericarditis (restricted filling of the heart because of surrounding rigid pericardium).

Acknowledgment   Contributors to the previous editions of this chapter were Angela Fowler, MD; Kathy Glatter, MD; Alan Braverman, MD; Thomas G. Roberts, MD; and Leonard S. Lilly, MD.

ADDITIONAL READING

Benoff LJ, Schweitzer P. Radiation therapy-induced cardiac injury. Am Heart J 1995;129:1193–1196.

Breen JF. Imaging of the pericardium. J Thorac Imaging 2001;16:47–54.

Koh KK, Kim EJ, Cho CH, et al. Adenosine deaminase and carcinoembryonic antigen in pericardial effusion diagnosis, especially in suspected tuberculous pericarditis. Circulation 1994;89:2728–2735.

Ling L, Oh J, Schaff HV, et al. Constrictive pericarditis in the modern era: evolving clinical spectrum and impact on outcome after pericardiectomy. Circulation 1999;100:1380–1386.

Oh JK, Hatle LK, Seward JB, et al. Diagnostic role of Doppler echocardiography in constrictive pericarditis. J Am Coll Cardiol 1994;23:154–162.

Sagrista-Sauleda J, Angel J, Permanyer-Miralda G, et al. Long-term follow-up of idiopathic chronic pericardial effusion. N Engl J Med 1999;341:2054–2059.

Sagrista-Sauleda J, Merce J, Permanyer-Miralda G, et al. Clinical clues to the causes of large pericardial effusions. Am J Med 2000;109:95–101.

Shabetai R. The effects of pericardial effusion on respiratory variations in hemodynamics and ventricular function. J Am Coll Cardiol. 1991;17:249–250.

Smith WH, Beacock DJ, Goddard AJ, et al. Magnetic resonance evaluation of the pericardium. Br J Radiol 2001;74:384–392.

Spodick DH. The Pericardium: A Comprehensive Textbook. New York: Marcel Dekker, 1997.

Diseases of the Peripheral Vasculature

*Mary Beth Gordon
and Mark A. Creager*

Diseases of the Aorta
  Aortic Aneurysms
  Aortic Dissection
Occlusive Arterial Diseases
  Peripheral Arterial Disease
  Acute Arterial Occlusion
  Vasculitic Syndromes

**Disease Causing Arterial Spasm: Raynaud's
  Phenomenon**
Venous Disease
  Varicose Veins
  Venous Thrombosis

Peripheral vascular disease is an umbrella term that includes a number of diverse pathologic entities that affect arteries, veins, and lymphatics. Although this terminology makes a distinction between the "central" coronary and "peripheral" systemic vessels, the vasculature as a whole comprises a dynamic, integrated, and multifunctional organ system that does not naturally comply with this semantic division.

Blood vessels serve many critical functions. First, they regulate the differential distribution of blood to tissues. Second, blood vessels actively synthesize and secrete vasoactive substances that regulate vascular tone, and antithrombotic substances that maintain the fluidity of blood and vessel patency (see Chapters 5 and 6). Third, the vessels play an integral role in the transport and distribution of immune cells to traumatized or infected tissues. Disease states of the peripheral vasculature interfere with these essential functions.

Peripheral vascular diseases result from many pathophysiologic processes that can be grouped into three categories: 1) *structural changes in the vessel wall* secondary to degenerative diseases, infection, or inflammation that lead to aneurysm, dissection, or rupture; 2) *narrowing of the vascular lumen* due to atherosclerosis, thrombosis, or in-flammation; and 3) *spasm* of vascular smooth muscle. These processes can occur in isolation or can potentiate one another.

DISEASES OF THE AORTA

The aorta is the largest conductance vessel of the vascular system. In adults, its diameter is approximately 3 cm at its origin at the base of the heart. The **ascending aorta,** 5–6 cm in length, leads to the **aortic arch,** from which arise three major branches: the brachiocephalic (which bifurcates into the right common carotid and subclavian arteries), the left common carotid, and the left subclavian arteries. As the **descending aorta** continues beyond the arch, its diameter narrows to approximately 2–2.5 cm in healthy adults. As the aorta pierces the diaphragm, it becomes the **abdominal aorta,** which provides arteries to the abdominal viscera before bifurcating into the left and right common iliac arteries, which supply the pelvic organs and lower extremities.

The aorta, like other arteries, is composed of three layers, as shown in Figure 5.1, page 112. At the luminal surface, the intima is composed of endothelial cells overlying the internal elastic lamina. The endothelial layer is a functional interface between the vasculature and the circulating blood cells and plasma. The media is composed of smooth muscle cells and a matrix that includes collagen and elastic fibers. Collagen provides tensile strength, a stiffness that allows the vessels to withstand high-pressure loads. Elastin, capable of stretching to 250% of its original length, confers a distensible quality on vessels that allows them to recoil under pressure. The adventitia is made up primarily of collagen fibers, perivascular nerves, and vasa vasorum. The vasa vasorum is a rich vascular network that supplies oxygenated blood to the aorta, particularly in its thoracic portion.

The predominance of elastin in the media (2:1 over collagen) allows the aorta to expand during systole and then to recoil during diastole. This recoil against the closed aortic valve contributes to the distal propagation of blood flow during the phase of left ventricular relaxation. With advancing age, the elastic component of the aorta and its branches degenerates, collagen becomes more prominent, and the arteries stiffen. Systolic blood pressure therefore tends to rise with age because less energy is dissipated into the aorta during left ventricular contraction. The aorta is subject to injury from mechanical trauma because it is continuously exposed to high pulsatile pressure and shear stress.

Diseases of the aorta most commonly appear as one of three clinical conditions: aneurysm, dissection, or obstruction.

Aortic Aneurysms

An aneurysm is an abnormal, localized dilatation of an artery. In the aorta, aneurysms are distinguished from *diffuse ectasia*, which is a generalized yet lesser increase of the aortic diameter. Ectasia develops in older individuals as elastic fibers fragment, smooth muscle cells decrease in number, and acid mucopolysaccharide ground substance accumulates within the vessel wall.

The term aneurysm is applied when the diameter of a portion of the aorta has increased by 50% or more or if a portion of the abdominal aorta has enlarged to greater than 3.5–4 cm in diameter. A **true aneurysm** represents a dilatation of all three layers of the aorta, creating a large bulge of the vessel wall. True aneurysms are characterized as either *fusiform* or *saccular,* depending on the extent of the vessel's circumference within the aneurysm (Fig. 15.1). A fusiform aneurysm, the more common type, is one in which the entire circumference of a segment of the aorta is dilated, whereas a saccular aneurysm is a localized outpouching involving only a portion of the circumference.

In distinction, a **pseudoaneurysm,** or **false aneurysm,** is a contained *rupture* of the vessel wall that may mimic the appearance of a true aneurysm. A pseudoaneurysm develops when blood leaks out of the vessel lumen through a hole in the intimal and medial layers and is contained merely by the layer of adventitia or perivascular organized thrombus (see Fig. 15.1). Such a lesion may develop at sites of vessel injury caused by infection or trauma, such as puncture of the vessel during surgery or percutaneous catheterization. Pseudoaneurysms are very unstable lesions that are prone to rupture.

Aneurysms may be confined to the abdominal aorta (most common), the thoracic aorta, or both locations. They may also appear in peripheral and cerebral arteries.

Etiology and Pathogenesis of True Aortic Aneurysms

The etiology of aortic aneurysm formation is multifactorial and may vary depending on the location of the lesion. Atherosclerosis is an important contributor, implicated in approximately 90% of abdominal aortic aneurysms (Fig. 15.2). Within the thoracic aorta, atherosclerotic aneurysms are more common in the descending, compared with the ascending, portions. Atherosclerotic aneurysms rarely develop before age 50, they are more common in men, and their development is accelerated by other risk factors that predispose to atherosclerosis (e.g., smoking, hypertension, dyslipidemia).

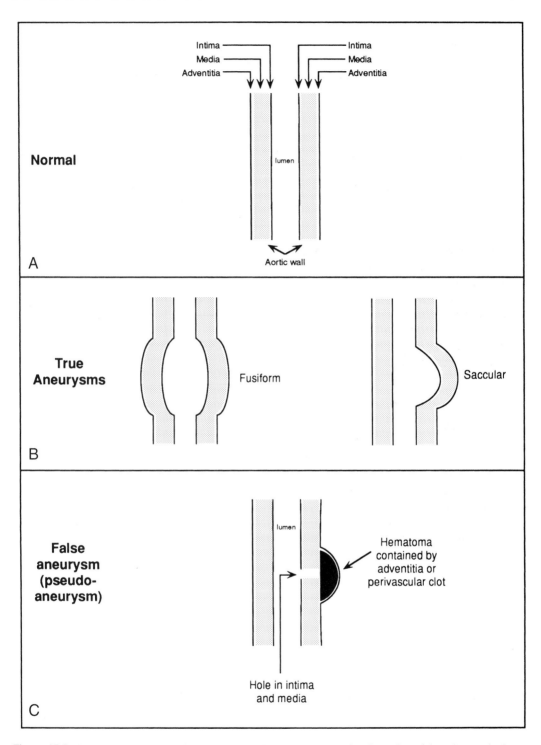

Figure 15.1. **Classification of aortic aneurysms. A.** The normal arterial wall consists of three layers: the intima, media, and adventitia. **B.** True aneurysms represent localized dilatation of all three layers of the arterial wall. Fusiform aneurysms involve the entire circumference of the aorta, whereas saccular aneurysms are a localized bulge of only a portion of the circumference. **C.** A false aneurysm (or pseudoaneurysm) is actually a hole in the intima and media, with hematoma contained by a thin layer of adventitia or perivascular clot.

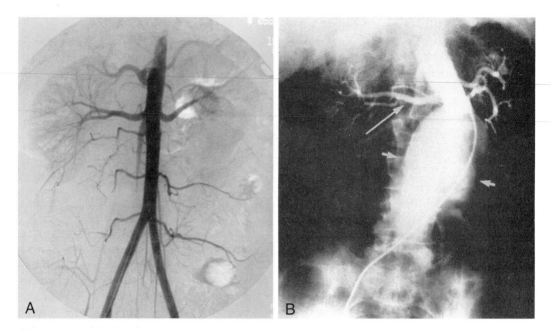

Figure 15.2. Abdominal aortic angiograms A. Angiogram of the abdominal aorta in a normal individual (vascular structures appear black in this digital subtraction image). Note the renal arteries and the outline of the kidneys. **B.** Angiographic demonstration of an abdominal aortic aneurysm (short arrows). The aorta is dilated below the level of the renal arteries (long arrow). Blood vessels containing the injected contrast agent appear white on this conventional angiogram.

Aneurysms of the ascending thoracic aorta are *uncommonly* atherosclerotic in origin. Rather, degenerative changes in the media appear to play an important role. This process, termed **cystic medial degeneration** (or **cystic medial necrosis**), involves the degeneration and fragmentation of elastic fibers, with subsequent accumulation of collagenous and mucoid material within the medial layer. When present, cystic medial degeneration often affects the ascending aorta because it is subjected to the greatest pulsatile expansion and shear stress. Medial degeneration may occur in association with connective tissue disorders (e.g., Marfan syndrome or Ehlers-Danlos syndrome) or in response to hypertension and aging.

Less common causes of aortic aneurysms are listed in Table 15.1. For example, weakness of the media and aneurysm formation may result from certain infections of the arterial wall, such as syphilis, tuberculosis, staphylococcus, streptococcus, or salmonella. Inflammatory diseases such as Takayasu's arteritis and giant cell arteritis (described below) may similarly weaken the vessel wall and result in an aneurysm. Recently, an increasing number of genetic defects in the connective tissue fibers that make up the medial layer of the arterial wall have been observed in patients with aortic aneurysms, suggesting a familial basis for the disease. Approximately 5–10% of patients have a first-degree relative in whom aortic aneurysm has been diagnosed.

TABLE 15.1. Some Causes of True Aortic Aneurysms

- Atherosclerosis

- Cystic medical necrosis
  Idiopathic
  Marfan syndrome
  Ehlers-Danlos syndrome

- Infectious aortitis
  Syphilitic aortitis
  Mycotic aneurysms (primary or embolic infection of vessel wall)

- Vasculitis
  Takayasu's arteritis
  Giant cell arteritis

- Familial aneurysms

Clinical Presentation and Diagnosis

Aortic aneurysms are often asymptomatic, but occasionally patients are aware of a pulsatile mass, particularly when the abdominal aorta is involved. More often, when symptoms occur, it is because of compression of neighboring structures by the expanding aneurysm. For example, erosion of vertebrae by a large abdominal aneurysm may cause back pain. Compression of the esophagus or trachea by a thoracic aneurysm may cause dysphagia, hemoptysis, or respiratory symptoms such as dyspnea, wheezing, or cough. Enlargement of the aorta may also stretch the left recurrent laryngeal nerve as it passes around the ligamentum arteriosum (the embryonic remnant of the ductus arteriosus, located between the pulmonary artery and distal aortic arch), resulting in hoarseness. Aneurysms of the ascending thoracic aorta may dilate the aortic ring, resulting in aortic regurgitation, with subsequent symptoms of heart failure.

Aortic aneurysms are often first suspected when aortic dilatation is observed as an incidental finding on chest or abdominal radiographs, particularly if the aneurysmal walls are calcified. Aneurysms of the abdominal aorta or of the large peripheral arteries may also be discovered by careful palpation during physical examination. The diagnosis is confirmed by ultrasonography, computed tomography, magnetic resonance imaging, or conventional arteriography.

The most devastating consequence of aortic aneurysms is rupture, which is often fatal. An aneurysm may rupture suddenly, or it may leak slowly—extravasating blood into the vessel wall, causing pain and local tenderness. Thoracic aortic aneurysms may rupture into the pleural space, mediastinum, or bronchi. Abdominal aortic aneurysms may rupture into the retroperitoneal space or abdominal cavity, or they may erode into the intestines, resulting in massive gastrointestinal bleeding. Natural history studies have shown that the risk of rupture is related to the size of the aneurysm, as predicted by the law of LaPlace (i.e., wall tension is proportional to the product of pressure and radius). The 5-year risk of rupture of an abdominal aortic aneurysm <5 cm in diameter is 1–2%. Conversely, the risk is 20–40% if the aneurysm exceeds 5 cm in diameter.

Treatment

Several options exist for the treatment of aortic aneurysms. Transabdominal surgical repair with placement of a prosthetic graft is the gold standard for most abdominal aortic aneurysms exceeding 4.5–5 cm in diameter or for those expanding in diameter at a rate exceeding 1 cm per year. Alternatively, percutaneous deployment of an endovascular graft shows promise as a less invasive, cost-effective technique with morbidity and mortality rates at least comparable to those of open repair. Surgical repair is generally recommended for thoracic aortic aneurysms that exceed 6 cm in diameter or that cause symptoms due to compression of adjacent structures. In patients with Marfan syndrome, in whom the complication rate of aneurysms is very high, surgical repair is often recommended at a lower threshold, when thoracic aortic aneurysms are greater than 5 cm in diameter.

Aortic Dissection

Aortic dissection is a life-threatening condition in which a blood-filled channel divides the medial layers of the aorta, splitting (or "dissecting") the intima from the adventitia along various lengths of the vessel.

Etiology, Pathogenesis, and Classification

Aortic dissection is thought to arise from a tear in the intimal layer of the vessel wall that allows blood from the lumen, under the driving force of the systemic pressure, to enter into the media and propagate along the plane of the muscle layer. Another postulated origin of aortic dissection relates to rupture of vasa vasorum with hemorrhage into the media, forming a hematoma in the arterial wall that subsequently tears through the intima and into the vessel's lumen.

Any condition that interferes with the normal integrity of the elastic or muscular components of the medial layer can predispose to aortic dissection. Such degeneration may arise from chronic hypertension, aging, and/or cystic medial degeneration (which, as described above, is a feature of certain hereditary connective tissue disorders, such as the Marfan and Ehlers-Danlos syndromes). In addition, traumatic insult to the aorta (e.g., blunt chest trauma or accidental vessel damage during intra-arterial catheterization or cardiac surgery) can also incite dissection.

Aortic dissection is most common in the sixth and seventh decades of life and occurs more frequently in men. More than two-thirds of patients have a history of hypertension.

Dissection most commonly involves the ascending thoracic aorta (65%) and descending thoracic aorta (20%), whereas the aortic arch (10%) and abdominal aortic (5%) segments are less commonly affected.

Dissections are commonly classified into two types (types A and B), depending on their location and extent (Fig. 15.3). Type A, or proximal dissections, are those in which the ascending aorta is involved. They may be confined to the ascending aorta or may extend into the arch and descending portion of the vessel. Type B, or distal dissections, do not involve the ascending aorta or arch and are confined to the descending thoracic and abdominal aorta. This distinction is important, because treatment strategies and prognosis are determined by location. Proximal aortic involvement tends to be the more devastating form due to its potential for extension into the coronary and arch vessels, into the support structures of the aortic valve, or into the pericardial space. Approximately two-thirds of dissections are type A, and one-third are type B. Dissections may also be classified as acute or chronic. Acute dissections present with symptoms of less than 2 weeks' duration.

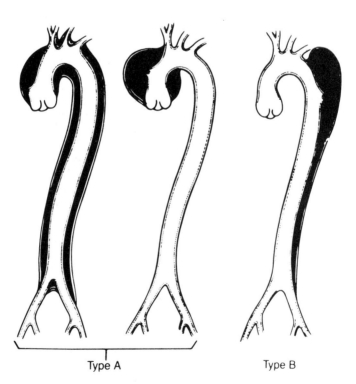

Type A   Type B

Figure 15.3. Aortic dissection. Type A involves the ascending aorta, whereas type B does not. (Reprinted with permission from Cotran RS, Kumar V, Robbins SL. Robbin's Pathologic Basis of Disease. Philadelphia: WB Saunders, 1989.)

Clinical Presentation and Diagnosis

The most common symptom of aortic dissection is sudden, severe pain with a "tearing" or "ripping" quality in the anterior chest (typical of type A dissections) or between the scapulae (in type B dissections). Classically, this pain then travels as the dissection propagates along the aorta. Other symptoms relate to the catastrophic complications that can occur at the time of presentation or thereafter (Table 15.2) and include: 1) rupture through the adventitia anywhere along the aorta (often into the left pleural space or pericardium); 2) occlusion of major branches of the aorta by the propagating hematoma within the vessel wall, which compresses the lumen and can result in myocardial infarction (coronary artery involvement), stroke (carotid artery involvement), visceral ischemia, renal failure, or loss of pulse in an extremity; and 3) extension into the aortic root with disruption of the aortic valve support apparatus causing aortic regurgitation.

Several important physical findings may be present. Hypertension is frequently detected, either as an underlying cause of dissection, a result of diminished renal vascular flow (with activation of the renin-angiotensin system), or because of the sympathetic nervous system response to severe pain. However, if the dissection has occluded flow to one of the subclavian arteries, a difference in systolic blood pressure between the arms is noted. Neurologic deficits may accompany dissection into the carotid vessels. If a type A dissection results in aortic regurgitation, an early diastolic murmur is present on auscultation. Leakage from a type A dissection into the pericardial sac may produce signs of cardiac tamponade (see Chapter 14).

The diagnosis of aortic dissection must not be delayed, because catastrophic complications or death may rapidly ensue. The confirmatory imaging techniques most useful in detecting dissection include transesophageal echocardiography, magnetic resonance imaging, and contrast angiography. In many hospital settings, transesophageal echocardiography is the initial diagnostic test because of its availability, excellent sensitivity and specificity, and reasonable cost.

Treatment

Treatment of acute aortic dissection is designed to arrest progression of the dissecting channel. Suspicion of acute aortic dissection warrants immediate medical therapy to reduce systolic blood pressure and decrease the force of left ventricular contraction to minimize aortic wall shear stress. Useful pharmacologic agents in this regard include β-blockers (to reduce the force of contraction and heart rate as well as to lower blood pressure) and vasodilators such as sodium-nitroprusside (to rapidly reduce blood pressure). In proximal (type A) dissections, early surgical correction has been shown to improve the outcome compared with medical therapy alone. Surgical therapy involves repairing the intimal tear, suturing the edges of the false channel and, if necessary, inserting a synthetic aortic graft.

Conversely, patients with uncomplicated, subacute type B dissections are initially managed with aggressive medical therapy alone; early surgical intervention does not improve the outcome in such patients. Surgery is warranted, however, if there is clinical evidence of propagation of the dissection, compromise of major branches of the aorta, impending rupture, or continued pain. Catheter-based repair with endovascular stent-grafts is being explored as an alternative to surgery.

TABLE 15.2. Complications of Aortic Dissection

Rupture
- Pericardial tamponade
- Hemomediastinum
- Hemothorax (usually left-sided)

Occlusion of aortic branch vessels
- Carotid (stroke)
- Coronary (myocardial infarction)
- Splanchnic (organ infarction)
- Renal (acute renal failure)

Distortion of aortic annulus
- Aortic regurgitation

OCCLUSIVE ARTERIAL DISEASES

Arterial occlusion may result from atherosclerosis, thromboembolism, or vasculitis (inflammation of the vessel wall). The clinical presentation of these disorders results from decreased perfusion to the affected limb or organs.

Peripheral Arterial Disease

Etiology and Pathogenesis

The formation of atherosclerotic plaques in large- and medium-sized arteries may result in chronic occlusive arterial disease, with progressive stenosis and obstruction of blood flow. This disorder is often referred to as peripheral arterial disease (PAD), and although it may affect many vascular beds, it generally refers to atherosclerotic disease in arteries of the pelvis or lower limbs. Its complications result from ischemia distal to the stenosis. It is the most prevalent vascular disorder, with a symptomatic incidence of 0.3% of the entire population and 5.2% of individuals older than 70 years of age.

The pathology of PAD is identical to that of atherosclerotic coronary artery disease, and the major coronary risk factors (e.g., cigarette smoking, dyslipidemia, diabetes mellitus, and hypertension) are also associated with PAD. Approximately 45% of patients with symptomatic PAD have concurrent clinically significant CAD.

The pathophysiology of PAD is also similar to that of CAD (as described in Chapter 6). Ischemia of the affected region occurs when there is an imbalance between oxygen supply and demand: exercise raises the demand for blood flow in the tissues, and a stenosed or obstructed artery is unable to provide an adequate supply. Conversely, rest improves symptoms as the balance between oxygen supply and demand is restored.

Recall from Chapter 6 that the amount of blood flow reduction relates closely to the extent of vessel narrowing, the length of the stenosis, and the blood viscosity. Pouseille's equation describes this relationship:

$$Q = \frac{\Delta P \pi r^4}{8 \eta L}$$

in which Q = flow; ΔP = pressure drop across the stenosis; r = vessel radius; η = blood viscosity; and L = length of stenosis. Thus, the degree of vessel narrowing by the stenosis (i.e., the change in r) has the greatest impact on flow. For example, if the radius is reduced by $\frac{1}{2}$, the flow will be reduced by $\frac{1}{16}$. The equation also indicates that for stenoses of the same length and radius, higher flow rates correspond to greater pressure drops across the stenosis. That is, as the flow velocity increases across a stenotic vessel, the blood turbulence results in a loss of kinetic energy. The result is a decline in perfusion pressure distal to the stenosis.

Furthermore, during exercise products of skeletal muscle metabolism (e.g., adenosine) act locally to dilate arterioles. The resultant decrease in vascular resistance serves to increase blood flow to the active muscle (recall that flow = pressure/resistance). In turn, the increased flow stimulates healthy arterial endothelium to release vasodilating factors such as nitric oxide, thereby increasing the radii of upstream vessels to become appropriate conduits. However, in PAD, obstructed arteries cannot respond to the vasodilating stimuli, thereby limiting flow increases. In addition, dysfunctional atherosclerotic endothelium does not release normal amounts of vasodilating substances (see Chapter 6). Thus, both the physical properties of a stenosis and the reduced vasodilator activity imposed by diseased endothelium prevent adequate blood flow from reaching distal tissues, thereby contributing to ischemia.

Hemodynamic changes alone cannot account for the dramatic reductions in exercise capacity experienced by PAD patients; changes in muscle structure and function are also seen. One such change is the denervation and dropout of muscle fibers, thought to occur as an adaptation to intermittent ischemia. The loss of such fibers can explain the reduced muscle strength and atrophy that occur in PAD patients. Even viable muscle fibers in affected limbs may show abnormalities of mitochondrial oxidative metabolism.

To summarize this section, atherosclerotic lesions produce stenoses in peripheral conduit vessels, thereby limiting blood flow to the affected extremity. Mechanisms normally in place to compensate for increased demand, such as endogenous release of vasodilators during exercise and recruitment of microvessels, fail in the face of endothelial dysfunction and diminished flow velocity. Thus, states of increased oxygen demand are not met with adequate supply, producing limb ischemia. Adaptations to ischemia include changes in muscle fiber metabolism and muscle fiber dropout. Together, these physical and biochemical changes result in weak lower limbs that suffer ischemic discomfort during exercise. *Severe* peripheral atherosclerosis may reduce limb blood flow to such an extent that it cannot satisfy even resting metabolic requirements. This results in critical limb ischemia, which may progress to tissue necrosis and gangrene and may threaten viability of the limb.

Clinical Presentation and Diagnosis

PAD may affect the aorta or the iliac, femoral, popliteal, and tibioperoneal arteries (Fig. 15.4). Patients with PAD may thus develop buttock, thigh, or calf discomfort precipitated by walking and relieved by rest. This classic symptom of exertional limb fatigue and pain is known as **claudication.** In severe PAD, patients may experience pain *at rest,* usually affecting the feet or toes. The chronically reduced blood flow in this case predisposes the extremity to ulceration, infection, and skin necrosis (Fig. 15.5). Patients with diabetes mellitus and those who smoke are at high risk of these complications.

The location of claudication corresponds to the diseased artery, with the femoral and popliteal arteries being the most common sites (Table 15.3). The arteries of the upper extremities are less frequently affected, but brachiocephalic or subclavian artery disease can cause arm claudication.

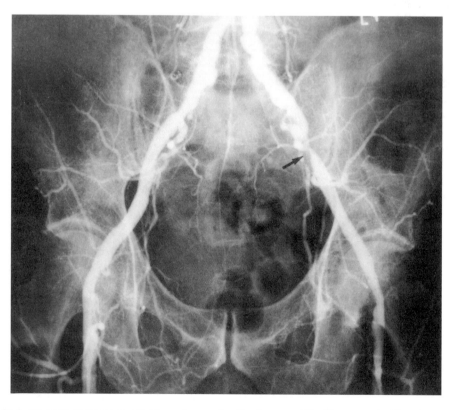

Figure 15.4. An angiogram demonstrating atherosclerotic disease of the iliac vessels. Note the severe stenosis of the left external iliac artery (arrow).

TABLE 15.3. Relation of Stenotic Site to Claudication Symptoms

Site	Location of Claudication Symptoms
Distal aorta or iliac arteries	Buttocks, hips, thighs, or calves
Femoral-popliteal arteries	Calves
Subclavian or axillary arteries	Arms

toms of claudication, whereas an index <0.5 is often observed in patients with rest pain and severe arterial compromise of the affected extremity. Duplex ultrasonography may also be used to visualize and assess the extent of arterial stenoses and the corresponding reductions in blood flow.

Physical examination generally reveals loss of pulses distal to the stenotic segment. Bruits (swishing sound auscultated over a region of turbulent blood flow) may be audible in the abdomen (because of stenoses within the mesenteric or renal arteries) or over iliac, femoral, or subclavian arterial stenoses. In patients with chronic severe ischemia, the lack of blood perfusion results in muscle atrophy, pallor, cyanotic discoloration, hair loss, and occasionally gangrene and necrosis of the foot and digits.

Ischemic ulcers resulting from PAD often begin as small traumatic wounds in areas of increased pressure or in regions prone to injury, such as the tips of toes and lateral malleolus (see Fig. 15.5A). These often painful ulcers fail to heal due to the inadequate blood supply. Diabetic patients with peripheral sensory neuropathies are particularly susceptible to ulcers at sites of trauma or pressure from ill-fitting footwear. Ischemic ulcers can be distinguished from venous insufficiency ulcers, which develop more proximally and on the medial portion of the leg. Venous ulcers are also associated with reddish-brown pigmentation and varicose veins. (see Fig. 15.5B).

In the evaluation of PAD, it is helpful to measure the ratio of blood pressure in the ankles to that in the arms (termed the ankle-brachial index [ABI]) using sphygmomanometer cuffs and a Doppler instrument to detect blood flow. A normal ABI is ≥1.0 (i.e., the ankle pressure is equal to or slightly greater than that in the arms). An index <0.9 may be associated with symp-

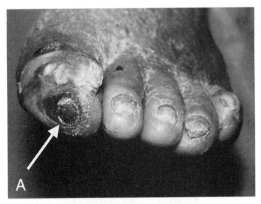

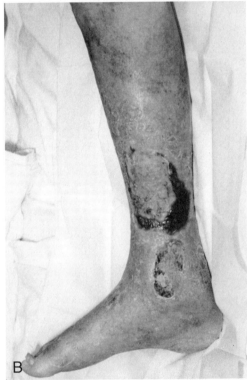

Figure 15.5. Ulcerations caused by vascular insufficiency A. Arterial insufficiency. Ulceration (arrow) affecting the great toe in a patient with severe peripheral arterial disease. **B.** Venous insufficiency ulcer near the medial malleolus of the right leg. Note the pigmentation of the surrounding skin.

Treatment

For all patients with PAD, anti-platelet therapy and risk factor modification (including smoking cessation, lipid-lowering, and control of diabetes and hypertension) are important in reducing the likelihood of coronary events. However, it has not been established if anti-platelet agents actually reduce symptoms or prevent thrombotic complications of PAD itself.

Specific goals of PAD treatment include symptomatic relief and improvement of exercise capacity. In severe cases, therapy is directed at healing ischemic ulcerations and preventing limb loss. Exercise, particularly walking, improves endurance by increasing oxygen extraction and metabolic efficiency in the legs. Formal exercise programs are thus considered first-line therapy for PAD.

Other useful medical therapies include *cilostazol*, a selective phosphodiesterase inhibitor, which increases cAMP and is thought to improve intermittent claudication by inducing vasodilatation and inhibition of platelet aggregation. Cilostazol has been shown to improve exercise capacity and results in small increases in the ABI. Agents that improve the deformability of red and white blood cells (e.g., *pentoxifylline*) may improve symptoms in some patients. Conversely, most vasodilator drugs are not helpful in relieving claudication.

New and more effective medical therapies for PAD are needed and are on the horizon. For example, exciting advances in angiogenesis research and ongoing clinical trials provide hope that pharmacologic revascularization with angiogenic growth factors, such as vascular endothelial growth factor (VEGF) and basic fibroblast growth factor (bFGF), may soon become part of medical treatment.

Mechanical revascularization is indicated when medical therapy has failed for patients with disabling claudication and as first-line therapy in cases of severe limb ischemia. Catheter-based interventions such as percutaneous transluminal angioplasty and stent implantation can be performed on selected patients with low morbidity. Surgical procedures include bypass operations to circumvent the occluded arteries using prosthetic or saphenous vein grafts. However, in severe cases of limb ischemia, amputation is sometimes necessary if blood flow cannot be satisfactorily reestablished.

Acute Arterial Occlusion

Acute arterial occlusion is caused either by embolization from a cardiac or vascular site or by thrombus formation in situ. The origin of arterial emboli is most often the heart, usually due to disorders in which there is intracardiac stasis of flow (Table 15.4). Emboli may also originate from thrombus or atheromatous material overlying an atherosclerotic segment of the aorta itself. Rarely, arterial emboli may originate from the *venous* circulation. If a venous clot travels to the right-heart chambers and is able to pass through an abnormal intracardiac communication (e.g., an atrial septal defect), it would then enter into the systemic arterial circulation (a condition known as a **paradoxical embolism**). Primary arterial thrombus formation may appear at sites of endothelial damage or atherosclerotic stenoses, or within bypass grafts.

The extent of tissue damage from thromboembolism relates to the site of the occluded artery and the degree of collateral circulation serving the tissue beyond the

---

TABLE 15.4. Origins of Arterial Emboli

- Cardiac origin
  Stagnant left atrial flow (e.g., atrial fibrillation, mitral stenosis)
  Left ventricular miral thrombus (e.g., dilated cardiomyopathy, myocardial infarction, ventricular aneurysm)
  Valvular lesions (endocarditis, mitral stenosis, thrombus on prosthetic valve)
  Left atrial myxoma (mobile tumor in left atrium)
- Aortic origin
  Thrombus material overlying atherosclerotic segment
- Venous origin
  Paradoxical embolism travels through intra-cardiac shunt

obstruction. Common symptoms and signs that may develop from reduced blood supply include pain, pallor, paralysis, paresthesia, and pulselessness (termed the "five P's"). A sixth "P," poikilothermia (coolness), is also often manifest.

Therapy includes an anticoagulant agent (e.g., heparin) to prevent propagation of the clot and to reduce the likelihood of additional embolic events. Intra-arterial thrombolysis (e.g., using tissue plasminogen activator) or catheter-based thrombectomy are used in selected cases to eliminate acute thrombi. Surgical techniques to improve severely compromised blood flow include removal of the thrombus or arterial bypass surgery.

Vasculitic Syndromes

Vasculitis (inflammation of the vessel wall) results from immune complex deposition or from cell-mediated immune reactions directed against the vessel wall. Immune complexes activate the complement cascade with subsequent release of chemoattractants and anaphylatoxins that direct neutrophil migration to the vessel wall and increase vascular permeability. Neutrophils injure the vessel by releasing their lysosomal contents and by producing toxic oxygen-derived free radicals. In cell-mediated immune reactions, T lymphocytes bind to vascular antigens and release lymphokines, which attract additional lymphocytes and macrophages to the vessel wall. These inflammatory processes can cause end-organ ischemia because of either vascular necrosis or local thrombosis.

The cause of most of the vasculitic syndromes is unknown, but they often can be distinguished from one another by the pattern of involved vessels and by histologic characteristics (Table 15.5).

Polyarteritis nodosa (PAN) is a necrotizing systemic vasculitis of small- and medium-sized arteries. The name is derived from the many nodules that are found along the course of these vessels. It has a prevalence of approximately 6 per 100,000 and a male-to-female ratio of 1.6:1. Histologic examination of affected arteries reveals polymorphonuclear infiltration in all three vessel layers, intimal proliferation and degeneration, and fibrinoid necrosis with occlusion of the lumen. The vessel wall and elastic lamina are disrupted, leading to aneurysmal dilatation of the vessel. PAN may be idiopathic but can also be seen in the setting of hepatitis B infection (accounting for 30% of PAN cases). The resultant ischemia distal to the involved vessel damages tissues and visceral organs, the most commonly affected of which are the kidney, heart, and liver. Patients may experience generalized inflammatory symptoms such as fever, malaise, and musculoskeletal pains. Alternatively, symptoms may relate to decreased organ blood flow. For example, the presentation may be one of hyper-

TABLE 15.5. Vasculitic Syndromes

Type	Arteries Commonly Affected	Histology
Polyarteritis nodosa	Small to medium size (especially renal, coronary, hepatic, skeletal muscle)	PMN infiltration, acute fibrinoid necrosis, aneurysmal dilatation
Takayasu's arteritis	Aorta and its branches	Granulomatous arteritis with fibrosis; significant luminal narrowing
Giant cell arteritis	Medium to large size (especially cranial vessels as well as aortic arch and its branches)	Lymphocyte infiltration, intimal fibrosis, granuloma formation
Thromboangiitis obliterans (Buerger's disease)	Small size (especially distal arteries of extremities)	Inflammation and thrombosis without necrosis

PMN, polymorphonuclear leukocyte.

tension due to reduced flow into the renal arteries with subsequent activation of the renin-angiotensin system.

The presence of antineutrophil cytoplasmic antibodies (ANCAs) in the circulation is highly suggestive of necrotizing vasculitis, but the diagnosis of PAN is established by biopsy of involved vessels. The prognosis is poor if the disease remains unrecognized. The 5-year survival rate for untreated patients is as low as 15% but may improve to 80% if the diagnosis is established and therapy with prednisone and other immunosuppressive agents is instituted.

Takayasu's arteritis is a disease of unknown cause that targets the aorta and its major branches. It most often occurs in women younger than age 40. The majority of cases have been reported from Asia and Africa, but it occurs worldwide. General symptoms include malaise and fever, but focal symptoms are related to inflammation of the affected vessel and include cerebrovascular ischemia (brachiocephalic or carotid artery), myocardial ischemia (coronary artery), arm claudication (brachiocephalic or subclavian artery), or hypertension (renal artery). The carotid and limb pulses are diminished or absent in nearly 85% of patients at the time of diagnosis; hence, this condition is often termed "pulseless" disease. It is also an uncommon cause of aortic aneurysm or aortic dissection. Histologic examination of affected vessels reveals infiltration of plasma cells and lymphocytes into the media and adventitia, giant cells, intimal proliferation, disruption of the elastic lamina, and fibrosis. Steroid and cytotoxic drugs may reduce vascular inflammation and alleviate symptoms of Takayasu's arteritis. Surgical bypass of obstructed vessels may be helpful in severe cases.

Giant cell arteritis (also termed **temporal arteritis**) is a disease of medium-sized to large arteries that most commonly involves the cranial vessels, the aortic arch, and its branches. It is an uncommon disease, with an incidence of 24 per 100,000, and can be associated with the inflammatory condition known as polymyalgia rheumatica. In distinction to PAN, renal, hepatic, and coronary vessels are usually spared in this condition. It occurs most often in patients older than 55, and 65% of patients are female. Histologic findings in infected vessels include lymphocyte infiltration, intimal fibrosis, and focal necrosis, with granulomas containing multinucleated giant cells.

Symptoms and signs of giant cell arteritis depend on the distribution of affected arteries and may include diminished temporal pulses, prominent headache (from temporal artery involvement) or facial pain, and claudication of the jaw while chewing (facial artery involvement). Nearly 50% of patients experience visual impairment due to ophthalmic artery giant cell arteritis; irreversible blindness can follow. In giant cell arteritis, the erythrocyte sedimentation rate and C-reactive protein are invariably elevated as markers of inflammation. An ultrasound examination can support the diagnosis by demonstrating a hypoechoic halo around the arterial lumen with arterial stenosis and/or occlusion. The diagnosis can be confirmed by biopsy of an involved vessel, usually a temporal artery, but treatment should not wait for biopsy results. High-dose systemic steroids are effective in treating vasculitis and preventing visual complications. Giant cell arteritis usually runs a self-limited course of 1–5 years.

Thromboangiitis obliterans (Buerger's disease) is an inflammatory disease of small- and medium-sized arteries, veins, and nerves involving the distal vessels of the upper and lower extremities. It has a very strong association with cigarette smoking and is most common in men younger than 40. Fewer than 2% of patients are female. There is an increased incidence of HLA-A9 and HLA-B5 in affected individuals.

Buerger's disease presents with a triad of symptoms and signs: distal arterial occlusion, Raynaud's phenomenon (described below), and migrating superficial vein thrombophlebitis. As a result of arterial occlusion, patients develop arm and foot claudication as well as ischemia of the digits. Traditional laboratory markers of inflammation and autoimmune disease are usually not detected. Arteriographic features of involved arteries include areas of stenosis interspersed with normal-appearing vessels with more severe disease distally, collateral vessels with a "corkscrew" appearance around the stenotic regions, and lack of atherosclerosis in proximal arteries. The diagnosis can be established by tissue biopsy, although this is rarely needed. Biopsy specimens of affected vessels (Fig. 15.6) reveal an occlusive, highly cellular, inflammatory thrombus, with limited involvement of the vessel wall and preservation of the internal elastic lamina. The only treatment for Buerger's disease is smoking cessation, which usually prevents progression of the disease and its complications.

DISEASE CAUSING ARTERIAL SPASM: RAYNAUD'S PHENOMENON

Raynaud's phenomenon is a vasospastic disease of the digital arteries (most often the fingers) that occurs in susceptible individuals when exposed to cool temperatures or sometimes emotional stress. Vasospasm is an extreme vasoconstrictor response that temporarily obliterates the vascular lumen, inhibiting blood flow. Typically, episodes of vasospasm are characterized by a triphasic color response. First, the fingers and/or toes blanch to a distinct white as blood flow

is interrupted (Fig. 15.7). The second phase is characterized by cyanosis, related to local accumulation of desaturated hemoglobin, followed by the third phase—a ruddy color as blood flow begins to resume. Accompanying the color response may be numbness, paresthesias, or pain of the affected digits.

This condition may occur as an isolated disorder, termed *primary Raynaud's phenomenon* or *Raynaud's disease.* Such patients are predominantly female and between the ages of 20 and 40; genetic factors do not appear to play a predisposing role. Primary Raynaud's phenomenon most often manifests in the fingers, but 40% of patients also have involvement of their toes. The prognosis of primary Raynaud's phenomenon is relatively benign, with only 16% of patients reporting a worsening of their symptoms over time.

Secondary Raynaud's phenomenon may appear as a component of other conditions. Common causes include connective tissue diseases (e.g., scleroderma, systemic lupus erythematosus) and arterial occlusive disorders. Other causes of secondary Raynaud's phenomenon include carpal tunnel syndrome, thoracic outlet syndrome, blood dyscrasias, certain drugs, and thermal or vibration injury.

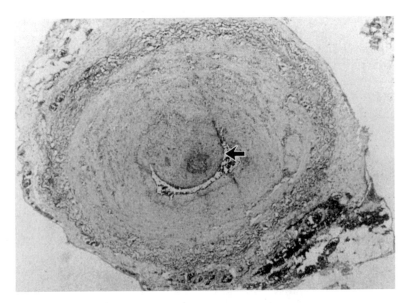

Figure 15.6. **Histologic section of an artery displaying thromboangiitis obliterans.** There is endothelial cell and fibroblast proliferation in the vessel wall, and thrombus is present in the vessel lumen (arrow).

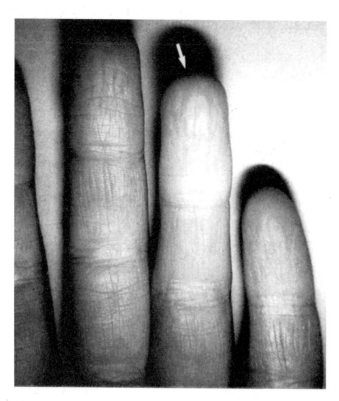

Figure 15.7. **Raynaud's phenomenon.** The fourth digit (arrow) is blanched (phase 1 of the tricolor response).

Even in healthy vessels, cold exposure normally produces a vasoconstrictor response. Cooling stimulates the sympathetic nervous system, resulting in local discharge of norepinephrine. Norepinephrine binds to vascular adrenergic receptors. In the fingers and toes, only vasoconstricting α-receptors are present; other regional circulations have both constrictor and dilator adrenergic responses. Thus, a modest vasoconstriction results when healthy people are exposed to cooling. In contrast, in Raynaud's phenomenon cold exposure induces *severe* vasoconstriction.

A variety of mechanisms have been proposed to explain the vasospastic response to cold and stress in patients with primary Raynaud's phenomenon, including an exaggerated sympathetic discharge in response to cold, heightened vascular sensitivity to adrenergic stimuli, or excessive release of vasoconstrictor stimuli, such as serotonin, thromboxane, and endothelin. In patients with secondary Raynaud's phenomenon caused by connective tissue dis-eases or arterial occlusive disease, the digital vascular lumen is largely obliterated by sclerosis or inflammation, resulting in lower intraluminal pressure and greater susceptibility to sympathetically mediated vasoconstriction.

Treatment of Raynaud's phenomenon involves avoiding cold environments, dressing in warm clothes, and using insulated gloves or footwear during such exposure. There has also been some success in preventing vasospasm with pharmacologic agents that relax vascular tone, including calcium channel blockers and α-adrenergic blockers (described in Chapter 17).

VENOUS DISEASE

Veins are high-capacitance vessels that contain more than 70% of the total blood volume. In contrast to the muscular structure of arteries, the subendothelial layer of veins is thin, and the tunica media comprises fewer, smaller bundles of smooth muscle cells intermixed with reticular and elastic fibers. Whereas veins of the extremities possess intrinsic vasomotor activity, transport of blood back to the heart relies greatly on external compression by the surrounding skeletal muscles and on a series of one-way endothelial valves.

Veins of the extremities are classified as either deep or superficial. In the lower extremity, where most peripheral venous disorders occur, the deep veins generally course along the arteries, whereas the superficial veins are located subcutaneously. The superficial vessels drain into deeper veins via a series of perforating connectors, ultimately returning blood to the heart.

Varicose Veins

Varicose veins (Fig. 15.8) are dilated, tortuous superficial vessels that often develop in the lower extremities. Clinically apparent varicose veins occur in 10–20% of the general population. They affect women two to three times more frequently than men, and

roughly half of patients have a family history of this condition. Varicosities can occur in any vein in the body but are most common in the saphenous veins of the leg and their tributaries. They may also develop in the anorectal area (hemorrhoids), in the lower esophageal veins (esophageal varices), and in the spermatic cord (varicocele).

Varicosity is thought to result from intrinsic weakness of the vessel wall, from increased intraluminal pressure, or from congenital defects in the structure and function of the valves that severely impair flow toward the heart. Varicose veins in the lower extremity are classified as either primary or secondary. *Primary* varicose veins originate in the superficial system, and factors that contribute to their development include pregnancy, prolonged standing, and obesity. During pregnancy or prolonged standing, the high venous pressure within the legs contributes to the development of varicosities in individuals with inherent weakness of the vessel walls. In obese patients,

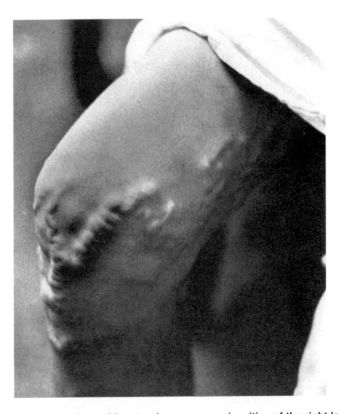

Figure 15.8. **A patient with extensive venous varicosities of the right leg.**

the adipose tissue surrounding vessel walls offers less structural support to veins than lean mass. *Secondary* varicose veins occur when an abnormality in the deep venous system is the cause of superficial varicosities. These may develop in the setting of deep venous insufficiency or occlusion, or when the perforating veins are incompetent. In such cases, deep venous blood is shunted retrograde via perforating channels into superficial veins, increasing intraluminal pressure and volume, and causing dilatation and varicosity formation.

Many individuals with varicose veins are asymptomatic but seek treatment for cosmetic reasons. When symptoms do develop, they include a dull ache or pressure sensation in the legs after prolonged standing. Superficial venous insufficiency may result when venous valves are unable to function normally in the dilated veins. This can cause swelling and skin ulceration that is particularly severe near the ankle. Stasis of blood within varicose veins can promote superficial vein thrombosis, and varicosities can also rupture, causing a localized hematoma.

Varicose veins are usually treated conservatively. Patients should elevate their legs while supine, avoid prolonged standing, and wear external compression stockings that counterbalance the increased venous hydrostatic pressure. Small symptomatic varicose veins are sometimes treated by injection of a sclerosing solution into the vein. Laser treatments can be used to improve the cosmetic appearance of small affected vessels. Surgical therapy includes vein ligation and removal and is reserved for patients who are very symptomatic, suffer recurrent superficial vein thrombosis, or develop skin ulcerations.

Venous Thrombosis

The terms venous thrombosis or thrombophlebitis are used to describe thrombus within a superficial or deep vein and the inflammatory response in the vessel wall that it incites. Thrombi in the lower extremities are classified by location as either deep venous thrombi or superficial venous thrombi.

Initially, the venous thrombus is composed principally of platelets and fibrin. Later, red blood cells become interspersed within the fibrin, and the thrombus tends to propagate in the direction of blood flow. The changes in the vessel wall can be minimal or can include granulocyte infiltration, loss of endothelium, and edema. Thrombi may diminish or obstruct vascular flow or they may dislodge, forming thromboemboli.

Deep Venous Thrombosis

Epidemiology, Etiology, and Pathogenesis

Deep venous thrombosis (DVT) occurs most commonly in the veins of the calves but may also develop initially in more proximal veins such as the popliteal, femoral, and iliac vessels. If left untreated, 20–30% of DVTs that occur in the calves may propagate to these proximal veins. The two major consequences of deep venous thrombosis are pulmonary embolism and postphlebitic syndrome. Pulmonary embolism can supervene when a clot, most often from a DVT in the proximal veins of the lower extremities, dislodges and travels through the inferior vena cava and right heart chambers, finally reaching and obstructing a portion of the pulmonary vasculature (Fig. 15.9). This complication may be heralded by pleuritic chest pain, tachypnea, cough, and/or dyspnea. Pulmonary embolism is common (incidence of approximately 600,000 per year in the United States) and is often fatal, with an untreated mortality rate of 30–40%.

Postphlebitic syndrome, or chronic deep venous insufficiency, results from valvular damage and/or persistent occlusion by deep venous thrombosis. This may lead to chronic leg swelling, stasis pigmentation, and skin ulcerations.

In 1856, Virchow described a triad of factors that predispose to venous thrombosis: 1) stasis of blood flow, 2) hypercoagulability, and 3) vascular damage. Stasis disrupts laminar flow and brings platelets into contact with the endothelium. This allows coagulation factors to accumulate and retards the influx of clotting inhibitors. Factors that slow venous flow and induce stasis include

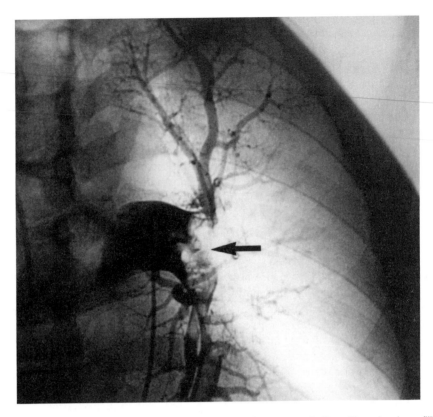

Figure 15.9. Pulmonary angiogram displaying a massive pulmonary embolism. There is a large filling defect in the left main pulmonary artery (arrow), additional filling defects in the lower pulmonary artery branches, and a paucity of vessels in the left mid-lung region (due to obstructed flow).

TABLE 15.6. Conditions that Predispose to DVT

Stasis of blood flow
- Prolonged inactivity (following surgery, long travel by car or plane)
- Immobilized extremity (following bone fracture)
- Heart failure (with systemic venous congestion)
- Hyperviscosity syndromes (e.g., polycythemia vera)

Hypercoagulable states
- Inherited disorders of coagulation
  Resistance to activated protein C (factor V Leiden)
  Prothrombin gene mutation (prothrombin 20210)
  Antithrombin III deficiency
  Deficiency of protein C or protein S
- Antiphospholipid antibodies/lupus anticoagulant
- Neoplastic disease (e.g., pancreatic, lung, stomach, or breast cancers)
- Pregnancy and oral contraceptive use (or other high estrogen states)
- Myeloproliferative diseases
- Smoking

Vascular damage
- Instrumentation (e.g., intravenous catheters)
- Trauma

immobilization (e.g., prolonged bed rest after surgery, or sitting in a car or an airplane for a long trip), cardiac failure, and hyperviscosity syndromes (Table 15.6).

A variety of clinical disorders cause systemic hypercoagulability, including resistance of factor V to activated protein C, a prothrombin gene mutation, and inherited deficiencies of antithrombin III, protein C, and protein S (see Chapter 7). Pancreatic, lung, stomach, breast, and genitourinary tract adenocarcinomas are associated with a high prevalence of venous thrombosis. This is thought to occur in part because necrotic tumor cells release thrombogenic factors. Other conditions that contribute to hypercoagulability are listed in Table 15.6.

Vascular damage, either by external injury or intravenous catheters, can denude the endothelium and expose subendothelial collagen. Exposed collagen acts as a substrate for the binding of von Willebrand's factor and platelets and initiates the clotting cascade, leading to clot formation. Less severe damage can cause endothelial dysfunction rather than denudation and also contributes to thrombosis. This is because normal endothelium secretes vasodilating substances (e.g., nitric oxide and prostacyclin) and antithrombotic molecules such as thrombomodulin and heparan sulfate. When the endothelium is damaged, synthesis of these factors is diminished and thrombosis can occur more easily.

The risk of venous thrombosis is particularly high after fractures of the spine, pelvis, and bones of the lower extremities. The risk following bone fracture may be related to stasis of blood flow, increased coagulability, and possibly traumatic endothelial damage. In addition, venous thrombosis occurs frequently in patients following surgical procedures, particularly major orthopedic operations.

During late pregnancy and the early postpartum period, women have a several-fold increase in the incidence of venous thrombus formation. In the third trimester, the fetus compresses the inferior vena cava and can cause stasis of blood flow, and a hypercoagulable state may be induced by high levels of circulating estrogens. Oral contraceptives and other pharmacologic estrogen products may also predispose to thrombus formation.

Clinical Presentation

Patients with DVT may be asymptomatic. Symptomatic patients often describe calf or thigh discomfort, particularly on standing or walking, or report unilateral leg swelling. The physical signs of proximal DVT include edema of the involved leg and occasionally localized warmth and erythema. Tenderness may be present over the course of the phlebitic vein, and a deep venous cord (induration along the thrombosed vessel) is occasionally palpable. Calf pain produced by dorsiflexion of the foot (Homan's sign) is a nonspecific and unreliable sign of DVT.

Diagnosis

The primary laboratory tests used to diagnose DVT include measurement of the serum D-dimer level and venous compression ultrasonography. *D-dimer* is a byproduct of fibrin degradation that can be measured from a peripheral blood sample. Using an enzyme-linked immunoassay, the D-dimer assay is highly sensitive for the diagnosis of DVT and/or acute pulmonary embolism. As D-dimer may also be elevated in many other conditions (such as cancer, inflammation, infection, or necrosis), a positive test result is not *specific* for DVT. Thus, a normal D-dimer value can help exclude the presence of DVT, but an elevated level does not confirm the diagnosis.

Venous compression duplex ultrasonography is a readily available, noninvasive technique that is 97% sensitive and 97% specific for the diagnosis of symptomatic DVT in a proximal vein, but it is less sensitive for diagnosing calf vein thrombi. This technique uses real-time ultrasound scanning to image the vein and pulsed Doppler ultrasound to assess blood flow within it (Fig. 15.10). Criteria used for diagnosis of DVT with duplex ultrasonography include the inability to compress the vein with direct pressure (suggesting the presence of an intraluminal thrombus), direct visualization of the thrombus, and absence of blood flow within the vein.

Other diagnostic techniques are sometimes used. For example, *magnetic resonance venography* can aid in the diagnosis of proximal DVT, particularly pelvic vein thrombi, which are difficult to detect using ultrasound. *Contrast venography* is an invasive imaging technique that can provide a definitive diagnosis. Radiocontrast material is administered into a foot vein, and images are obtained as the contrast ascends through the venous system of the leg. DVT is diagnosed if a filling defect is present (Fig. 15.10).

Treatment

The most important reason for treating patients with proximal DVT is to prevent pulmonary embolism. Elevation of the affected extremity above the level of the heart is implemented to help reduce edema and tenderness, and anticoagulation is begun to prevent extension of the thrombus. Initial

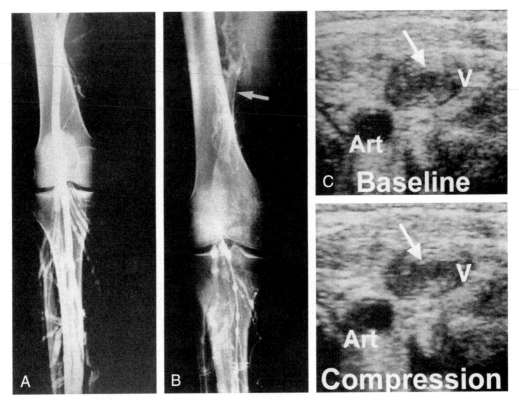

Figure 15.10. Diagnostic imaging of deep venous thrombosis. A. Normal venogram. Contrast material was injected into a foot vein and fills the leg veins in this radiograph. **B.** Venogram demonstrating extensive thrombosis of the deep calf veins, popliteal vein, and superficial femoral vein. Arrow indicates a filling defect in the superficial femoral vein (which is actually a *deep* vein despite its name) due to the presence of thrombus. The deep calf veins are filled with thrombus and cannot be visualized. **C.** Ultrasound indicating deep venous thrombosis. The thrombus appears as an echogenic area (arrow) within the femoral vein (V). A healthy vein would be easily compressible by the ultrasound transducer. This vein, however, has the same diameter at baseline (top panel) and after compression (bottom panel), confirming the presence of thrombus within it. Art, artery.

treatment of DVT is usually with subcutaneous low-molecular-weight heparin to prevent thrombus progression and recurrent thromboembolism. Intravenous unfractionated heparin is a cost-effective alternative that has been used successfully for this purpose for many years, although some studies have shown superior outcomes with low-molecular-weight heparin (which is also more convenient to administer—see Chapter 17). Warfarin, an oral anticoagulant, is prescribed for long-term management and is usually continued for 6 months or more, depending on the underlying cause of DVT. Catheter-based thrombolysis is useful in selected patients with ileofemoral deep vein thrombosis. In patients with proximal DVT who cannot be treated with anticoagulant medication because of a bleeding disorder, an intravascular filter can be inserted into the inferior vena cava to prevent emboli from reaching the lungs.

Treatment of patients with calf vein thrombosis is more controversial because pulmonary emboli from that site are uncommon. Some physicians advocate serial noninvasive monitoring to determine if the thrombus propagates into proximal veins, whereas others treat such thrombosis with intravenous heparin followed by warfarin for 3–6 months.

Prophylaxis against DVT is mandatory in clinical situations in which the risk of deep venous thrombosis is high, such as during bed rest following surgery. Prophylactic measures include subcutaneous unfractionated heparin or low-molecular-weight heparin, low-dose oral warfarin, compression stockings, and/or intermittent external pneumatic compression of the legs to prevent venous stasis.

Superficial Thrombophlebitis

Much less serious than DVT, this is a benign disorder associated with inflammation and thrombosis of a superficial vein, just below the skin. Superficial thrombophlebitis may occur, for example, as a complication of an indwelling intravenous catheter. It is characterized by erythema, tenderness, and edema over the involved vein. Treatment consists of local heat and rest of the involved extremity. Aspirin or other anti-inflammatory medications may relieve the associated discomfort. Unlike DVT, superficial thrombophlebitis does not lead to pulmonary embolism.

SUMMARY

1. Aortic aneurysms are of two types: true aneurysms and false (pseudo) aneurysms. True aneurysms are most commonly related to atherosclerosis, especially in the abdominal and descending thoracic aorta. In the ascending aorta, cystic medial necrosis is an important contributor. A false aneurysm is actually a hole in the arterial intima and media contained by a layer of adventitia or perivascular clot.

2. Symptoms of aortic aneurysms relate to compression of adjacent structures (back pain, dysphagia, respiratory symptoms) or blood leakage. The most severe consequence is aneurysm rupture. Aneurysms can be repaired either with an open surgical procedure or by insertion of an endovascular graft.

3. Aortic dissections result from a splitting apart of a weakened medial layer of the aorta, often in the setting of advanced age, hypertension, or other causes of medial degeneration (cystic medial necrosis). Type A (proximal) aortic dissections involve the ascending aorta, whereas type B dissections are confined to the descending aorta. The former are more common, more

devastating, and require surgical treatment. Type B dissections are often managed by medical therapy alone.

4. PAD is a common atherosclerotic disease of large and medium-sized arteries, often resulting in claudication of the limbs. PAD is treated by risk factor modification, anti-platelet agents, exercise, and sometimes cilostazol, a selective phosphodiesterase inhibitor.

5. Acute arterial occlusion results from thrombus formation in situ or from arterial embolism. The latter arises from thrombus within the heart, from proximal arterial sites, or paradoxically from the systemic veins if an intracardiac shunt (e.g., atrial septal defect) is present. Therapeutic options include anticoagulation, thrombolysis, and surgical or endovascular interventions.

6. Vasculitic syndromes are inflammatory diseases of blood vessels that impair arterial blood flow and result in localized and systemic symptoms. They are distinguished from one another by the pattern of vessel involvement and morphologic findings (see Table 15.5). Most can be treated effectively with systemic corticosteroids.

7. Raynaud's phenomenon is an episodic vasospasm of arteries that supply the digits of the upper and lower extremities. It may be a primary condition (Raynaud's disease) or may appear in association with other disorders such as connective tissue diseases or blood dyscrasias.

8. Varicose veins are dilated tortuous vessels, which may present cosmetic problems. Occasionally they cause discomfort, become thrombosed, or lead to venous insufficiency. Initial management is conservative, with periodic leg elevation and compression stockings.

9. Venous thrombosis results from stasis of blood flow, hypercoagulability, and vascular damage. The major complication of deep venous thrombosis is pulmonary embolism. A chronic complication is venous insufficiency causing chronic leg swelling and skin ulceration.

10. D-dimer assay and venous compression ultrasonography are the primary tools used to diagnose deep venous thrombosis. Anticoagulation therapy with low-molecular-weight heparin or unfractionated intravenous heparin, followed by oral warfarin, is the usual treatment.

Acknowledgment   Contributors to the previous editions of this chapter were C. Geoffrey McDonough, MD; Michael Diminick, MD; Stuart Kaplan, MD; Jesse Salmeron, MD; and Mark A. Creager, MD.

ADDITIONAL READING

Breddin HK, Hach-Wunderle V, Nakov R, et al. Effects of a low-molecular-weight heparin on thrombus regression and recurrent thromboembolism in patients with deep-vein thrombosis. N Engl J Med 2001;344:626–631.

Creager MA, ed. Management of Peripheral Arterial Disease: Medical, Surgical and Interventional Aspects. London: Remedica, 2000.

Creager MA, Dzau VJ. Vascular diseases of the extremities. In: Braunwald E, Fauci AS, Kasper D, et al., eds. Harrison's Principles of Internal Medicine. 15th Ed. New York: McGraw-Hill, 2001.

Dake MD, Katon N, Mitchell RS, et al. Endovascular stent-graft placement for the treatment of acute aortic dissection. N Engl J Med 1999;340:1546–1552.

Dormandy JA, Rutherford RB. Management of peripheral arterial disease: TransAtlantic InterSociety Consensus (TASC). J Vasc Surg 2000;31:S1–S296.

Dzau VJ, Creager MA. Diseases of the aorta. In: Braunwald E, Fauci AS, Kasper D, et al., eds. Harrison's Principles of Internal Medicine. 15th Ed. New York: McGraw-Hill, 2001.

Fuster V, Halperin JL. Aortic dissection: a medical perspective. J Card Surg 1994;9:713–728.

Gerhard M, Creager MA. Raynaud's phenomenon: vasospastic disease and current therapy. In: Advances in Vascular Surgery, vol 2. St. Louis: Mosby-Year Book: 1994:245–275.

Hiatt WR. Medical treatment of peripheral arterial disease and claudication. N Engl J Med 2001;344: 1608–1621.

Loscalzo J, Creager MA, Dzau VJ, eds. Textbook of Vascular Medicine and Biology. Boston: Little, Brown & Co., 1996.

Nienaber CA, Fattori R, Lund G, et al. Nonsurgical reconstruction of thoracic aortic dissection by stent-graft placement. N Engl J Med 1999;340:1539–1545.

Olin JW. Thromboangiitis obliterans (Buerger's disease). N Engl J Med 2000;343:864–869.

Perrier A, Bounameaux H. Cost-effective diagnosis of deep-vein thrombosis and pulmonary embolism. Thromb Haemost 2001;86:475–487.

Congenital Heart Disease

Yi-Bin Chen, Richard R. Liberthson, and Michael D. Freed

Chapter
16

Normal Development of the Cardiovascular System
  Development of the Heart Tube
  Formation of the Heart Loop
  Septation
  Development of the Cardiac Valves

Fetal and Transitional Circulations
  Fetal Circulation
  Transitional Circulation
Common Congenital Heart Lesions
  Acyanotic Lesions
  Cyanotic Lesions
Eisenmenger Syndrome

Congenital heart diseases affect 8 of every 1000 live births. Some abnormalities are severe and require immediate medical attention, whereas many are less pronounced and have minimal clinical consequences. Although congenital heart defects are present at birth, milder defects may remain inapparent for weeks, months, or years and, not infrequently, may escape detection until adulthood.

The past half-century has seen tremendous growth in the understanding of the pathophysiology of congenital heart disease and substantial improvement in the ability to evaluate and treat those afflicted. Research has shown that single gene defects, environmental factors, maternal ingestion of toxic substances, and maternal sickness can all contribute to cardiac malformations. However, specific etiologies remain unknown in the majority of cases.

The survival of children with congenital heart disease has also improved dramatically in recent decades, due in large part to better diagnostic and surgical techniques. However, the lifelong needs of these patients include guidance regarding physical activity, pregnancy, endocarditis prophylaxis, insurance, and employment.

Formation of the cardiovascular system begins during the third week of embryonic development. Soon thereafter, a unique circulation develops that allows the fetus to mature in the uterus, using the placenta as the primary organ of gas, nutrient, and waste exchange. At birth, the fetal lungs inflate and become functional, making the placenta unnecessary and dramatically altering circulation patterns to allow the neonate to adjust to life outside the womb. Given the remarkable complexity of these processes, it is easy to envision ways that cardiovascular malfunctions could develop.

This chapter begins with an overview of fetal cardiovascular development and then describes the most common forms of congenital heart disease.

NORMAL DEVELOPMENT OF THE CARDIOVASCULAR SYSTEM

By the middle of the third week of gestation, the nutrient and gas exchange needs of the rapidly growing embryo can no longer be met by diffusion alone, and the tissues begin to rely on the developing cardiovascular system to deliver these substances over long distances.

Development of the Heart Tube

At approximately day 17 of embryogenesis, mesenchymal cells proliferate at the cranial end of the early embryonic disc. They eventually form two longitudinal cell clusters known as angioblastic cords. These cords canalize and become paired endothelial heart tubes (Fig. 16.1). Lateral embryonic folding gradually causes these two tubes to oppose one another and allows them to fuse in the ventral midline, forming a single endocardial tube by day 22. From inside to outside, the layers of this primitive heart tube are an endothelial lining that becomes the endocardium, a layer of gelatinous connective tissue (cardiac jelly), and a thick muscular layer derived from the splanchnic mesoderm which develops into

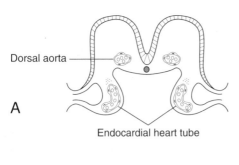

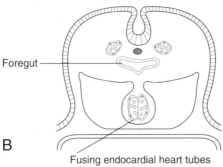

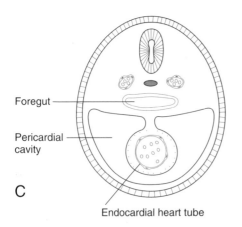

Figure 16.1. **Embryonic transverse sections illustrating fusion of the two heart tubes into a single endocardial heart tube. A.** 18 days. **B.** 21 days. **C.** 22 days.

the myocardium. The endocardial tube is continuous with the aortic arch system rostrally and with the venous system caudally. The primitive heart begins to beat around day 22–23, causing blood to circulate by the beginning of the fourth week. The space overlying the developing cardiac area eventually becomes the pericardial cavity, housing the future heart.

Formation of the Heart Loop

As the tubular heart grows and elongates, it develops a series of alternate constrictions and dilations, creating the first sign of the primitive heart chambers—the truncus arteriosus, the bulbus cordis, the primitive ventricle, the primitive atrium, and the sinus venosus (Fig. 16.2). Continued growth and elongation within the confined pericardial cavity force the heart tube to bend upon itself, eventually forming a U-shaped loop with the round end pointing ventrally and to the right. The result of this looping is placement of the atrium and sinus venosus above and behind the truncus arteriosus, bulbus cordis, and ventricle (Fig. 16.3). At this point, neither definitive septa between the developing chambers nor definitive valvular tissue have formed. The connection between the primitive atrium and ventricle is termed the **atrioventricular (AV) canal.** In time, the AV canal becomes two separate canals, one housing the tricuspid valve and the other the mitral valve. The sinus venosus is eventually incorporated into the right atrium, forming both the coronary sinus and a portion of the right atrial wall. The bulbus cordis and truncus arteriosus contribute to the future ventricular outflow tracts, forming parts of the proximal aorta and pulmonary artery.

Septation

Septation of the developing atrium, AV canal, and ventricle occurs between the fourth and sixth weeks. Although these events are described separately here, they actually occur simultaneously.

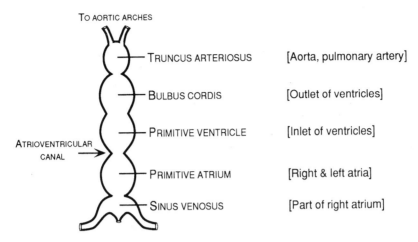

Figure 16.2. **The straight heart tube at approximately 22 days.** The structures that will ultimately form from each segment are listed in brackets.

Septation of the Atria

The primary atrial septum, also known as the **septum primum,** begins as a ridge of tissue on the roof of the common atrium that grows downward into the atrial cavity (Fig. 16.4). As the septum primum advances, it leaves a large opening known as the **ostium primum** between the crescent-shaped leading edge of the septum and the endocardial cushions (discussed below) surrounding the AV canal. The ostium primum allows passage of blood between the forming atria. Eventually, the septum primum fuses with the superior aspect of the endocardial cushions, obliterating the ostium primum. However, before closure of the ostium primum is complete, small perforations appear in the center of the septum primum that ultimately coalesce to form the **ostium secundum,** preserving a

pathway for blood flow between the atria (see Fig. 16.4). Following closure of the ostium primum, a second, more muscular membrane, the **septum secundum,** begins to develop immediately to the right of the superior aspect of the septum primum. This septum grows downward and overlaps the ostium secundum. The septum secundum eventually fuses with the endocardial cushions, although only in a partial fashion, leaving an oval-shaped opening known as the **foramen ovale.** The superior edge of septum primum then gradually regresses, leaving the lower edge to act as a "flap-like" valve that allows only right-to-left flow through the foramen ovale (Fig. 16.5). During gestation, blood passes from the right atrium to the left atrium because the pressure in the fetal right atrium is greater than that of the left atrium. This pressure gradient changes direction post-

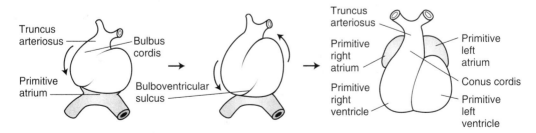

Figure 16.3. **Formation of the heart loop. Left, middle.** By day 24 continued growth and elongation within the confined pericardial space necessitate bending of the heart tube upon itself, forming a U-shaped loop that points ventrally and to the right. **Right.** Looping eventually places the atria above and behind the primitive ventricles.

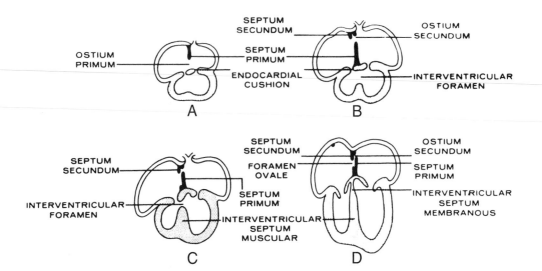

Figure 16.4. **Atrial septal formation at 30 days (A), 33 days (B), and 37 days (C) of development as well as in the newborn (D).** As the septum primum grows toward the ventricles, the opening between it and the AV canal is the ostium primum. Before the ostium primum completely closes, perforations within the upper portion of the septum primum form the ostium secundum. A second ridge of tissue, the septum secundum, grows downward to the right of the septum primum, partially covering the ostium secundum. The foramen ovale is an opening of the septum secundum that is covered by the "flap-valve" of the lower septum primum. (Modified from Moss AJ, Adams FH. Heart Disease in Infants, Children, and Adolescents. Baltimore: Williams & Wilkins, 1968:16.)

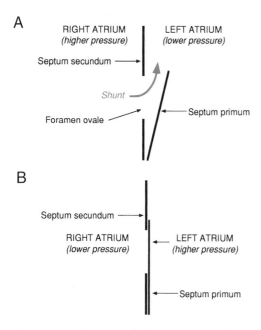

Figure 16.5. **Diagrammatic depiction of the flap-type valve of the foramen ovale. A.** Before birth, the valve permits only right-to-left flow of blood from the higher-pressured right atrium (RA) to the lower-pressured left atrium (LA). **B.** Following birth, the pressure in the LA becomes greater than that in the RA, causing the septum primum to close firmly against the septum secundum. (Modified from Moore KL, Persaud TVN. The Developing Human. Philadelphia: WB Saunders, 1993:318.)

natally, causing the valve to close, as described below.

Septation of the Atrioventricular Canal

Growth of the **endocardial cushions** contributes to atrial septation, and as described later, to the membranous portion of the interventricular septum. Endocardial cushions initially begin as swellings of the gelatinous connective tissue layer within the AV canal. They are then populated by migrating cells from the primitive endocardium which subsequently transform into mesenchymal tissue. The majority of tissue growth is in the horizontal plane, resulting in septation of the AV canal through the continued growth of the lateral, superior, and inferior endocardial cushions (Fig. 16.6). Septation creates separate right and left canals that give rise to the tricuspid and mitral orifices, respectively.

Septation of the Ventricles and Ventricular Outflow Tracts

At the end of the fourth week, the primitive ventricle begins to grow, leaving a me-

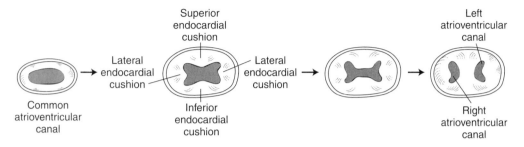

Figure 16.6. **The progression of septal formation in the atrioventricular canal through successive stages.** The septum forms through growth of the superior, inferior, and lateral endocardial cushions. The endocardial cushions are masses of mesenchymal tissue that surround the atrioventricular canal and aid in the formation of the orifices of the mitral and tricuspid valves, as well as the upper interventricular septum and lower interatrial septum.

dian muscular ridge, the primitive interventricular septum. The majority of the early increase in height of the septum is due to dilation of the two new ventricles forming on either side of it. Only later does new cell growth in the septum itself contribute to its size. The free edge of the muscular interventricular septum does not fuse with the endocardial cushions; the opening that remains and allows communication between the right and left ventricles is the interventricular foramen (Fig. 16.7). This remains open until the end of the seventh week of gestation, at which time fusion of tissue from the right and left bulbar ridges (see below) and the endocardial cushions forms the membranous portion of the interventricular septum.

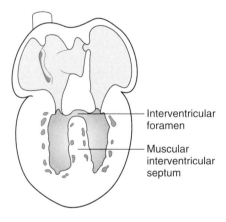

Figure 16.7. **The interventricular septum and the interventricular foramen.** (Modified from Moore KL, Persaud TVN. The Developing Human. Philadelphia: WB Saunders, 1993:325.)

During the fifth week, neural crest-derived mesenchymal proliferation occurring in the bulbus cordis and truncus arteriosus creates a pair of protrusions known as the bulbar ridges (Fig. 16.8). These ridges fuse in the midline and undergo a 180° spiraling process, forming the aorticopulmonary septum. This septum divides the bulbus cordis and the truncus arteriosus into two separate arterial channels, the pulmonary artery and the aorta, the former continuous with the right ventricle (RV) and the latter with the left ventricle (LV).

Development of the Cardiac Valves

Semilunar Valve Development (Aortic and Pulmonary Valves)

The semilunar valves start to develop just before the completion of the aorticopulmonary septum. The process begins when three outgrowths of subendocardial mesenchymal tissue form around both the aortic and pulmonary orifices. These growths are ultimately shaped and excavated by the joint action of programmed cell death and blood flow to create the three thin-walled cusps of both the aortic and pulmonary valves.

Atrioventricular Valve Development (Mitral and Tricuspid Valves)

After the endocardial cushions fuse to form the septa between the right and left AV canals, the surrounding subendocardial mesenchymal tissue proliferates and devel-

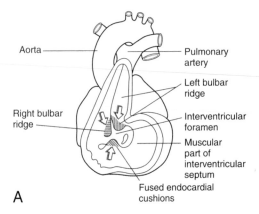

A

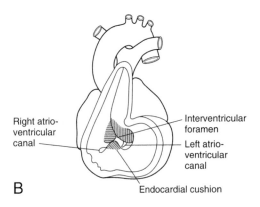

B

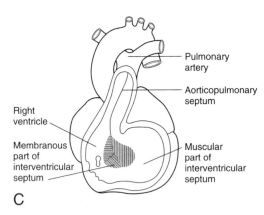

C

Figure 16.8. **Formation of the aorticopulmonary septum occurs via fusion of the bulbar ridges, resulting in division of the bulbus cordis and truncus arteriosus into the aorta and pulmonary artery (A, 5 weeks; B, 6 weeks; C, 7 weeks).** The bulbus cordis becomes the right ventricular outflow tract. Fusion of tissue from the endocardial cushions, the aorticopulmonary septum, and the muscular interventricular septum creates the membranous interventricular septum. (Modified from Moore KL, Persaud TVN. The Developing Human. Philadelphia: WB Saunders, 1993:322.)

ops outgrowths similar to those of the semilunar valves. These are also sculpted by programmed cell death that occurs within the inferior surface of the nascent leaflets and in the ventricular wall. This process leaves behind only a few, fine muscular strands to connect the valves to the ventricular wall (Fig. 16.9). The superior portions of these strands eventually degenerate and are replaced by strings of dense connective tissue, becoming the chordae tendineae.

FETAL AND TRANSITIONAL CIRCULATIONS

The fetal circulation is elegantly designed to serve the needs of in utero development. At the time of birth, the circulation automatically undergoes modifications that establish the normal blood flow pattern of a newborn infant.

Fetal Circulation

In fetal life, oxygenated blood leaves the placenta through the umbilical vein (Fig. 16.10). Approximately half of this blood is shunted through the fetal **ductus venosus,** bypassing the hepatic vasculature, and proceeding directly into the inferior vena cava (IVC). The remaining blood passes through the portal vein to the liver and then into the IVC through the hepatic veins. IVC blood is therefore composed of a mixture of *well-oxygenated* umbilical venous blood and the blood of *low oxygen tension* returning from the systemic veins of the fetus. Because of this mixture, the oxygen tension of inferior vena caval blood is higher than that of blood returning to the fetal right atrium from the superior vena cava. This distinction is important because these two streams of blood are partially separated within the right atrium to follow different circulatory paths. The consequence of this separation is that the fetal brain and myocardium receive blood of relatively higher oxygen content, whereas the more poorly oxygenated blood is diverted to the placenta (via the descending aorta and umbilical arteries) for subsequent oxygenation.

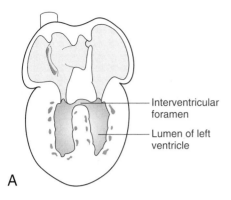

Interventricular foramen

Lumen of left ventricle

A

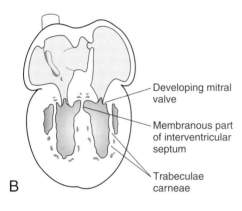

Developing mitral valve

Membranous part of interventricular septum

Trabeculae carneae

B

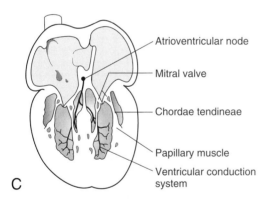

Atrioventricular node

Mitral valve

Chordae tendineae

Papillary muscle

Ventricular conduction system

C

Figure 16.9. Proliferation of mesenchymal tissue surrounding the atrioventricular canals forms the atrioventricular valves. Degeneration of myocardium and replacement by connective tissue forms the chordae tendineae; their muscular attachments to the ventricular wall are the papillary muscles. (Modified from Moore KL, Persaud TVN. The Developing Human. Philadelphia: WB Saunders, 1993:325.)

The majority of IVC blood entering the right atrium is directed to the left atrium through the foramen ovale. This intracardiac shunt of relatively well-oxygenated blood is facilitated by the inferior border of

the septum secundum, termed the crista dividens, which is positioned such that it overrides the opening of the IVC into the right atrium. This shunted blood then mixes with the small amount of poorly oxygenated blood returning to the left atrium through the fetal pulmonary veins (remember that the lungs are not ventilated in utero; the developing pulmonary tissues actually *remove* oxygen from the blood). From the left atrium, blood flows into the LV and is then pumped into the ascending aorta. This well-oxygenated blood is distributed primarily to three territories: 1) approximately 9% enters the coronary arteries and perfuses the myocardium, 2) 62% travels in the carotid and subclavian vessels to the upper body and brain, and 3) 29% passes into the descending aorta to the rest of the fetal body.

The remaining well-oxygenated inferior vena caval blood entering the right atrium mixes with poorly oxygenated blood from the superior vena cava and passes to the RV. In the fetus, the RV is the actual "workhorse" of the heart, providing two-thirds of the total cardiac output. This output flows into the pulmonary artery and from there through either the **ductus arteriosus** into the descending aorta (88% of RV output) or through the pulmonary arteries and into the lungs (12% of RV output). This unequal distribution of right ventricular outflow is actually quite efficient. Bypassing the lungs is desired because the fetal lungs are filled with amniotic fluid and are incapable of gas exchange. The low oxygen tension of this fluid causes constriction of the pulmonary vessels, which increases pulmonary vascular resistance and facilitates shunting of blood through the ductus arteriosus to the systemic circulation. From the descending aorta, there is distribution of blood to the lower body and to the umbilical arteries, leading back to the placenta for gas exchange.

Transitional Circulation

Immediately following birth, the neonate rapidly adjusts to life outside the womb. The newly functioning lungs replace the

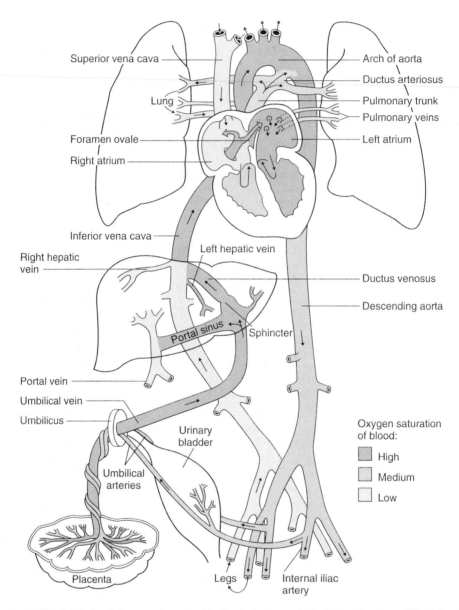

Figure 16.10. The fetal circulation, as described in the text. Arrows indicate the direction of blood flow. Three shunts (ductus venosus, foramen ovale, and ductus arteriosus) allow the majority of the blood to bypass the lungs and liver during fetal life, but cease to function shortly after birth. (Modified from Moore KL, Persaud TVN. The Developing Human. Philadelphia: WB Saunders, 1993:344.)

placenta as the organ of gas exchange, and the three shunts (ductus venosus, foramen ovale, and ductus arteriosus) that operated during gestation close. This shift in the site of gas exchange and the resulting changes in cardiovascular architecture allow the newborn to survive independently.

As the umbilical cord is clamped, or constricts naturally, the low-resistance placental flow is removed from the arterial sys-

tem, resulting in an increase in vascular resistance. There is also an accompanying fall in pulmonary vascular resistance for two reasons: 1) the mechanical inflation of the lungs after birth stretches the lung tissues, causing pulmonary artery expansion and wall thinning, and 2) vasodilatation of the pulmonary vasculature in response to the rise in blood oxygen tension accompanying aeration of the lungs. This reduction in pulmonary resistance results in a dramatic rise in pulmonary blood flow. It is most marked within the first day after birth but continues for the next several weeks until adult levels of pulmonary resistance are achieved.

As pulmonary resistance falls and more blood travels to the lungs via the pulmonary artery, venous return from the pulmonary veins to the left atrium also increases, causing left atrial pressure to rise. At the same time, cessation of umbilical venous flow and constriction of the ductus venosus cause a fall in IVC and right atrial pressures. As a result, the left atrial pressure becomes greater than that in the right atrium, and the valve of the foramen ovale is forced against the septum secundum, eliminating the previous flow between the atria (see Fig. 16.5).

With oxygenation now occurring in the newborn lungs, the ductus arteriosus becomes superfluous and begins to constrict. During fetal life, a high circulating level of prostaglandin E_1 (PGE_1) is generated in response to relative hypoxia, which causes the smooth muscle of the ductus arteriosus to relax, keeping it patent. After birth, PGE_1 levels decline as oxygen tension rises and the ductus constricts. The responsiveness of the ductus to vasoactive substances depends on the gestational age of the fetus. The ductus often fails to constrict in premature infants, resulting in a congenital anomaly, patent ductus arteriosus (discussed below).

With the anatomic separation of the circulatory paths of the right and left sides of the heart now complete, the cardiac output of the LV increases, while that of the RV decreases such that the output of each becomes equal. The augmented pressure and volume load placed on the LV induces the myocardial cells of that chamber to hypertrophy, while the decreased pressure and volume loads on the RV result in gradual regression of RV wall thickness.

COMMON CONGENITAL HEART LESIONS

Congenital heart defects are generally well tolerated before birth. In utero, the fetus benefits from shunting of blood through the ductus arteriosus and the foramen ovale, allowing the bypass of most defects. It is only after birth, when the neonate has been separated from the maternal circulation and the oxygenation it provides and the fetal shunts have closed, that congenital heart defects usually become manifest.

Congenital heart lesions can be categorized as "cyanotic" or "acyanotic." Cyanosis refers to a blue-purple discoloration of the skin and mucous membranes due to an elevated blood concentration of deoxygenated hemoglobin (at least 4 g/dL, which corresponds to an arterial O_2 saturation of approximately 80–85%). In congenital heart disease, cyanosis results from defects that allow poorly oxygenated blood from the right side of the heart to be shunted to the left side, bypassing the lungs.

Acyanotic lesions include intracardiac or vascular stenoses, valvular regurgitation, and defects which result in *left-to-right* shunting of blood. Large left-to-right shunts at the atrial, ventricular, or great vessel level (all described below) cause the pulmonary artery volume and pressure to increase, and can be associated with the later development of pulmonary arteriolar hypertrophy and increased resistance to flow. Over time, the elevated pulmonary resistance may force the direction of the original shunt to reverse, that is, causing *right-to-left* flow to supervene, accompanied by the physical findings of hypoxemia and cyanosis. The development of such pulmonary vascular disease as a result of a chronic large left-to-right shunt is known as *Eisenmenger syndrome* and is described in greater detail below.

Acyanotic Lesions

Atrial Septal Defect

An atrial septal defect (ASD) is a persistent opening in the interatrial septum after birth that allows direct communication between the left and right atria. ASDs are relatively common, occurring with an incidence of 1 in every 1500 live births. They can occur anywhere along the atrial septum, but the most common site is at the region of the foramen ovale, termed an *ostium secundum* ASD (Fig. 16.11). This defect arises from excessive resorption or inadequate development of the septum primum, inadequate formation of the septum secundum, or a combination. Less commonly, an ASD appears in the inferior portion of the interatrial septum, adjacent to the AV valves. Named an *ostium primum* defect, this abnormality results from failure of the septum primum to fuse with the endocardial cushions and is typically associated with abnormal development of the mitral and tricuspid valves. A third type of ASD occurs in the superior portion of the atrial septum near the entry of the superior vena cava and is termed a *sinus venosus* ASD. It results from incomplete absorption of the sinus venosus into the right atrium and is often accompanied by the anomalous drainage of pulmonary veins from the right lung into the right atrium.

In distinction, a *patent foramen ovale (PFO)*, which is thought to be present in approximately 20% of the general population, is not a true ASD. As described above, the foramen ovale functionally shuts in the days after birth, and anatomically closes by the age of 6 months through fusion of the atrial septa. PFOs arise when there is failure of this fusion to occur.

A PFO is usually clinically silent because the one-way valve, while not sealed, remains functionally closed due to the higher LA pressure compared with that in the right atrium. However, a PFO takes on added significance if the right atrial pressure becomes elevated (e.g., in states of pulmonary hypertension or right-heart failure), resulting in pathologic *right-to-left* intracardiac shunting. In that case, deoxygenated blood passes directly into the arterial circulation. Occasionally, a PFO can be implicated in a patient who has suffered a systemic embolism (e.g., a stroke). This situation, termed *paradoxical embolism*, occurs when thrombus in a systemic vein breaks loose, travels to the right atrium, passes across the PFO to the left atrium (*if* right-to-left shunting is present because of elevated right-heart pressures), and passes into the systemic arterial circulation.

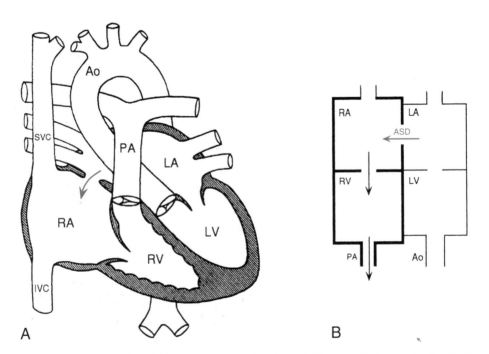

Figure 16.11. Atrial septal defect (ASD), ostium secundum type. A. The arrow indicates shunted flow from the left atrium (LA) toward the right atrium (RA). **B.** Schematic representation of blood flow through an uncomplicated ASD, resulting in enlargement of the RA, right ventricle (RV), and pulmonary artery (PA). Ao, aorta; IVC, inferior vena cava; SVC, superior vena cava.

Pathophysiology

In the uncomplicated case of an ASD, oxygenated blood from the left atrium is shunted into the right atrium, but not vice versa. Flow through the defect is a function of its size and the filling properties (compliance) of the ventricles into which the atria pass their contents. Normally after birth, right ventricular compliance becomes greater than that of the LV due to the regression of right ventricular wall thickness, facilitating a left-to-right directed shunt. The result is volume overload and enlargement of the right atrium and RV (see Fig. 16.11B). If right ventricular compliance decreases over time (because of the excessive load), the left-to-right shunt may become less. Occasionally, if severe pulmonary vascular disease develops (Eisenmenger syndrome), the direction of the shunt may actually reverse (causing right-to-left flow), such that desaturated blood enters the systemic circulation, resulting in hypoxemia and cyanosis.

Symptoms

The great majority of infants with an ASD are asymptomatic. Frequently, the condition is detected by a murmur on routine physical examination when they are school-aged children. If symptoms do occur, they include dyspnea on exertion, fatigue, and recurrent lower respiratory tract infections. The most common symptoms in adults are decreased stamina and palpitations due to atrial tachyarrhythmias resulting from right atrial enlargement.

Physical Examination

A prominent systolic impulse may be palpated along the lower left sternal border, representing contraction of the dilated RV (RV "heave"). The second heart sound (S_2) demonstrates a widened, fixed splitting pattern (see Chapter 2), because the normal respiratory variation in systemic venous return is countered by reciprocal changes in the volume of blood shunted across the ASD. The increased volume of blood flowing across the pulmonary valve often creates a systolic murmur at the upper left sternal border. A mid-diastolic murmur may also be present at the lower left sternal border due to the increased flow across the tricuspid valve. Blood traversing the ASD itself does not produce a murmur because of the absence of a significant pressure gradient between the two atria.

Laboratory Studies

On *chest radiographs*, the heart is usually enlarged due to right atrial and right ventricular dilatation, and there is prominence of the pulmonary artery with increased pulmonary vascular markings. The *ECG* shows right ventricular hypertrophy, often with right atrial enlargement and incomplete or complete right bundle branch block. In patients with the ostium primum type of ASD, left axis deviation is common and is thought to be due to displacement and hypoplasia of the left anterior fascicle. *Echocardiography* demonstrates right atrial and right ventricular enlargement; the ASD may be visualized directly, or its presence implied by the demonstration of a transatrial shunt by Doppler flow interrogation. The magnitude and direction of shunt flow and an estimation of right ventricular systolic pressure can be determined.

Given the high sensitivity of echocardiography, it is rarely necessary to perform *cardiac catheterization* to confirm the presence of an ASD. However, catheterization may be useful to assess the pulmonary vascular resistance and to diagnose concurrent coronary artery disease in older adults. In a normal individual undergoing cardiac catheterization, the oxygen saturations measured in the right atrium and superior vena cava are approximately equal, but in the presence of an ASD with left-to-right flow, the oxygen saturation of the right atrium is greater, because of shunting of oxygenated left atrial blood into the right atrium.

Treatment

Most patients with an ASD remain active and asymptomatic. However, if the volume of shunted blood is large (even in the absence of symptoms), elective surgical repair is recommended to prevent the development of heart failure or pulmonary vascular disease. The defect is repaired via direct suture closure or with a pericardial or a synthetic patch. In children and young adults, morphologic changes in the right heart often return to normal after repair. Catheter-based interventions (i.e., devices that close the defect, deployed via an intravenous catheter) are still under study but will likely allow safe and effective repair for many patients.

Ventricular Septal Defect

A ventricular septal defect (VSD) is an abnormal opening in the interventricular septum (Fig. 16.12). VSDs are relatively common and have an incidence of 1.5–3.5 per every 1000 live births. They are most often located in the membranous (70%) and muscular (20%) portions of the septum with a small minority of defects occurring just below the aortic valve or adjacent to the AV valves.

Pathophysiology

The hemodynamic changes that accompany VSDs depend on the size of the defect and the relative resistances of the pulmonary and systemic vasculatures. In small VSDs, the defect itself offers more resistance to flow than the pulmonary or systemic vasculature, so that the magnitude of the shunt depends on the size of the hole. Conversely, with larger "nonrestrictive" defects, the volume of the shunt is determined by the relative pulmonary and systemic vascular resistances. In the perinatal period, the pulmonary vascular resistance approximates the systemic vascular resistance, and minimal shunting occurs between the two ventricles. After birth, how-

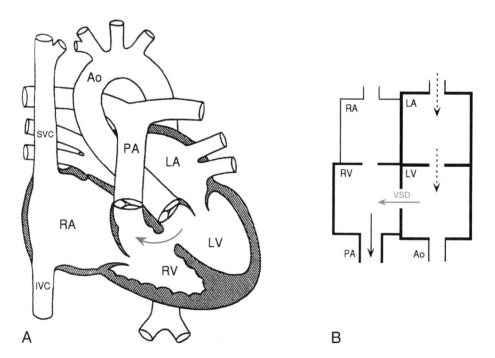

Figure 16.12. Ventricular septal defect (VSD). A. The arrow indicates shunted flow from the left ventricle (LV) toward the right ventricular (RV) outflow tract. **B.** Schematic representation of blood flow through an uncomplicated VSD. The dashed lines represent increased blood return to the left side of the heart as a result of the shunt, which causes enlargement primarily of the left atrium (LA) and left ventricle (LV). Ao, aorta; IVC, inferior vena cava; PA, pulmonary artery; RA, right atrium; SVC, superior vena cava.

ever, as the pulmonary vascular resistance falls, an increasing left-to-right shunt through the defect develops. When this shunt is large, the RV, pulmonary circulation, left atrium, and LV all experience a relative volume overload. Initially, the increased blood return to the LV augments stroke volume (via the Frank-Starling mechanism), but over time the increased volume load can result in chamber dilatation, systolic dysfunction, and symptoms of heart failure. In addition, the augmented circulation through the pulmonary vasculature can cause pulmonary vascular disease as early as 2 years of age. As pulmonary vascular resistance increases, the intracardiac shunt may reverse its direction (Eisenmenger syndrome) with the development of systemic hypoxemia and cyanosis.

Symptoms

Patients with a small VSD typically remain symptom free. Conversely, 10% of infants with a VSD have a large defect and will develop early symptoms of congestive heart failure which include tachypnea, poor feeding, failure to thrive, and frequent lower respiratory tract infections. Patients with VSDs complicated by pulmonary vascular disease and reversed shunts may present with dyspnea and cyanosis. Bacterial endocarditis can develop regardless of the size of the VSD.

Physical Examination

The most common physical finding is a harsh holosystolic murmur that is best heard at the left sternal border. Smaller defects tend to have the loudest murmurs, owing to the great turbulence of flow that they cause. A systolic thrill can commonly be palpated in the region of the murmur. In addition, a mid-diastolic rumble can often be heard at the apex due to the increased flow across the mitral valve. If pulmonary vascular disease develops, the holosystolic murmur diminishes as flow decreases through the defect. In these patients, an RV heave, a loud pulmonic closure sound (P_2), and cyanosis may be evident.

Laboratory Studies

On *chest radiographs*, the cardiac silhouette may be normal in patients with small defects, but in those with large shunts, cardiomegaly and prominent pulmonary vascular markings are present. If there is pulmonary vascular disease, enlarged pulmonary arteries with peripheral tapering may be evident. The *ECG* shows left atrial enlargement and left ventricular hypertrophy in those with a large shunt. If pulmonary vascular disease develops, right ventricular hypertrophy usually becomes evident. *Echocardiography* with Doppler studies can accurately determine the location of the VSD, identify the direction and magnitude of the shunt, and provide an estimate of right ventricular systolic pressure. *Cardiac catheterization* demonstrates increased oxygen saturation in the RV compared with the right atrium, due to shunting of highly oxygenated blood from the LV into the RV.

Treatment

By the age of 2, at least 50% of small- and moderate-sized VSDs undergo sufficient partial or complete spontaneous closure to make intervention unnecessary. Surgical correction of the defect is recommended in the first few months of life for children with congestive heart failure or pulmonary vascular disease. Moderate-sized defects without pulmonary vascular disease, but with significant volume overload, can be corrected later in childhood. Less invasive catheter-based treatments are still investigational. Medical management includes endocarditis prophylaxis for all VSD patients.

Patent Ductus Arteriosus

The ductus arteriosus is the vessel that connects the left pulmonary artery to the descending aorta during fetal life. Patent ductus arteriosus (PDA) results when the ductus fails to close after birth, resulting in a persistent connection between the great vessels (Fig. 16.13). It has an overall incidence of about 1 in every 2500–5000 live births. Risk factors for its presence include

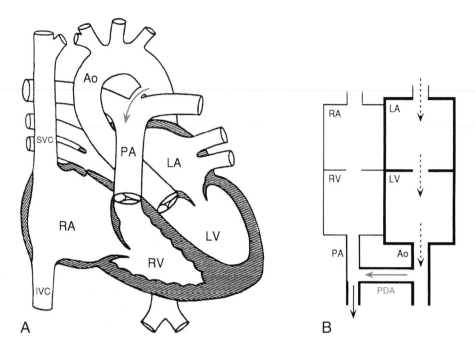

Figure 16.13. **Patent ductus arteriosus (PDA). A.** The arrow indicates shunted flow from the descending aorta (Ao) toward the pulmonary artery (PA). **B.** Schematic representation of blood flow through an uncomplicated PDA. The dashed lines represent increased blood return to the left side of the heart as a result of the shunt, which causes enlargement of the left atrium (LA), left ventricle (LV), and Ao. IVC, inferior vena cava; RA, right atrium; RV, right ventricle; SVC, superior vena cava.

first trimester maternal rubella infection, prematurity, and birth at high altitudes.

Pathophysiology

As described above, the smooth muscle of the ductus arteriosus usually constricts after birth due to the sudden rise in blood oxygen tension and a reduction in the level of circulating prostaglandins. Over the next several weeks, intimal proliferation and fibrosis result in permanent closure. Failure of the ductus to close results in a persistent shunt between the descending aorta and the left pulmonary artery. The magnitude of flow through the shunt depends on the cross-sectional area and length of the ductus itself as well as the relative resistances of the systemic and pulmonary vasculatures. Prenatally, when the pulmonary vascular resistance is high, the blood is diverted away from the immature lungs to the aorta. As the pulmonary resistance drops postnatally, the shunt reverses direction and blood flows from the aorta into the

pulmonary circulation instead. Due to this left-to-right shunt, the pulmonary circulation, left atrium, and LV become volume overloaded. This can lead to left ventricular dilatation and left-sided heart failure, whereas the right heart remains normal unless pulmonary vascular disease ensues. If the latter does develop, Eisenmenger physiology results with reversal of the shunt, such that blood flows from the pulmonary artery, through the ductus, to the descending aorta. In that case, the flow of desaturated blood to the lower extremities causes cyanosis of the feet; the upper extremities are not cyanotic, because they receive normally saturated blood from the proximal aorta.

Symptoms

Children with a small PDA are generally asymptomatic. Those with a large left-to-right shunt develop early congestive heart failure with tachycardia, poor feeding, slow growth, and recurrent lower respiratory tract infections. Moderate-sized lesions can present with fatigue, dyspnea, and palpitations in adolescence and adult life. Atrial fibrillation may occur owing to left atrial dilatation. Turbulent blood flow across the defect can set the stage for endovascular infection (similar to endocarditis [Chapter 8] but more accurately termed "endarteritis").

Physical Examination

The most common finding in patients with left-to-right shunting through a PDA is a *continuous, machine-like* murmur (see Fig. 2.10, page 41), heard best at the left subclavicular region. The murmur is present throughout the cardiac cycle because a pressure gradient exists between the aorta and pulmonary artery in both systole and diastole. However, if pulmonary vascular disease develops, the gradient between the aorta and the pulmonary artery decreases, leading to diminished flow through the PDA, and the murmur becomes shorter (the diastolic component may disappear). If Eisenmenger physiology develops, lower extremity cyanosis and clubbing may be present on examination due to shunting of poorly oxygenated blood to the descending aorta.

Laboratory Studies

With a large PDA, the *chest radiograph* shows an enlarged cardiac silhouette (left atrial and left ventricular enlargement) with prominent pulmonary vascular markings. In adults, calcification of the ductus may be visualized. The *ECG* shows left atrial enlargement and left ventricular hypertrophy when a large shunt is present. *Echocardiography* with Doppler imaging can visualize the defect, demonstrate flow through it, and estimate right-sided systolic pressures. *Cardiac catheterization* is usually unnecessary. When performed in patients with a left-to-right shunt, it demonstrates a step-up in oxygen saturation in the pulmonary artery compared with the RV, and angiography shows the abnormal flow of blood through the PDA.

Treatment

In the absence of other congenital cardiac abnormalities or severe pulmonary vascular disease, PDA should generally be occluded. Although many spontaneously close during the first months after birth, this rarely occurs later. Given the constant risk of endarteritis and minimal complications of current corrective procedures, even a small asymptomatic PDA is commonly referred for closure. For neonates and premature infants with congestive heart failure, a trial of prostaglandin synthesis inhibitors (e.g., indomethacin) can be administered to encourage constriction of the ductus. Definitive closure can be accomplished by surgical division or ligation of the ductus or by transcatheter techniques in which an occluding coil is placed.

Congenital Aortic Stenosis

Congenital aortic stenosis (AS) is most often caused by abnormal development of the aortic valve (Fig. 16.14). It is four times as common in males as in females, and 20% of patients have an additional abnormality, most commonly coarctation of the aorta (see below). The aortic valve in congenital AS usually has a bicuspid leaflet structure, instead of the normal tricuspid configuration, causing an eccentric stenotic opening through which blood is ejected. Bicuspid aortic valves are common, appearing in approximately 2% of the population. Although they only rarely result in congenital AS, they are a common cause of AS in adults as the leaflets fibrose and calcify over time (see Chapter 8).

Pathophysiology

Because the valvular orifice is narrowed, left ventricular systolic pressure must increase to pump blood across the valve into the aorta. In response to this increased pressure load, the LV hypertrophies. The high-velocity jet of blood that passes through the stenotic valve may impact on the proximal aortic wall and contribute to dilatation of that vessel as well.

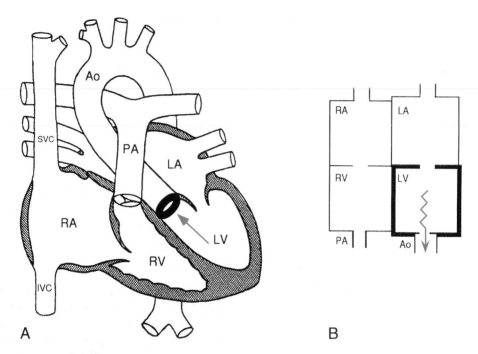

Figure 16.14. Congenital valvular aortic stenosis. A. The arrow points to the narrowed aortic valve. **B.** Schematic representation of obstructed flow through the narrowed aortic valve (jagged arrow). Left ventricular (LV) hypertrophy results from the chronic increased pressure load. Poststenotic dilatation of the aorta (Ao) is common. IVC, inferior vena cava; LA, left atrium; PA, pulmonary artery; RA, right atrium; RV, right ventricle; SVC, superior vena cava.

Symptoms

The clinical picture of AS depends on the severity of the lesion. Fewer than 10% of infants experience symptoms of heart failure before the age of 1, but if they do, they manifest tachycardia, tachypnea, failure to thrive, and poor feeding. Most older children with congenital AS are asymptomatic and develop normally. When symptoms do occur, they are similar to those of adult AS and include easily being fatigued, exertional dyspnea, angina pectoris, and syncope (see Chapter 8).

Physical Examination

Auscultation reveals a harsh crescendo-decrescendo systolic murmur, loudest at the base of the heart with radiation to the neck. It is often preceded by a systolic ejection click (see Chapter 2), especially when a bicuspid valve is present. Unlike the murmurs of ASD, VSD, or PDA, the murmur of congenital AS is characteristically present from birth as it is not dependent on a decline in pulmonary vascular resistance. With advanced disease, the ejection time becomes longer, causing the peak of the murmur to occur later in systole. In severe disease, the significantly prolonged ejection time causes a delay in closure of the aortic valve such that A_2 occurs *after* closure of the pulmonary valve (P_2)—a phenomenon known as reversed splitting of S_2 (see Chapter 2).

Laboratory Studies

The *chest radiograph* of an infant with AS may show an enlarged LV and a dilated ascending aorta. The *ECG* often shows left ventricular hypertrophy. *Echocardiography* can identify the structure of the aortic valve and the degree of left ventricular hypertrophy. Doppler assessment can accurately estimate the pressure gradient across the stenotic valve and measure the reduced valve area. *Cardiac catheterization* confirms the pressure gradient across the valve.

Treatment

In its milder forms, AS does not need to be corrected, but endocarditis prophylaxis should be followed (see Chapter 8). Severe obstruction of the aortic valve during infancy may mandate immediate surgical or transcatheter balloon valvuloplasty. Generally, valvuloplasty in infancy is only palliative and future surgical revision is usually needed.

Pulmonic Stenosis

Isolated pulmonic stenosis (Fig. 16.15) may occur at the level of the pulmonic valve (e.g., from congenitally fused valve commissures), within the body of the RV (due to obstruction in the RV outflow tract), or in the pulmonary artery itself. Valve stenosis is the most common form (>90% of cases).

Pathophysiology

The result of pulmonic stenosis is obstruction to right ventricular systolic ejection, which leads to increased right ventricular pressures and chamber hypertrophy. The clinical course is determined by the severity of the obstruction. In the setting of a normal cardiac output, a peak systolic transvalvular pressure gradient <50 mm Hg is considered *mild* pulmonic stenosis, between 50 and 80 mm Hg is *moderate* stenosis, and *severe* stenosis is defined by a peak gradient >80 mm Hg.

Symptoms

Children with mild or moderate pulmonary stenosis are asymptomatic. The diagnosis is often first made on discovery of a murmur heard during a routine physical examination. Severe stenosis may cause manifestations such as dyspnea with exertion, exercise intolerance and, with decom-

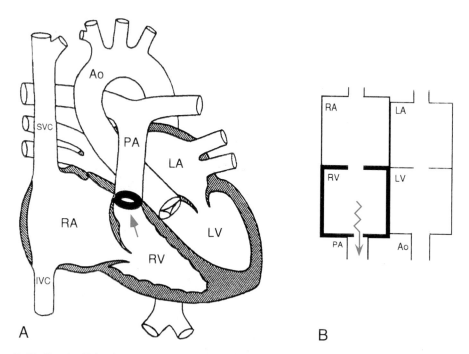

Figure 16.15. **Congenital pulmonary valve stenosis. A.** The arrow points to the narrowed pulmonary valve. **B.** Schematic representation of obstructed flow through the narrowed pulmonary valve (jagged arrow). Right ventricular hypertrophy results from the chronically increased pressure load. Ao, aorta; IVC, inferior vena cava; LA, left atrium; LV, left ventricle; PA, pulmonary artery; RA, right atrium; RV, right ventricle; SVC, superior vena cava.

pensation, symptoms of right-sided heart failure such as abdominal fullness and pedal edema.

Physical Examination

The physical findings in pulmonic stenosis depend on the severity of the obstruction. If the stenosis is severe with significant right ventricular hypertrophy, a prominent jugular venous "a" wave can be observed (see Chapter 2) and an RV heave is palpated over the sternum. A loud, late-peaking, crescendo-decrescendo systolic ejection murmur is heard at the upper left sternal border, often associated with a palpable thrill. Widened splitting of the S_2 with a soft P_2 component is caused by the delayed closure of the stenotic pulmonary valve.

In more moderate stenosis, a pulmonic ejection sound (a high-pitched "click") follows S_1 and precedes the systolic murmur. It occurs during the early phase of right ventricular contraction as the stenotic valve leaflets suddenly reach their maximum level of ascent into the pulmonary artery, just before blood ejection. Unlike other sounds and murmurs produced by the right side of the heart, the pulmonic ejection sound *diminishes* in intensity during inspiration. With inspiration, augmented right ventricular filling prematurely elevates the bodies of the leaflets into the pulmonary artery, preempting the rapid tensing that is thought to produce the sound when the RV contracts.

Laboratory Studies

The *chest radiograph* may demonstrate an enlarged right atrium and ventricle with poststenotic pulmonary artery dilation (due to the impact of the high-velocity jet of blood against the wall of the pulmonary artery). The *ECG* shows right ventricular hypertrophy and right axis deviation. *Echocardiography* with Doppler imaging assesses the pulmonary valve morphology, the presence of right ventricular hypertrophy, and the magnitude of obstruction.

Treatment

Mild pulmonic stenosis usually does not progress or require treatment. Moderate or severe valvular obstruction at the valvular level is treated by dilating the stenotic valve by transcatheter balloon valvuloplasty. Results after late follow-up for this procedure have uniformly been excellent, and right ventricular hypertrophy usually regresses after intervention. Antibiotic prophylaxis for endocarditis is required even after valvuloplasty.

Coarctation of the Aorta

Coarctation of the aorta is typically a discrete narrowing of the aortic lumen. This anomaly has an incidence of 1 in every 6000 live births and often occurs in patients with Turner's syndrome (45,XO). Two types of coarctation are distinguished according to the location of the aortic narrowing in relation to the ductus arteriosus: preductal (2%) and postductal (98%) (Fig. 16.16). *Preductal* coarctation, in which narrowing occurs proximal to the ductus, occurs when an intracardiac anomaly during fetal life de-

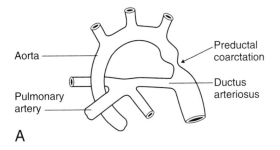

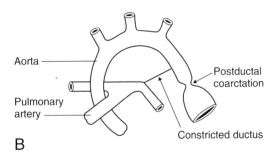

Figure 16.16. **Coarctation of the aorta. A.** Preductal coarctation. **B.** Postductal coarctation.

creases blood flow through the left side of the heart, resulting in hypoplastic development of the aorta. *Postductal* coarctation is most likely the result of muscular ductal tissue extending into the aorta during fetal life. When ductal tissue constricts following birth, the ectopic tissue within the aorta also constricts, creating an obstruction.

Pathophysiology

In both types of coarctation, the LV faces an increased pressure load. Blood flow to the head and upper extremities is preserved as the vessels supplying these areas usually branch off the aorta before the obstruction, while flow to the descending aorta and lower extremities may be diminished. If coarctation is not corrected, compensatory alterations include 1) the development of left ventricular hypertrophy, and 2) dilatation of compensatory collateral blood vessels from the intercostal arteries that bypass the coarctation and provide blood to the descending aorta. Eventually, these collateral vessels enlarge and can erode the undersurface of the ribs.

Symptoms

Patients with preductal and severe postductal coarctation usually present very shortly after birth with symptoms of heart failure. Infants with preductal coarctation may also exhibit *differential cyanosis* if the ductus arteriosus remains open. The upper half of the body, supplied by the LV and the ascending aorta, is perfused with well-oxygenated blood; however, the lower half appears cyanotic, as it is largely supplied by right-to-left flow (poorly oxygenated blood) from the pulmonary artery, across the ductus arteriosus into the descending aorta.

When the coarctation is less severe, as in most postductal cases, it may be suspected by finding hypertension on physical examination during childhood.

Physical Examination

On physical examination, the femoral pulses are weak and delayed. An elevated

blood pressure in the upper body is the most common presentation. If the coarctation occurs distal to the takeoff of the left subclavian artery, the systolic pressure in the arms is greater than that in the legs. If the coarctation occurs *proximal* to the takeoff of the left subclavian artery, the systolic pressure in the right arm may exceed that in the left arm. A systolic pressure in the right arm that is 15–20 mm Hg greater than that in a leg is sufficient to suspect coarctation because, normally, the systolic pressure in the leg is *higher* than that in the arm. A midsystolic ejection murmur (due to flow through the coarctation) may be audible over the chest and/or back. A prominent tortuous collateral arterial circulation may create continuous murmurs over the chest in adults.

Laboratory Studies

In adults in whom this anomaly is uncorrected, *chest radiography* generally reveals notching of the inferior surface of the posterior ribs due to enlarged intercostal vessels supplying collateral circulation to the descending aorta. An indented aorta at the site of coarctation may also be visualized. The *ECG* shows left ventricular hypertrophy due to the pressure load placed on that chamber. *Echocardiography* confirms the diagnosis of coarctation and assesses the pressure gradient across the lesion. *Magnetic resonance imaging (MRI)* demonstrates in detail the length and severity of coarctation. Diagnostic *catheterization* and angiography are rarely necessary.

Treatment

In neonates with severe obstruction, prostaglandin infusion is administered to keep the ductus arteriosus patent to maintain blood flow to the descending aorta before surgery is undertaken. In children, elective repair is usually performed to prevent systemic hypertension. There are several surgical procedures that have been used, including excision of the narrowed aortic segment with end-to-end reanastomosis and repair using a synthetic patch. For older children, adults, and patients with recurrent coarctation after previous repair, transcatheter interventions (balloon dilatation with or without stent placement) is usually successful. Antibiotic prophylaxis to prevent endarteritis (just like prophylaxis against endocarditis described in Chapter 8) is necessary even after repair.

Cyanotic Lesions

Tetralogy of Fallot

Tetralogy of Fallot results from a single developmental defect: an abnormal anterior and cephalad displacement of the infundibular (ventricular outflow tract) portion of the septum. As a consequence, four anomalies arise that characterize this condition (Fig. 16.17): 1) a VSD due to septal malalignment, 2) subvalvular pulmonic stenosis because of obstruction from the infundibular septum, 3) an overriding aorta that receives blood from both ventricles, and 4) right ventricular hypertrophy due to the high pressure load placed on the RV by the pulmonic stenosis. Tetralogy of Fallot is the most common form of cyanotic congenital heart disease seen after infancy and is often associated with other cardiac defects, such as a right-sided aortic arch (25% of patients), ASD (10% of patients), and less often anomalous origin of the left coronary artery.

Pathophysiology

Increased resistance by the subvalvular pulmonic stenosis causes deoxygenated blood returning from the systemic veins to be diverted from the RV, through the VSD, to the LV, and into the systemic circulation, resulting in systemic hypoxemia and cyanosis. The magnitude of shunt flow across the VSD is primarily a function of the severity of the pulmonary stenosis, but acute changes in the relative systemic and pulmonary vascular resistances can affect it as well.

Symptoms

Children with tetralogy of Fallot often experience dyspnea on exertion. *"Spells"* may occur following exertion, feeding, or crying when systemic vasodilatation results in an increased right-to-left shunt. Manifestations of such spells include irritability, cyanosis, hyperventilation, and occasionally syncope or convulsions. Children learn to alleviate their symptoms by squatting down, which is thought to increase systemic vascular resistance by "kinking" the femoral arteries, thereby decreasing the right-to-left shunt and directing more blood from the RV to the lungs.

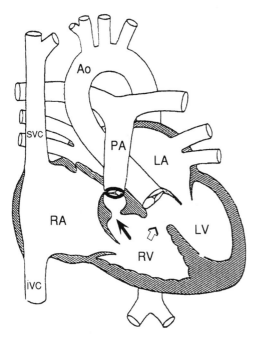

Figure 16.17. **Tetralogy of Fallot is characterized by four associated anomalies.** 1) A ventricular septal defect (hollow arrow), 2) obstruction to right ventricular outflow (solid arrow), 3) an overriding aorta that receives blood from both ventricles, and 4) right ventricular hypertrophy. Ao, aorta; IVC, inferior vena cava; LA, left atrium; LV, left ventricle; PA, pulmonary artery; RA, right atrium; RV, right ventricle; SVC, superior vena cava.

Physical Examination

Children with moderate pulmonary stenosis often have mild cyanosis, most notably of the lips, mucous membranes, and the digits. Those with severe pulmonary stenosis may present with profound cyanosis in the first few days of life. Chronic hypoxemia caused by the right-to-left shunt commonly results in clubbing of the fingers and toes. Right ventricular hypertrophy may be appreciated on physical examination as a palpable heave along the left sternal border. The S_2 is single, composed of a normal aortic component; the pulmonary component is soft and usually inaudible. A systolic ejection murmur heard best at the left upper sternal border is created by turbulent blood flow through the stenotic right ventricular outflow tract. There is usually no distinct murmur related to the VSD, as it is typically large and thus creates little turbulence.

Laboratory Studies

Chest radiography demonstrates prominence of the RV and a decrease in the size of the main pulmonary artery segment giving the appearance of a "boot-shaped" heart. Pulmonary vascular markings are typically diminished due to the decreased flow through the pulmonary circulation. The *ECG* shows evidence of right ventricular hypertrophy and right axis deviation. *Echocardiography* details the right ventricular outflow tract anatomy, the malaligned VSD, right ventricular hypertrophy, and other associated defects, as does *cardiac catheterization.*

Treatment

Before definitive surgical correction of tetralogy of Fallot was developed, several forms of palliative therapy were used. These involved creating anatomic communications between the aorta (or one of its major branches) to the pulmonary artery, creating a left-to-right shunt to increase pulmonary blood flow. Such procedures are occasionally used today for infants in whom definitive repair is planned at an older age. Complete surgical correction of tetralogy of Fallot involves closure of the VSD and enlargement of the subpulmonary infundibulum with the use of a pericardial

patch. Elective repair is usually recommended around age 1 to decrease the likelihood of future complications. Most patients who have undergone successful repair grow to become asymptomatic adults. However, antibiotic prophylaxis to prevent endocarditis is still required.

Transposition of the Great Arteries

Transposition of the great arteries (TGA) is present when the great vessels inappropriately arise from the opposite ventricle; that is, the aorta originates from the RV and the pulmonary artery originates from the LV (Fig. 16.18). This anomaly accounts for approximately 7% of congenital heart defects. Whereas tetralogy of Fallot is the most common etiology of cyanosis after infancy, TGA is the most common cause of cyanosis in the neonatal period.

The precise cause of transposition remains unknown. Historically, it was thought that failure of the aorticopulmonary septum to spiral in a normal fashion during fetal de-

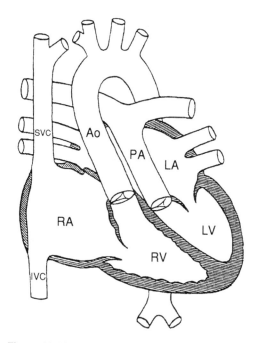

Figure 16.18. Transposition of the great arteries. The aorta (Ao) and pulmonary artery (PA) arise abnormally from the right ventricle (RV) and left ventricle (LV), respectively. IVC, inferior vena cava; LA, left atrium; RA, right atrium; SVC, superior vena cava.

velopment was the underlying problem. Recently, it has been suggested that the defect may be the result of abnormal growth and absorption of the subpulmonary and subaortic infundibuli during the division of the truncus arteriosus. Normally, reabsorption of the subaortic infundibulum places the forming aortic valve posterior and inferior to the pulmonary valve and in continuity with the LV. In TGA, the process of infundibular reabsorption is perhaps reversed, placing the pulmonary valve over the LV instead.

Pathophysiology

TGA separates the pulmonary and systemic circulations by placing the two circulations in parallel rather than in series. This arrangement forces desaturated blood from the systemic venous system to pass through the RV and then return to the systemic circulation through the aorta without undergoing normal oxygenation in the lungs. Similarly, oxygenated pulmonary venous return passes through the LV and then back through the pulmonary artery to the lungs without imparting oxygen to the systemic circulation. The end result is an extremely hypoxic, cyanotic neonate. Without intervention to create mixing between the two circulations, TGA is a lethal condition.

TGA is compatible with life in utero because flow through the ductus arteriosus and foramen ovale allows communication between the two circulations. Oxygenated fetal blood flows from the placenta through the umbilical vein to the right atrium, where the majority travels into the left atrium through the foramen ovale. The oxygenated blood in the left atrium then passes into the LV and is pumped out the pulmonary artery. The majority of pulmonary artery flow traverses the ductus arteriosus into the aorta instead of the high resistance pulmonary vessels, whereupon oxygen is provided to the developing tissues.

After birth, normal physiologic closure of the ductus and the foramen ovale eliminates the shunt between the parallel circulations and, without intervention, would result in death as oxygenated blood does not reach

the systemic tissues. However, if the ductus arteriosus and foramen ovale remain patent (either naturally, or with exogenous prostaglandins or surgical intervention), communication between the parallel circuits is maintained, and sufficiently oxygenated blood may be provided to the brain and other vital organs.

Symptoms and Physical Examination

Infants with transposition appear blue, with the intensity of the cyanosis dependent on the degree of intermixing between the parallel circuits. In most cases, generalized cyanosis is apparent on the first day of life and progresses rapidly as the ductus arteriosus closes. Palpation of the chest reveals a right ventricular impulse at the lower sternal border as the RV faces systemic pressures. Auscultation may reveal an accentuated S_2, which reflects closure of the anteriorly placed aortic valve just under the chest wall. Prominent murmurs are uncommon and may signal an additional defect.

Laboratory Studies

Chest radiography is usually normal, although the base of the heart may be narrow due to the more anterior-posterior orientation of the aorta and pulmonary artery. The *ECG* demonstrates right ventricular hypertrophy, reflecting the fact that the RV is the systemic "high-pressure" pumping chamber. The definitive diagnosis of transposition can be made by *echocardiography*, which demonstrates the abnormal orientation of the great vessels.

Treatment

TGA is a medical emergency. Initial treatment includes maintenance of the ductus arteriosus by prostaglandin infusion and creation of an interatrial communication using a balloon catheter (Rashkind procedure). These procedures allow adequate mixing of the two circulations until definitive corrective surgery can be performed. The current corrective procedure of choice is the "arterial-switch" operation (Jatene procedure), which involves transection of the great vessels above the semilunar valves and origin of the coronary arteries. The great vessels are then switched to the natural configuration, so the aorta arises from the LV and the pulmonary artery arises from the RV. The coronary arteries are then relocated to the new aorta.

EISENMENGER SYNDROME

Eisenmenger syndrome is the condition of severe pulmonary vascular obstruction that results from chronic left-to-right shunting through a congenital cardiac defect. The elevated pulmonary vascular pressure causes reversal of the original shunt (to the right-to-left direction) resulting in systemic cyanosis.

The mechanism by which increased pulmonary flow causes this condition is unknown. Histologically, the pulmonary arteriolar media hypertrophies and the intima proliferates, reducing the cross-sectional area of the pulmonary vascular bed. Ultimately, the vessels become thrombosed, and the resistance of the pulmonary vasculature rises, causing the left-to-right shunt to decrease. Eventually, if the resistance of the pulmonary circulation exceeds that of the systemic vasculature, the direction of shunt flow reverses.

With reversal of the shunt to the right-to-left direction, symptoms arise from hypoxemia, including exertional dyspnea and fatigue. Reduced hemoglobin saturation stimulates the bone marrow to produce more red blood cells (erythrocytosis), which can lead to hyperviscosity, symptoms of which include fatigue, headaches, and stroke (due to cerebrovascular occlusion). Infarction or rupture of the pulmonary vessels can result in hemoptysis.

On examination, a patient with Eisenmenger syndrome appears cyanotic with digital clubbing. A prominent "a" wave in the jugular venous pulsation represents elevated right-sided pressure during atrial contraction. A loud pulmonic closure sound (P_2) is common. The murmur of the inciting left-to-right shunt is usually *absent,* because the original pressure gradient across the lesion is negated by the elevated right-heart pressures.

Chest radiography in Eisenmenger syndrome is notable for proximal pulmonary artery dilatation with peripheral tapering. Calcification of the pulmonary vasculature may be seen. The *ECG* demonstrates right ventricular hypertrophy and right atrial enlargement. *Echocardiography* with Doppler studies can usually identify the underlying cardiac defect and quantitate the pulmonary artery systolic pressure.

Treatment includes the avoidance of activities that can exacerbate the right-to-left shunt. These include strenuous physical activity, high altitude, and the use of peripheral vasodilator drugs. Pregnancy is especially dangerous. The rate of spontaneous abortion is 20–40%, whereas the incidence of maternal mortality is 45%.

There is no reliably effective medical therapy to reduce the elevated pulmonary vascular resistance. Supportive measures include endocarditis prophylaxis, management of rhythm disturbances, and phlebotomy for patients with symptomatic erythrocytosis. The only effective long-term strategy for severely affected patients is lung or heart-lung transplantation.

SUMMARY

1. The significance of congenital heart lesions can be predicted from an understanding of cardiovascular embryonic development and the necessary transition to postnatal circulatory pathways.
2. Cardiac malformations occur in 0.8% of births. Such lesions can be grouped into cyanotic or acyanotic defects, depending on whether the abnormality results in pulmonary-to-systemic (right-to-left) shunting of blood.
3. Acyanotic defects often result in volume (ASD, VSD, PDA) or pressure (AS, pulmonic stenosis, coarctation of the aorta) overload. Chronic volume overload due to a large left-to-right shunt can ultimately result in increased pulmonary

vascular resistance, reversal of the direction of shunt flow, and subsequent cyanosis (Eisenmenger syndrome).

4. Among the most common cyanotic defects are tetralogy of Fallot and TGA.

Acknowledgment   The authors thank Emily McIntosh for her assistance. Contributors to the previous editions of this chapter were Lakshmi Halasyamani, MD; Andrew Karson, MD; Douglas W. Green, MD; Raymond Tabibiazar, MD; and Michael Freed, MD.

ADDITIONAL READING

Allen HD, Gutgesell HP, Clark EB, et al., eds. Moss and Adams' Heart Disease in Infants, Children and Adolescents. 6th Ed. Baltimore: Lippincott Williams & Wilkins, 2001.

Brickner ME, Hillis LD, Lange RA. Congenital heart disease in adults, part I of II. N Engl J Med 2000;342(4):256–263.

Brickner ME, Hillis LD, Lange RA. Congenital heart disease in adults, part II of II. N Engl J Med 2000;342(5):334–342.

Driscoll DJ. Left-to-right shunt lesions. Pediatr Clin North Am 1999;46(2):355–368.

Fedderly RT. Left ventricular outflow obstruction. Pediatr Clin North Am 1999;46(2):369–384.

Fyler DC, ed. Nadas' Pediatric Cardiology. Philadelphia: Hanley & Belfus, 1992.

Grifka RG. Cyanotic congenital heart disease with increased pulmonary blood flow. Pediatr Clin North Am 1999;46(2):405–425.

Kerut EK, Norfleet WT, Plotnick GD, et al. Patent foramen ovale: a review of associated conditions and the impact of physiological size. J Am Coll Cardiol 2001;38:613–623.

Ledesma M, Alva C, Gomez FD, et al. Results of stenting for aortic coarctation. Am J Cardiol 2001;88: 460–462.

Liberthson RR. Congenital heart disease diagnosis and management in children and adults. Boston: Little, Brown & Co., 1989.

Moodie DS. Diagnosis and management of congenital heart disease in the adult. Cardiol Rev 2001;9: 276–281.

Moore KL, Persaud TVN, Schmitt W. The Developing Human. 6th Ed. Philadelphia: WB Saunders, 1998.

Park MK, Troxler RG. Pediatric Cardiology for Practitioners. 4th Ed. St. Louis: Mosby, 2002.

Perloff JK. The Clinical Recognition of Congenital Heart Disease. 4th Ed. Philadelphia: WB Saunders, 1994.

Rudolph AM. Congenital Diseases of the Heart: Clinical-Physiological Considerations. 2nd Ed. New York: Futura, 2001.

Vongpatanasin W, Brickner ME, Hillis LD, et al. The Eisenmenger syndrome in adults. Ann Intern Med 1998;128:745–755.

Waldman JD, Wernly JA. Cyanotic congenital heart disease with decreased pulmonary blood flow in children. Pediatr Clin North Am 1999;46(2): 385–404.

Cardiovascular Drugs

Chiadi E. Ndumele, Mark Friedberg, Elliott M. Antman, Gary R. Strichartz, and Leonard S. Lilly

Chapter
17

Inotropic Drugs
Digitalis Glycosides
Sympathomimetic Amines
Phosphodiesterase Inhibitors
Vasodilator Drugs
Angiotensin-Converting Enzyme Inhibitors
Angiotensin II Type 1 Receptor Antagonists
Direct-Acting Vasodilators
Calcium Channel Blockers
Organic Nitrates
Antiadrenergic Drugs
Central Adrenergic Inhibitors
Sympathetic Nerve-Ending Antagonists
Peripheral α-Adrenergic Receptor Antagonists
β-Adrenergic Receptor Antagonists
Antiarrhythmic Drugs
Class IA Antiarrhythmics
Class IB Antiarrhythmics

Class IC Antiarrhythmics
Class II Antiarrhythmics
Class III Antiarrhythmics
Class IV Antiarrhythmics
Adenosine
Diuretics
Loop Diuretics
Thiazide Diuretics
Potassium-Sparing Diuretics
Antithrombotic Drugs
Platelet Inhibitors
Anticoagulant Drugs
Lipid-Regulating Drugs
HMG CoA Reductase Inhibitors
Bile-Acid Binding Agents
Niacin
Fibrates

This chapter reviews the physiologic basis and clinical use of cardiovascular drugs. Although a multitude of drugs is available to treat cardiac disorders, these agents can fortunately be grouped by their pharmacologic actions into a small number of categories. Additionally, many drugs are useful in more than one form of heart disease.

INOTROPIC DRUGS

Inotropic drugs are used to increase the force of ventricular contraction when myocardial systolic function is impaired. The pharmacologic agents in this category include the cardiac glycosides, sympathomimetic amines, and phosphodiesterase inhibitors. Although they work through different mechanisms, they are all thought to improve cardiac contraction by increasing the intracellular calcium concentration, thus augmenting actin and myosin interactions. The hemodynamic effect is to shift a depressed ventricular performance curve (Frank-Starling curve) in an upward direction (Fig. 17.1), so that for a given ventricular filling pressure, stroke volume and cardiac output are increased.

Digitalis Glycosides

The cardiac glycosides are often called "digitalis" because commonly used drugs of this class are based on extracts of the foxglove plant, *Digitalis purpurea*. In this discussion, the term digitalis is used to describe the entire group of cardiac glycosides, including digoxin, digitoxin, and ouabain. These compounds are composed of an aglycone ring (steroid nucleus and lactone ring) that confers the pharmacologic activity and a varying number of sugar residues that contribute to the drug's pharmacokinetics.

371

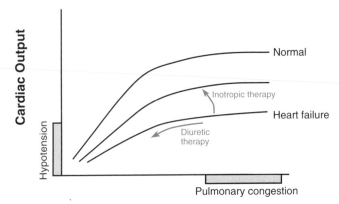

Left ventricular end-diastolic pressure

Figure 17.1. **Ventricular performance (Frank-Starling) curve.** In heart failure, the curve is displaced downward, so that at a given left ventricular end-diastolic pressure (LVEDP), the cardiac output is lower than in a normal individual. Diuretics reduce LVEDP but do not change the position of the curve; thus, pulmonary congestion improves but cardiac output may fall. Inotropic drugs displace the curve upward, toward normal, so that at any LVEDP, the cardiac output is higher.

Mechanism of Action

There are two desired effects of digitalis: 1) to improve contractility of the failing heart (mechanical effect), and 2) to prolong the refractory period of the atrioventricular (AV) node in patients with supraventricular arrhythmias (electrical effect).

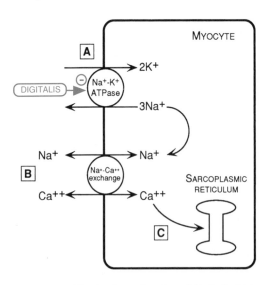

Figure 17.2. **Mechanism of action of digitalis (inotropic effect). A.** Digitalis inhibits the sarcolemmal Na^+-K^+ ATPase, causing intracellular $[Na^+]$ to rise. **B.** Increased cytosolic $[Na^+]$ reduces the transmembrane Na^+ gradient; thus, the Na^+/Ca^{++} exchanger drives less Ca^{++} out of the cell. **C.** The increased $[Ca^{++}]$ is stored in the sarcoplasmic reticulum, such that with subsequent action potentials, greater than normal Ca^{++} is released to the contractile elements in the cytoplasm, intensifying the force of contraction.

Mechanical Effect

The action by which digitalis improves contractility appears to be inhibition of the sarcolemmal Na^+/K^+-ATPase pump, normally responsible for maintaining transmembrane Na^+ and K^+ gradients. By binding to and inhibiting this pump, digitalis causes the intracellular $[Na^+]$ to rise. As shown in Figure 17.2, an increase in intracellular sodium content reduces Ca^{++} extrusion from the cell by the Na^+/Ca^{++} exchanger. Consequently, more Ca^{++} is pumped into the sarcoplasmic reticulum. As a result, when subsequent action potentials excite the cell, a greater than normal amount of Ca^{++} is released to the myofilaments, thereby enhancing the force of contraction. The magnitude of the positive inotropic effect correlates with the degree of Na^+/K^+-ATPase inhibition.

Electrical Effect

Digitalis affects the electrical properties of cardiac tissue directly. More importantly, it modifies autonomic nervous system influences on conduction by enhancing vagal tone and reducing sympathetic activity.

In the normal heart, the most important therapeutic electrical effect of digitalis occurs at the AV node (Table 17.1), where it slows conduction velocity and increases re-

TABLE 17.1. Electrophysiologic Effects of Digitalis

Region	Mechanism of Action	Effect
Therapeutic effects		
AV node	Vagal effect ↓ Conduction velocity ↑ Effective refractory period	1. ↓ Rate of transmission of atrial impulses to the ventricles in supraventricular tachyarrhythmias 2. ↓ Conduction velocity and ↑ refractory period may interrupt reentrant circuits passing through the AV node
Toxic effects		
Sinoatrial node	↑ Vagal and direct suppression	1. Sinus bradycardia 2. Sinoatrial block (impulse not transmitted from SA node to atrium)
Atrium	Delayed afterdepolarizations (triggered activity), ↑ slope of phase 4 depolarization (↑ automaticity) Variable effects on conduction velocity and ↑ refractory period (can fragment conduction and lead to reentry)	1. Atrial premature beats 2. Nonreentrant SVT (ectopic rhythm) 3. Reentrant PSVT
AV node	Direct and vagal-mediated conduction block	1. AV block (first, second or third degree)
AV junction (between AV node and His bundle)	Delayed afterdepolarizations (triggered activity), ↑ slope of phase 4 depolarization (↑ automaticity)	1. Accelerated junctional rhythm
Purkinje fibers and ventricular muscle	Delayed afterdepolarizations (triggered activity), ↓ conduction velocity and ↑ refractory period (can lead to reentry) ↑ slope of phase 4 depolarization (↑ automaticity)	1. Ventricular premature beats 2. Ventricular tachycardia

PSVT, paroxysmal supraventricular tachycardia; *AV*, atrioventricular.

fractoriness, mostly via augmenting vagal activity. As a result, digitalis decreases the frequency of transmission of atrial impulses through the AV node to the ventricles. This is beneficial in reducing the rate of ventricular stimulation in patients with rapid supraventricular tachycardias such as atrial fibrillation or atrial flutter. In addition, by enhancing the refractoriness of the AV node, digitalis may convert supraventricular reentrant arrhythmias to a normal rhythm.

However, if digitalis concentrations rise into the toxic range, further enhancement of vagal tone and more extreme inhibition of the Na^+/K^+-ATPase pump can result in adverse electrophysiologic effects. For example, in atrial and ventricular Purkinje fibers, a high digitalis concentration has three important actions that may lead to dangerous arrhythmias (Fig. 17.3):

1. *Less negative resting potential.* Inhibition of the Na^+/K^+-ATPase causes the resting potential to become less negative. Recall

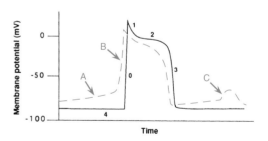

Figure 17.3. Direct effects of digitalis on the Purkinje cell action potential. The solid tracing represents depolarization and repolarization of a normal cell; the dashed tracing demonstrates the effects of digitalis. The maximum diastolic potential is less negative, and there is an increase in the slope of phase 4 depolarization (**A**), endowing the cell with intrinsic automaticity, and the potential for ectopic rhythms. Because depolarization of the cell occurs at a more positive voltage, the rate of rise of phase 0 is decreased (**B**), and conduction velocity is slowed, which, if present heterogeneously among neighboring cells, can produce conditions for reentry. Delayed afterdepolarizations may develop at high concentrations of digitalis (**C**) in association with an increased intracellular calcium concentration and can result in triggered tachyarrhythmias.

from Chapter 1 that the Na^+/K^+-ATPase normally removes three Na^+ ions from the cell in exchange for two inwardly moving K^+ ions; inhibition of the pump results in a decrease of this pump-mediated outward current and a resulting depolarization of the cell. Consequently, there is a voltage-dependent partial inactivation of the fast Na^+ channels, which leads to a slower rise of phase 0 depolarization and reduction in conduction velocity (see Fig. 1.17). The slowed conduction, if present heterogeneously among neighboring cells, enhances the possibility of reentrant arrhythmias.

2. *Decreased action potential duration.* At high digitalis concentrations, the cardiac action potential shortens. This relates in part to the digitalis-induced elevated intracellular $[Ca^{++}]$, which increases the activity of a Ca^{++}-dependent K^+ channel. The opening of this channel promotes K^+ efflux and more rapid *repolarization.* In addition, high intracellular $[Ca^{++}]$ inactivates the Ca^{++} channels, decreasing the inward *depolarizing* Ca^{++} current. The decrease in action potential duration and the associated shortened refractory period increase the time during which cardiac fibers are responsive to external stimulation, allowing greater opportunity for propagation of arrhythmic impulses.

3. *Enhanced automaticity.* Digitalis enhances cellular automaticity and may generate ectopic rhythms by two mechanisms:

   a. The less negative membrane resting potential may induce phase 4 gradual depolarization, even in non-pacemaker cells (see Chapter 11), and an action potential is triggered each time the threshold voltage is reached.

   b. The digitalis-induced increase in intracellular $[Ca^{++}]$ may trigger delayed afterdepolarizations (see Fig. 17.3). If an afterdepolarization reaches the threshold voltage, an action potential (ectopic beat) is generated. Ectopic beats may lead to additional afterdepolarizations and self-sustaining arrhythmias such as ventricular tachycardia.

Thus, digitalis in toxic concentrations may lead to several types of ectopic or reentrant rhythms (see Table 17.1). In addition, the augmented direct and indirect vagal effects of toxic doses of digitalis slow conduction through the AV node, such that high degrees of AV block, including complete heart block, can occur.

Clinical Uses

The most common use of digitalis is as an inotropic agent to treat heart failure caused by decreased ventricular contractility (see Chapter 9). Digitalis increases the force of contraction, augments cardiac output, and thereby improves left ventricular emptying, reduces LV size, and decreases the elevated ventricular filling pressures typical of patients with systolic dysfunction. Digitalis is *not* beneficial in forms of heart failure associated with normal ventricular contractility (e.g., high-output failure associated with thyrotoxicosis, pulmonary congestion due to mitral stenosis, or in the setting of pure *diastolic* dysfunction).

Once the mainstay of therapy in congestive heart failure (CHF), the use of digitalis has waned in the face of newer therapies (see Chapter 9 and below). Nonetheless, digitalis continues to be useful in treating patients with CHF complicated by atrial fibrillation (it has the added benefit of slowing the ventricular heart rate), or when symptoms do not respond adequately to angiotensin-converting enzymes (ACE) inhibitors, β-blockers, and diuretics. Unlike ACE inhibitors and β-blockers, digitalis does not prolong the life expectancy of patients with chronic heart failure.

The second common use of digitalis is as an antiarrhythmic agent in the treatment of atrial fibrillation, atrial flutter, and paroxysmal supraventricular tachycardia (PSVT). In atrial fibrillation and flutter, digitalis reduces the number of impulses transmitted across the AV node, thereby slowing the ventricular rate. Digitalis may terminate reentrant supraventricular tachycardias, likely through enhancement of vagal tone, which slows impulse conduction, prolongs the effective refractory period, and can therefore interrupt reentrant circuits that pass through the AV node.

The use of digitalis as an antiarrhythmic has also become less frequent in recent years, because other agents such as β-blockers, calcium channel blockers, and adenosine are more effective and work more rapidly. Nonetheless, for the treatment of supraventricular tachyarrhythmias in the presence of CHF, digitalis remains an important option.

Pharmacokinetics

Digitalis has an oral availability ranging from 75–100% and has a large volume of distribution. The most commonly used form of digitalis is digoxin, which is excreted unchanged by the kidney. A series of loading doses of digoxin is necessary to raise the drug's concentration into the therapeutic range. If a loading dose is not given, the steady-state concentration is established in approximately 7 days. The maintenance dosage depends on the ability to excrete the drug (i.e., the patient's age and renal function).

Toxicity

The potential for digitalis toxicity is significant because of a low toxic-to-therapeutic drug concentration ratio. Although many side effects are minor, life-threatening arrhythmias may also result.

Extracardiac signs of acute digitalis toxicity are often gastrointestinal (nausea, vomiting, anorexia), thought to be mediated by the action of digoxin on the area postrema of the medulla. Cardiac toxicity includes a host of arrhythmias (see Table 17.1) that may precede extracardiac warning symptoms. The most frequently encountered rhythm disturbance is the development of ventricular extrasystoles. In addition, various degrees of AV block may occur because of the direct and vagal effects on AV nodal conduction. Digitalis toxicity is the most common cause of nonreentrant types of supraventricular tachycardia (due to enhanced automaticity or delayed afterdepolarizations).

Many factors may contribute to digitalis intoxication, the most common of which is hypokalemia, often caused by the concurrent administration of diuretics. Hypokalemia exacerbates digitalis toxicity as it further inhibits the Na^+/K^+-ATPase pump. Other conditions that promote digitalis toxicity include hypomagnesemia and hypercalcemia. In addition, the concurrent administration of other drugs (e.g., quinidine) may raise the serum digoxin concentration by decreasing its excretion and reducing its volume of distribution.

The treatment of digitalis-induced tachyarrhythmias includes administration of potassium (if hypokalemia is present) and often intravenous lidocaine (see below). High-grade AV block may require temporary pacemaker therapy. In patients with severe intoxication, administration of Fab fragments of antidigitalis antibodies may be life-saving.

Sympathomimetic Amines

Sympathomimetic amines are inotropic drugs that bind to cardiac $β_1$-receptors. Stimulation of these receptors increases the activity of adenylate cyclase, causing increased cAMP formation (Fig. 17.4). Increased cAMP activates protein kinases, which promote intracellular calcium influx by phosphorylating the slow calcium channels. The increased calcium entry triggers a corresponding rise in Ca^{++} release from the sarcoplasmic reticulum, which enhances the force of contraction. Intravenous dopamine and dobutamine are commonly used sympathomimetic amines in the treatment of acute heart failure. Norepinephrine, epinephrine, and isoproterenol are used in special circumstances as described below. Table 17.2 summarizes the receptor actions and major hemodynamic effects of these agents.

Dopamine is an endogenous catecholamine and the precursor of norepinephrine. It possesses an unusual combination of actions that make it attractive in the treatment of heart failure associated with hypotension and poor renal perfusion. There are several types of receptors with

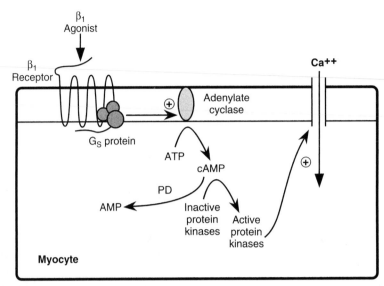

Figure 17.4. Mechanism by which β-adrenergic stimulation increases intracellular Ca++. β₁-receptor stimulation acts through G proteins (guanine nucleotide regulatory proteins) to activate adenylate cyclase. The latter increases cAMP production, which mediates protein kinase phosphorylation of cellular proteins, including ion channels. Phosphorylation of the slow Ca++ channel increases calcium influx. cAMP is degraded by phosphodiesterase (PD).

different affinities for dopamine. At *low dosages,* <2 μg/kg/min, dopamine interacts primarily with dopaminergic receptors that are distributed in the renal and mesenteric vascular beds. Stimulation of these receptors causes local vasodilation and increases renal blood flow and glomerular filtration, facilitating diuresis.

Medium dosages of dopamine, 2–10 μg/kg/min, increase inotropy by stimulation of cardiac β₁-receptors directly and indirectly by promoting release of norepinephrine from sympathetic nerve terminals. This action increases heart rate, cardiac contractility, and stroke volume, all of which augment cardiac output.

At *high dosages,* >10 μg/kg/min, dopamine also stimulates systemic α-receptors, thereby causing vasoconstriction and elevating systemic resistance. High-dose dopamine is indicated in hypotensive states such as shock. However, such doses are inappropriate in most patients with cardiac failure because the peripheral vasoconstriction increases the resistance against which the heart must contract (i.e., higher afterload), further impairing left ventricular output.

The major toxicity of dopamine arises in patients who are treated with high-dose therapy. The most important side effects are acceleration of the heart rate (which in-

TABLE 17.2. Sympathomimetic Drug Effects

Drug	Receptor Stimulation			
	D_1 (↑ *renal perfusion*)	α (*vasoconstriction*)	$β_1$ (↑ *contractility*)	$β_2$ (*vasodilatation*)
Dopamine	+	++++	++++	++
	(low dose)	(high dose)	(mid or high dose)	(mid dose)
Dobutamine	0	+	++++	+
Norepinephrine	0	++++	++++	0
Epinephrine	0	++++	++++	++
Isoproterenol	0	0	++++	++++

creases oxygen consumption) and stimulation of tachyarrhythmias.

Dobutamine is a synthetic analog of dopamine that stimulates β_1-, β_2-, and α-receptors. It increases cardiac contractility by virtue of the β_1 effect but does not increase peripheral resistance because of the balance between α-mediated vasoconstriction and β_2-mediated vasodilation. Thus, it is useful in the treatment of heart failure not accompanied by hypotension. Unlike dopamine, dobutamine does not stimulate dopaminergic receptors (i.e., no renal vasodilating effect), nor does it facilitate the release of norepinephrine from peripheral nerve endings. Like dopamine, it is useful for short-term therapy (>1 week), after which time it loses its efficacy, presumably because of down-regulation of adrenergic receptors. The major adverse effect is the provocation of tachyarrhythmias.

Norepinephrine is an endogenous catecholamine synthesized from dopamine in adrenergic postganglionic nerves and in adrenal medullary cells (where it is both a final product and the precursor of epinephrine). Via its β_1 activity, norepinephrine has positive inotropic and chronotropic effects. Acting at peripheral α receptors, it is also a potent vasoconstrictor. The increase in total peripheral resistance causes the mean arterial blood pressure to rise.

With this combination of effects, norepinephrine is useful in patients suffering from "warm shock," in which the combination of cardiac contractile dysfunction and peripheral vasodilatation lower blood pressure. However, the intense vasoconstriction elicited by this drug makes it less attractive than others in treating most cases of shock. Norepinephrine's side effects include precipitation of myocardial ischemia (due to the augmented afterload and force of contraction) and tachyarrhythmias.

Epinephrine, the predominant endogenous catecholamine produced in the adrenal medulla, is formed by the decarboxylation of norepinephrine. As indicated in Table 17.2, epinephrine is an agonist of α, β_1-, and β_2-receptors. Administered as an intravenous infusion at low doses (<0.01 μg/kg/min) epinephrine's stimulation of the β_1-receptor increases ventricular contractility and speeds impulse generation (e.g., by enhancing phase 4 depolarization in sinoatrial [SA] nodal cells). As a result, stroke volume, heart rate, and cardiac output all increase. However, at this dose range β_2-mediated vasodilation may reduce total peripheral resistance and blood pressure.

At *higher doses* (>0.2 μg/kg/min), epinephrine is a very potent vasopressor because α-mediated constriction dominates over β_2-mediated vasodilation. In this case, the effects of positive inotropy, positive chronotropy, and vasoconstriction act together to raise the arterial blood pressure.

Epinephrine is therefore used most often when the combination of inotropic and chronotropic stimulation is desired, such as in the setting of cardiac arrest. The α-associated vasoconstriction may also help support blood pressure in that setting. The most common toxic effect is the precipitation of tachyarrhythmias. Epinephrine should be avoided in patients receiving β-blocker therapy, because unopposed α—mediated vasoconstriction could produce acute severe hypertension and its complications (see Chapter 13).

Isoproterenol is a synthetic epinephrine analog. Unlike norepinephrine and epinephrine, it is a "pure" β agonist, having activity almost exclusively at β_1- and β_2-receptors, with almost no α-receptor effect. In the heart, isoproterenol has positive inotropic and chronotropic effects, thereby increasing cardiac output. In peripheral vessels, stimulation of β_2-receptors results in vasodilation and reduced peripheral resistance, which may cause blood pressure to fall.

Isoproterenol is sometimes used in emergency circumstances to increase the heart rate in patients with bradycardia or heart block (e.g., as a temporizing measure before pacemaker implantation). It may also be useful in patients with systolic dysfunction and slow heart rates with high systemic vascular resistance (a situation sometimes encountered after cardiac surgery in patients who had previously been receiving β-blocker therapy). Isoproterenol should be avoided in patients with myocardial ischemia in whom the increased heart rate and inotropic stimulation would further increase myocardial oxygen consumption.

Phosphodiesterase Inhibitors

Amrinone and **milrinone** are nondigitalis, noncatecholamine inotropic agents. They exert their positive inotropic actions by inhibiting phosphodiesterase in cardiac myocytes (see Fig. 17.4). This inhibition reduces the breakdown of intracellular cAMP, the ultimate result of which is enhanced Ca^{++} entry into the cell and increased force of contraction. These agents also have vasodilating properties.

Amrinone and milrinone are used in the treatment of heart failure only if there has been insufficient improvement with conventional vasodilators, digitalis, and diuretics. This is because of the high incidence of adverse effects, including serious ventricular arrhythmias. Amrinone has not been shown to improve the clinical state with chronic use in heart failure patients, and chronic milrinone therapy has actually demonstrated an *increase* in mortality rates. Roles for these agents are limited to short-term therapy in hospitalized patients.

The most important effects of the inotropic drugs are summarized in Table 17.3.

VASODILATOR DRUGS

Vasodilator drugs play a central role in the treatment of heart failure and hypertension. As described in Chapter 9, the fall in cardiac output in heart failure triggers important compensatory pathways, including the adrenergic nervous system and the renin-angiotensin system (see Fig. 9.9). As a result of activating these pathways, two potent vasoconstrictors are released into the circulation: norepinephrine and angiotensin II. These hormones bind to receptors in arterioles and veins, where they cause vasoconstriction. Initially, vasoconstriction is beneficial in heart failure because it maximizes left ventricular preload (through venous constriction) and maintains systemic blood pressure (by arterial constriction).

However, venous constriction may ultimately cause excessive venous return to the heart, with a rise in the pulmonary capillary hydrostatic pressure and development of pulmonary congestion. In addition, excessive arteriolar constriction increases the resistance against which the left ventricle must contract and therefore ultimately impedes forward cardiac output. Vasodilator therapy is directed at modulating the exces-

TABLE 17.3. Inotropic Drugs

Drug	Mechanism of Action	Major Adverse Effects
Cardiac glycosides Digoxin	Inhibition of sarcolemmal Na^+/K^+ ATPase Enhanced vagal tone	**Gastrointestinal:** nausea, vomiting **Cardiac:** atrial, nodal, and ventricular tachyarrhythmias; high-degree AV block
Sympathomimetic amines Dopamine	Low dose (<2 μg/kg/min): D_1 receptor stimulation results in mesenteric and renal arterial dilatation (facilitates diuresis) Medium dose (2–10 μg/kg/min): β_1-receptor stimulation and release of norepinephrine from sympathetic nerve terminals (inotropic effect) High dose (>10μg/kg/min): α-receptor stimulation (peripheral vasoconstriction)	Tachycardia, arrhythmias, hypertension, drug tolerance
Dobutamine	β_1, β_2, and α receptor stimulation	Tachyarrhythmias, drug tolerance
Phosphodiesterase inhibitors Amrinone Milrinone	Increased intracellular cAMP due to inhibition of its breakdown by phosphodiesterase	**Gastrointestinal:** nausea, vomiting **Cardiac:** arrhythmias (Amrinone only): thrombocytopenia

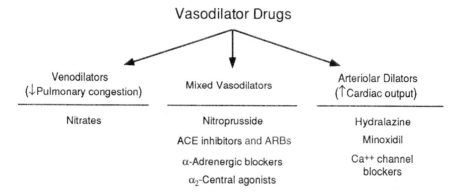

Figure 17.5. **Examples of vasodilator drugs and their sites of action: the venous bed, the arteriolar bed, or both.** ACE, angiotensin converting-enzyme; ARB, angiotensin receptor blocker.

sive constriction of veins and arterioles, thus reducing pulmonary congestion and augmenting forward cardiac output (see Fig. 9.10).

Vasodilators are also useful antihypertensive drugs. Recall from Chapter 13 that blood pressure is the product of cardiac output and systemic vascular resistance. Vasodilator drugs decrease arteriolar resistance and therefore lower elevated blood pressure.

Individual vasodilator drug classes act at specific vascular sites (Fig. 17.5). Nitrates, for example, are primarily venodilators, whereas hydralazine is a pure arteriolar dilator. Some drugs, such as the ACE inhibitors, α-blockers, and sodium nitroprusside, are balanced vasodilators that act on both sides of the circulation. Nesiritide, an important balanced vasodilator used in the management of decompensated heart failure, is described in Chapter 9.

Angiotensin-Converting Enzyme Inhibitors

The renin-angiotensin system plays an intricate role in cardiovascular homeostasis. The major effector of this pathway (Fig. 17.6) is angiotensin II (AII), which is formed by the cleavage of angiotensin I by angiotensin-converting enzyme (ACE). All the actions of AII known to affect blood pressure control are mediated by its binding to angiotensin II receptors of the AT_1 subtype (see Fig. 13.6). Interaction with this receptor generates a series of intracellular

reactions that cause, among other effects, vasoconstriction and the adrenal release of aldosterone, which promotes Na^+ reabsorption from the distal nephron. As a result of these actions on vascular tone and sodium homeostasis, AII plays a major role in blood pressure and blood volume regulation. By blocking the formation of AII, ACE inhibitors decrease the systemic arterial pressure (decreased vasoconstriction), facilitate natriuresis (e.g., decreased aldosterone and reduced Na^+ reabsorption from the distal nephron), and reduce adverse ventricular remodeling (see Chapter 9).

Another action of ACE inhibitors, which likely contributes to their hemodynamic effects, is related to bradykinin (BK) metabolism, as shown in Figure 17.6. The natural vasodilator BK is normally degraded to inactive metabolites by ACE, such that ACE inhibitors prevent that degradation. As a result, BK accumulates and contributes to the antihypertensive effect, likely by stimulating the endothelial release of nitric oxide and biosynthesis of vasodilating prostaglandins.

Clinical Uses

Hypertension

In hypertensive patients without CHF, ACE inhibitors lower blood pressure with little change in cardiac output or heart rate. One might assume that because this class of drug interferes with the renin-angiotensin system, it would be effective only in patients with "high-renin" hypertension, but that is not the case. Rather, they are effec-

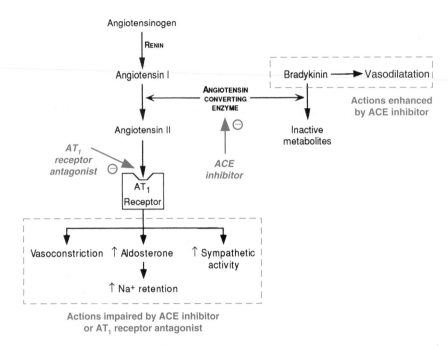

Figure 17.6. **The renin-angiotensin system.** Angiotensin-converting enzyme (ACE) generates angiotensin II, which results in actions including vasoconstriction, sodium retention, and increased sympathetic activity. ACE inhibitors and angiotensin II type 1 (AT$_1$) receptor antagonists impair these effects. ACE also promotes the degradation of the natural vasodilator bradykinin; thus, ACE inhibition—but not AT$_1$ receptor inhibition—results in accumulation of bradykinin and enhanced vasodilatation.

tive in most hypertensive patients, regardless of serum renin levels. The reason for this is not clear but may relate to the additional antihypertensive effects of BK and vasodilatory prostaglandins discussed above. In addition, several researchers have demonstrated the presence of renin-angiotensin activity within tissues outside the circulation, including the walls of the vasculature, where ACE inhibitors may exert an effect regardless of circulating renin concentrations.

ACE inhibitors increase renal blood flow in hypertensive patients, usually without altering glomerular filtration rate (GFR), because of dilation of both the afferent and efferent glomerular arterioles. Used alone in hypertension, ACE inhibitors show similar efficacy compared with diuretics and β-blockers. They do not adversely affect serum glucose or lipid concentrations; they do not result in hypokalemia, as do diuretics. Studies have shown that ACE inhibitors are preferred therapy in diabetic hypertensive patients, because they slow the devel-

opment of diabetic nephropathy (a syndrome of progressive renal deterioration, proteinuria, and hypertension) through favorable effects on intraglomerular pressure.

Heart Failure

In heart failure, ACE inhibitors reduce peripheral vascular resistance (decrease afterload), reduce cardiac filling pressures (decrease preload), and increase cardiac output. The rise in cardiac output usually matches the fall in peripheral resistance such that blood pressure tends not to fall (remember: BP = CO × TPR), except in those patients who are intravascular volume depleted, as might result from too vigorous diuretic therapy. The augmented cardiac output reduces the drive for neurohormonal stimulation in CHF (see Chapter 9), such that elevated levels of norepinephrine fall. In addition, clinical trials have shown that ACE inhibitors significantly increase survival in patients with chronic heart failure (see Chapter 9) and following myocardial infarction (see Chapter 7). ACE inhibition also reduces the risk of myocardial infarction and death in patients with chronic vascular disease, including coronary artery disease (CAD).

The available agents are listed in Table 17.4. The primary excretory pathway of most ACE inhibitors is via the urine, so their dosages should generally be reduced in patients with renal dysfunction.

Toxicity

Serious side effects of ACE inhibitors, described here, are not common.

Hypotension

This is a rare side effect when ACE inhibitors are used to treat hypertension. It is more likely to occur in heart failure patients in whom intravascular volume depletion has resulted from vigorous diuretic use. Such patients have significant activation of the renin-angiotensin system; therefore, blood pressure is largely maintained by the vasoconstricting actions of circulating AII. The administration of an ACE inhibitor in that setting may result in hypotension due

to the sudden reduction of AII levels. This side effect is avoided by temporarily reducing the diuretic regimen and starting the ACE inhibitor at low dosage.

Hyperkalemia

Because ACE inhibitors indirectly reduce serum aldosterone concentrations, the serum potassium concentration may rise, but only rarely into the clinically important hyperkalemic range. Conditions that can further increase serum potassium levels and *may* result in dangerous hyperkalemia during ACE inhibitor use include renal insufficiency, diabetes (due to hyporeninemic hypoaldosteronism often present in elderly diabetics), and concomitant use of potassium-sparing diuretics.

Renal Insufficiency

As described above, administration of an ACE inhibitor to individuals with intravascular volume depletion may result in hypotension as well as decreased renal perfusion and azotemia. Correction of the volume depletion or reduction of the ACE inhibitor dosage usually corrects this complication.

ACE inhibitor therapy can also precipitate renal failure in patients with *bilateral renal artery stenosis* because such patients rely on high efferent glomerular arteriolar resistance (which is highly dependent on AII) to maintain intraglomerular pressure and filtration. Administration of an ACE inhibitor abruptly decreases efferent arteriolar tone and glomerular hydrostatic pressure and may therefore worsen GFR in this setting.

Cough

Irritation of the upper airways resulting in a dry cough has been reported in up to 15% of patients receiving ACE inhibitor therapy. Its mechanism has not been established but may relate to the increased BK concentration provoked by ACE inhibitor therapy. This side effect may last several weeks after the drug is discontinued.

TABLE 17.4. Drugs that Interfere with the Renin-Angiotensin System

Drug	Major Elimination Pathway
ACE inhibitors	
Benazepril	Renal
Captopril	Renal
Enalapril	Renal
Fosinopril	Hepatic/renal
Lisinopril	Renal
Moexipril	Hepatic/renal
Perindopril	Renal
Quinapril	Renal
Ramipril	Renal
Trandolapril	Hepatic/renal
Angiotensin II receptor antagonists	
Candesartan	Hepatic/renal
Eprosartan	Hepatic/renal
Irbesartan	Hepatic/renal
Losartan	Hepatic/renal
Olmesartan	Hepatic/renal
Telmisartan	Hepatic
Valsartan	Hepatic/renal

Other Effects

Very rare adverse reactions to the ACE inhibitors include angioedema and agranulocytosis.

Angiotensin II Type 1 Receptor Antagonists

Angiotensin II type 1 (AT$_1$) receptor antagonists (also termed angiotensin receptor blockers [ARBs]) are a more recent addition to the list of drugs that interfere with the renin-angiotensin system. There are at least two distinct types of AII receptors: AT$_1$ and AT$_2$. All the actions of AII known to affect blood pressure control (e.g., vasoconstriction, aldosterone release, renal Na$^+$ reabsorption, and increased sympathetic nervous system activity) are mediated by its binding to receptors of the AT$_1$ subtype. The AT$_2$ receptor subtype is abundant during fetal development and has been located in some adult tissues, but its precise actions are unknown.

ARBs are nonpeptide drugs that compete with AII for AT$_1$ receptors. ARBs therefore inhibit AII-mediated effects, such as vasoconstriction, aldosterone secretion, and renal sodium ion reabsorption (see Fig. 17.6), thus lowering the blood pressure of hypertensive individuals. ARBs provide a more substantial blockade of the renin-angiotensin system than ACE inhibitors, because the latter do not completely block formation of AII (some AI is converted to AII by circulating enzymes other than ACE). Unlike ACE inhibitors, the AT$_1$ receptor antagonists do not affect serum BK levels (see Fig. 17.6).

The available ARBs are listed in Table 17.4. Each of these is excreted primarily in the bile but also partly in the urine. Trials have demonstrated that ARBs are as effective as ACE inhibitors in treating hypertension, and they are among the best-tolerated antihypertensive drugs. As with the ACE inhibitors, the antihypertensive effect of the ARBs is enhanced by concurrent use of a thiazide diuretic. Also like ACE inhibitors, hypotension and hyperkalemia (due to reduced aldosterone levels) are potential side effects. Unlike ACE inhibitors, cough is not a common side effect.

In the setting of moderate to severe heart failure, ARBs display hemodynamic benefits similar to those of ACE inhibitors, but have not demonstrated superiority over the latter (see Chapter 9). Thus, ARBs are currently recommended in heart failure only for patients who are intolerant of ACE inhibitors (e.g., because of ACE inhibitor-induced cough).

Recent studies in patients with type 2 diabetes showed that ARBs slow the progression of kidney disease, an effect that has been also demonstrated with ACE inhibitors.

Direct-Acting Vasodilators

Hydralazine, minoxidil, sodium nitroprusside, and diazoxide are examples of direct-acting vasodilators (Table 17.5). Hydralazine and minoxidil are primarily used as long-term oral vasodilators, whereas nitroprusside and diazoxide are administered intravenously in more acute settings. Fenoldopam is a newer arterial vasodilator administered intravenously for severe hypertension.

Hydralazine acts as a potent and direct arteriolar dilator at the level of the precapillary arterioles and has no effect on systemic veins. The cellular mechanism of its effect is unknown. The fall in blood pressure following arteriolar dilation results in a baroreceptor-mediated increase in sympathetic outflow and cardiac stimulation (e.g., reflex tachycardia), which could precipitate myocardial ischemia in patients with underlying CAD. Therefore, hydralazine is often combined with a β-blocker to blunt this undesired response.

As newer drugs have emerged, hydralazine is now only occasionally used as an antihypertensive, often in combination with other drugs. It is also sometimes prescribed concurrently with the venodilator isosorbide dinitrate to treat heart failure in patients with systolic dysfunction. This combination improves symptoms in patients with mild to moderate heart failure and has been shown to reduce long-term mortality rates in that setting, but not as effectively as ACE inhibitors.

Hydralazine possesses low bioavailability because of its extensive first-pass he-

TABLE 17.5. Direct Vasodilators

Drug	Clinical Use	Route of Administration	Major Adverse Effects
Hydralazine	• Hypertension (chronic and acute therapy) • CHF	Oral, intravenous bolus, intramuscular	• Hypotension, tachycardia • Headache, flushing • Angina • Drug-induced lupus
Minoxidil	• Chronic therapy of hypertension	Oral	• Reflex tachycardia • Na$^+$ retention • Hypertrichosis
Nitroprusside	• Hypertensive emergencies • Acute CHF	Intravenous infusion	• Hypotension • Cyanide and thiocyanate toxicity
Fenoldopam	• Hypertensive emergencies	Intravenous infusion	• Hypotension • Increased intraocular pressure
Diazoxide	• Hypertensive emergencies	Intravenous bolus	• Hypotension • Na$^+$ retention • Hyperglycemia

CHF, congestive heart failure.

patic metabolism. However, its metabolism depends on whether the patient displays fast or slow acetylation; on average, 50% of Americans are fast and 50% are slow hepatic acetylators. Slow acetylators show less hepatic degradation, higher bioavailability, and increased antihypertensive effects, whereas fast acetylators demonstrate the opposite. Hydralazine has a short half-life (2–4 hours) in the circulation, but its effect persists as long as 12 hours because most of the drug is avidly bound to vascular tissue.

The most common side effects of hydralazine include headache (increased cerebral vasodilatation), palpitations (reflex tachycardia), flushing (increased systemic vasodilatation), nausea, and anorexia. As indicated above, tachycardia due to reflex adrenergic stimulation may precipitate anginal attacks in patients with CAD if hydralazine is not jointly administered with a β-blocker. Finally, a systemic lupus-like syndrome (characterized by arthralgias, myalgia, skin rashes, and fever) may develop, especially in slow acetylators.

Minoxidil also results in arteriolar vasodilatation without significant venodilation. Its mechanism of action may involve an increase in potassium channel permeability, which results in smooth muscle cell hyperpolarization and relaxation. Like other agents that selectively cause arteriolar dilation, reflex adrenergic stimulation leads to increased heart rate and contractility, an undesired effect that can be blunted by coadministration of a β-blocker. In addition, decreased renal perfusion often results in fluid retention, so that a diuretic must usually be administered concurrently.

Minoxidil's primary clinical indication is in the treatment of severe or intractable hypertension. It is especially useful in patients with renal failure who are often refractory to other antihypertensive regimens. It is well absorbed from the gastrointestinal tract and is metabolized primarily by hepatic glucuronidation, but approximately one-fifth is excreted unchanged by the kidney. Although it has a short half-life, its pharmacologic effects persist even after serum drug concentration falls, probably because, like hydralazine, the drug is avidly bound to vascular tissue.

Side effects of minoxidil, in addition to reflex sympathetic stimulation and fluid retention, include hypertrichosis (excessive hair growth) and occasional pericardial effusion (mechanism unknown).

Sodium nitroprusside, a potent dilator of *both* arterioles and veins, is used to treat hypertensive emergencies and in intensive care units for intravenous control of blood

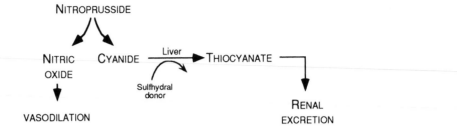

Figure 17.7. **Sodium nitroprusside is a complex of iron, cyanide (CN), and a nitroso group.** Erythrocyte metabolism liberates CN and the active vasodilator nitric oxide. The CN is metabolized in the liver to thiocyanate, which is eliminated by the kidneys.

pressure. It is also used for preload and afterload modulation in severe CHF. Sodium nitroprusside is a complex of iron, cyanide groups, and a nitroso moiety, and its metabolism by red blood cells results in the liberation of nitric oxide (Fig. 17.7). Nitric oxide causes vasodilation through activation of guanylate cyclase in vascular smooth muscle (see Chapter 6 and below).

Sodium nitroprusside's hemodynamic effects result from its ability to decrease arterial resistance and to increase venous capacitance. In patients with normal left ventricular function, it can actually decrease cardiac output because of the reduction in venous return (see Fig. 9.10). However, in a patient with impaired left ventricular contractile function, the decreased systemic resistance induced by sodium nitroprusside leads to an increase in forward cardiac output, while venous dilation reduces return of blood to the heart. The latter decreases pulmonary capillary hydrostatic pressure and improves symptoms of pulmonary congestion.

Sodium nitroprusside is often the treatment of choice for hypertensive emergencies because of its great potency and rapid action. A β-blocker is often administered concurrently to counteract the reflex increase in sympathetic outflow that may accompany the use of this drug.

Sodium nitroprusside is administered by continuous intravenous infusion. Its onset of action begins within 30 seconds; the peak effect is achieved in 2 minutes and dissipates within minutes of its discontinuation. After sodium nitroprusside is metabolized into nitric oxide and cyanide, the liver, in

the presence of a sulfhydryl donor, transforms cyanide into thiocyanate; the thiocyanate, in turn, is excreted by the kidney. *Thiocyanate accumulation and toxicity,* manifested by blurred vision, tinnitus, disorientation, and/or nausea, may occur with continued use, especially in the setting of renal impairment. Thus, it is important to monitor serum levels of thiocyanate if sodium nitroprusside is administered for more than 24 hours. In addition, excessive infusion rates of sodium nitroprusside, or a deficiency in hepatic thiosulfate stores, can result in lethal *cyanide toxicity,* the early signs of which include metabolic acidosis, headache, and nausea, followed by loss of consciousness.

Fenoldopam is a rapidly acting potent arteriolar vasodilator used intravenously to treat episodes of severe hypertension. It is a selective agonist of peripheral dopamine-1 (DA1) receptors, whose activation results in arteriolar vasodilatation through a cAMP-dependent mechanism. Unlike other intravenous antihypertensive agents, it beneficially maintains or enhances renal perfusion. In addition, fenoldopam's activation of renal tubular DA1 receptors facilitates natriuresis. Unlike dopamine, fenoldopam does not stimulate α- or β-adrenergic receptors.

Fenoldopam is administered by continuous intravenous infusion. Its onset of action is rapid, achieving 50% of maximal effect within 15 minutes and steady-state in 30–60 minutes. It is metabolized by the liver to inactive substances that are excreted through the kidney. It has a rapid offset of action after discontinuation (an elimination half-life of <10 min), which is a desirable effect that minimizes the risk of excessive blood pressure reduction during the treatment of hypertensive emergencies. These pharmacologic properties also make fenoldopam useful for controlling hypertension in the postoperative setting. However, nitroprusside works even faster and remains more popular for this purpose. Unlike nitroprusside, fenoldopam does not cause thiocyanate toxicity. The most common side effects are headache, dizziness, and tachycardia. Fenoldopam also increases intraocular pressure (probably by slowing aqueous humor drainage) and should be avoided in patients with glaucoma.

Diazoxide is a potent arteriolar dilator that is now infrequently used. Its mechanism of action involves activation of ATP-sensitive potassium channels, leading to arteriolar smooth muscle hyperpolarization and vasodilatation. The fall in resistance leads to a reflex activation of the adrenergic nervous system with tachycardia, and to fluid retention because of activation of the renin-angiotensin system. It also inhibits pancreatic insulin secretion and can result in hyperglycemia. This drug is administered intravenously and has been used primarily for hypertensive emergencies. However, its use has declined in favor of newer and better tolerated agents.

Calcium Channel Blockers

The calcium channel blockers (CCBs) are discussed here as a group, but differences exist among the drugs of this class. The common property of CCBs is their ability to impede the influx of Ca^{++} through membrane channels in cardiac and smooth muscle cells. Two principal types of voltage-gated Ca^{++} channels have been identified in cardiac tissue, termed L and T. The L-type channel is responsible for the Ca^{++} entry that maintains phase 2 of the action potential (the "plateau" in Fig. 1.14, p. 18). The T-type Ca^{++} channel likely plays a role in the initial depolarization of nodal tissues. It is the L-channel that is antagonized by current CCBs.

The cellular mechanism of CCBs has been partly delineated. Increased concentrations of intracellular Ca^{++} lead to augmented contractile force in both myocardium and vascular smooth muscle. At both sites, the net effect of Ca^{++} channel blockade is to decrease the amount of Ca^{++} available to the contractile proteins within these cells, which translates into vasodilatation of vascular smooth muscle and a negative inotropic effect in cardiac muscle.

Vascular Smooth Muscle

Contraction of vascular smooth muscle depends on the cytoplasmic Ca^{++} concentration, which is regulated by the transmembrane flow of Ca^{++} through the voltage-gated channels during depolarization. Intracellular Ca^{++} interacts with calmodulin to form a Ca^{++}-calmodulin complex. This complex stimulates myosin light chain kinase, which phosphorylates myosin light chains and allows myosin and actin to interact and cause contraction. CCBs promote relaxation of vascular smooth muscle by inhibiting Ca^{++} entry through the voltage-gated channels. Other organs possessing smooth muscle (including gastrointestinal, uterine, and bronchiolar tissues) are also susceptible to this relaxing effect.

Cardiac Cells

Cardiac muscle also depends on Ca^{++} influx during depolarization for contractile protein interactions, but by a different mechanism than that in vascular smooth muscle. Ca^{++} entry into the cardiac cell upon depolarization triggers additional intracellular Ca^{++} release from the sarcoplasmic reticulum, leading to contraction (see Chapter 1). By blocking Ca^{++} entry, CCBs therefore interfere with excitation-contraction coupling and decrease the force of contraction. Because the pacemaker tissues of the heart (e.g., SA and AV node) are the most dependent on the inward Ca^{++} current for their depolarization, one would expect that CCBs would reduce the rate of sinus firing and AV nodal conduction. Some, but not all, CCBs have this property (Table 17.6). The effect on cardiac conduction appears to depend not only on whether the

TABLE 17.6. Calcium Channel Blockers

Drug	Vasodilation	Negative Inotropic Effect	Suppress AV Node Conduction	Major Adverse Effects
Verapamil	+	+++	+++	• Hypotension • Bradycardia, AV block • CHF • Constipation
Diltiazem	++	++	++	• Hypotension • Peripheral edema • Bradycardia
Dihydropyridines Amlodipine Felodipine Isradipine Nicardipine Nifedipine Nisoldipine	+++	0 to +	0	• Hypotension • Headache, flushing • Peripheral edema

AV, atrioventricular; *CHF*, congestive heart failure.

specific CCB reduces the inward Ca^{++} current, but also on whether it delays recovery of the Ca^{++} channel to its preactivated state. **Verapamil** and **diltiazem** have this property, whereas **nifedipine** and the other dihydropyridine CCBs do not (see below).

Clinical Uses

As a result of their actions on vascular smooth muscle and cardiac cells, CCBs are useful in several cardiovascular disorders through the mechanisms summarized in Table 17.7. In angina pectoris, they exert beneficial effects by reducing myocardial oxygen consumption as well as by potentially increasing oxygen supply through coronary dilatation. The latter effect is also useful in the management of coronary artery vasospasm.

CCBs are often used to treat hypertension. More so than β-blockers or ACE inhibitors, they are particularly effective in elderly patients. Nifedipine and the other dihydropyridines are the most potent vasodilators of this class.

CCBs are usually administered orally, and once-a-day formulations are available for most of these agents. Routes of excretion vary. For example, nifedipine and verapamil are eliminated primarily in the urine, whereas diltiazem is excreted via the liver. Common side effects (see Table 17.6) include the development of hypotension (due

TABLE 17.7. Clinical Effects of Calcium Channel Blockers

Condition	Mechanism
Angina pectoris	↓Myocardial oxygen consumption ↓ blood pressure ↓ contractility ↓ heart rate (verapamil and diltiazem) ↑ Myocardial oxygen supply ↑ coronary dilatation
Coronary artery spasm	Coronary artery vasodilatation
Hypertension	Arteriolar smooth muscle relaxation
Supraventricular arrhythmias	(Verapamil and diltiazem): Decrease conduction velocity and increase refractoriness of atrioventricular node via blockade of slow inward Ca^{++} current

to excessive vasodilatation) and ankle edema (presumably caused by local vasodilatation of peripheral vascular beds). Verapamil and diltiazem may result in bradyarrhythmias and should be used with caution (or not at all) in patients already receiving β-blocker therapy.

The safety of *short-acting* CCBs has been called into question in recent years. In several observational studies, a higher incidence of myocardial infarction or death has been reported in patients with hypertension or coronary disease taking such agents. In contrast, such adverse outcomes have not been demonstrated with long-acting CCBs (i.e., formulations meant for once-a-day ingestion). Thus, only the long-acting versions should be used in most cases. Also, recall from Chapter 6 that β-blockers and/or nitrates are preferred over CCBs for initial therapy in patients with CAD.

Organic Nitrates

The nitrates constitute one of the oldest treatments of angina pectoris. They are also used in other ischemic syndromes and in heart failure. The main physiologic action of the nitrates is vasodilatation, particularly of the systemic veins.

Mechanism of Action

Nitrates produce vascular smooth muscle relaxation. The proposed mechanism involves the conversion of the administered drug to nitric oxide at or near the plasma membrane of vascular smooth muscle cells (Fig. 17.8). Nitric oxide, in turn, activates guanylate cyclase to produce cyclic GMP (cGMP), and the intracellular accumulation of cGMP leads to smooth muscle relaxation. This mechanism of vascular smooth muscle relaxation is similar to that associated with nitroprusside and endogenous endothelial-derived nitric oxide.

Hemodynamic and Antianginal Effects

At low doses, nitroglycerin, the prototypical organic nitrate, produces greater dilation of veins than of arterioles. The resulting venodilation causes venous pooling, diminished venous return, and hence decreased right and left ventricular filling. Systemic arterial resistance is generally unaffected, but cardiac output may fall because of the diminished preload, especially in patients with intravascular volume depletion (see Fig. 9.10). *Arterial* dilation occurs to some extent in the coronary arteries and may also occur in the facial vessels and the meningeal

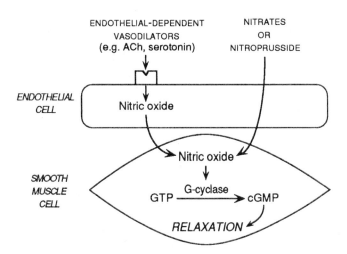

Figure 17.8. Organic nitrates incite vascular smooth muscle (SM) relaxation by conversion to nitric oxide (NO) at or near the cell membrane. Nitroprusside and endothelial-dependent vasodilators also promote NO delivery to vascular smooth muscle and cause relaxation. In the SM, NO stimulates formation of cyclic GMP (cGMP), which mediates relaxation.

arterioles, giving rise to the side effects of flushing and headache, respectively.

At *high* doses, nitrates result in widespread arteriolar dilation and venodilation. Arteriolar dilation may result in systemic hypotension and reflex tachycardia. However, the increase in heart rate is not typically manifest in patients with heart failure, because decreasing afterload in that situation may actually improve cardiac output and reduce the sympathetic drive.

The major use of nitrates is in the treatment of angina pectoris, in which the reduction of left ventricular filling reduces preload. The smaller left ventricular size lowers ventricular wall stress and myocardial oxygen consumption, which alleviates the oxygen imbalance in ischemic states. Nitrates are also useful in patients with coronary artery spasm (Prinzmetal's variant angina) by dilating the coronary arterioles.

Agents and Pharmacokinetics

There are many available formulations of nitrates. When the relief of acute angina is the objective, rapid onset of action is essential. However, in the long-term prevention of anginal attacks in a patient with chronic CAD, duration of action and predictability of effect are more crucial than the speed of drug effect.

Sublingual **nitroglycerin tablets** or **spray** are used in the treatment of acute angina attacks. The peak action of these agents occurs within 3 minutes, because they are rapidly absorbed into the bloodstream via the oral mucosa; their effect, however, diminishes rapidly, falling off within 15–30 minutes, as the drug is deactivated in the liver. These forms of nitroglycerin are also effective when taken prophylactically, immediately before situations known by the patient to produce angina (e.g., before walking up a hill).

The "long-acting" nitrates are used to prevent chest pain in the chronic management of angina and must be given in sufficient dosage to saturate the liver's deac-

tivating capacity. In this situation, high oral doses of **sustained-release nitroglycerin, isosorbide dinitrate,** or **isosorbide mononitrate** are routinely used. These agents have a duration of action of 2–14 hours. **Transdermal nitroglycerin patches** or **nitroglycerin paste** applied to the skin also deliver a sustained release of nitroglycerin. However, the efficacy of long-acting nitrate therapy is attenuated by the rapid development of drug tolerance with continuous use. For this reason, it is important that the dosing regimens allow a drug-free interval of several hours each day to maintain drug efficacy.

Intravenous nitroglycerin is administered by continuous infusion. This route is most useful in the treatment of hospitalized patients with unstable angina or acute heart failure.

Adverse Effects

The most common adverse effects of the nitrates include hypotension, reflex tachycardia, headache, and flushing.

ANTIADRENERGIC DRUGS

Drugs that interfere with the sympathetic nervous system are used commonly to treat cardiovascular disorders. These agents act at different loci (Fig. 17.9), including the central nervous system (CNS), postganglionic sympathetic nerve endings, and peripheral α- and β-receptors.

Normally, when a sympathetic nerve is stimulated, norepinephrine is released, traverses the synapse, and stimulates postsynaptic α- and β-receptors. The consequences of receptor stimulation depend on the organ involved (Table 17.8). The effect of α-receptor stimulation on vascular smooth muscle is vasoconstriction, whereas β_2 stimulation causes vasodilatation. In the CNS, β_2 stimulation *inhibits* sympathetic outflow to the periphery, thereby contributing to vasodilatation.

In addition, norepinephrine within the synapse can bind to *presynaptic* β- and α_2-receptors, which provides a feedback

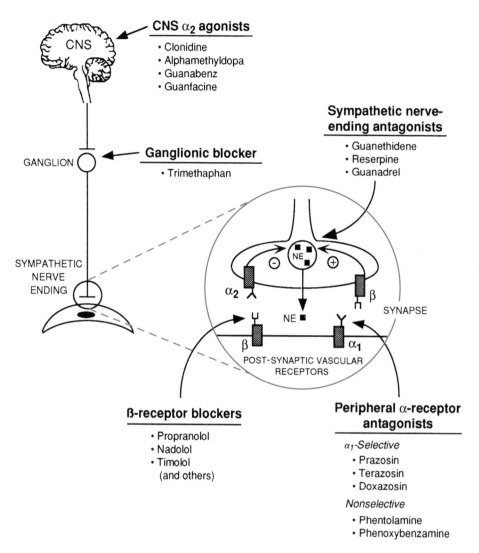

Figure 17.9. Sites of action of the antiadrenergic drugs. Note that receptors at the sympathetic nerve ending bind norepinephrine (NE) and provide feedback: the β-receptor stimulates, and the α₂-receptor inhibits, further NE releases. CNS, central nervous system.

mechanism that modulates further release of the hormone. The β-receptor increases, and the α₂ inhibits, further norepinephrine release.

Central Adrenergic Inhibitors

Alpha₂-receptors are located in the presynaptic neurons of the CNS. When stimulated by an α₂-agonist, they lead to *diminished* sympathetic outflow from the medulla. This action reduces peripheral vascular resistance and decreases cardiac stimulation, resulting in a fall in blood pressure and heart rate. Thus, drugs known as "central adrenergic inhibitors" are actually agonists of the CNS α₂-receptors. They were once among the most commonly used antihypertensive drugs, but have largely

TABLE 17.8. Responses to Adrenergic Receptor Stimulation

Receptor Type	Distribution	Response
α_1	Vascular smooth muscle (arterioles and veins)	Vasoconstriction
α_2	Presynaptic adrenergic nerve terminals	Inhibition of NE release
	Vascular smooth muscle (coronary and renal arterioles)	Vasoconstriction
β_1	Heart	Increases heart rate
		Increases contractility
		Speeds AV node conduction
	Kidney (JG cells)	Increases renin release
	Presynaptic adrenergic nerve terminals	Increases NE release
	Adipose tissue	Stimulates lipolysis
β_2	Vascular smooth muscle (arterioles, except skin and cerebral)	Vasodilation
	Bronchial smooth muscle	Bronchodilation
	Liver	Stimulates glycogenolysis

AV, atrioventricular; *NE*, norepinephrine.

given way to better tolerated agents. They are not sufficiently potent to serve as vasodilators in the treatment of heart failure.

The common drugs in this group are listed in Figure 17.9. They are all available as oral preparations, and clonidine can also be prescribed as a skin patch that is applied and left in place for 1 week at a time, facilitating drug compliance in the treatment of hypertension. Side effects of CNS α_2-agonists include sedation, dry mouth, bradycardia, and if the drug is stopped suddenly, the possibility of a sudden, paradoxical rise in blood pressure.

Sympathetic Nerve-Ending Antagonists

This group includes guanethidine, reserpine, and guanadrel. **Guanethidine** and **guanadrel** are actively transported into the postganglionic neuron via the norepinephrine reuptake pump. Once inside, they bind to norepinephrine vesicles and prevent the release of norepinephrine upon nerve stimulation.

Early in the course of therapy, guanethidine decreases blood pressure and cardiac output by slowing the heart rate and increasing venous capacitance, via the reduction of norepinephrine. There is no compensatory rise in peripheral resistance, because the drug effectively blocks sympathetically mediated reflex vasoconstriction. Guanethidine was once used extensively as an antihypertensive, but its side effects

(primarily postural hypotension) and the development of better tolerated agents have demoted it to "rarely used" status. Guanadrel has a shorter duration of action and somewhat fewer side effects than guanethidine.

Reserpine was the first drug found to interfere with the sympathetic nervous system, and its use ushered in many of the concepts used today in hypertension management. It inhibits the uptake of norepinephrine into storage vesicles in postganglionic and central neurons, leading to norepinephrine degradation. The antihypertensive effect is due to the depletion of catecholamines, which causes the force of myocardial contraction and total peripheral resistance to decrease.

Reserpine's CNS toxicity represents its chief drawback. It often produces sedation and can impair concentration. The most serious potential toxicity is psychotic depression, and patients with a history of depressive disorders should not receive this drug. Newer, better tolerated antihypertensive agents have largely supplanted the use of reserpine.

Peripheral α-Adrenergic Receptor Antagonists

Peripheral α antagonists (Table 17.9) are divided into those that act on both α_1- and α_2-receptors, and those that inhibit α_1 alone. Alpha$_1$-selective receptor antagonists (**prazosin, terazosin, doxazosin**) are

TABLE 17.9. α-Receptor Blockers

Mechanism/Drug	Indications	Major Adverse Effects
Selective peripheral α₁ blockade Prazosin Terazosin Doxazosin	• Hypertension • Benign prostatic hyperplasia	• Postural hypotension • Headache, dizziness • [No reflex tachycardia]
Nonselective α blockade Phentolamine Phenoxybenzamine	• Pheochromocytoma	• Postural hypotension • Reflex tachycardia • Arrhythmias

used in the treatment of hypertension. Their selectivity for the α₁-receptor explains their ability to produce less reflex tachycardia than nonselective agents. Normally, drug-induced vasodilatation results in baroreceptor-mediated stimulation of the sympathetic nervous system (see Chapter 13) and an undesired increase in heart rate. This effect is amplified by drugs that block the presynaptic α₂-receptor, as feedback inhibition of norepinephrine release is prevented. However, α₁ selective agents do not block the negative feedback on the α₂-receptor. Thus, further norepinephrine release and reflex sympathetic side effects are blunted.

The principal indication for α₁ antagonists has been in the treatment of hypertension. One of their advantages is that they do not adversely affect the serum concentrations of cholesterol and triglycerides as can other antihypertensives such as diuretics and β-blockers. However, in one recent large trial, patients treated with the α₁ antagonist doxazosin experienced more adverse cardiac outcomes than those treated with a diuretic. Thus α₁ antagonists are falling out of favor in the management of hypertension. They have also been evaluated in the treatment of heart failure, but lose their effectiveness over time (i.e., they display drug tolerance), and unlike other vasodilator regimens (e.g., ACE inhibitors or hydralazine plus nitrates), do not reduce mortality rates in chronic CHF. Terazosin and doxazosin are often used to treat the symptoms of benign prostatic hyperplasia, as they beneficially relax prostatic smooth muscle tone.

Phentolamine and **phenoxybenzamine** are nonselective α-blockers. They are used primarily in the treatment of pheochromocytoma, a tumor that abnormally secretes catecholamines into the circulation (see Chapter 13). Otherwise, these drugs are rarely used, as the α₂ blockade impairs normal feedback inhibition of norepinephrine release, an undesired effect, as indicated above.

β-Adrenergic Receptor Antagonists

The β-adrenergic antagonists are used for a number of cardiovascular conditions, including ischemic heart disease, hypertension, heart failure, and tachyarrhythmias.

Because catecholamines increase inotropy, chronotropy, and conduction velocity of the heart, it follows that β-receptor antagonists decrease inotropy, slow the heart rate, and decrease conduction velocity. When stimulation of the β-receptors is low, as in a normal resting individual, the effect of blocking agents is likewise mild. However, when the sympathetic nervous system is activated (e.g., during exercise), these antagonists can substantially diminish catecholamine-mediated effects.

The β-blockers can be distinguished from one another by specific properties (Table 17.10): 1) the relative affinity of the drug for β₁- and β₂-receptors, 2) whether partial β-*agonist* activity is present, 3) whether α₁-receptors are also blocked, and 4) differences in pharmacokinetic properties. The goal of β₁-*selective* agents is to achieve myocardial receptor blockade, with less effect on bronchial and vascular smooth muscle (tissues that exhibit β₂-receptors), so as to produce less bronchospasm and vasoconstriction in susceptible individuals. Agents with partial β-agonist effects (also termed *intrinsic*

TABLE 17.10. β-Adrenergic Blockers

	Nonselective β-blockers	β₁-selective β-blockers
No β-agonist activity	Carvedilol[a] Labetalol[a] Propranolol Nadolol Timolol	Atenolol Betaxolol Bisoprolol Esmolol[b] Metoprolol
β-agonist activity	Carteolol Penbutolol Pindolol	Acebutolol

[a]Also has α_1-adrenergic blocking properties.
[b]Administered intravenously only.

sympathomimetic activity [ISA]) tend to slow the heart rate less than other β-blockers.

During short-term use, nonselective β antagonists tend to reduce cardiac output because they decrease heart rate and contractility as well as slightly increase peripheral resistance (via β_2-receptor blockade). β antagonists that have partial agonist activity (such as pindolol), or those that possess some α-blocking activity (such as labetalol), can actually lower peripheral resistance by interacting with their respective β_2- and α-receptors.

Clinical Uses

Ischemic Heart Disease

The beneficial effects of β-blockers in ischemic heart disease are related to their ability to decrease myocardial oxygen demand (see Chapter 6). They reduce the heart rate, blood pressure (afterload), and contractility. The negative inotropic effect is directly related to blockade of the cardiac β-receptor, which results in decreased calcium influx into the myocyte (Fig. 17.4). β-blockers also improve survival and reduce the rate of reinfarction following an acute myocardial infarction. Agents with intrinsic sympathomimetic activity are less beneficial in this regard than β-blockers without ISA.

Hypertension

β-blocking agents reduce the blood pressure in hypertensives but often do not display this effect in normotensive individu-

als. Despite their widespread use as antihypertensives, the mechanisms responsible for this effect are not well understood. With initial use, the antihypertensive action is thought to result from a decrease in cardiac output, in association with slowing of the heart rate and mild decrease in contractility. However, with chronic administration, other mechanisms are likely at work, including reduced renal secretion of renin and possibly CNS actions.

Heart Failure

The negative inotropic effect of beta blockade would be expected to worsen heart failure symptoms in patients with underlying left ventricular systolic dysfunction. However, recent trials in patients with all classes of clinically stable heart failure have actually shown a survival benefit with chronic β-blocker administration using carvedilol, metoprolol, or bisoprolol (see Chapter 9). The mechanism of this benefit is unclear but may relate to blunting of the cardiotoxic effects of excessive circulating catecholamines. Because of the potential risk of actually transiently *worsening* heart failure, β-blocker therapy should be started at low dosage, augmented slowly, and carefully monitored.

Other conditions that benefit from β-blocker therapy include tachyarrhythmias (see below) and hypertrophic cardiomyopathy (see Chapter 10).

Toxicity

Fatigue may occur during β-blocker therapy and is most likely a CNS side effect. β-blockers with less lipid solubility (e.g., nadolol) do not penetrate the blood–brain barrier and may have fewer CNS adverse effects than more lipid-soluble drugs, such as propranolol. Other potential adverse effects relate to the predictable consequences of β blockade:

1. β_2 blockade associated with use of nonselective agents (or large doses of β_1-selective blockers) can exacerbate *bronchospasm*, worsening preexisting asthma or chronic obstructive lung disease.

2. The impairment of AV nodal conduction by β_1 blockade can provoke conduction blocks.

3. β_2 blockade can precipitate arterial *vasospasm*, which can result in Raynaud's phenomenon or worsen symptoms of peripheral vascular disease (see Chapter 15).

4. Abrupt withdrawal of a β antagonist after chronic use could precipitate myocardial ischemia in patients with CAD ("rebound ischemia").

5. Undesirable reduction of high-density lipoprotein (HDL) cholesterol and elevation of triglycerides can occur through an unknown mechanism. This effect appears to be less pronounced with blockers that have partial β-agonist activity, or combined β- and α-blocking properties.

6. β_2 blockade may impair recovery from hypoglycemia in diabetics suffering an insulin reaction. In addition, β-blockers may mask the sympathetic warning signs of hypoglycemia, such as tachycardia. If β-blockers are used in diabetics, β_1-selective agents are generally preferred.

Other potential side effects include insomnia, depression, and impotence. Finally, β antagonists should be used with caution in combination with certain CCBs (verapamil or diltiazem) because both types of drugs can impair myocardial contractility and AV nodal conduction, and could precipitate heart failure or AV conduction blocks.

ANTIARRHYTHMIC DRUGS

Drug therapy is a common approach to treat cardiac tachyarrhythmias. However, despite their benefits, antiarrhythmic drugs are among the most dangerous pharmacologic agents because of their frequent serious adverse effects. Therefore, a thorough understanding of their mechanisms of action, indications, and toxicities is of particular importance.

Although a number of classification systems for these agents exist, antiarrhythmic drugs are commonly separated into four groups based on their mechanisms of action (Table 17.11):

1. *Class I* drugs block the fast sodium channel responsible for phase 0 depolarization of the action potential. They are further divided into three subtypes based on the degree of sodium channel blockade and the effect of the drug on the cell's refractory period.

TABLE 17.11. Classification of Antiarrhythmic Drugs

Class		General Mechanism		Examples
I		**Na⁺ channel blockade**		
	IA	Moderate block	↓↓Phase 0 upstroke rate Prolong repolarization	Quinidine Procainamide Disopyramide
	IB	Mild block	↓Phase 0 upstroke rate Shorten repolarization	Lidocaine Tocainide Mexiletine Phenytoin (DPH)
	IC	Marked block	↓↓↓Phase 0 upstroke rate No change in repolarization	Flecainide Propafenone
II		**β-blockers**		Propranolol Esmolol Metoprolol and many others
III		**Marked prolongation of repolarization**		Amiodarone Sotalol Bretylium Ibutilide Dofetilide
IV		**Ca⁺⁺ channel blockers**		Verapamil Diltiazem

2. *Class II* drugs are β-adrenergic receptor blockers.
3. *Class III* drugs are those that significantly prolong the action potential with little effect on the rise of phase 0 depolarization. The main mechanism of action is blockade of the repolarizing K⁺ current (during phases 2 and 3 of the action potential).
4. *Class IV* drugs block the slow L-type calcium channel.

Drugs that do not conveniently fit into these classes, and are discussed separately, include adenosine and the digitalis glycosides.

Regardless of the class, the goal of antiarrhythmic therapy is to abolish the mechanisms by which tachyarrhythmias occur. These mechanisms (as described in Chapter 11) are 1) increased automaticity of pacemaker or non-pacemaker cells, 2) reentrant pathways, and 3) triggered activity.

In the case of arrhythmias due to *increased automaticity*, treatment is aimed at lowering the maximum frequency at which cardiac action potentials can occur by 1) reducing the slope of spontaneous phase 4 diastolic depolarization, and/or 2) prolonging the effective refractory period. These actions reduce or extinguish abnormally high rates of firing.

Antiarrhythmic drugs inhibit *reentrant* rhythms by a different mechanism. Recall that the initiation of a reentrant circuit relies on a region of unidirectional block and slowed conduction (Fig. 17.10). For a reentrant rhythm to sustain itself, the length of time it takes for an impulse to propagate around the circuit must exceed the effective refractory period of the tissue. If an impulse returns to an area of myocardium that was depolarized moments earlier but has not yet recovered excitability, it cannot restimulate that tissue. Thus, one strategy to stop reentry is to lengthen the tissue's refractory period. When the refractory period is pharmacologically prolonged, a propagating impulse confronts inactive sodium channels, cannot conduct further, and is extinguished.

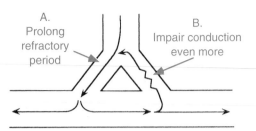

Figure 17.10. **Two strategies to interrupt reentry are (A) to prolong the tissue refractory period, so that returning impulses find the tissue unexcitable, or (B) to further reduce conduction, so that the impulse "dies out" in the slow retrograde limb of the circuit.**

A second means to interrupt reentrant circuits is to *additionally impair* impulse propagation within the already slowed retrograde limb. This is accomplished via pharmacologic blockade of the Na⁺ channels responsible for phase 0 depolarization. Such blockade fully abolishes the compromised impulse conduction within the retrograde limb and breaks the self-sustaining loop.

The elimination of the third type of tachyarrhythmia, *triggered activity*, requires suppression of early and delayed afterdepolarizations.

An ideal pharmacologic agent would suppress ectopic foci and interrupt reentrant loops without affecting normal conduction pathways. Unfortunately, when the concentrations of antiarrhythmic drugs exceed their narrow therapeutic ranges, even normal electrical activity may become suppressed. In addition, most antiarrhythmic drugs have the potential to aggravate rhythm disturbances (termed *proarrhythmic effect*). For example, this may occur when an antiarrhythmic drug prolongs the action potential, and induces early afterdepolarizations, resulting in a triggered-type of arrhythmia, such as torsades de pointes (see Chapter 11). Drug-induced proarrhythmia occurs most often in patients with left ventricular dysfunction or in those with an increased QT interval (a sign that the action potential is prolonged).

Class IA Antiarrhythmics

Mechanisms of Action

Effect on Arrhythmias due to Increased Automaticity

Class IA agents produce moderate blockade of the fast sodium channels, thus raising the threshold potential and slowing the upstroke of the action potential (phase 0). In addition, perhaps by inhibition of pacemaker channels, the slope of phase 4 depolarization is depressed (Fig. 17.11) so that it takes longer to reach threshold and fire the action potential. These effects are most pronounced at Purkinje fibers and abnormal ectopic pacemakers. Because IA agents have little effect on the automaticity of the SA node, it can resume its function as the cardiac pacemaker after ectopic foci are suppressed.

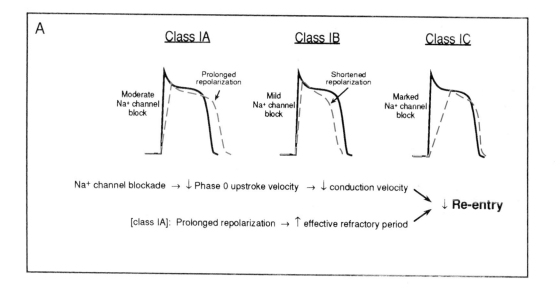

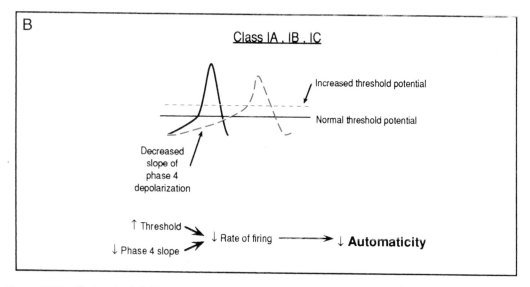

Figure 17.11. **Electrophysiologic effects of the class I antiarrhythmic drugs on the (A) Purkinje cell action potential and (B) pacemaker cell action potential.**

Effect on Reentrant Arrhythmias

Because sodium channel blockade slows the rate of phase 0 depolarization by reducing the magnitude of the inward current, it reduces cellular and tissue conduction velocities. If impaired sufficiently within a reentrant circuit, the impulse will die out within the already slowed retrograde limb, aborting the rhythm. In addition, class IA agents prolong the cell's refractory period, both by lengthening the action potential and by dissociating relatively slowly from Na^+ channels after repolarization (see Fig. 17.11). Thus, an impulse traveling in the reentrant loop encounters unexcitable tissue and is extinguished.

Effect on the Electrocardiogram

Because the conduction velocity is decreased and the action potential duration and repolarization are prolonged, the effect of class IA agents is to mildly prolong the QRS and QT intervals (Table 17.12). At higher dosage, these intervals may become substantially lengthened, potentially setting the stage for afterdepolarizations and drug-induced arrhythmias.

Clinical Uses

Class IA drugs are effective in treating a wide variety of reentrant and ectopic supraventricular and ventricular tachycardias (Table 17.13). However, their use has declined because of the development of more effective and less proarrhythmic strategies discussed below.

TABLE 17.12. Effect of Antiarrhythmic Drugs on Electrocardiographic Intervals

Class	PR	QRS	QT
IA	0	↑	↑
IB	0	0	0 or ↓
IC	↑	↑	0 or ↑
II	0 or ↑	0	0 or ↓
III	0 or ↑	↑	↑
IV	↑	0	0

TABLE 17.13. Common Clinical Uses of Antiarrhythmic Drugs

Class	Use
IA	• Atrial fibrillation and flutter • Paroxysmal SVT • Ventricular tachycardia
IB	• Ventricular tachycardia • Digitalis-induced arrhythmias
IC	• Atrial fibrillation and paroxysmal SVT
II	• Atrial or ventricular premature beats • Paroxysmal SVT • Atrial fibrillation and flutter • Ventricular tachycardia (ischemia-related)
III	• Ventricular tachycardia (amiodarone and sotalol) • Atrial fibrillation and flutter • Bypass-tract mediated paroxysmal SVT (amiodarone)
IV	• Paroxysmal SVT • Atrial fibrillation and flutter (↓ VR) • Multifocal atrial tachycardia (↓ VR)

SVT, supraventricular tachycardia; *VR*, ventricular rate.

Specific Class IA Drugs

Quinidine displays the electrophysiologic effects inherent to class IA agents but also has anticholinergic properties that may *augment* conduction at the AV node, thus antagonizing its direct suppressant effect. Quinidine also displays an α-adrenergic blocking action that may cause hypotension, especially with parenteral intravenous administration. Therefore, it is administered only by the oral route. Because quinidine is metabolized primarily by the liver, its dosage must be reduced in patients with hepatic dysfunction.

Cardiac and noncardiac side effects occur frequently during quinidine therapy. The most common are related to the gastrointestinal tract, including diarrhea in one-third of patients. Cardiac toxicities are serious and potentially fatal. For example, excessive prolongation of the QT interval (usually >0.5 sec) can lead to the life-threatening ventricular tachyarrhythmia torsades de pointes, described in Chapter 12.

Quinidine raises blood digoxin levels by decreasing the body's clearance and volume of distribution of the latter. Thus, it is important to prevent drug toxicity by reducing the dose of digoxin if quinidine is added.

Finally, the anticholinergic effect of quinidine may actually *speed* AV nodal conduction, in contrast to its direct effect on tissue excitability, and cause an *acceleration* of the ventricular rate in patients with atrial fibrillation or flutter. This response is avoided by combining quinidine with a negative chronotropic agent such as digitalis, a β-blocker, verapamil, or diltiazem.

The electrophysiologic effects of **procainamide** are similar to those of quinidine. However, procainamide does not prolong the action potential (and therefore QT interval) as much as quinidine, although dangerous arrhythmias such as torsades de pointes can still be provoked. Procainamide also has less pronounced anticholinergic effects than quinidine, so that facilitation of AV nodal conduction is less significant.

Procainamide has mild ganglionic blocking effects that may cause peripheral vasodilatation and a negative cardiac inotropic effect, particularly when the drug is administered intravenously. However, because hypotension associated with intravenous procainamide is much less common than with quinidine, it is used when an intravenous class IA agent is desired.

Procainamide can be administered by mouth, intramuscularly, or intravenously. More than 50% of the drug is excreted unchanged in the urine; the remainder undergoes acetylation by the liver to form N-acetyl procainamide (NAPA), which is subsequently excreted by the kidneys. In renal failure, or in "rapid acetylators," high serum levels of NAPA may accumulate. NAPA shares procainamide's ability to prolong the action potential and refractory period, but it does not alter the rate of phase 4 depolarization or the slope of phase 0 upstroke of the action potential.

Noncardiac side effects are common and include fever and rash. Approximately one-third of patients develop a systemic lupus-like syndrome after 6 months of therapy, manifested by arthralgias, rash, and connective tissue inflammation. It most often occurs among slow acetylators and is reversible upon cessation of drug therapy.

Disopyramide's electrophysiologic and antiarrhythmic effects are similar to those of quinidine. However, the two drugs have four main differences:

1. Gastrointestinal side effects are much less common with disopyramide.
2. Disopyramide does not increase serum digoxin levels.
3. Disopyramide has a much greater anticholinergic effect, so that common side effects include constipation, urinary retention (bladder sphincter tone is acetylcholine-dependent), and exacerbation of glaucoma (intraocular pressure is increased by the anticholinergic action).
4. Disopyramide, more so than quinidine or procainamide, has a pronounced negative inotropic effect and must be used with caution in patients with left ventricular systolic dysfunction.

Disopyramide is administered orally. The primary excretory pathway is via the kidneys, and toxic levels may accumulate in patients with renal insufficiency. QT prolongation and precipitation of ventricular arrhythmias (including torsades de pointes) can occur, similar to the other type IA agents.

Class IB Antiarrhythmics

Class IB drugs inhibit the fast sodium channel. Unlike IA agents, they typically *shorten* the action potential duration and the refractory period. Such shortening is attributed to blockade of small sodium currents that normally continue through phase 2 of the action potential.

Class IB drugs at therapeutic concentrations do not substantially alter the electrical activity of normal tissue; rather, they preferentially act on diseased or ischemic cells. Conditions present during ischemia, such as acidosis, faster rates of cell stimulation, and increased extracellular potassium concentration (and consequently less negative diastolic membrane potential), all increase the ability of class IB drugs to block the sodium channel. Such blockade promotes conduction block in ischemic cells by reducing the slope of phase 0 depolarization and slowing the conduction velocity, thus inhibiting reentrant arrhythmias (see Fig. 17.11). Similar to other class I drugs, the automaticity of ectopic pacemakers is also suppressed by decreasing phase 4 spontaneous depolarization and (in the case of some drugs of this class) by raising the threshold potential. In addition, intravenous lidocaine, a member of this class, suppresses delayed afterdepolarizations.

The most common use of class IB drugs is in the suppression of ventricular arrhythmias, especially those that appear in association with ischemia or digitalis toxicity. Conversely, they have little effect on *atrial* tissue at therapeutic concentrations, due to the shorter action potential duration of atrial cells, which allows less time for the drug to bind and block the Na$^+$ channel. Thus, these drugs are ineffective in atrial fibrillation, atrial flutter, and supraventricular tachycardias.

Because the QT interval is not prolonged by class IB drugs, early afterdepolarizations do not occur, and torsades de pointes is not an expected complication.

Specific Class IB Drugs

Lidocaine is an antiarrhythmic drug commonly used acutely to suppress ventricular arrhythmias in hospitalized patients. It is administered intravenously only, because oral administration results in unpredictable plasma levels. As a result of rapid distribution and hepatic metabolism, lidocaine must be administered as a continuous infusion following two or three loading boluses. The half-life of the drug depends greatly on hepatic blood flow. Reduced flow (as in heart failure or in older individuals) or intrinsic liver disease can greatly increase serum lidocaine concentrations and toxic effects; therefore, the infusion rate should be lowered in such patients.

The most common side effects of lidocaine are not cardiac; rather, they are related to the CNS and include confusion, dizziness, and seizures. These effects are dose-related and can be prevented by monitoring serum levels of the drug or preemptively reducing the infusion rate when liver disease or decreased hepatic blood flow is suspected.

Tocainide is an analog of lidocaine whose structure protects it from first-pass hepatic metabolism, so it can be administered orally. Its electrophysiologic effects are similar to those of lidocaine. Toxic effects are common and include those related to the CNS (dizziness, tremor, numbness) and to the gastrointestinal tract (nausea, diarrhea). The potential for serious blood disorders, including a severely reduced white blood cell count (agranulocytosis), has limited the usefulness of this drug. Approximately half of the dose of tocainide is excreted unchanged in the urine, so administration must be reduced in patients with renal dysfunction.

Mexiletine is structurally similar to lidocaine and shares its electrophysiologic properties. Similar to tocainide, it is administered orally. Ninety percent of mexiletine is metabolized in the liver to inactive products, and the dosage of the drug should be reduced in patients with hepatic dysfunction.

Dose-related side effects of mexiletine are common, especially of the CNS (dizziness, tremor, slurred speech) and the gastrointestinal tract (nausea, vomiting). The toxic hematologic effects seen with tocainide do not occur with mexiletine.

Diphenylhydantoin is an antiseizure medication that also has class IB antiarrhythmic properties. It is only occasionally used as an antiarrhythmic, generally limited to the treatment of digitalis-induced arrhythmias, in which it inhibits triggered automaticity (digitalis-induced delayed afterdepolarizations) without worsening digitalis-induced AV block.

Diphenylhydantoin can be administered by the intravenous or oral routes. It is primarily metabolized in the liver, and its degradation is slowed by hepatic disease. Serious adverse effects of diphenylhydantoin are related to the CNS (ataxia, drowsiness, nystagmus) and gastrointestinal tract (nausea, anorexia). Protracted use may cause hyperplasia of the gums and lymph nodes.

Class IC Antiarrhythmics

The class IC drugs are the most potent sodium channel blockers. They markedly decrease the upstroke of the action potential and conduction velocity in atrial, ventricular, and Purkinje fibers (see Fig. 17.11). Although they have little effect on the duration of the action potential, repolarization, or refractory period of Purkinje fibers, they significantly prolong the refractory period within the AV node and in accessory bypass tracts.

The group IC agents were originally developed to treat ventricular arrhythmias. However, that use has diminished, as studies have shown an *increased* mortality rate in patients taking class IC drugs for ventricular ectopy following myocardial infarction and in patients who have survived cardiac arrest. In patients with underlying left ventricular dysfunction, class IC drugs can precipitate heart failure. Thus, drugs of this subclass should be avoided in patients who have other underlying heart abnormalities, such as CAD or ventricular dysfunction. Class IC drugs *have* been shown to be beneficial (and reasonably safe) in preventing *supraventricular* arrhythmias in patients who have otherwise healthy hearts (see Table 17.13).

Flecainide is well absorbed after oral administration. Approximately 40% of the drug is excreted unchanged in the urine, and the remainder is converted to inactive metabolites by the liver. As indicated above, cardiac toxicities include the aggravation of ventricular arrhythmias and precipitation of CHF in patients with underlying left ventricular dysfunction. Noncardiac side effects are referable to the CNS and include confusion, dizziness, and blurred vision.

The electrophysiologic properties of **propafenone** are similar to those of flecainide, but in addition, it has a weak β-adrenergic blocking action. It is metabolized by the liver, but there is much genetic variation, such that an individual's dosage must be carefully titrated by observing the drug's effect. Extracardiac side effects are not common and include dizziness and disturbances of taste.

Class II Antiarrhythmics

The class II drugs are β-adrenergic receptor blockers, which are used in the management of both supraventricular and ventricular arrhythmias. Most of their antiarrhythmic properties can be attributed to inhibition of cardiac sympathetic activity. Additional actions of some β-blockers, such as β_1 cardioselectivity or a "membrane stabilizing effect," seem to make no contribution to antiarrhythmic activity.

Chapter 11 described how β-adrenergic stimulation results in a more rapid upslope of phase 4 depolarization and an increased firing rate of the SA node. β-adrenergic blockers inhibit these effects, thus reducing automaticity (Fig. 17.12). This action extends to the cardiac Purkinje fibers, where arrhythmias due to enhanced automaticity are inhibited. In addition, because afterdepolarizations may be caused by excessive catecholamines, β-blockers may prevent triggered arrhythmias induced by that mechanism. All β-blockers increase the effective refractory period of the AV node; therefore, these drugs are effective at interrupting reentrant rhythms that pass through it. β-blockers may also have a beneficial antiarrhythmic effect by decreasing myocardial oxygen demand, thus reducing myocardial ischemia. Several drugs from this group have been shown to reduce mortality following myocardial infarction (see Chapter 7), which may in part relate to their antiarrhythmic effect.

Since the AV nodal conduction time is prolonged by β-blockers, the PR interval on the ECG may become prolonged (see Table 17.12). The QRS and QT intervals are usually unaffected.

Clinical Uses

β-blockers are most useful in suppressing tachyarrhythmias induced by excessive catecholamines (e.g., during exercise or emotional stimulation). They are also frequently used to slow the ventricular rate in atrial flutter and fibrillation by impairing conduction and increasing the refractoriness of the AV node. In addition, β-blockers may terminate reentrant supraventricular arrhythmias in which the AV node constitutes one limb of the reentrant pathway.

β-blockers are effective in suppressing ventricular premature beats and other ventricular arrhythmias, especially when in-

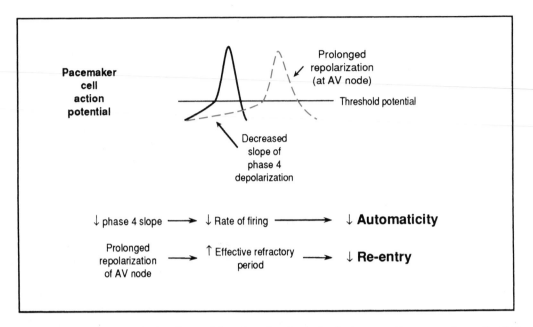

Figure 17.12. **Electrophysiologic effects of the class II antiarrhythmic drugs on the pacemaker cell action potential.**

duced by exercise. They are also effective in treating ventricular arrhythmias related to prolongation of the QT interval because, unlike group IA agents, they do not pathologically prolong that interval.

Class III Antiarrhythmics

Class III drugs are structurally dissimilar from one another, but share the property of significantly prolonging the action potential and refractoriness of Purkinje and ventricular muscle fibers (Fig. 17.13). In distinction to class I agents, they generally have little effect on phase 0 depolarization or conduction velocity.

Amiodarone is a powerful antiarrhythmic with many potential adverse reactions. Its major therapeutic effect is to prolong the action potential duration and refractoriness of all cardiac fibers. However, it also shares actions with each of the other antiarrhythmic classes. The slope of phase 0 depolarization may be depressed through sodium channel blockade (class I effect), it exerts a β-blocking effect (class II), and also demonstrates weak calcium channel blockade (class IV). As a result, the electrophysiologic effects of amiodarone are to decrease the si-

nus node firing rate, suppress automaticity, interrupt reentrant circuits, and prolong the PR, QRS, and QT intervals on the ECG.

In addition, amiodarone is a vasodilator (because of α-receptor and calcium channel blocking effects) and a negative inotrope (β-blocker and CCB effects). The resultant vasodilatation is more prominent than the negative inotropic effect, so that cardiac output does not usually suffer in patients treated with this drug.

Amiodarone is more effective than most other antiarrhythmic drugs for a wide spectrum of ventricular and supraventricular tachyarrhythmias. These include atrial fibrillation, atrial flutter, ventricular tachycardia, ventricular flutter, and supraventricular tachycardias, including those involving bypass tracts. It is a first-line agent for the emergency treatment of ventricular arrhythmias during cardiac resuscitation (including ventricular fibrillation and ventricular tachycardia refractory to electrical shocks), and is more effective than lidocaine for this purpose. It is a commonly used drug to treat arrhythmias in patients with ventricular systolic dysfunction because it causes fewer proarrhythmic complications in that population than other agents. In addition, low-dose amiodarone is very effective for long-term suppression of atrial fibrillation and flutter.

Amiodarone is absorbed slowly from the gastrointestinal tract, requiring 5–6 hours to reach peak plasma concentrations. It is highly lipophilic, is extensively sequestered in tissues, and undergoes very slow hepatic metabolism. Its elimination half-life is long and variable, averaging 25–60 *days*. The drug is excreted by the biliary tract, lacrimal glands, and skin but not by the kidney; thus, its dosage does not need to be adjusted in patients with renal failure. However, the delayed onset of action and very long duration of action make amiodarone a difficult drug to regulate if side effects ensue.

There are numerous potential side effects associated with amiodarone. The most serious is pulmonary toxicity, manifested as pneumonitis leading to pulmonary fibrosis. Its origin is unclear but may represent a hy-

persensitivity reaction and, if recognized early, is reversible.

Other life-threatening side effects of amiodarone relate to cardiac toxicity: symptomatic bradycardia and aggravation of ventricular arrhythmia each occur in approximately 2% of patients. As amiodarone significantly prolongs the QT interval, early afterdepolarizations and torsades de pointes can occur, but this happens only rarely. Intravenously administered amiodarone occasionally precipitates heart failure.

Abnormalities of thyroid function are common during amiodarone treatment, because the drug contains a significant iodine load and because it inhibits the peripheral conversion of T_4 to T_3. During the first few weeks of therapy, it is common to observe transient abnormalities of thyroid biochemical tests without clinical findings of thyroid disease: the serum TSH and T_4 rise, and serum T_3 falls. Over time, some patients develop overt hypothyroidism (due

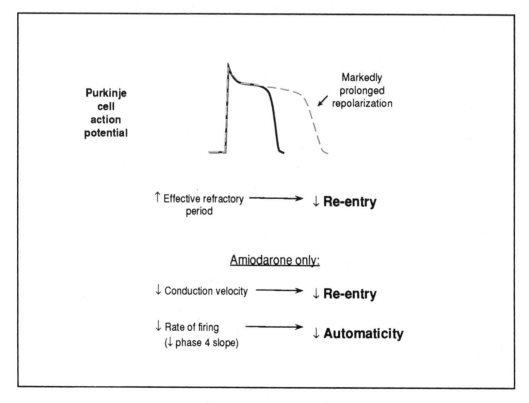

Figure 17.13. **Electrophysiologic effects of the class III antiarrhythmic drugs on the Purkinje cell action potential.**

mostly to the antithyroid effects of iodine) or hyperthyroidism (either because of an iodine effect in iodine-deficient communities, or because of a direct inflammatory thyroid process incited by amiodarone in susceptible individuals).

Gastrointestinal side effects of amiodarone include anorexia, nausea, and elevation of liver function tests, all of which improve with lower doses of the drug. Neurologic side effects include proximal muscle weakness, peripheral neuropathy, ataxia, tremors, and sleep disturbances. Commonly, corneal microdeposits can be detected in patients receiving chronic amiodarone therapy but these rarely affect vision.

As a result of the potential adverse effects, ECGs, chest radiographs, and thyroid and liver function blood tests are performed on a regular basis in patients receiving chronic therapy. Amiodarone interacts with, and increases the activity of, certain drugs including warfarin and digoxin, such that the dosages of those agents must be adjusted. Because amiodarone prolongs the QT interval, other drugs that do the same should be used with great caution or not at all. Other drugs that possess negative chronotropic or negative inotropic effects (β-blockers, verapamil, diltiazem) should also generally be avoided.

Sotalol is actually a nonselective β-blocker, but it is used in practice because of its additional class III antiarrhythmic properties. It prolongs the duration of the action potential, increases the refractory period of atrial and ventricular tissue, and inhibits conduction in accessory bypass tracts. The phase 0 upstroke velocity is not altered in the usual dosage range. It is effective in the treatment of both supraventricular and ventricular arrhythmias.

Sotalol is excreted exclusively by the kidneys, and its dosage should be adjusted in the presence of renal disease. Potential side effects include those of β-blockers described above. Since it prolongs the QT interval, the most serious potential adverse effect is provoking the ventricular arrhythmia torsades de pointes. This complication occurs in approximately 2% of patients and is more common in patients with a history

of heart failure and in women (for unclear reasons).

Bretylium tosylate is an intravenously administered class III drug used on occasion to treat life-threatening ventricular tachycardia or fibrillation, when all other attempts at resuscitation have failed. Its mechanism of action is different from that of other antiarrhythmic agents in that it acts at postganglionic adrenergic nerve terminals, where it initially releases norepinephrine but then inhibits subsequent release. Thus, after initial stimulation, sympathetic activity of the heart decreases. The initial catecholamine release can transiently aggravate arrhythmias, but continued therapy lengthens the action potential duration and refractoriness of atrial, ventricular, and Purkinje fibers. As a result, the threshold for ventricular fibrillation is substantially raised.

Immediately after bretylium administration, blood pressure may rise because of the catecholamine release. However, significant orthostatic *hypotension* may follow because of the drug's antiadrenergic actions.

Ibutilide is an intravenous antiarrhythmic agent used for the acute conversion of atrial fibrillation or atrial flutter of recent onset. This agent prolongs the action potential duration and increases atrial and ventricular refractoriness. The mechanism relates to activation of a slow inward current that prolongs the plateau (phase 2) of the action potential, rather than the effect of blocking outward potassium currents that is typical of other class III drugs. In clinical trials, the success rate for conversion of atrial flutter is approximately 60%, but only 30% for those in atrial fibrillation.

Because ibutilide prolongs the QT interval, the potentially fatal arrhythmia torsades de pointes can be precipitated, especially in patients with underlying ventricular dysfunction. Therefore, careful electrocardiographic monitoring is necessary for several hours after drug administration.

Dofetilide is the newest class III antiarrhythmic drug. It acts by blocking the outward potassium current, causing prolongation of the action potential duration and an increase in the effective refractory period. It is used orally for the conversion of atrial fibrillation and atrial flutter into sinus rhythm as well as for the maintenance of sinus rhythm after conversion. QT prolongation complicated by torsades de pointes is the major potential adverse effect. Thus, like most antiarrhythmics, drug administration should be initiated in the hospital with electrocardiographic monitoring. Dofetilide is excreted by the kidney, and its dose should be adjusted in patients with renal failure.

Class IV Antiarrhythmics

Class IV drugs exert their electrophysiologic effects by selective blockade of the slow L-type cardiac calcium channels and include **verapamil** and **diltiazem,** but not nifedipine or the other dihydropyridine CCBs. They are most potent in tissues in which the action potential depends on calcium currents, such as the SA and AV nodes. Within nodal tissue, calcium channel blockade decreases phase 4 spontaneous depolarization (resulting in decreased automaticity), elevates the threshold potential, decreases the rate of rise of phase 0 depolarization and conduction ve-

locity, and lengthens the refractory period of the AV node (Fig. 17.14). These electrophysiologic actions translate into their clinical effects: 1) the heart rate slows; 2) transmission of rapid atrial impulses through the AV node to the ventricles decreases, thus slowing the ventricular rate in atrial fibrillation and atrial flutter; and 3) reentrant rhythms traveling through the AV node may terminate.

A primary antiarrhythmic use of class IV drugs is in the treatment of reentrant PSVT. Formerly, intravenous verapamil was the treatment of choice for acute episodes of this rhythm, but intravenous adenosine (which is not a Ca^{++} channel blocker; see below) has subsequently assumed that role. The class IV antiarrhythmics are also often used clinically to slow the ventricular rate in patients with atrial fibrillation or flutter.

The pharmacology and toxicities of CCBs were presented earlier in this chapter. The most important side effect of verapamil and diltiazem, when administered intravenously as antiarrhythmics, is hypotension. In addition, these agents should be avoided in patients receiving β-blocker

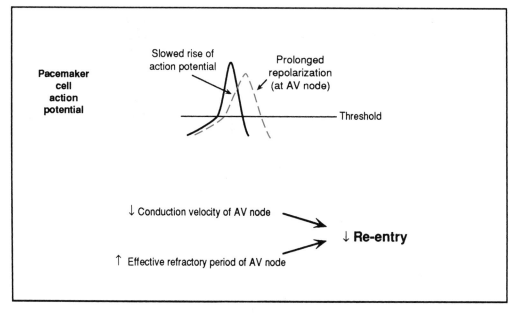

Figure 17.14. **Electrophysiologic effects of the class IV antiarrhythmic drugs on the pacemaker cell action potential.**

therapy, because the additive negative inotropic and chronotropic effects may precipitate heart failure.

Adenosine

Adenosine is an endogenous nucleoside with a very short half-life. Administered intravenously, it is the most effective drug for the rapid termination of reentrant PSVT.

Adenosine has substantial electrophysiologic effects on specialized conduction tissues, especially the SA and AV nodes. By binding to specific adenosine receptors, it activates potassium channels (Fig. 17.15). The resultant increase in the outward potassium current hyperpolarizes the membrane, and therefore suppresses spontaneous depolarization of the SA node, and slows conduction through the AV node.

In addition, adenosine decreases intracellular cyclic AMP (cAMP) concentrations by inhibiting adenylate cyclase. The result is a decrease in the inward pacemaker current (I_f) and a decrease in the calcium inward current (see Fig. 17.15). Thus, the net

effect of adenosine is to slow the SA node firing rate and to decrease AV nodal conduction. By inducing transient AV nodal block, adenosine terminates reentrant pathways that include the AV node as part of the circuit. Ventricular myocytes are relatively immune to these effects, at least in part because the specific potassium channels responsive to adenosine are not present in those cells.

Because the half-life of adenosine is only 10 sec, side effects (headache, chest pain, flushing, bronchoconstriction) are very transient. Because methylxanthines (caffeine, theophylline) competitively antagonize the adenosine receptor, higher doses of adenosine may be necessary in patients using those substances. Conversely, dipyridamole inhibits the breakdown of adenosine and amplifies its effect.

In summary, antiarrhythmic drugs have complex actions and display multiple cardiac and noncardiac toxicities. The potential of inducing dangerous arrhythmias exists with most agents. Whenever antiarrhythmic drugs are used, patients must be followed

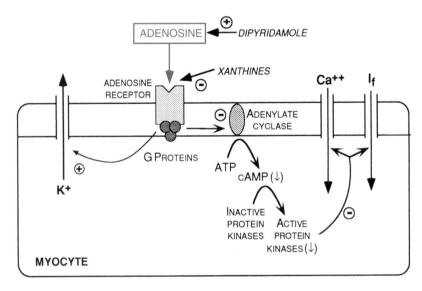

Figure 17.15. Mechanism of antiarrhythmic action of adenosine. Stimulation of the myocyte adenosine receptor activates potassium channels, and the resultant outward K^+ current hyperpolarizes the membrane (resulting in decreased automaticity). Adenosine also inhibits membrane adenylate cyclase activity; the subsequent reduction in active protein kinases decreases the inward pacemaker (I_f) and Ca^{++} currents (resulting in decreased automaticity and decreased conduction through the AV node). Xanthines compete for the adenosine receptor, blocking these effects. Dipyridamole interferes with cellular uptake and degradation of adenosine and therefore amplifies its effect.

closely, the effectiveness of the drug demonstrated, and surveillance for toxicity continued over the long term.

DIURETICS

Diuretics are most often used to treat heart failure and hypertension. In heart failure, enhanced renal reabsorption of sodium and water, with subsequent expansion of the extracellular volume, contributes to peripheral edema and pulmonary congestion. Diuretics eliminate excess sodium and water through renal excretion and are therefore the cornerstone of therapy to relieve congestive symptoms (see Chapter 9). In the treatment of hypertension, diuretics act in part by elimination of intravascular volume and in some cases through vascular dilatation.

In the kidney, the rate of glomerular filtration typically averages 135–180 L/day in normal adults. Most of the filtered Na^+ is reabsorbed by the renal tubules, leaving only a small quantity in the final urine (Fig.

17.16). Approximately 65–70% of the filtered Na^+ is reabsorbed isosmotically in the proximal tubule by active transport. In the thick ascending limb of the loop of Henle, an additional 25% of the filtered sodium is reabsorbed, through a Na^+/K^+ cotransport system coupled to the uptake of two Cl^- ions. Because this region is impermeable to the reabsorption of water, hypotonic tubular fluid is formed here, and the surrounding interstitium becomes hypertonic. In the distal convoluted tubule, an additional small fraction of NaCl is reabsorbed (approximately 5%). In the cortical collecting duct, Na^+ permeability is modulated by an aldosterone-sensitive mechanism, such that Na^+ is reabsorbed into the tubular cells in the presence of aldosterone, creating a lumen negative potential difference that enhances K^+ and H^+ excretion. Approximately 1–2% of sodium reabsorption takes place at this location.

All but the terminal segment of the distal tubule is impermeable to water. In the col-

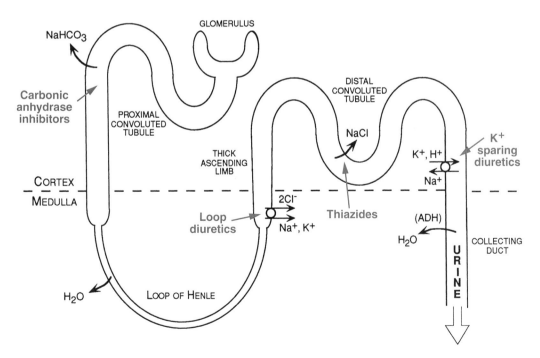

Figure 17.16. Schematic diagram of the renal tubules. Approximately 70% of filtered sodium is reabsorbed in the proximal convoluted tubule, 25% in the thick ascending limb of the loop of Henle, 5% in the distal convoluted tubule, and 1–2% in the cortical collecting tubule (mediated by the action of aldosterone). Antidiuretic hormone (ADH) increases the permeability of the distal nephron for water. Diuretics are secreted into the proximal convoluted tubule and act at the sites shown.

TABLE 17.14. Commonly Used Diuretics

Diuretic		Onset of Action (hours)	Duration of Action (hours)	Potential Adverse Effects
Thiazides				Hypokalemia, hypomagnesemia,
Chlorothiazide	PO	1	6–12	hyponatremia, hypercalcemia,
	IV	0.25	2	hyperglycemia, hyperuricemia,
Hydrochlorothiazide	PO	2	12	hypercholesterolemia,
Chlorthalidone	PO	2	24	hypertriglyceridemia, metabolic
Metolazone	PO	1	12–24	alkalosis
Indapamide	PO	1–2	16–36	
Loop diuretics				Hypotension, hypokalemia,
Furosemide	PO	1	6	hypomagnesemia,
	IV	5 min	2	hyperglycemia, hyperuricemia,
Bumetanide	PO	0.5–1	4–6	metabolic alkalosis
	IV	0.25	0.5–1	
Torsemide	PO	<1	6–8	
	IV	10 min	6–8	
Ethacrynic acid	IV	0.25	3	
Potassium-sparing diuretics				Hyperkalemia, gastrointestinal disturbances
Spironolactone	PO	1–2 days	2–3 days	(spironolactone only):
Triamterene	PO	2	12–16	gynecomastia
Amiloride	PO	2	24	

lecting tubule, however, water permeability and reabsorption are promoted by antidiuretic hormone and driven by the osmotic gradient between the tubule and the hypertonic interstitium. Substances that interfere with antidiuretic hormone, such as ethanol consumption, therefore have diuretic actions.

The three most commonly used groups of diuretics are the loop diuretics, thiazide diuretics, and potassium-sparing diuretics (Table 17.14 and Fig. 17.16). These three classes are generally distinguished by the site of the kidney tubule where they act, and their potency. Loop diuretics impair absorption in the thick ascending limb of the loop of Henle, thiazide diuretics act on the distal tubule and collecting segment, and potassium-sparing diuretics act on the aldosterone-sensitive region of the cortical collecting tubule. A fourth group, the carbonic anhydrase inhibitors, are weak diuretics rarely used in the treatment of hypertension or heart failure. They act at the proximal convoluted tubule, resulting in a loss of bicarbonate (and sodium) in the urine.

Diuretics, as active pharmacologic agents, are secreted into the proximal renal tubule, and their major sites of action are shown schematically in Figure 17.16.

Loop Diuretics

These agents are so named because they act principally on the thick ascending limb of the loop of Henle. They are powerful diuretics that result in the excretion of 20–25% of the filtered Na^+ load through inhibition of the $Na^+/2Cl^-/K^+$ cotransport system. Because inhibition at this site impairs the generation of a hypertonic interstitium, the gradient for passive water movement out of the collecting duct is diminished and water diuresis results.

Loop diuretics are of great importance in the acute management of pulmonary edema (administered intravenously) and in the treatment of chronic heart failure or peripheral edema (taken orally). Unlike other diuretics, they tend to be effective even in the setting of impaired renal function. In addition to the diuretic effect, and even preceding it, drugs of this class may induce venodilatation, which is also beneficial in reducing venous return and pulmonary congestion (see Chapter 9). The mechanism of venodilatation appears to involve drug-induced prostaglandin and nitric oxide generation from endothelial cells, which act to relax vascular smooth muscle.

The most common side effects of the loop diuretics are intravascular volume depletion, hypokalemia, and metabolic alkalosis. *Hypokalemia* arises because 1) these agents impair the reabsorption of sodium in the loop of Henle, such that an increased amount of Na^+ is delivered to the distal tubule, where it prompts greater-than-usual exchange for potassium (and therefore more K^+ excretion into the urine); and 2) diuretic-induced intravascular volume depletion activates the renin-angiotensin system. The subsequent rise in aldosterone promotes additional Na^+/K^+ exchange and hence potassium loss into the urine.

Metabolic alkalosis during loop diuretic therapy results from two mechanisms: 1) increased H^+ secretion into the distal tubule (and therefore into the urine) due to the secondary hyperaldosteronism described above, and 2) contraction alkalosis—increased sodium bicarbonate reabsorption by the proximal tubule (see Fig. 17.16) is promoted by the reduced intravascular volume.

Additional side effects may also occur during continued loop diuretic therapy. *Hypomagnesemia* may result, because magnesium reabsorption depends on NaCl transport in the thick ascending limb of the loop of Henle, the action blocked by these drugs. *Ototoxicity* (eighth cranial nerve toxicity) occasionally develops, impairing hearing and vestibular function. It is thought to arise from electrolyte disturbances of the endolymphatic system, most likely because of $Na^+/2Cl^-/K^+$ cotransport inhibition by the loop diuretic at that site.

The most commonly used loop diuretic is **furosemide,** the oral form of which demonstrates reliable gastrointestinal absorption but a short duration of action (4–6 hours) that limits its usefulness in the chronic treatment of hypertension. **Bumetanide** is similar to furosemide and shares its actions and adverse effects but has greater potency and bioavailability. It also appears to have a lower incidence of ototoxicity than the other drugs of this class. Bumetanide is sometimes

useful in CHF when edema is refractory to other agents and in some individuals allergic to furosemide. **Torsemide** also has actions similar to those of furosemide, with more complete bioavailability. **Ethacrynic acid** is the only nonsulfonamide loop diuretic, so it can be prescribed to patients who cannot tolerate sulfonamide compounds. However, ethacrynic acid is not widely used because of its high incidence of ototoxicity.

Thiazide Diuretics

Thiazides and related compounds (chlorthalidone, indapamide, and metolazone) are commonly used diuretics because they demonstrate excellent gastrointestinal absorption when administered orally and are usually well tolerated. They are less potent than the loop diuretics, but because of their sustained actions, are useful in chronic conditions such as hypertension and mild CHF.

This class of drugs acts at the distal tubule, where they block the reabsorption of approximately 3–5% of the filtered sodium (see Fig. 17.16). Na^+ reabsorption at this site is mediated through a Na^+/Cl^- cotransporter on the luminal membrane. The thiazides inhibit this carrier by a mechanism that has not been elucidated but may involve competition for the Cl^- site. The antihypertensive effect is initially associated with a decrease in cardiac output, due to reduced intravascular volume, and unchanged peripheral resistance. With long-term thiazide use, however, cardiac output often returns to normal as total peripheral resistance becomes reduced by an unexplained vascular dilatation. **Indapamide** is unique among this class in that it displays a particularly prominent vasodilating effect.

Thiazides are most often administered orally. Diuresis occurs after 1–2 hours, but the full antihypertensive effect of continued therapy may not become manifest for up to 12 weeks (possibly related to the vasodilator mechanism alluded to above). **Chlorothiazide,** the parent compound, has a low lipid solubility and hence low bioavailability: higher doses are therefore required to achieve therapeutic levels compared with the more commonly used **hydrochloro-thiazide. Chlorthalidone** is slowly absorbed and hence has a long duration of action. **Metolazone,** unlike other drugs of this class, is sometimes effective in patients with reduced renal function.

Clinically, the thiazides differ from the loop diuretics in that they are less potent, have a longer duration of action, and (with the exception of metolazone) demonstrate poor diuretic efficacy in the setting of impaired renal function: They are generally not effective when the GFR is <25 ml/min.

Thiazides serve as the cornerstone of antihypertensive therapy because of their low cost, effectiveness, and proven benefits in reducing the risk of stroke and cardiac events. They are sometimes used in heart failure, generally for patients with mild chronic congestive symptoms. In addition, they can be combined with a loop diuretic for patients who have become refractory to the diuretic effect of the latter. The combination of the two classes lowers the dose-dependent adverse effects that accompany each drug; because they act on sequential segments of the renal tubule, a more profound natriuretic effect ensues than with either agent used alone.

Among the most important potential adverse effects of thiazides are 1) *hypokalemia* and *metabolic alkalosis,* which result in part from increased Na^+ delivery to the distal tubule, where exchange for K^+ and H^+ takes place, and partly from volume contraction and secondary hyperaldosteronism, as described for the loop diuretics above; 2) *hyponatremia,* during prolonged treatment because of continued Na^+ excretion in the setting of chronic free water consumption; 3) *hyperuricemia* (and possible precipitation of gout) due to decreased clearance of uric acid; 4) *hyperglycemia,* because of either impaired pancreatic insulin release or decreased peripheral glucose utilization; 5) *alterations in serum lipids (at least transiently),* characterized by increased low-density lipoprotein (LDL) cholesterol and triglycerides; and 6) *weakness, fatigability,* and *paresthesias,* which can occur with long-term use because of volume depletion and hypokalemia. Also, serum calcium levels often rise slightly during thiazide therapy, but this is rarely clinically significant.

In past decades, the standard thiazide dosage was excessive compared with current practice. By using lower dosages, it is possible to accrue the benefits of this class of diuretics while minimizing the adverse effects.

Potassium-Sparing Diuretics

These agents are relatively weak diuretics that antagonize physiologic Na^+ reabsorption at the distal convoluted tubule and cortical collecting tubule. Potassium-sparing diuretics reduce K^+ excretion; thus, unlike with diuretics, hypokalemia is not a side effect. They are used when maintenance of serum potassium levels is crucial and in states characterized by aldosterone excess (e.g., primary or secondary hyperaldosteronism). Two types of drugs make up this group: 1) aldosterone antagonists (e.g., spironolactone) and 2) direct inhibitors of Na^+ permeability in the collecting duct, which act independently of aldosterone (e.g., triamterene and amiloride).

Na^+ and K^+ exchange in the collecting tubules accounts for only a small percentage of sodium reuptake, so that a clinically important diuresis does not occur with these agents when used alone. Rather, they are often used in combination with the loop or thiazide classes for additive diuretic effect and to prevent clinically important hypokalemia.

Spironolactone is a synthetic steroid that competes for the cytoplasmic aldosterone receptor, thereby inhibiting the aldosterone-sensitive Na^+ channel in the kidney. Because Na^+ reabsorption through the sodium channel is inhibited, no lumen-negative potential exists to drive K^+ and H^+ ion excretion at the distal nephron sites; thus, K^+ and H^+ ions are retained in the circulation. Spironolactone also displays anti-remodeling effects in the heart that appear to be of special benefit (see Chapter 9). In a trial of patients with severe heart failure, spironolactone (added to an ACE-inhibitor and a loop diuretic, with or without digoxin) improved heart failure symptoms and reduced mortality rates.

The most serious complication of spironolactone is the development of hyperkalemia, resulting from impaired excretion of that ion. Thus, one should be cautious about administration of K^+ supplements, or ACE inhibitors or angiotensin receptor blockers when potassium-sparing diuretics are used, as they could contribute to this complication. Spironolactone also displays antiandrogenic activity that may produce gynecomastia in men and menstrual irregularities in women.

Triamterene and **amiloride** are structurally related potassium-sparing diuretics that act independently of aldosterone. At the distal tubules, they inhibit the Na^+ channel; therefore, the excretion of K^+ and H^+ is diminished. Triamterene is metabolized by the liver, and its active product is secreted into the proximal tubule by the organic cation transport system. Amiloride is secreted directly into the proximal tubule and appears unchanged in the urine. As with spironolactone, the most important potential adverse effect of these drugs is the development of hyperkalemia.

ANTITHROMBOTIC DRUGS

Platelets and the coagulation proteins play a key role in the pathogenesis of many cardiovascular disorders, including the acute coronary syndromes (unstable angina, acute myocardial infarction), deep venous thrombosis, and thrombi that may complicate atrial fibrillation, dilated cardiomyopathy, or mechanical prosthetic heart valves. Therefore, the modulation of platelet function and of the coagulation pathway is often critically important in cardiovascular therapeutics.

The formation of a thrombus, whether in normal hemostasis or in pathologic clot formation, requires three events: 1) exposure of circulating blood elements to thrombogenic material (e.g., unmasking of subendothelial collagen after atherosclerotic plaque rupture), 2) activation of platelets, and 3) triggering of the coagulation cascade, ultimately resulting in a fibrin clot. Hemostasis effected by platelets and the coagulation system are closely interlinked—

activated platelets accelerate the coagulation pathway, and certain coagulation proteins (e.g., thrombin) contribute to platelet aggregation.

This section focuses first on drugs that interfere with platelet function and then on those that inhibit the coagulation cascade. Thrombolytic agents, which dissolve clots that have already formed, are described in Chapter 7.

Platelet Inhibitors

Platelets are responsible for primary hemostasis by a three-part process: 1) adhesion to the site of injury, 2) release reaction (secretion of platelet products and activation of key surface receptors), and 3) aggregation. For example, following blood vessel injury, platelets quickly adhere to exposed subendothelial collagen by means of membrane glycoprotein receptors, a process that is dependent on von Willebrand factor. Following adhesion to the vessel wall, platelets release the preformed contents of their granules in response to agonists (including collagen and thrombin) that bind to platelet receptors. Prepackaged substances that are released from the platelet cytoplasmic granules include ADP, serotonin, fibrinogen, growth factors, and procoagulants. Concurrently within the activated platelet, there is de novo synthesis and secretion of thromboxane A_2 (TXA_2), a powerful vasoconstrictor (Fig. 17.17).

Certain agonists, including ADP, thrombin, and TXA_2, then stimulate platelets to aggregate and form the primary hemostatic plug, as additional platelets are recruited from the circulation. During this process, there is a critical conformational change in the platelet membrane glycoprotein (GP) IIb/IIIa receptors. This alteration allows the previously inactive IIb/IIIa receptor to bind fibrinogen molecules, an action that tightly links platelets to one another and constitutes the final common pathway of platelet aggregation. The developing clump of platelets is stabilized and tethered to the site of injury by a developing mesh of fibrin, which is produced by the simultaneous activation of the coagulation protein cascade.

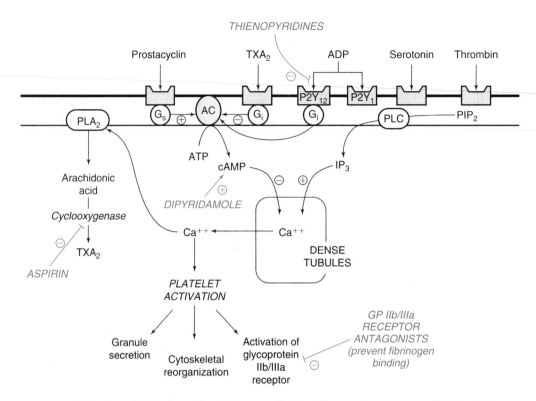

Figure 17.17. **Platelet activation is mediated by cytosolic Ca^{++}.** Factors that promote and inhibit calcium release from the platelet-dense tubules are shown. Thrombin and serotonin, acting at their specific receptors, stimulate the formation of inositol triphosphate (IP$_3$) from phosphatidylinositol diphosphate (PIP$_2$) by phospholipase C (PLC). IP$_3$ subsequently enhances the intracellular release of calcium. Thromboxane A$_2$ (TXA$_2$) also facilitates calcium release. It inhibits adenyl cyclase (AC) and reduces cyclic AMP (cAMP) formation. Since cAMP normally *prevents* Ca^{++} release from the ER, the reduction of this effect by TXA$_2$ *increases* Ca^{++} release into the cytosol. Conversely, endothelial-derived prostacyclin has the opposite effect. It reduces intraplatelet calcium release because it *stimulates* AC activity and cAMP formation. ADP also stimulates calcium release via its two receptors (see text for details). Calcium promotes the action of phospholipase A$_2$ (PLA$_2$), which generates the precursors of TXA$_2$ from the cell membrane. Platelet activation modulated by [Ca^{++}] ultimately results in granule secretion, cytoskeletal reorganization, and the critical conformational change in glycoprotein IIb/IIIa receptors that is necessary for platelet aggregation. The sites of action of commonly used antiplatelet drugs are shown in color.

Platelet activation is regulated to a great extent by release of stored Ca^{++} from the platelet-dense tubular system. This action results in an increase in the cytosolic calcium concentration, with activation of protein kinases and phosphorylation of intraplatelet regulatory proteins. The increase in cytosolic Ca^{++} also stimulates phospholipase A$_2$, causing the release of arachidonic acid, the precursor of TXA$_2$ (see Fig. 17.17).

The critical release of calcium is modulated by several factors. Acting at their respective platelet membrane receptors, thrombin and other agonists generate intermediaries that *stimulate* the release of cal-

cium from the dense tubules. TXA$_2$ increases the intracellular Ca^{++} by binding to its platelet receptor, which inhibits the activity of adenylate cylase and thereby reduces cAMP formation, an action that augments the release of Ca^{++} from the dense tubules (see Fig. 17.17). Conversely, endothelial cell-derived prostacyclin (PGI$_2$) *stimulates* adenylate cyclase activity and increases platelet cAMP concentration, which *inhibits* Ca^{++} release from the dense tubular system.

Antiplatelet drugs interfere with platelet function at various points along the sequence of activation and aggregation (see Fig. 17.17). The most commonly used antiplatelet drug is aspirin, but the roles of newer antiplatelet drugs, especially the thienopyridines and GP IIb/IIIa inhibitors, have rapidly expanded.

Aspirin

As described in the previous section, TXA_2 is an important mediator of platelet activation and clot formation. Aspirin (acetylsalicylic acid) acts by irreversibly acetylating (and thus blocking the action of) cyclooxygenase, an enzyme essential to thromboxane production from arachidonic acid (see Fig.17-17). The form of the enzyme found in platelets is cyclooxygenase-1 (COX-1), which is effectively inhibited by the nonselective action of aspirin (but it is *not* inhibited by selective COX-2 antagonists, such as celecoxib or rofecoxib). Because platelets lack nuclei and therefore cannot synthesize new proteins (including cyclooxygenase), aspirin *permanently* disables TXA_2 production in exposed platelets.

The prostaglandin PGI_2, a major antagonist of TXA_2 that is produced by endothelial cells, shares a dependency on cyclooxygenase activity for its formation, and aspirin, at high dosage, impairs its synthesis as well. Unlike platelets, however, endothelial cells *are* able to generate new cyclooxygenase to replace what has been deactivated by acetylation. Thus, when used in low dosage, aspirin effectively inhibits platelet TXA_2 synthesis without significantly interfering with the presence and beneficial actions of PGI_2.

Since the antiplatelet effect of aspirin is limited to inhibition of TXA_2 formation, platelet aggregation induced by other factors (e.g., ADP) is not significantly impeded. Thus, aspirin is not a "complete" antithrombotic agent.

Clinical Uses

Aspirin therapy has many proven clinical benefits in patients with cardiovascular disease (Table 17.15). In individuals with unstable angina, acute myocardial infarction, or a history of myocardial infarction, aspirin conclusively reduces the incidence of future fatal and nonfatal coronary

TABLE 17.15. Cardiovascular Uses of Antithrombotic Drugs

Drug	Chronic Angina	Unstable Angina/ NSTEMI	Acute MI	Post- MI	DVT	Mechanical Heart Valve	Atrial Fibrillation	PCI	HIT
Platelet inhibitors									
Aspirin	+	+	(1)	+		(2)	(3)	+	
Thienopyridines		+						(4)	
GP IIb/IIIa inhibitors		(5)						(5)	
Dipyridamole						(6)			
Anticoagulants									
UFH		+	(7)		+	(8)	(8)	+	
LMWH		+	(9)		+				
Direct thrombin inhibitors								+	+
Warfarin			(10)	+		+	+		

(1) Chewed or crushed non–enteric-coated aspirin preferred.
(2) Sometimes used in combination with warfarin.
(3) If patient has a low risk of stroke, or if warfarin is contraindicated.
(4) When intracoronary stent is implanted.
(5) In combination with aspirin and heparin.
(6) Sometimes used in combination with warfarin for recurrent embolism, but combination of aspirin and warfarin is better.
(7) After thrombolytic therapy (with tPA, rPA, or TNK-tPA), or if large akinetic segment develops.
(8) For hospitalized patients unable to take warfarin.
(9) Emerging use, following newer thrombolytic agents (e.g., TNK-tPA).
(10) For 3–6 months if large akinetic segment present.
NSTEMI, non-ST-elevation myocardial infarction; *MI,* myocardial infarction; *DVT,* deep venous thrombosis; *PCI,* percutaneous coronary interventions; *HIT,* heparin-induced thrombocytopenia; *UFH,* unfractionated heparin; *LMWH,* low-molecular-weight heparin.

events. Similarly, in patients with chronic stable angina *without* a history of myocardial infarction, aspirin lessens the occurrence of subsequent myocardial infarction and mortality. In patients who have suffered a minor stroke or transient cerebral ischemic attacks, aspirin reduces the rate of future stroke and cardiovascular events. In patients who have undergone coronary artery bypass surgery, aspirin lowers the likelihood of graft occlusion.

The use of aspirin for *primary* prevention (i.e., for individuals without a history of cardiovascular events or symptoms) is of less clear benefit. When tested in a large cohort of healthy, American, middle-aged men, aspirin was associated with a reduced incidence of nonfatal myocardial infarction, but an increased rate of nonfatal hemorrhagic stroke and gastrointestinal bleeding; there was no effect on total vascular mortality. Subsequent meta-analyses of clinical trials have similarly concluded that aspirin is effective for primary prevention of myocardial infarction in patients with coronary risk factors, but it also increases the risk of hemorrhagic stroke. Thus, whereas aspirin plays an extremely important role in patients with known cardiovascular disease, it is not evident that otherwise healthy people should routinely take aspirin for cardiovascular "protection."

It is currently recommended that aspirin (at a low dosage of 75–325 mg/d) be administered to patients with clinical manifestations of coronary disease in the absence of contraindications (i.e., aspirin allergy or complications described below). It should not be prescribed routinely for primary prevention purposes in healthy individuals. However, pending the results of ongoing research, many physicians believe it is appropriate to recommend aspirin use in men and women older than age 50 who have at least one major cardiac risk factor (as described in Chapter 5). In addition, the American Diabetes Association recommends that all diabetics with at least one other coronary risk factor take aspirin for cardiovascular protection. Finally, aspirin is not as beneficial as warfarin (described below) for the prevention of stroke in high-risk patients with atrial fibrillation and should only be used in that setting when warfarin cannot be safely administered.

Side Effects

The most common adverse effects of aspirin are related to the gastrointestinal system, including dyspepsia and nausea, which often can be ameliorated by lowering the dosage and/or using enteric-coated or buffered tablets. More serious potential side effects include gastrointestinal bleeding, hemorrhagic strokes, allergic reactions, and asthma exacerbation in aspirin-allergic patients. Because aspirin is excreted by the kidneys and competes with uric acid for the renal proximal tubule organic anion transporter, it may also occasionally exacerbate gout.

Thienopyridines

The thienopyridines inhibit ADP-mediated activation of platelets (see Fig. 17.17). Normally, extracellular ADP activates platelets by binding to two types of surface purinoceptors. The first (termed $P2Y_1$) acts through phospholipase C to increase intraplatelet $[Ca^{++}]$ and potentiates platelet activation. The second, recently characterized purinoceptor ($P2Y_{12}$) is linked to an inhibitory G-protein and reduces cAMP production when activated, thus also raising intraplatelet $[Ca^{++}]$ (see Fig. 17.17). ADP-induced platelet aggregation requires that ADP simultaneously activate *both* $P2Y_1$ and $P2Y_{12}$ purinoceptors. The thienopyridines (or their metabolites) irreversibly block the $P2Y_{12}$ purinoceptor by binding directly to it or to a nearby membrane protein. As a result, platelet aggregation is inhibited.

Ticlopidine and **clopidogrel** are the thienopyridines approved for clinical use. Both are well absorbed orally and have good bioavailability. Their onset of action is delayed (2–4 days), so they are generally used for long-term, rather than acute, antiplatelet effect. Meta-analyses of ticlopidine or clopidogrel in patients prone to coronary syndromes have concluded that these drugs are modestly superior to aspirin in reducing the risk of myocardial infarction, stroke, or vascular deaths, but at an increased risk of side effects and at a much higher economic cost. A recent study evaluated the *combination* of aspirin plus clopidogrel in patients with unstable angina or non-ST-elevation myocardial infarction and found a small benefit in cardiovascular outcomes compared with aspirin alone, but with an increased bleeding risk.

The main uses of the thienopyridines (especially clopidogrel) are as an antiplatelet substitute in patients allergic to aspirin and for short-term therapy to prevent thrombotic complications following percutaneous coronary stenting (see Chapter 6). The combination of clopidogrel plus aspirin is also approved for use in patients with unstable angina or non-ST-elevation myocardial infarction.

The most common side effects of the thienopyridines are dyspepsia and diarrhea. However, the use of ticlopidine has been limited by potentially life-threatening side effects: severe neutropenia (occurring in 0.8–2.5% of patients) and thrombotic thrombocytopenic purpura (in approximately 0.02% of treated patients). These hematologic effects are much rarer with clopidogrel, which is therefore now the preferred agent of this class.

Glycoprotein (GP) IIb/IIIa Receptor Antagonists

The GP IIb/IIIa receptor antagonists constitute one of the most potent classes of antiplatelet agents. This group reversibly inhibits the critical and final common pathway of platelet aggregation—the binding of activated platelet GP IIb/IIIa receptors to fibrinogen and von Willebrand factor. As a result, platelets are inhibited from "sticking" to one another, impairing the formation of a hemostatic plug. Three types of GP IIb/IIIa receptor antagonists have been developed: 1) monoclonal antibodies (e.g., **abciximab**), 2) synthetic peptide antagonists (e.g., **eptifibatide**), and 3) synthetic nonpeptide antagonists (e.g., **tirofiban**). As described in Chapters 6 and 7, the GP IIb/IIIa antagonists represent a major advance in improving outcomes of patients undergoing percutaneous coronary interventions and in high-risk acute coronary syndromes.

All the GP IIb/IIIa receptor inhibitors in current clinical use must be given intravenously. Oral GP IIb/IIIa receptor inhibitors have been developed but have not demonstrated beneficial outcomes in clinical trials.

The major side effects of the GP IIb/IIIa receptor inhibitors are bleeding (in 1–10% of patients) and thrombocytopenia (in approximately 2% of patients treated with abciximab and less commonly with the other agents). Because abciximab has a short plasma half-life (30 minutes), its effects can be reversed (e.g., if bleeding occurs) by discontinuing infusion of the drug or by administering a platelet transfusion. The other GP IIb/IIIa receptor antagonists have longer half-lives and may continue to inactivate transfused platelets. However, bleeding complications are infrequent using current protocols and careful dosing of concurrent heparin therapy.

Dipyridamole

Dipyridamole, another antiplatelet agent, is occasionally prescribed for patients who are intolerant to aspirin, but it is not as effective. Its mechanism of antiplatelet action is unclear, but it may act, in part, by increasing platelet cAMP levels, either by inhibiting phosphodiesterase or by blocking cellular uptake and destruction of adenosine. As a result, cytosolic [Ca^{++}] falls, which inhibits platelet aggregation (see Fig. 17.17). By itself, dipyridamole has no proven benefits. It is used sometimes in combination with warfarin for an augmented antithrombotic effect in patients with recurrent thromboembolism from prosthetic heart valves, but the combination of aspirin plus warfarin is more effective. Its most common current use is actually as a pharmacologic stress testing agent (see Chapter 3).

Anticoagulant Drugs

Anticoagulant drugs interfere with the coagulation cascade and impair secondary hemostasis. Since the final step in both the intrinsic and extrinsic coagulation pathways is the formation of a fibrin clot by the action of thrombin, major goals of anticoagulant therapy are to inhibit thrombin activation from prothrombin (e.g., using unfractionated or low-molecular-weight forms of heparin), to inhibit thrombin itself (e.g., with unfractionated heparin or direct thrombin inhibitors), or to decrease the production of functional prothrombin (e.g., using warfarin).

Unfractionated Heparin

Unfractionated heparin (UFH) is a heterogeneous mixture of highly charged mucopolysaccharide polymers. Although it has little anticoagulant action by itself, it associates with antithrombin III (AT III) in the circulation, greatly increasing its effect. AT III is a natural protein that inhibits the action of thrombin and other clotting factors. When UFH complexes with AT III, the affinity of AT III for thrombin increases 1000-fold. As a result, thrombin's ability to produce fibrin from fibrinogen is significantly reduced. The UFH-AT III complex also inhibits activated factor X, additionally contributing to the anticoagulant action. Furthermore, UFH has antiplatelet properties by binding to, and blocking the action of, von Willebrand factor.

UFH is administered parenterally, as it is not absorbed from the gastrointestinal tract. For most acute indications, an intravenous bolus is followed by a continuous infusion of the drug. The bioavailability of UFH varies from patient to patient since it is a heterogeneous collection of molecules that bind to plasma proteins, macrophages, and endothelial cells. Since the dose–effect relationship is often not predictable, frequent blood samples are required to monitor the degree of anticoagulation (most commonly, measurement of the activated partial thromboplastin time [aPTT]), so that the infusion rate can be adjusted properly.

The usual cardiovascular settings in which intravenous UFH is indicated include the following: 1) *unstable angina* (Chapter 6), 2) *acute myocardial infarction* af-

ter thrombolytic therapy or if an extensive wall motion abnormality is present (Chapter 7), 3) *pulmonary embolism* or *deep venous thrombosis* (DVT) (Chapter 15), and 4) when a patient receiving chronic anticoagulation therapy is unable to ingest the oral drug (e.g., in the perioperative setting). Among hospitalized or bed-ridden patients not receiving intravenous heparin, fixed low dosages of *subcutaneous* UFH are often administered to prevent DVT.

The most important side effect of heparin is *bleeding*. An overdose of UFH can be treated with intravenous protamine sulfate, which forms a stable complex with UFH and immediately reverses the anticoagulation effect.

Heparin-induced thrombocytopenia (HIT) is another potential adverse effect and can occur in two forms. The more common type, thought to result from direct heparin-induced platelet aggregation, occurs in up to 15% of patients and is usually asymptomatic, dose-dependent, and self-limited. This mild HIT rarely causes severe reductions in platelet counts and usually does not require cessation of heparin.

The less common, much more dangerous form of HIT is immune-mediated, a condition that affects 3% of UFH-treated patients. It can lead to life-threatening bleeding and, paradoxically, to thrombosis. Thrombosis is produced by the formation of antibodies directed against heparin-platelet complexes, resulting in platelet activation, aggregation, and clot production. In the immune-mediated form of HIT, the platelet count can fall markedly and is not dependent on the dose of heparin. Therapy requires immediate cessation of heparin and substitution by alternate antithrombotic therapy to prevent further thrombosis (e.g., direct thrombin inhibitors, described below).

Patients receiving long-term UFH therapy are also prone to a dose-dependent form of osteoporosis, through an unclear mechanism.

Low-Molecular-Weight Heparins

Some of the shortcomings of UFH (e.g., short half-life and unpredictable bioavailability) have been addressed by the development of low-molecular-weight heparins (LMWH). As the name implies, LMWH molecules are approximately one-third the size of UFH molecules. They also interact with AT III. Unlike UFH, the LMWH-AT III complex preferentially inhibits factor Xa more potently than it inhibits thrombin (thrombin inhibition requires heparin molecules larger than those in LMWH).

Advantages of LMWH over UFH include 1) inhibition of platelet-bound factor Xa, contributing to a more prominent anticoagulant effect; 2) less binding to plasma proteins and endothelial cells, resulting in more predictable bioavailability and a longer half-life; 3) fewer bleeding complications; and 4) a lower incidence of immune-mediated HIT.

From a practical standpoint, the major advantage of LMWH formulations is the ease of use. They can be administered as subcutaneous injections once or twice a day in fixed doses, without the frequent blood monitoring required for UFH. In rare cases in which monitoring the anticoagulant effect *is* necessary (e.g., in patients with renal dysfunction, since LMWH is cleared via the kidneys), a factor Xa inhibition assay is used.

In clinical trials, LMWH therapy is at least as effective as UFH in preventing DVT and treating unstable angina. It also has a better safety profile than UFH, with lower rates of bleeding, thrombocytopenia, and osteoporosis. LMWH should not, however, be used in patients with a history of HIT, and unlike UFH, the effects of LMWH cannot be completely reversed by protamine. Current clinical indications for LMWH are 1) prophylaxis against DVT following hip, knee, or abdominal surgery; 2) treatment of DVT (with or without pulmonary embolism); and 3) management of acute coronary syndromes.

Direct Thrombin Inhibitors

The anticoagulation effects of UFH and LMWH are limited because their activity depends, at least in part, on AT III, and they inhibit only *circulating* thrombin. The large heparin-AT III complex cannot inactivate thrombin that is already bound to fibrin within a clot. In distinction, the direct thrombin inhibitors (**lepirudin, bivalirudin, argatroban,** and others) inhibit thrombin activity independently of AT III and are effective against both circulating and clot-bound thrombin. They do not cause thrombocytopenia and are used to maintain anticoagulation and prevent thrombosis in the setting of heparin-induced thrombocytopenia. However, these are potent anticoagulants and the major side effect is bleeding.

Warfarin

Warfarin is an oral agent prescribed for long-term anticoagulation. It acts by antagonizing an enzyme (vitamin K epoxide reductase) that is required for proper vitamin K metabolism. Normally, the reduced form of vitamin K promotes the carboxylation of a glutamic acid residue within specific coagulation factors (factors II, VII, IX, and X), an action that is necessary for the factors to subsequently bind calcium, become functional, and participate in coagulation (Fig. 17.18). By interfering with the formation of

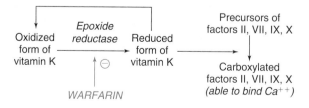

Figure 17.18. Mechanism of action of warfarin. Normally, coagulation factors II, VII, IX, and X are converted to functional forms by carboxylation in the liver, in the presence of reduced vitamin K. During this reaction, vitamin K undergoes oxidation and must be regenerated back to the reduced state for the sustained synthesis of functional clotting factors. Warfarin inhibits the formation of reduced vitamin K by antagonizing the enzyme epoxide reductase, such that the conversion of the coagulation factors does not occur and they remain nonfunctional.

reduced vitamin K, warfarin indirectly inhibits carboxylation of the coagulation factors, rendering them inactive. Since certain natural coagulation inhibitors (protein C and protein S) are also vitamin-K–dependent, warfarin impairs their functions as well, which in some cases may counteract the drug's anticoagulant effect.

Warfarin's anticoagulation action has a delayed onset of 2–7 days, so that if immediate effect is needed, UFH or LMWH must be used concurrently at first. The half-life of warfarin is long (37 hours), and the drug's dosage must be individualized to achieve a therapeutic effect while minimizing the risk of bleeding complications. The extent of anticoagulation is monitored by measuring the prothrombin time in blood samples, reported as an International Normalized Ratio (INR). There are two "target" ranges of anticoagulant intensity. For patients at greatest risk of pathologic thrombosis (e.g., mechanical heart valve), the desired INR is 2.5–3.5. In less thrombogenic circumstances (e.g., atrial fibrillation), the target INR is 2.0–3.0.

Many factors can influence the anticoagulation effect of warfarin and require alterations in its dosage. For example, liver disease or heart failure reduces the warfarin requirement, whereas a high dietary ingestion of vitamin-K–containing foods (e.g., green leafy vegetables) increases the dosage need. Similarly, many pharmaceuticals alter warfarin's anticoagulation effect, examples of which are shown in Table 17.16. Finally, the combined use of warfarin with aspirin or other antiplatelet agents increases the risk of a bleeding complication.

If serious bleeding arises during warfarin therapy, the drug's effect can be reversed within hours by the administration of vitamin K (or even more quickly by transfusing fresh-frozen plasma, which directly replenishes functional circulating clotting factors). In patients with mechanical heart valves, vitamin K should be avoided unless life-threatening bleeding occurs, because of the possibility of rebound valve thrombosis.

Warfarin is teratogenic and should not be taken during pregnancy, especially in the first trimester.

TABLE 17.16. Drugs that Alter the Anticoagulation Effect of Warfarin

Reduced Anticoagulation Effect	Increased Anticoagulation Effect
Hepatic enzyme induction	Hepatic enzyme inhibition
Barbiturates	Amiodarone
Rifampin	Cephalosporin
Carbamazepine	antibiotics
Nafcillin	Cimetidine
Warfarin malabsorption	Erythromycin
Cholestyramine	Fluconazole
Sucralfate	Isoniazid
	Ketoconazole
	Metronidazole
	Propafenone
	Trimethoprim-sulfamethoxazole
	Protein displacement
	Allopurinol
	Phenytoin
	Altered vitamin K production by gut flora
	Ciprofloxacin
	Piperacillin

LIPID-REGULATING DRUGS

As described in Chapter 5, serum lipids play a critical role in the pathogenesis of atherosclerosis. Drugs that improve lipid abnormalities are cardioprotective; they inhibit the progression of atherosclerosis, improve cardiovascular outcomes, and in high-risk individuals, reduce mortality rates. The most commonly used lipid-regulating drugs are HMG CoA reductase inhibitors, bile-acid binding agents, and niacin and fibric acid derivatives.

HMG CoA Reductase Inhibitors

The HMG CoA reductase inhibitors, commonly known as the "statins," are the most effective drugs for reducing LDL cholesterol. By virtue of their potency, excellent tolerability, and mortality benefits, they are the most widely prescribed anti-lipid drugs. The available agents of this group, in increasing order of potency, are **fluvastatin, lovastatin, pravastatin, simvastatin,** and **atorvastatin** (Table 17.17).

The statins are competitive inhibitors of the enzyme HMG CoA reductase, a rate-controlling step in cholesterol biosynthesis (Fig. 17.19). As these drugs inhibit cholesterol

TABLE 17.17. Lipid-Regulating Drugs

Class	LDL Effect	HDL Effect	Triglyceride Effect	Side Effects
HMG CoA reductase inhibitors (in increasing order of potency) Fluvastatin Lovastatin Pravastatin Simvastatin Atorvastatin	↓18–55%	↑5–15%	↓7–30%	↑Transaminases Myopathy
Bile-acid binding agents Cholestyramine Colestipol Colesevelam	↓15-30%	↑3-5%	May ↑	Constipation Bloating
Niacin	↓5–25%	↑15–35%	↓20–50%	Flushing Hepatotoxicity Hyperglycemia Hyperuricemia Exacerbates peptic ulcer disease
Fibric acid derivatives Fenofibrate Gemfibrozil	↓0–20% or ↑0–10%	↑10–20%	↓20–50%	Nausea Gallstones

Modified from Expert Panel on Detection, Evaluation, and Treatment of High Blood Cholesterol in Adults. Executive summary of the Third Report of the National Cholesterol Education Program (NCEP) Expert Panel on Detection, Evaluation, and Treatment of High Blood Cholesterol in Adults (Adult Treatment Panel III). JAMA 2001;285:2486–2497.

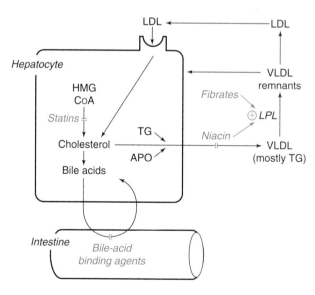

Figure 17.19. Major sites of action of lipid-regulating drugs. The *statins* inhibit cholesterol biosynthesis in the liver by competing with the enzyme HMG CoA reductase. This action depletes intrahepatic cholesterol stores and results in increased expression of surface LDL receptors, which enhance clearance of LDL and VLDL remnants from the circulation. Due to the lower intrahepatic cholesterol content, VLDL synthesis is also reduced. *Bile-acid binding agents* interrupt the enterohepatic circulation of bile acids in the intestine, causing more hepatic cholesterol to be converted to new bile acids. In response to reduced availability of intrahepatic cholesterol, LDL receptor expression and LDL clearance increase. *Niacin* inhibits VLDL production. It also increases lipoprotein lipase (LPL) activity, thus promoting triglyceride (TG) clearance from circulating VLDL particles. Niacin raises circulating HDL by impairing hepatic uptake of apo-AI, an HDL apoprotein (not shown). *Fibrates* enhance VLDL catabolism by increasing the synthesis of lipoprotein lipase. They also raise HDL by stimulating the production of HDL-associated apoproteins (not shown). Apo, apoproteins.

production in the liver, serum LDL cholesterol falls because of three mechanisms: 1) the reduced intrahepatic cholesterol level induces increased expression of the LDL receptor gene, causing a greater number of LDL receptors to appear on the surface of the hepatocyte, which facilitates the binding and clearance of LDL from the circulation; 2) circulating LDL precursors (known as very-low-density lipoprotein [VLDL] remnants and intermediate-density lipoprotein [IDL] particles) are cleared more rapidly from the circulation because of their cross-recognition with the hepatic LDL receptor; and 3) hepatic VLDL production falls due to the reduced availability of intracellular cholesterol for lipoprotein assembly. Since it is the catabolism of VLDL in the circulation that ultimately forms LDL, this too decreases circulating LDL levels. The reduced production of VLDL is also likely responsible for the triglyceride-lowering effect of statins, since this lipoprotein is the major carrier of triglycerides in the circulation.

The overall effect is that statins reduce serum LDL levels by 18–55%, depending on which agent is used. Statins also decrease plasma triglyceride levels by 7–30%, and by an unclear mechanism, HDL levels increase by 5–15%.

The lowering of LDL reduces the lipid content of atherosclerotic lesions and promotes plaque stability. This lessens the vulnerability of plaque to rupture, thus decreasing the likelihood of thrombus formation and vascular occlusion. In addition to their lipid-modulating properties, statins have other potentially cardioprotective effects. They improve endothelial function as evidenced by enhanced synthesis of nitric oxide. They further promote plaque stability by inhibiting monocyte penetration into the arterial wall and reducing macrophage secretion of metalloproteinases, enzymes that degrade and weaken the fibrous caps of plaques. Statins also diminish the vulnerability of lipoproteins to oxidation, thus inhibiting the unregulated uptake of modified LDL cholesterol by macrophages. Finally, they appear to suppress inflammation, thought to be a key aspect of atherogenesis.

Statins are widely prescribed for patients with CAD, because major trials have shown that they substantially reduce mortality, cardiac events, and strokes in this population, whether LDL cholesterol is elevated or even average. In studies of patients not known to have CAD, statin therapy has been shown to reduce coronary events in high-risk individuals—those with elevated LDL cholesterol levels, or those with average total cholesterol but low HDL values.

Statins are usually well tolerated. Mild gastrointestinal upset or sleep disturbances occasionally occur. The major potential adverse effects are hepatotoxicity and myotoxicity, and these are rare. Hepatotoxicity is dose related and occurs in fewer than 1% of patients. Those affected may experience fatigue, anorexia, and weight loss. More commonly, the patient is asymptomatic, but results of routine laboratory studies show an increase in transaminase levels (ALT, AST) to more than three times the normal values. Symptoms disappear almost immediately after the drug is discontinued, but transaminase levels may remain elevated for weeks. The risk of statin-associated hepatic toxicity is higher in patients who drink excessive amounts of alcohol.

Myopathy is characterized by intense myalgias and muscle weakness, and can lead to rhabdomyolysis (destruction of muscle) with myoglobinuria and renal failure. When this occurs, muscle-derived creatine kinase levels in the serum rise to more than 10 times the upper limit of normal. This severe complication occurs in fewer than 0.1% of patients taking statins alone. However, the incidence is increased significantly by concomitant therapy with certain other drugs, including other lipid-lowering agents (i.e., niacin and the fibric acid derivatives).The incidence is also increased by concurrent administration of drugs that inhibit the 3A4 isoform of cytochrome P-450, which is responsible for hepatic metabolism of most statins. Such drugs include macrolide antibiotics (e.g., erythromycin, clarithromycin), azole antifungal agents (e.g., ketoconazole, itraconazole), cyclosporine, and many HIV protease inhibitors. Notably, pravastatin and fluvastatin are not substantially dependent on the cytochrome P-450 3A4 isoform for their metabolism and appear to be less likely to cause myopathy in combination with these other drugs.

Bile-Acid Binding Agents

The bile-acid binding agents are among the safest anti-lipid agents, as they are not absorbed into the circulation. This group includes the resins **cholestyramine** and **colestipol** as well as the newer hydrophilic polymer **colesevelam.** These drugs are large, highly positively charged molecules that bind bile acids (which are negatively charged) in the intestine and prevent their normal reabsorption back to the liver through the enterohepatic circulation (see Fig. 17.19). To make up for the loss, more hepatic cholesterol is converted into newly produced bile acids. This action decreases the intrahepatic cholesterol stores, which stimulates the production of more LDL receptors. Similar to the effect of the statins, an increased number of hepatic LDL receptors binds a greater amount of circulating LDL, reducing the circulating concentration of the lipoprotein. However, unlike statins, *new* hepatic cholesterol production is also stimulated by the reduced intrahepatic cholesterol content. The boost in cholesterol synthesis augments VLDL production, which explains the commonly observed rise in serum triglyceride levels during bile-acid binding agent therapy.

In one of the first drug trials of men with hypercholesterolemia, cholestyramine significantly reduced the risk of fatal and nonfatal myocardial infarctions. However, because of their side effects and inferior potency compared with statins, the bile-acid binding agents are now used mainly as second-line lipid-regulating drugs, often in combination with statins. This combination allows the use of lower dosages of each type of drug to minimize side effects, yet results in powerful (up to 60%) reductions in LDL cholesterol levels. The combination also prevents the increase in hepatic cholesterol synthesis that occurs when bile-acid binding agents are used alone.

Cholestyramine and colestipol can cause elevations in the serum triglyceride level and should be avoided in patients with hypertriglyceridemia at baseline. These resins also interfere with the absorption of several other drugs (e.g., warfarin, digoxin, propranolol, thyroid hormones). Thus, other medications should be given 1 hour before, or 3–4 hours after resin administration. The main side effects of these drugs are bloating, constipation, and nausea.

Preliminary studies of the newer bile-acid binding agent, colesevelam, have demonstrated similar improvements in LDL cholesterol but less tendency to raise the triglyceride level compared with the other agents of this group. In addition, it is administered as an anhydrous capsule that absorbs water and seems to cause substantially fewer gastrointestinal side effects.

Niacin

Niacin is one of the oldest lipid-regulating drugs and has favorable effects on all the circulating lipid fractions. It is the most effective agent for raising HDL cholesterol (by 15–35%), and it also reduces LDL cholesterol (by 5–25%) and triglyceride levels (by 20–50%). Furthermore, unlike most other anti-lipid drugs, niacin substantially reduces the circulating level of lipoprotein (a), an LDL-like lipoprotein that carries an independent risk of cardiovascular disease (see Chapter 5).

Niacin modifies lipid levels through multiple mechanisms. It inhibits the release of fatty acids from adipose tissue. As a result, fewer fatty acids are transported to the liver, such that hepatic triglyceride synthesis declines. Impaired triglyceride production by the liver reduces VLDL secretion into the circulation; consequently, less LDL is formed (see Fig. 17.19). Niacin also enhances the clearance of triglycerides from circulating VLDL by promoting the activity of lipoprotein lipase, the enzyme that processes VLDL particles by hydrolyzing the triglyceride core at adipose and muscle cells. The net effect of these actions is a reduction in serum triglyceride and LDL levels. In addition, the drug reduces the proportion of small, dense LDL particles (which are thought to promote atherogenesis) in favor of larger and more buoyant forms. Niacin raises circulating HDL cholesterol levels by decreasing the hepatic uptake of its apoprotein, apo-A1, thus reducing clearance of HDL particles from the circulation. However, hepatic retrieval (and disposal) of cholesterol from HDL is not disturbed.

In one major study of niacin in men who had experienced a prior myocardial infarction, niacin reduced the risk of future cardiac events and lowered the mortality rate in long-term follow-up. That study was performed before the better-tolerated and more effective statin drugs were available. Niacin is now mainly used to treat patients with low serum HDL levels and/or elevated serum triglycerides.

Niacin has several common side effects. Transient cutaneous flushing episodes occur in most patients. They are prostaglandin mediated and can be minimized by taking daily aspirin. Gastrointestinal side effects include nausea and exacerbation of peptic ulcer disease. Hepatotoxicity can occur, manifested by fatigue, weakness, and elevated serum transaminases (ALT, AST). Niacin should be used cautiously in diabetic patients because it can induce insulin resistance and contribute to hyperglycemia. Niacin also raises serum uric acid levels and can reactivate gout.

Rare cases of myopathy have been reported with niacin therapy. The incidence is increased when niacin is prescribed concurrently with a statin.

Fibrates

The fibric acid derivatives, or "fibrates," include **gemfibrozil** and **fenofibrate**. They are the most powerful agents to reduce serum triglyceride levels (by up to 50%). They also raise HDL cholesterol levels (by up to 20%), but their effect on LDL cholesterol levels is more variable. Fibrate therapy may lower LDL cholesterol. However, in patients with baseline hypertriglyceridemia, fibrate therapy can actually increase LDL cholesterol levels. Fibrates shift

the proportion of LDL from smaller and denser sizes to more buoyant, larger, and less atherogenic particles.

A large study of men who had hypercholesterolemia but were not known to have coronary disease showed that gemfibrozil reduced the number of subsequent myocardial infarctions (without affecting the total death rate). In another study of men with known CAD, normal LDL levels, and low HDL levels, the rate of coronary events was decreased, but again total mortality was not significantly affected. In a study of patients with diabetes who also had CAD, fenofibrate slowed the progression of coronary narrowings but did not significantly reduce the rate of coronary events.

Fibrates are thought to exert their antilipid effects through interactions with peroxisome proliferator-activated receptor (PPAR)-α, which regulates gene transcription. Activation of PPAR-α leads to a decrease in triglycerides, at least in part, by augmenting fatty acid oxidation and by increasing the synthesis of lipoprotein lipase (see Fig. 17.19). The latter results in increased VLDL catabolism, which may *augment* the circulating LDL level, especially in patients with baseline hypertriglyceridemia. Fibrates raise HDL cholesterol levels via PPAR-α gene stimulation of the apoproteins A-I and A-II, which are key constituents of HDL particles.

Fibrates are primarily used to lower triglyceride levels and raise HDL cholesterol levels. They are metabolized by hepatic glucuronidation with subsequent renal excretion. Thus, they should be avoided or prescribed at lower doses for patients with impaired liver or kidney function.

Fibrates are generally well tolerated. Potential side effects include dyspepsia, gallstones, and myalgias. When used in combination with a statin, the risk of rhabdomyolysis is increased. Therefore, if these drugs are prescribed concurrently, it is recommended that the serum creatine kinase (derived from muscle) be monitored every several months. Fibrates augment the effect of warfarin by displacing it from albumin binding sites, such that the anticoagulant dosage may need to be decreased. In a similar fashion, fibrates also enhance the effects of oral hypoglycemic drugs.

Table 17.17 summarizes the expected results and potential side effects of the commonly used lipid-altering drugs.

SUMMARY

This chapter presented an overview of the most commonly used cardiovascular drugs. These agents are covered in greater detail in the following references. It is hoped that the tables, figures, and brief explanations presented here will be useful to the reader when the basic pathophysiology of heart disease is considered while caring for patients.

Acknowledgment   The authors thank Dr. Robert Handin for his helpful suggestions. Contributors to the previous editions of this chapter were Andrew C. Hecht, MD; Steven P. Leon, MD; Steven N. Kalkanis, MD; David Sloane, MD; Ralph A. Kelly, MD; Gary R. Strichartz, MD; and Leonard S. Lilly, MD.

ADDITIONAL READING

Abrams J. The role of nitrates in coronary heart disease. Arch Intern Med 1995;155:357–364.

Antithrombotic Trialists' Collaboration. Collaborative meta-analysis of randomised trials of antiplatelet therapy for prevention of death, myocardial infarction, and stroke in high risk patients. BMJ 2002;324:71–86.

Antman EM. Cardiovascular Therapeutics: A Companion to Braunwald's Heart Disease. Philadelphia: WB Saunders, 2001.

Bhatt DL, Topol EJ. Current role of platelet glycoprotein IIb/IIIa inhibitors in acute coronary syndromes. JAMA 2000;284:1549–1558.

Brater DC. Drug therapy: diuretic therapy. N Engl J Med 1998;339:387–395.

Brouwer MA, Verheugt FWA. Oral anticoagulation for acute coronary syndromes. Circulation 2002;105: 1270–1274.

Burnier M, Brunner HR. Angiotensin II receptor antagonists. Lancet 2000;355:637–645.

Cleland JGF. Preventing atherosclerotic events with aspirin. BMJ 2002;324:103–105.

Digitalis Investigation Group. The effect of digoxin on mortality and morbidity in patients with heart failure. N Engl J Med 1997;336:525–533.

Expert Panel on Detection, Evaluation, and Treatment of High Blood Cholesterol in Adults. Executive summary of the Third Report of the National Cholesterol Education Program Expert Panel on Detection, Evaluation, and Treatment of High Blood Cholesterol in Adults (Adult Treatment Panel III). JAMA 2001;285:2486–2497.

Felker GM, O'Connor CM. Inotropic therapy for heart failure: an evidence-based approach. Am Heart J 2001;142:393–401.

Foody JM, Farrell MH, Krumholz HM. β-Blocker therapy in heart failure: scientific review. JAMA 2002;287:883–889.

Hirsh J, Anand SS, Halperin JL, et al. Guide to anticoagulant therapy: heparin. Circulation 2001;103: 2994–3018.

Hollopeter G, Jantzen HM, Vincent D. Identification of the platelet ADP receptor targeted by antithrombotic drugs. Nature 2001;409:202–207.

Khalil ME, Basher AW, Brown EJ, et al. A remarkable medical story: benefits of angiotensin-converting enzyme inhibitors in cardiac patients. J Am Coll Cardiol 2001;37:1757–1764.

Kizer RJ, Kimmel SE. Epidemiologic review of the calcium channel blocker drugs. Arch Intern Med 2001;161:1145–1158.

Knopp RH. Drug therapy: drug treatment of lipid disorders. N Engl J Med 1999;341:498–511.

Messerli FH. Cardiovascular Drug Therapy. Philadelphia: WB Saunders, 1996.

Murphy MB, Murray C, Shorten GD. Fenoldopam—a selective peripheral dopamine-receptor agonist for the treatment of severe hypertension. N Engl J Med 2001;345:1548–1557.

Opie LH, Gersh BJ, eds. Drugs for the Heart. 5th Ed. Philadelphia: WB Saunders, 2001.

Parmley WW, Chatterjee K. Cardiovascular Pharmacology. London: Mosby-Year Book Europe, Ltd., 1994.

Quinn MJ, Fitzgerald DJ. Ticlopidine and clopidogrel. Circulation 1999;100:1667–1672.

Sicilian Gambit Members. New approaches to antiarrhythmic therapy: emerging therapeutic applications of the cell biology of cardiac arrhythmias. Circulation 2001;104:2865–2873 and 2990–2994.

Weitz JI, Buller HR. Direct thrombin inhibitors in acute coronary syndromes. Circulation 2002;105: 1004–1011.

Index

Page numbers in *italics* denote figures; those followed by "t" denote tables; those followed by "b" denote boxes.

Abciximab, 413
Abdominal aortic aneurysm, 303
Acetylcholine, 25, 134b
Actin, 23
Action potential
  cardiac cells, 11–12, *18,* 18–19
  digitalis effects, 374
  early afterdepolarization-triggered, 261
  pacemaker cells, *20, 254*
  refractory periods, 21
  spontaneous, 253
  triggered activity, 260
  unidirectional block of, 262
Acute arterial occlusion, 335–336
Acute bacterial endocarditis, 204
Acute coronary syndromes
  angina pectoris (*see* Angina pectoris)
  clinical features of, 167
  cocaine abuse and, 163
  description of, 157
  diagnosis of
    creatine kinase levels, 172
    echocardiography, 172
    electrocardiography, 170, *170–171*
    findings to support, 169–170
    lactate dehydrogenase, 172
    troponin levels, 171–172
  differential diagnosis, 169t
  frequency of, 157
  hemostasis, 158
  ischemic heart disease (*see* Ischemic heart disease)
  myocardial infarction (*see* Myocardial infarction)
  nonatherosclerotic causes of, 162–163
  pathogenesis of, 157–163
  pathologic and pathophysiologic findings
    contractility and compliance impairments, 166
    description of, 163
    early changes, 163–165
    functional changes, 166–167
    gross changes, 165
    ischemic preconditioning, 166–167
    late changes, 166, 166t
    ventricular remodeling, 167
  thrombosis
    antithrombotic mechanisms, 158–160
    consequences of, *162*
    formation of, 161
    partially occlusive, 157
    pathogenesis of, *160,* 160–162
    significance of, 161–162, *162*
  treatment of
    description of, 173
    in-patient measures, 173
    schematic diagram of, *173*
  triggers for, 161
  vasoconstriction associated with, 139
Acute pulmonary edema, 234–235
Acute rheumatic fever, 185–186, 186t
Adenosine, 133, 148, 280, 404–405

Adenosine diphosphate, 24, 133
Adenosine triphosphate, 24, 133, 140, 164
β_2-Adrenergic receptors, 151
β-Adrenergic signaling, 24–25, *26*
Adventitia, 111, *112*
Afterdepolarizations, 260–261
Afterload
  definition of, 213–214, 214t
Aggregation of platelets, 139–140
Alcoholic cardiomyopathy, 238
Amiloride, 406t, 409
Amiodarone, 234, 400–402
Amlodipine, 152
Amrinone, 378, 378t
Aneurysms, aortic
  classification of, *327*
  definition of, 326
  description of, 206, 326
  false
    definition of, 326
    illustration of, *327*
  true
    characteristics of, 326
    clinical presentation of, 329
    etiology of, 326, 328t
    familial factors, 328
    illustration of, *327*
    rupture of, 329
    treatment of, 329
Angina pectoris
  aortic stenosis-related, 197
  congestive heart failure caused by, 197
  definition of, 132t
  differential diagnosis, 169t
  discovery of, 131
  "fixed-threshold," 142
  hypertrophic cardiomyopathy and, 247
  natural history of, 149, 149t
  prevention of, 150–152
  Prinzmetal's (*see* Angina pectoris, variant)
  stable
    causes of, 142
    coronary angiography evaluations, 148–149
    definition of, 132t
    diagnostic studies for, 145–149
    differential diagnosis, 144–145, 145t
    electrocardiographic findings, 145–146
    exercise echocardiography evaluations, 148
    exercise stress test for, 146–147
    history-taking findings, 143–145
    location of, 144
    natural history of, 149, 149t
    nitroglycerin for, 144
    nuclear studies for, 147
    oxygen supply inadequacies associated with, 142
    pathophysiologic findings, *141*
    physical examination findings, 145, *146*
    precipitants of, 144
    quality of, 143–144

Angina pectoris *(continued)*
  stable *(continued)*
    risk factors, 144
    signs and symptoms of, 143–144
    treatment of, 149–150
  treatment of
    acute episodes, 149–150, 150t
    atherectomy, 154
    coronary artery bypass graft, 154, *154*, 155t
    percutaneous coronary interventions, 153, 155t
    percutaneous transluminal coronary angioplasty,
      153
    revascularization, 153–155
  unstable
    characteristics of, 142
    clinical presentation of, 167–168
    complications of, 178–179
    definition of, 132t
    diagnosis of, 169–170
    pathophysiologic findings, *141*
    "variable-threshold," 142
  variant
    characteristics of, 142–143
    definition of, 132t
    pathophysiologic findings, *141*
Angioblastic cords, 347, *348*
Angiography
  contrast, 62–64, *63*
  coronary, 148–149
  magnetic resonance, 71
Angiotensin II, 223, 297, 378
Angiotensin II receptor blockers
  characteristics of, 382
  heart failure treated using, 232
  hypertension treated using, 309
  indications, 382
  renin-angiotensin system interactions, 381t
  types of, 381t
Angiotensin-converting enzyme, 223
Angiotensin-converting enzyme inhibitors
  description of, 379
  indications
    dilated cardiomyopathy, 242
    heart failure, 231–233, 380–381
    hypertension, 308–309, 379–380
    myocardial infarction, 152–153, 178
    renovascular hypertension, 298
  renal blood flow effects, 380
  renin-angiotensin system interactions, 381t
  side effects of, 381–382
  sites of action, *379*
Ankle-brachial index, 334
Anterior interventricular groove, *3*
Antiadrenergic drugs
  β-blockers *(see* β-Blockers)
  central adrenergic inhibitors, 389–390
  description of, 388, *389*, 390t
  indications, 388
  peripheral α-adrenergic receptor antagonists,
    390–391, 391t
  sympathetic nerve-ending antagonists, 390
Antiarrhythmic drugs
  adenosine, 404–405
  class IA
    clinical uses of, 396, 396t
    disopyramide, 397
    electrocardiogram effects, 396, 396t
    electrophysiologic effects of, *395*
    mechanism of action, 393t, 395–396

    procainamide, 313, 397
    quinidine, 396–397
    types of, 393t
  class IB
    clinical uses of, 396t, 398
    diphenylhydantoin, 398
    electrophysiologic effects of, *395*
    lidocaine, 398
    mechanism of action, 393t, 397–398
    mexiletine, 398
    tocainide, 398
    types of, 393t
  class IC
    clinical uses of, 396t, 399
    electrophysiologic effects of, *395*
    flecainide, 399
    mechanism of action, 393t
    propafenone, 399
    types of, 393t
  class II *(see also* β-Blockers)
    clinical uses of, 396t, 399–400
    electrocardiogram effects, 399
    mechanism of action, 393t, 399
    types of, 393t
  class III
    amiodarone, 234, 400–402
    bretylium tosylate, 402
    clinical uses of, 396t
    dofetilide, 402–403
    electrophysiologic effects of, *401*
    ibutilide, 402
    mechanism of action, 393t
    sotalol, 402
    types of, 393t
  class IV *(see also* Calcium channel blockers)
    clinical uses of, 396t, 403–404
    diltiazem, 403–404
    electrophysiologic effects of, *403*
    mechanism of action, 393t
    types of, 393t
    verapamil, 403–404
  description of, 393
  mechanism of action, 393–394
  reentrant rhythms inhibited by, 394
  triggered activity treated using, 394
Anticoagulants
  description of, 413–414
  dilated cardiomyopathy treated using, 242
  direct thrombin inhibitors, 415
  low-molecular-weight heparin, 414–415
  unfractionated heparin, 414
  warfarin, 415–416, 416t
Antidiuretic hormone, 223–224
Antihypertensive therapy, 126–127, 306–309
Antineutrophil cytoplasmic antibodies, 337
Antiplatelet drugs
  aspirin
    acute coronary syndromes treated using, 173
    clinical uses of, 411t, 411–412
    myocardial infarction treated using, 173
    side effects of, 412
    ST-segment elevation myocardial infarction
      treated using, 177
  description of, 174, 409–411
  dipyridamole, 148, 413
  glycoprotein IIb/IIIa receptor antagonists, 174, 409,
    413
  thienopyridines, 412–413
Antithrombin III, 158, *159*, 174

Antithrombotic drugs
  anticoagulants
    description of, 413–414
    direct thrombin inhibitors, 415
    low-molecular-weight heparin, 414–415
    unfractionated heparin, 414
    warfarin, 415–416, 416t
  clinical uses of, 411t
  description of, 409
  platelet inhibitors
    aspirin, 411–412
    description of, 409–411
    dipyridamole, 148, 413
    glycoprotein IIb/IIIa receptor antagonists, 174,
      409, 413
    thienopyridines, 412–413
Aorta
  abdominal, 325
  anatomy of, 325–326, 327
  ascending, 325
  coarctation of
    clinical features of, 364, 364
    hypertension caused by, 298–299
    incidence of, 364
    laboratory studies, 365
    pathophysiology of, 365
    physical examination, 365
    postductal, 365
    preductal, 364–365
    symptoms of, 365
    treatment of, 365–366
  descending, 325
  dilatation of, 47, 48
  diseases of, 325–331
  hypertension effects, 303
Aortic aneurysms
  classification of, 327
  definition of, 326
  description of, 206, 326
  false
    definition of, 326
    illustration of, 327
  true
    characteristics of, 326
    clinical presentation of, 329
    definition of, 326
    diagnosis of, 329
    etiology of, 326, 328t
    familial factors, 328
    illustration of, 327
    rupture of, 329
    treatment of, 329
Aortic arch, 3
Aortic dissection
  classification of, 330, 330
  clinical presentation of, 331
  complications of, 331t
  definition of, 329
  differential diagnosis, 169t
  etiology of, 329–330
  hypertension effects, 303
  mortality rate, 303
  pathogenesis of, 329–330
  treatment of, 331
  type A, 330, 330
  type B, 330, 330
Aortic insufficiency
  radiographic findings, 48
  types of, 198t

Aortic regurgitation
  acute, 199
  assessment of, 200
  characteristics of, 208t
  chronic, 199
  clinical manifestations of, 200
  echocardiographic findings, 57t
  etiology of, 198
  murmur caused by, 39
  pathophysiology of, 198–200, 199
  radiographic findings, 50t, 200
  severity of, 198
  treatment of, 200, 202
Aortic stenosis
  cardiac catheterization findings, 64t, 198
  characteristics of, 208t
  clinical manifestations of, 197–198, 361, 362
  continuous murmur caused by, 41, 193
  echocardiographic findings, 57t
  electrocardiographic findings, 198
  etiology of, 195–196
  evaluation of, 197–198
  hemodynamic profile of, 196
  incidence of, 361
  laboratory studies, 362–363
  pathology of, 196
  pathophysiology of, 196, 196–197, 361
  physical examination, 197–198, 362
  radiographic findings, 48, 50t
  symptoms of, 197, 362
  systolic ejection murmur caused by, 37–38, 38
  treatment of, 198, 363
Aortic valve
  anatomy of, 5
  area of, 197
  development of, 351
  replacement of, 198
Apo B-100, 117b, 128
Apolipoproteins, 115, 116b
Apoptosis
  in heart failure, 225
  in myocardial infarction, 164
Argatroban, 415
Arrhythmias
  anticholinergic drugs for, 265
  atrial fibrillation
    cardioversion for, 278
    definition of, 277
    electrocardiographic findings, 277
    in heart failure, 233
    in hypertrophic cardiomyopathy, 248–249
    mechanism of, 277
    mitral stenosis effects, 188
    myocardial infarction-related, 180
    treatment of, 277–278
  atrial flutter, 276–277
  atrial premature beats, 180, 274 275
  atrioventricular nodal reentrant tachycardia, 279–281
  atrioventricular reentrant tachycardia, 281
  conduction block and, 261
  definition of, 253, 269, 274
  differential diagnosis, 275
  in dilated cardiomyopathy, 242
  ectopic atrial tachycardia, 284
  electronic pacemakers for, 266
  escape rhythms
    definition of, 259, 271
    junctional, 271, 271
    ventricular, 271

Arrhythmias (continued)
  heart failure secondary to, 225
  in hypertrophic cardiomyopathy, 247
  impulse formation and conduction alterations,
      254
  mechanisms of, 265t
  multifocal atrial tachycardia, 282–284, 283
  myocardial infarction-related, 179–180
  paroxysmal supraventricular tachycardia, 278–279
  reentrant, 396
  sick sinus syndrome, 270, 270–271
  sinus bradycardia
    benign, 269
    definition of, 86, 269
    etiology of, 269
    management of, 269
    myocardial infarction-related, 180
  sinus tachycardia
    characteristics of, 274
    definition of, 86
    electrocardiographic findings, 274, 275
    in heart failure, 228
    myocardial infarction-related, 180
  supraventricular, 180
  torsades de pointes, 286, 286
  types of, 270t
  ventricular fibrillation, 286–287, 287
  ventricular tachycardia, 285–286
  wide complex tachycardias, 287t, 287–288
Arterial insufficiency, 334
Arteries (see also specific artery)
  acute occlusion of, 335–336
  coronary (see Coronary arteries)
  emboli of, 335t
  nitrate-induced dilation of, 387–388
  occlusive disease of (see Occlusive arterial
      disease)
  Raynaud's phenomenon, 338–339, 339
  wall of
    anatomy of, 111–112, 112
    endothelial cells, 112–113, 113t
    endothelium of, 112, 113t
    extracellular matrix, 113
    leukocyte adherence to, 112
    vascular smooth muscle cells, 113
Arterioles
  constriction of, 223
  description of, 111
  dilation of, 332
Arteriovenous oxygen difference, 61
Aspirin
  acute coronary syndromes treated using, 173
  clinical uses of, 411t, 411–412
  description of, 411
  myocardial infarction treated using, 173
  side effects of, 412
  ST-segment elevation myocardial infarction treated
      using, 177
Atherectomy, 154
Atherosclerosis
  arterial wall
    anatomy of, 111–112, 112
    endothelial cells, 112–113, 113t
    endothelium of, 112, 113t
    extracellular matrix, 113
    leukocyte adherence to, 112
    vascular smooth muscle cells, 113
  causes of, 111
  complications of, 111, 120–122, 121t

  definition of, 111
  Framingham Heart Study, 122
  monoclonal hypothesis of, 120
  pathogenesis of
    endothelial dysfunction, 114–115
    fatty streak, 118, 119
    leukocytes, 118, 119
    lipoproteins, 115t, 115–118
    smooth muscle cells, 118–120
  physical activity effects, 127
  plaque formation (see Atherosclerotic plaque)
  risk factors
    C-reactive protein, 128–129
    description of, 122–123
    diabetes mellitus, 127
    dyslipidemia, 123–126
    estrogen status, 127–128
    homocystinemia, 128
    hypertension, 115, 126–127
    infection, 129
    inflammatory markers, 128–129
    lipoprotein (a), 128
    nonmodifiable, 122–123
    tobacco smoking, 126
  schematic diagram of, 114
  thrombus formation caused by, 160
Atherosclerotic plaque
  cellular debris in, 119–120
  characteristics of, 119–120, 120
  complications of, 120–121, 121t
  description of, 111
  fatty streak transition into, 118–119, 119
  foam cells, 118–120
  formation of, 160
  renovascular hypertension caused by, 298
  rupture of, 121, 122, 160–161
  schematic diagram of, 114
Atorvastatin, 417t
ATP binding cassette 1, 123
Atria
  contraction of, 31
  digitalis effects, 373t
  dilatation of, 46
  left
    anatomy of, 5, 6
    compliance of, 191–192, 214t
    mitral stenosis pathophysiology, 188
    pressure measurements, 58, 192
  right
    anatomy of, 2, 4, 4
    pressure measurements, 58, 58, 60t
  septation of, 349–350, 350
Atrial fibrillation
  cardioversion for, 278
  definition of, 277
  electrocardiographic findings, 277
  in heart failure, 233
  in hypertrophic cardiomyopathy, 248–249
  mechanism of, 277
  mitral stenosis effects, 188
  myocardial infarction-related, 180
  treatment of, 277–278
Atrial flutter, 276–277
Atrial gallop, 35
Atrial premature beats, 180, 274, 275
Atrial septal defect
  incidence of, 355
  laboratory studies of, 357
  ostium primum, 356

ostium secundum, 355–356, *356*
pathophysiology of, 357
physical examination, 357
sinus venosus, 356
site of, 355–356
symptoms of, 357
treatment of, 357–358
Atrioventricular block
first-degree, 272, *272*
high-grade, 273, *273*
second-degree, 272, *272–273*
third-degree, *273*, 273–274
Atrioventricular canal
definition of, 348
septation of, 350, *351*
Atrioventricular dissociation, 274
Atrioventricular nodal artery, 8, *9*
Atrioventricular nodal cells, 255
Atrioventricular nodal reentrant tachycardia,
279–281
Atrioventricular node
anatomy of, 6, *7*
cells of, 20
digitalis effects, 372–373, 373t
Atrioventricular reentrant tachycardia, 281, 374
Atrioventricular valve development, 351–352
Atropine, 265
Auscultation of heart
technique for, 30, *30*
Austin Flint murmur, 200
Automaticity
abnormal, 259–260
arrhythmias caused by increases in, 394–396
depressed, 269
description of, 20, 253
digitalis effects, 374
ionic basis of, 253–255
latent pacemaker, 259
sinoatrial node, 258–259
suppression of, 255–256
Autonomic nervous system, 258
Azygous vein, *3*

Bacterial pericarditis, 312
Barlow's syndrome, 195
Baroreceptor reflex, 292
Basic fibroblast growth factor, 335
Bernoulli equation, 55
Bile-acid binding agents, 419
Biliary colic, 145t
Bisferiens pulse, 200t
Bivalirudin, 415
Biventricular pacing, 234
β-Blockers (*see also* Antiarrhythmics, class II)
characteristics of, 391–392
contraindications, 151, 174
description of, 391
indications
angina pectoris, 151, 174–175
aortic dissection, 331
dilated cardiomyopathy, 242
heart failure, 233, 392
hypertension, 308, 392
hypertrophic cardiomyopathy, 248
ischemic heart disease, 392
myocardial infarction, 174–175
ST-segment elevation myocardial infarction, 177
side effects of, 151, 392–393
toxicity of, 392–393

types of, 392t
vasospasm precipitated by, 393
Blood, oxygen-carrying capacity of, 132, 353
Blood pressure
ankle-brachial index, 334
calculation of, 221, 290, 380
classification of, 291t
diastolic, 289, 290t
elevated (*see* Hypertension)
reflexes, 292
regulation of, 290–292, *291*
renal component of, 290
systolic, 289, *290*
variations of, 289
Blood vessels
acetylcholine effects, 134b
arteries (*see* Arteries)
arterioles
constriction of, 223
description of, 111
dilation of, 332
functions of, 325
peripheral vascular resistance-based hypertension
and, 293
veins, 339–341
Brachiocephalic artery, *3*
Bradyarrhythmias
anticholinergic drugs for, 265
conduction block and, 261
definition of, 269
electronic pacemakers for, 266
escape rhythms
definition of, 259, 271
junctional, 271, *271*
ventricular, 271
impulse formation and conduction alterations, *254*
mechanisms of, 265t
sick sinus syndrome, *270*, 270–271
sinus bradycardia
benign, 269
definition of, 86, 269
etiology of, 269
management of, 269
myocardial infarction-related, 180
treatment of, 265–266
types of, 270t
Bradycardia-tachycardia syndrome, 270, *270*
Bradykinin, 379
Bretylium tosylate, 402
Buerger's disease, 336t, 337–338, *338*
Bulbus cordis, 348
Bumetanide, 406t, 407
Bundle branches, 7
Bundle of His
description of, 7
firing rates of, 255
Bundle of Kent, 264, 281
Bypass tracts
concealed, 283–284
impulse conduction and, 264–265
types of, 281

Cachexia, 227
Calcium, intracellular, *376*
Calcium channel blockers (*see also* Antiarrhythmic
drugs, class IV)
cardiac cell effects, 385–386
cellular mechanism of, 385
description of, 385

Calcium channel blockers (*continued*)
  dihydropyridine, 152
  diltiazem, 152, 386–387
  indications
    angina pectoris, 151–152, 175
    description of, 386t, 386–387
    hypertension, 308
    hypertrophic cardiomyopathy, 248
    myocardial infarction, 175
  nondihydropyridine, 152
  side effects of, 386–387
  types of, 386t
  verapamil, 152, 386–387
Calcium channels, 24, 385
Carbonic anhydrase inhibitors, 406
Cardiac catheterization
  blood flow measurements using, 61–62
  catheter insertion and guidance, 57
  characteristics of, 72t
  complications associated with, 62, 64
  contrast angiography performed concurrently with, 62–64, *63*
  description of, 56–57
  history of, 57
  indications
    aortic regurgitation, 200
    aortic stenosis, 198, 363
    atrial septal defect, 357
    constrictive pericarditis, 322
    description of, 64t
    dilated cardiomyopathy, 241
    hypertrophic cardiomyopathy, 248
    mitral regurgitation, 194
    mitral stenosis, 190
    patent ductus arteriosus, 361
    tetralogy of Fallot, 367
    ventricular septal defect, 359
  pressure measurements using
    pulmonary artery pressure, 60, 60t
    pulmonary artery wedge pressure, 60t, 60–61, *61*
    right atrium, 58, *58*, 59b, 60t
    right ventricle, *58*, 59, 59b
    technique for, 57–58
    tracings, 59b
Cardiac cells (*see also* Myocytes)
  action potential of, 11–12, *18*, 18–19
  automaticity of, 253–255
  calcium channel blockers effect, 385–386
  contraction of, 23
  depolarization of, 18, 22, *22*, 75, 77–78
  impulse transport in, 75–78
  ion channels, 12–16
  pacemaker, 20
  potassium concentration in, 16
  repolarization of, 76–77, *77*
  resting potential of, 16–18, *17*
  resting state of, 14, 75
  types of, 12
Cardiac conduction system, 81–85, 179t
Cardiac cycle
  coronary artery compression during, 133
  description of, 29–30
Cardiac function determinants
  pressure-volume loops, 215–218
  stroke volume
    afterload, 214, 214t
    contractility, 214t, 214–215
    definition of, 214t
    preload, 213–214, 214t

Cardiac index, 62
Cardiac jelly, 348
Cardiac output
  calculation of, 61, 213, 290
  definition of, 214t
  dilated cardiomyopathy effects, 240
  Fick method for measuring, 61
  heart failure effects, 222, 378
  mediators of, *213*
  thermodilution method for measuring, 61
Cardiac rhythm, 86
Cardiac silhouette, 46–47
Cardiac tamponade
  clinical features of, 318–319
  diagnosis of, 319–320
  echocardiographic evaluations, 55–56, *56*
  etiology of, 318
  pathophysiology of, 318, *319*
  treatment of, 320, *321*
Cardiac transplantation
  dilated cardiomyopathy treated using, 243
  heart failure treated using, 234
Cardiogenic shock, 180–181
Cardiomyopathy
  alcoholic, 238
  dilated
    anatomic findings, *238*
    arrhythmias associated with, 242
    cardiac catheterization findings, 241
    cardiac enlargement in, 237
    cardiac output reductions, 240
    characteristics of, 237, 251t
    clinical findings of, 240–241
    diagnostic studies, 241
    echocardiographic findings, 57t, 241
    electrocardiographic findings, 241
    familial forms of, 239
    pathologic findings, 239, *239*
    pathophysiology of, 239–240, *240*
    physical examination findings, 241
    prognosis, 243
    signs and symptoms of, 240–241
    thromboembolic complications, 242–243
    treatment of
      angiotensin-converting enzyme inhibitors, 242
      β-blockers, 242
      cardiac transplantation, 243
      digitalis, 242
      diuretics, 241–242
      goals, 241
      implantable cardioverter-defibrillator, 242
    types of, 238t
    ventricular dilatation associated with, 239
    viral myocarditis and, 237
  echocardiographic findings, 55, *55*, 57t
  hypertrophic
    anatomic findings, *238*
    angina pectoris associated with, 247
    arrhythmias in, 247
    atrial fibrillation associated with, 248–249
    cardiac catheterization findings, 248
    characteristics of, 237, 243, 251t
    clinical findings of, 247
    diagnostic studies, 248
    echocardiography findings, 57t, 248
    electrocardiography findings, 248
    etiology of, 243–244
    familial, 243
    genetic counseling, 249

incidence of, 243
infective endocarditis in, 249
left ventricular outflow tract obstruction associated with, 246, *246*
pathologic findings, 244, *244–245*
pathophysiology of, 244, *245*
physical examination findings, 247–248
prognosis, 249
signs and symptoms of, 247
sudden death risks, 247, 249
syncope in, 247
treatment of
    myomectomy, 249
    pharmacologic, 248–249
two-dimensional echocardiography findings, 55
Valsalva maneuver, 247–248
ventricular hypertrophy associated with, 244, *245*
without outflow tract obstruction, 244, 246
restrictive
    anatomic findings, *238*
    characteristics of, 237, 249, 251t
    clinical findings of, 250
    diagnostic studies, 250–251
    echocardiographic findings, 57t
    pathophysiology of, 250, *250*
    physical examination findings, 250
    treatment of, 251
    types of, 250t
Cardio/thoracic ratio, 46
Cardiovascular system development
    description of, 347
    heart loop, 348, *349*
    heart tube, 347–348, *349*
    septation, 348–349
Cardioversion
    atrial fibrillation treated using, 278
    tachyarrhythmias treated using, 267
Carotid sinus massage, 267, 279
Catecholamines, 136–137, 299, 377
Catheter ablation, tachyarrhythmias treated using, 268
Cells (*see specific cell*)
Cell-surface adhesion molecules, 112
Central adrenergic inhibitors, 389–390
Cerebrovascular accident, 302
Cervical radiculitis, 145t
Chemokines, 112
Chest pain, 145t (*see also* Angina pectoris)
Chest radiography (*see* Radiography)
Cheyne-Stokes respiration, 227
Chlamydia pneumoniae, 129
Chlorothiazide, 406t, 407–408
Chlorthalidone, 406t, 408
Cholesterol
    functions of, 123
    intracellular content of, 123
    myocardial ischemia risks and, 123
    pathways of, 116b–117b
Cholesterol efflux regulatory protein, 117b, 123
Cholestyramine, 417t, 419
Cholinergic signaling, 25–26, *26*
Chordae tendineae
    anatomy of, 5
    rupture of, 191
Chylomicrons, 115t, 116b
Cigarette smoking
    atherosclerosis and, 126
    hypertension and, 306

Cilostazol, 335
Circulation
    fetal, 352–353, *354*
    transitional, 353–355
Claudication, 333, *334*
Clopidogrel, 412–413
Coagulation necrosis, 164, *165*
Coarctation of the aorta
    clinical features of, 364, *364*
    hypertension caused by, 298–299
    incidence of, 364
    laboratory studies, 365
    pathophysiology of, 365
    physical examination, 365
    postductal, 365
    preductal, 364–365
    symptoms of, 365
    treatment of, 365–366
Cocaine
    acute coronary syndromes and, 163
    hypertension and, 297
Colesevelam, 417t, 419
Colestipol, 417t, 419
Collagen, 113, 326
Compliance, 216
Computed tomography, 69–70, *69–70*, 72t, 322
Concentration gradient, 12
Conduction blocks
    definition of, 261
    myocardial infarction and, 180
Congenital heart disease
    acyanotic, 355–366
    aortic stenosis (*see* Aortic stenosis)
    atrial septal defect
        incidence of, 355
        laboratory studies of, 357
        ostium primum, 356
        ostium secundum, 355–356, *356*
        pathophysiology of, 357
        physical examination, 357
        sinus venosus, 356
        site of, 355–356
        symptoms of, 357
        treatment of, 357–358
    circulation
        fetal, 352–353, *354*
        transitional, 353–355
    classification of, 355
    coarctation of the aorta
        clinical features of, 364, *364*
        hypertension caused by, 298–299
        incidence of, 364
        laboratory studies, 365
        pathophysiology of, 365
        physical examination, 365
        postductal, 365
        preductal, 364–365
        symptoms of, 365
        treatment of, 365–366
    cyanotic, 366–369
    Eisenmenger syndrome, 369
    heart development
        aorticopulmonary septum, 352
        atrial septation, 349–350
        atrioventricular canal septation, 350, *351*
        heart loop formation, 348, *349*
        heart tube, 347–348, *349*
        septation, 348–349
        valves, 351–352

Congenital heart disease *(continued)*
  heart development *(continued)*
    ventricular outflow tract septation, 350–351
    ventricular septation, 350–351
  incidence of, 347
  patent ductus arteriosus
    incidence of, 359–360
    laboratory studies, 361
    pathophysiology of, 360
    physical examination, 361
    risk factors, 359–360
    symptoms of, 360–361
    treatment of, 361
  patent foramen ovale, 356
  pulmonic stenosis
    characteristics of, 202
    clinical features of, 363, *363*
    heart sounds associated with, 364
    laboratory studies, 364
    pathophysiology of, 363
    physical examination, 364
    radiographic findings, 50t, 364
    symptoms of, 363–364
    systolic ejection murmur caused by, 38
    treatment of, 364
  survival rates, 347
  tetralogy of Fallot, 366–367
  transposition of the great arteries, 367–369
  ventricular septal defect
    clinical features of, 358, *358*
    incidence of, 358
    laboratory studies, 359
    left-to-right shunting associated with, 359
    pansystolic murmurs caused by, 39
    pathophysiology of, 358–359
    physical examination, 359
    symptoms of, 359
    treatment of, 359
Congestive heart failure *(see* Heart failure)
Conn's syndrome, 299
Constrictive pericarditis
  cardiac catheterization evaluations, 322–323
  clinical features of, 322
  diagnostic approach, 322–323
  echocardiographic evaluations, 55–56
  etiology of, 320–321
  pathogenesis of, 320–321
  pathology of, 321
  pathophysiology of, *319*, 321–322
  treatment of, 323
Continuous murmurs, 40–41, *41*
Contractility
  alterations in, 218
  definition of, 214t
  digitalis effects, 372
  impairments in, *219*
  loss of, 218
  principles of, 136–137, 213–215
Contraction bands, 164, *165*
Contrast angiography, 62–64, *63*
Contrast echocardiography, 54
Coronary arteries
  anatomy of, 8, *9*, 137–138
  angiography of, 62, *63*
  external compression of, 133
  ischemic heart disease pathophysiology and, 137–138
  narrowing of, 137–138

  spasm of, 142
  stenosis of
    description of, 137–138
    revascularization of, 153
  tone of, 133, 135–137
  vasoconstriction of, 136, 138–139
  vasodilatation of, 137
Coronary artery bypass graft, 154, *154, * 155t
Coronary artery disease *(see also* Ischemic Heart Disease)
  cardiac catheterization findings, 64t
  contrast angiography findings, *63–64*
  coronary angiography evaluations, 148–149
  echocardiographic evaluations, 55
  endothelial-dependent vasodilation impairments, 139
  hypertension and, 302
  mortality rates, 149
  nitrates for, 151
  peripheral arterial disease and, 332
  radionuclide exercise tests for, 147
  statins for, 418
Coronary atherectomy, 154
Coronary blood flow
  determinants of, 133
  during systole, 133
  vasoconstriction effects, 161
Coronary stents, 153
Coronary vascular resistance
  description of, 132–133, 137
  neural factors that affect, 136
  regulation of, 133, 135–136
Coronary veins, 9
Corrigan's pulse, 200t
Costochondral syndrome, 145t
C-reactive protein, 128–129, 337
Creatine kinase, 172
Cushing's syndrome, 300
Cyclooxygenase-1, 411
Cytochrome P-450, 418
Cytokines, 128
Cytosol, 24

D-dimer, 343
de Musset's sign, 200t
Deep venous thrombosis
  calf vein, 344
  clinical presentation of, 343
  D-dimer measurements, 343
  description of, 341
  diagnosis of, 343
  epidemiology of, 341
  natural history of, 341
  pathogenesis of, 342–343
  postpartum, 343
  predisposing conditions, 341–342, 342t
  prophylaxis against, 344–345
  pulmonary embolism secondary to, 341, *342*
  risk factors, 343
  treatment of
    reasons for, 343–344
    thrombolysis, 344
    warfarin, 344
  venography evaluations, 343, *344*
  venous compression duplex ultrasonography for, 343
Defibrillation, 267
Delayed afterdepolarizations, 261

Depolarization
    cardiac cells, 18, 22, *22*, 75, 77–78
    diastolic, 258
    phase 4, 254
    ventricular, 81–85, *83–84*, 89
Diabetes mellitus
    atherosclerosis risks and, 127
    glucose assessments in, 127
Diagnostic imaging (*see* Imaging)
Diastole, 29, *30*
Diastolic current theory, 98
Diastolic depolarization, 258
Diastolic dysfunction
    heart failure caused by, 219–220
    hypertension and, 302
    treatment of, 234
Diastolic murmurs
    classification of, *40*
    early, 39, *40*, 42t
    grading of, 36
    mid to late, 39, *40*, 42t
Diazoxide, 383t, 385
Diet
    hypertension treated by, 305
    lipoprotein reductions, 124
Dietary Approaches to Stop Hypertension, 126–127
Digital subtraction angiography, 62
Digitalis
    action potential effects, 374
    atrial tachycardia and, 284
    atrioventricular node effects, 372–373, 373t
    automaticity effects, 374
    clinical uses of, 374–375
    contractility effects, 372
    electrical effects of, 372–374, 373t
    hypokalemia effects, 375
    indications
        arrhythmias, 374–375
        atrial fibrillation, 278, 374–375
        atrioventricular nodal reentrant tachycardia, 280–281
        dilated cardiomyopathy, 242
        heart failure, 232–233, 374
    mechanical effects of, 372
    mechanism of action, 372–374
    pharmacokinetics of, 375
    Purkinje cell effects, *373*
    sodium levels affected by, 372
    toxicity, 284, 374–375
Digoxin
    pharmacokinetics of, 375
Dilated cardiomyopathy
    anatomic findings, *238*
    arrhythmias associated with, 242
    cardiac catheterization findings, 241
    cardiac enlargement in, 237
    cardiac output reductions, 240
    characteristics of, 237, 251t
    clinical findings of, 240–241
    diagnostic studies, 241
    echocardiographic findings, 57t, 241
    electrocardiographic findings, 241
    familial forms of, 239
    pathologic findings, 239, *239*
    pathophysiology of, 239–240, *240*
    physical examination findings, 241
    prognosis, 243
    signs and symptoms of, 240–241

    thromboembolic complications, 242–243
    treatment of
        angiotensin-converting enzyme inhibitors, 242
        β-blockers, 242
        cardiac transplantation, 243
        digitalis, 242
        diuretics, 241–242
        goals, 241
        implantable cardioverter-defibrillator, 242
    types of, 238t
    ventricular dilatation associated with, 239
    viral myocarditis and, 237
Diltiazem, 152, 386–387
Diphenylhydantoin, 398
Dipyridamole, 148, 413
Disopyramide, 397
Diuretics
    description of, 405
    dilated cardiomyopathy treated using, 241–242
    heart failure treated using, 230–231
    hypertension treated using, 307–308
    loop, 406t, 406–407
    mechanism of action, 405–406
    potassium-sparing, 406t, 408–409
    thiazide, 230–231, 406t, 406–408
    types of, 406t
Dobutamine, 148, 376t, 377, 378t
Dofetilide, 402–403
Dopamine, 375–377, 378t
Doppler ultrasonography, 51, *52*
Doxazosin, 390–391, 391t
Dressler syndrome, 182, 313
Ductus arteriosus
    definition of, 353, 355, 359
    patent
        incidence of, 359–360
        laboratory studies, 361
        pathophysiology of, 360
        physical examination, 361
        risk factors, 359–360
        symptoms of, 360–361
        treatment of, 361
Ductus venosus, 352
Duroziez's sign, 200t
Dyspnea, 144, 189, 226, 247

Early afterdepolarizations, 260–261
ECG (*see* Electrocardiogram)
Echocardiography
    contrast, 54
    description of, 49
    Doppler
        description of, 51, *52*
    indications
        aortic regurgitation, 57t
        aortic stenosis, 57t, 198, 362–363
        atrial septal defect, 357
        cardiac tamponade, 319–320
        cardiomyopathy, 55, *55*, 57t
        coarctation of the aorta, 365
        constrictive pericarditis, 322
        coronary artery disease, 55
        dilated cardiomyopathy, 241
        Eisenmenger syndrome, 369
        hypertrophic cardiomyopathy, 248
        infective endocarditis, 206
        mitral regurgitation, 57t, 194
        mitral stenosis, 57t

Echocardiography *(continued)*
  indications *(continued)*
    myocardial infarction, 57t, 172
    patent ductus arteriosus, 361
    pericardial disease, 55–56
    pericardial effusion, 317, *317*
    pericarditis, 315
    pulmonic stenosis, 364
    tetralogy of Fallot, 367
    transposition of the great arteries, 368
    valvular lesions, 54–55
    ventricular septal defect, 359
  mechanism of action, 49–50
  M-mode, 50, *51*
  stress, 55
  transesophageal, 51, 53–54, *53–54*, 72t, 206
  transthoracic, 50–51, *52*, 72t, 206
  two-dimensional (2-D)
    description of, 50, *52*
    indications
      coronary artery disease, 55
      pericardial disease, 55–56
      ventricular assessments, 54, *55*
Ectopic atrial tachycardia, 284
Ectopic beat, 259
Ectopic pacemakers, 255
Ectopic rhythms
  description of, 259
  digitalis effects, 374
Edema
  acute pulmonary, 234–235
  peripheral, 227–228
Eisenmenger syndrome, 369
Ejection fraction, 214t
Elastin, 111, 113, 326
Electrocardiogram
  abnormal findings, *103–109*
  calibration of machine, 85–86, 101t
  cardiac cell impulse physiology, 75–78
  class IA antiarrhythmics effect, 396, 396t
  class II antiarrhythmics effect, 399
  description of, 75
  heart beat recordings, 81, *82*, 101t
  heart rate assessments, 86–88, *87*, 101t
  heart rhythm assessments, 86, 101t
  indications
    angina pectoris, 145–146, 170, *170*
    aortic stenosis, 198
    atrial fibrillation, 277
    atrial premature beats, 274, *275*
    atrioventricular nodal reentrant tachycardia,
      279
    coarctation of the aorta, 365
    dilated cardiomyopathy, 241
    Eisenmenger syndrome, 369
    hypertrophic cardiomyopathy, 248
    infective endocarditis, 206
    left bundle branch block, 93–94, *104*
    mitral regurgitation, 194
    mitral stenosis, 190
    mitral valve prolapse, 195
    myocardial infarction, 95–98, *99–100*, *105*
    patent ductus arteriosus, 361
    pericardial effusion, 317
    pericarditis, 315, *315*
    pulmonic stenosis, 364
    sinus bradycardia, *106–107*
    sinus tachycardia, 274, *275*
    transposition of the great arteries, 368

    ventricular hypertrophy, *107, 109*
    ventricular septal defect, 359
  leads
    bipolar, 78, *79*, 79t
    chest, 80–81, *81, 84,* 85
    electrical activity magnitude and direction, *80*
    placement positions for, 78, *78*
    unipolar, 78, *79*, 79t
  mean QRS axis, 88–91, *89–90*
  normal findings, *102–103*
  P wave
    abnormalities of, 91, *92,* 101t
    definition of, 81
  paper for, 85, *86*
  PR interval, 88, 88t, 101t
  QRS complex
    abnormalities of, 91–95, 101t
    atrioventricular node block, 273
    bundle branch block findings, 92–95, *94*
    description of, 81
    escape rhythm findings, 271
    myocardial infarction findings, 95–98
    shapes of, 81, *82*
    ventricular hypertrophy findings, 91–92, *93*
    ventricular tachycardia findings, 285
  QRS interval, 88, 88t, 101t
  QT interval, 88, 88t, 101t
  ST interval
    deviations of, 98–101, *100,* 101t
    elevations of, 146, 315
  T wave
    abnormalities of, 98–101, 101t
    definition of, 81
Electron beam computed tomography, 69–70, *70*
End-diastolic pressure, 214, 216
End-diastolic volume, 214, 216
Endocardial cushions, 350–351
Endocarditis *(see* Infective endocarditis)
Endocardium
  description of, 2
  injury of, 204
Endothelial cells
  dysfunction of, 114, 138–139
  functions of, 112–113, 113t
  ischemic heart disease pathophysiology, 137–138
  platelets and, interactions between, *139*
  vasoactive substances produced by, 133
Endothelin-1, 133, 135–136, 224
Endothelium
  acetylcholine effects, 135
  anatomy of, 112
  denuding of, 342
  dysfunction of, 114–115, 161
  functions of, 112t
  permeability of, 115
  vascular smooth muscle relaxation, 136
  vasoactive substances derived from, 135, *135*
Endothelium-derived hyperpolarizing factor, 133, 135
Endothelium-derived relaxing factor, 134b
End-systolic pressure, 217
End-systolic volume, 217
Epicardium, 2
Epinephrine, 376t, 377
Eptifibatide, 413
Escape beat, 259
Escape rhythms
  definition of, 259, 271
  junctional, 271, *271*
  ventricular, 271

Esophageal spasm, 145t, 169t
Essential hypertension
abnormalities in, *294*
definition of, 289
epidemiology of, 293
experimental findings, 293–294
genetics of, 293
hemodynamic progression of, 295, *295*
insulin and, 294
natural history of, 294–295
obesity and, 294
prevalence of, 292
severity of, 293
Estrogen
atherosclerosis risks and, 127–128
hormone replacement therapy, 127–128
Ethacrynic acid, 406t, 407
Excitation-contraction coupling
β-adrenergic signaling, 24–25, *26*
calcium ion movement during, *24*
cholinergic signaling, 25–26, *26*
description of, 22–23
Exercise
hypertension treated by, 305
lipoprotein reductions, 124
myocardial oxygen supply and demand during,
131
Exercise stress test, angina pectoris evaluations using,
146–147
Extra diastolic heart sounds, 34–36, 41t
Extra systolic heart sounds, 34, 41t
Extracellular matrix, 113
Extremities, 340

False aortic aneurysms
definition of, 326
illustration of, *327*
Familial hypercholesterolemia, 123
Fast sodium ion channels, 14–15, *17*
Fatty streak
description of, 118
fibrous plaque transition of, 118–119, *119*
illustration of, *119*
Fenfluramine, 201b
Fenofibrate, 417t, 420
Fenoldopam, 383t, 384–385
Fetal circulation
description of, 352–353
schematic diagram of, *354*
transition to normal circulation, 353–355
Fibrates, 417t, 420–421
Fibrin clot lysis, 159
Fibromuscular dysplasia, 298
Fibrosis, 166
Fick method, 61
First heart sound
characteristics of, 41t
description of, 29–30
intensity of, 31, 31t
production of, 30–31
First-degree atrioventricular block, 272, *272*
Fixed splitting, *32*, 33
Flecainide, 399
Fluvastatin, 417t
Foam cells, 118–119, *119*
Foramen ovale
definition of, 349, *350*
patent, 356
Fourth heart sound, 35

Framingham Heart Study, 122
Frank-Starling relationship
description of, 193, 213–214, *215*
heart failure
compensatory responses, 221
treatment effects, *230*
inotropic drugs effect, 371, *372*
Free fatty acids, 117b
Furosemide, 406t, 407

G proteins, 25–26
Gadolinium-enhanced magnetic resonance imaging,
71, 73, *73*
Gamma interferon, 121–122
Gap junctions, 255
Gastroesophageal reflux, 145t
Gemfibrozil, 417t, 420
Giant cell arteritis, 336t, 337
Glucocorticoids, 300
Glycoprotein IIb/IIIa receptor antagonists, 174, 409,
413
Great vessels
dilatation of, 46
transposition of, 367–369
Guanadrel, 390
Guanethidine, 390
Guanosine triphosphate, 134b
Guanylate cyclase, 387
Guanylyl cyclase, 134b

Heart
activation sequence for, 81–85
anteroposterior view of, 2
apex of, 1–2
atria of (*see* Atria)
auscultation of, 30, *30*
base of, 2
blood flow patterns, 5–6
cardiac skeleton of, 2, *3*
congenital disorders of (*see* Congenital heart disease)
electrophysiology of
description of, 11–12
ion channels, 12, 14
permeability, 14–16
embryologic development of
aorticopulmonary septum, 352
atrial septation, 349–350
atrioventricular canal septation, 350, *351*
heart loop formation, 348, *349*
heart tube, 347–348, *349*
septation, 348–349
valves, 351–352
ventricular outflow tract septation, 350–351
ventricular septation, 350–351
impulses (*see* Impulse)
innervation of, 7–8
intrapericardial pressure, 311
lymphatic vessels of, 9–10
myocardial cells of, 10–11
pericardium, 1
physiology of, 211–218
surface anatomy of, 1–2, *3*
ventricles of (*see* Ventricles of heart)
vessels of, 8–10
Heart failure
aortic stenosis-related, 197
apoptosis in, 225
atrial fibrillation associated with, 233
cardiac catheterization findings, 64t

Heart failure *(continued)*
  cardiac function determinants
    pressure-volume loops, 215–218
    stroke volume
      afterload, 214, 214t
      contractility, 214t, 214–215
      definition of, 214t
      preload, 213–214, 214t
  cardiac output decreases caused by, 222, 378
  Cheyne-Stokes respiration associated with, 227
  classification of, 227t
  clinical manifestations of, 226–229
  compensatory mechanisms
    adrenergic nervous system, 222–223
    antidiuretic hormone, 223–224
    description of, 221
    Frank-Starling mechanism, 221
    natriuretic peptides, 224
    neurohormonal alterations, 221–224, 222
    renin-angiotensin-aldosterone system, 223
    ventricular hypertrophy and remodeling, 224
  definition of, 211
  description of, 211
  laboratory tests and findings, 228–229
  left-sided
    acute pulmonary edema associated with, 234–235
    characteristics of, 228
  mitral regurgitation associated with, 228
  myocyte loss and dysfunction secondary to, 224–225
  New York Heart Association classification of, 227t
  orthopnea associated with, 226
  pathophysiology of
    description of, 218
    diastolic dysfunction, 219–220, 234
    systolic dysfunction, 218–219, *219*, 233
  physiology of, 211–218
  precipitating factors, 225t, 225–226
  prevalence of, 211
  prognosis, 229
  radiographic findings, *49*, 50t
  right-sided, 220–221, 227
  signs and symptoms of, 226t, 226–228
  sinus tachycardia findings, 228
  stages of, 227t
  tachyarrhythmias effect, 225
  treatment of, 233
    angiotensin-converting enzyme inhibitors, 231–233, 380–381
    β-adrenergic agonists, 232
    β-blockers, 233, 392
    biventricular pacing, 234
    cardiac transplantation, 234
    digitalis, 232–233, 374
    diuretics, 230–231
    goals, 229–230
    inotropic drugs, 232–233
    nitrates, 231
    phosphodiesterase inhibitors, 232
    resynchronization therapy, 234
    spironolactone, 233
    vasodilators, 231–232
  tricuspid regurgitation associated with, 228
  vasoconstriction, 378
  wall stress increases, 224
Heart loop, 348, *349*

Heart murmurs (*see* Murmurs)
Heart rate
  electrocardiogram assessments of, 86–88, *87*
  myocardial oxygen demand and, 136
  parasympathetic nervous system effects, 258
Heart sounds
  extra diastolic, 34–36, 41t
  extra systolic, 34, 41t
  first
    characteristics of, 41t
    description of, 29–30
    intensity of, 31, 31t
    production of, 30–31
  fourth, 35
  "gallops," 35–36
  myocardial infarction, 169
  pericardial knock, 36
  second
    abnormalities of, 33
    in atrial septal defect, 357
    characteristics of, 41t
    description of, 29–30
    production of, 31
    splitting of, 31–34, *32*, 362
  third, 35
Heart transplantation
  dilated cardiomyopathy treated using, 243
  heart failure treated using, 234
Heart valves
  anatomy of, 2, *3–4*
  aortic (*see* Aortic valve)
  embryologic development of, 351–352
  mitral (*see* Mitral valve)
  prosthetic, 53, 202–204
  pulmonary (*see* Pulmonary valve)
  tricuspid (*see* Tricuspid valve)
Heat shock protein 60, 129
Hemiblocks, 94
Hemorrhagic pericarditis, 314
Hemostasis, 158, 409
Heparan sulfate, 120, 158
Heparin
  low-molecular-weight, 174, 414–415
  myocardial infarction treated using, 174
  ST-segment elevation myocardial infarction treated using, 177
  unfractionated, 414
  unstable angina treated using, 174
Heparin-induced thrombocytopenia, 414
Hibernating myocardium, 68t, 141
High-density lipoproteins, 115t, 117b
Hill's sign, 200t
His-Purkinje system, 7
HMG CoA reductase, 123
HMG CoA reductase inhibitors (*see also* Statins)
  description of, 124, 129, 416
  mechanism of action, 416, *418*
  types of, 416, 417t
Homocystinemia, 128
Hormone replacement therapy, 127–128
Hydralazine, 308, 313, 382–383, 383t
Hydrochlorothiazide, 406t, 408
Hypercoagulability, 342
Hyperglycemia, 408
Hyperinsulinemia, 294
Hyperkalemia, 381
Hyperpolarization, 257

Hyperpolarizing current, 256–257
Hypertension
  accelerated-malignant, 305
  antihypertensive therapy, 126–127
  arterial narrowing associated with, 303
  atherosclerosis risks and, 126–127
  consequences of, *301*
  coronary artery disease caused by, 302
  definition of, 289–290
  essential
    abnormalities in, *294*
    definition of, 289
    epidemiology of, 293
    experimental findings, 293–294
    genetics of, 293
    hemodynamic progression of, 295, *295*
    insulin and, 294
    natural history of, 294–295
    obesity and, 294
    prevalence of, 292
    severity of, 293
  incidence of, 289
  mild, 305
  nephropathy induced by, 303
  organ damage caused by
    aorta, 303
    cerebrovascular system, 302–303
    description of, 300–302
    diastolic dysfunction, 302
    heart, 302
    kidneys, 303
    left ventricular hypertrophy, 302
    overview of, 301t
    retina, 303–304
    systolic dysfunction, 302
    vasculature abnormalities, 301
  renovascular, 298
  secondary
    causes of
      adrenocortical hormone excess, 299–300
      coarctation of the aorta, 298–299
      description of, 296t
      medications, 296–298
      pheochromocytoma, 299
      renal parenchymal disease, 298
      thyroid abnormalities, 300
    definition of, 289
    evaluation of, 296
    incidence of, 295
    laboratory tests, 296
    predisposing conditions, 295–296
  signs and symptoms of, 300
  strokes caused by, 302–303
  treatment of
    alcohol reduction, 306
    angiotensin II receptor blockers, 309
    angiotensin-converting enzyme inhibitors,
      308–309, 379–380
    antihypertensive medications, 306–309, 307t
    β-blockers, 308, 392
    calcium channel blockers, 308
    centrally acting α_2 adrenergic agonists, 309
    dietary changes, 305–306
    diuretics, 307–309
    exercise, 305
    hydralazine, 382
    nonpharmacologic, 305–306
    pharmacologic, 306–309

    potassium levels, 306
    relaxation therapy, 306
    salt restriction, 305–306
    smoking cessation, 306
    sympatholytic agents, 308
    vasodilators, 308
    weight reduction, 305
Hypertensive crises, 304–305
Hypertensive encephalopathy, 305
Hypertensive retinopathy, 303–304
Hypertrophic cardiomyopathy
  anatomic findings, *238*
  angina pectoris associated with, 247
  arrhythmias in, 247
  atrial fibrillation associated with, 248–249
  cardiac catheterization findings, 248
  characteristics of, 237, 243, 251t
  clinical findings of, 247
  diagnostic studies, 248
  echocardiography findings, 57t, 248
  electrocardiography findings, 248
  etiology of, 243–244
  familial, 243
  genetic counseling, 249
  incidence of, 243
  infective endocarditis in, 249
  left ventricular outflow tract obstruction associated
    with, 246, *246*
  pathologic findings, 244, *244–245*
  pathophysiology of, 244, *245*
  physical examination findings, 247–248
  prognosis, 249
  signs and symptoms of, 247
  sudden death risks, 247, 249
  syncope in, 247
  treatment of
    myomectomy, 249
    pharmacologic, 248–249
  two-dimensional echocardiography findings, *55*
  Valsalva maneuver, 247–248
  ventricular hypertrophy associated with, 244, *245*
  without outflow tract obstruction, 244, 246
Hypertrophy, ventricular
  compensatory, 224
  eccentric, 224
  hypertension and, 302
  in hypertrophic cardiomyopathy, 244, *245*
  left, 92
  QRS complex abnormalities associated with, 91–92,
    93, 107, 109
  radiographic findings, 46
  right, 91–92, *93*
  wall stress effects, 136, 224
Hyperuricemia, 408
Hypokalemia, 375, 407–408
Hyponatremia, 408
Hypotension, 381

Ibutilide, 402
Imaging
  cardiac catheterization (*see* Cardiac
    catheterization)
  computed tomography, 69–70, *69–70*, 72t
  echocardiography (*see* Echocardiography)
  magnetic resonance angiography, 71
  magnetic resonance imaging
    applications of, 71
    characteristics of, 72t

Imaging *(continued)*
  magnetic resonance imaging *(continued)*
    contrast-enhanced, 71, 73, *73*
    principles of, 70–71
  nuclear
    characteristics of, 72t
    description of, 64
    myocardial assessments
      metabolism, 68
      perfusion, 65–67
    pharmacologic agents, 66
    positron emission tomography, 68, 72t
    radioisotopes, 65–66
    radionuclide ventriculography, 67–68 *67*, 72t
    stress studies, 66
  radiography *(see* Radiography)
Immune response
  endothelial cell role in, 112, 113t
  T cell role in, 118
Implantable cardioverter-defibrillators
  dilated cardiomyopathy treated using, 242
  tachyarrhythmias treated using, 267–268
Impulse
  blockade of, 261
  conduction of
    altered, 261–265
    bypass tracts, 264–265
    process of, 21–22
    reentry, 261–262, *263*
  formation of
    abnormal automaticity, 259–260
    automaticity, 253–255
    description of, 253
    escape rhythms, 259
    latent pacemaker assumption of, 259
    overdrive suppression, 255–257
    pacemakers, 255
    triggered activity, 260–261
Indapamide, 406t, 407
Infarction *(see* Myocardial infarction)
Infective endocarditis
  acute, 205
  causes of, 205t
  classification of, 204
  clinical manifestations of, 205–207
  description of, 188, 203
  echocardiographic findings, 206
  electrocardiographic findings, 206
  in hypertrophic cardiomyopathy, 249
  inflammatory response to, 206
  microorganisms associated with, 205t, 207, 207t
  mortality rates, 204
  murmurs associated with, 206
  pathogenesis of, 204–205
  prophylaxis, 207, 209, 249
  prosthetic valves and, 203
  skin manifestations of, 206
  subacute, 205
  treatment of, 207, 209
Inferior vena cava, 1, 2–3, 352–353
Inflammatory mediators, 118
Inotropic drugs
  digitalis *(see* Digitalis)
  heart failure treated using, 232–233
  hemodynamic effects, 371, *372*
  mechanism of action, 371
  phosphodiesterase inhibitors, 378, 378t
  pulmonary edema treated using, 235

sympathomimetic agents
  cAMP formation effects, 375
  definition of, 375
  dobutamine, 376t, 377, 378t
  dopamine, 375–377, 376t, 378t
  epinephrine, 376t, 377
  isoproterenol, 376t, 377–378
  norepinephrine, 376t, 377
Insulin, 294
Insulin resistance, 294
Intercalated disk, 11
Intercellular adhesion molecule, 118
Interleukin-6, 113
Intermediate-density lipoproteins, 124
Internal mammary artery grafts, 154
Interventricular septum, *4, 5*–6
Intima
  anatomy of, 111, *112*, 325
  functions of, 112
  leukocyte adherence to, 118
  lipoprotein retention in, 115
Intra-aortic balloon pump, 181
Intrinsic sympathomimetic activity, 392
Ion channels
  description of, 12, 14
  fast sodium, 14–15, *17*
  gating, 14
  resting state of, 14
  selectivity, 14
  structure of, *15*
  voltage-sensitive, 14
Ischemic heart disease
  adaptations, 333
  angina pectoris *(see* Angina pectoris)
  chest pain associated with, 145t
  cholesterol levels and, 123
  consequences of, 140–141
  electrocardiographic findings, 145–146
  exercise stress test for, 146–147
  myocardial effects, 140
  nuclear imaging findings, 68t
  pathophysiology of
    endothelial cell dysfunction, 138–139
    fixed vessel narrowing, 137–138
    myocardial oxygen alterations, 140
  prevention of, 152–153
  recurrent, 150–152
  silent
    characteristics of, 143
    definition of, 132t
  treatment of
    acute episodes, 149–150, 150t
    atherectomy, 154
    β-blockers, 392
    coronary artery bypass graft, 154, *154*, 155t
    goals, 149–150
    percutaneous coronary interventions, 153, 155t
    percutaneous transluminal coronary angioplasty,
      153
    pharmacologic agents, 150–152
    revascularization, 153–155
Ischemic preconditioning, 166–167
Isoelectric complex, 89
Isoproterenol, 265, 376t, 377–378
Isosorbide dinitrate, 232, 388
Isosorbide mononitrate, 388
Jones' criteria for rheumatic fever, 186, 186t
Junctional escape rhythms, 271, *271*

Kerley lines, 228
Kidneys
  glomerular filtration rate, 405
  hypertension effects, 303
  tubules of, 405, *405*
Kussmaul's sign, 250, 322

Lactate dehydrogenase, 172, 320
LaPlace's relationship, 136, 214
Late systolic murmurs, 39
Latent pacemaker, 255
Lecithin cholesterol acyltransferase, 117b
Left anterior fascicular block, 94–95
Left atrial appendage, 3
Left atrium
  anatomy of, 5, *6*
  compliance of, 191–192, 214t
  mitral stenosis pathophysiology, 188
  pressure measurements, *58*, 192
Left bundle branch, 7
Left bundle branch block
  description of, 33
  electrocardiographic findings, 93–94, *104*
  QRS complex abnormalities associated with,
      93–94
Left posterior fascicular block, 95
Left ventricle
  anatomy of, 5, *6*
  aneurysm of, 182
  depolarization of, 94
  diastolic dysfunction, 166, 182
  dilatation of, 199
  dilated cardiomyopathy effects, 239–240
  enlargement of, 191, 193
  hypertrophy of, 302
  outflow tract obstruction, in hypertrophic
      cardiomyopathy, 246, *246*
Left-to-right shunting, 355
Lepirudin, 415
Leukocytes
  arterial wall adherence of, 112, 118
  pericarditis and, 314
  recruitment of, 118
Levine's sign, 144
Lidocaine, 398
Ligamentum arteriosum, 3
Lipid-regulating drugs
  bile-acid binding agents, 419
  description of, 416
  fibrates, 417t, 420–421
  HMG CoA reductase inhibitors
    description of, 124, 129, 416
    mechanism of action, 416, 418
    types of, 416, 417t
  niacin, 417t, 419–420
  sites of action, *389, 417*
Lipoprotein(s)
  atherosclerosis and, 115–118, 123–126
  characteristics of, 115t
  classification of, 115, 115t
  high-density, 115t, 117b
  intermediate-density, 124
  low-density
    atherosclerosis risks and, 123
    characteristics of, 115t, 115–116
    familial hypercholesterolemia, 123
    lowering of, 418
    serum levels of, 123
    statins effect, 418

  subclasses of, 123–124
  lowering of, 124–126, 125t
  oxidation of, 115
  reduction methods
    diet, 124
    exercise, 124
    lipid-regulating drugs (*see* Lipid-regulating
        drugs)
    statins, 124–126, 125t, 152
  transport of, 116b–117b
  very-low-density
    atherosclerosis risks and, 124
    characteristics of, 115t, 117b
    niacin effects, 419
Lipoprotein (a), 128
Lipoprotein lipase, 116b–117b
Local metabolites, 138–139
Lovastatin, 417t
Low-density lipoproteins
  atherosclerosis risks and, 123
  characteristics of, 115t, 115–116
  familial hypercholesterolemia, 123
  lowering of, 418
  serum levels of, 123
  statins effect, 418
  subclasses of, 123–124
Low-molecular-weight heparin, 174, 414–415
Lown-Ganong-Levine syndrome, 283
Lymphatic system, 9–10

Magnetic resonance angiography, 71
Magnetic resonance imaging
  applications of, 71
  characteristics of, 72t
  contrast-enhanced, 71, 73, *73*
  principles of, 70–71
Magnetic resonance venography, 343
Mean QRS axis, 88–91, *89–90*
Media
  anatomy of, 111, *112,* 326
  degeneration of, 328
Membrane potential, 13b, 255, 260
Mesenchymal tissue, *353*
Metabolic acidosis, 408
Metabolic syndrome, 124, 127
Metolazone, 406t, 408
Mexiletine, 398
Milrinone, 378, 378t
Mineralocorticoids, 299–300
Minoxidil, 308, 383, 383t
Mitral regurgitation
  acute, 192–193
  cardiac catheterization findings, 64t
  characteristics of, 208t
  chronic, 193
  clinical manifestations of, 193–194
  description of, 31
  Doppler color-flow mapping of, *52*
  echocardiographic findings, 57t, 194
  electrocardiographic findings, 194
  etiology of, 190–191, 191t
  evaluation of, 193–194
  in heart failure, 228
  hemodynamic profile of, *192*
  left ventricular enlargement and, 191
  natural history of, 194
  pansystolic murmurs caused by, 39
  pathophysiology of, 191–193, *192*
  physical examination findings, 193–194

Mitral regurgitation (*continued*)
  pulmonary capillary wedge pressure increases
      associated with, 61
  radiographic findings, 50t, 194
  regurgitant fraction, 191
  rheumatic fever and, 191
  treatment of, 194–195
Mitral stenosis
  acute rheumatic fever and, 186
  cardiac catheterization findings, 64t, 190
  characteristics of, 208t
  clinical manifestations of, 188–190
  complications of, 189
  description of, 31
  diagnostic findings, 189
  diastolic murmurs caused by, 40
  dyspnea associated with, 189
  echocardiographic findings, 57t, 190
  electrocardiographic findings, 190
  etiology of, 186
  evaluation of, 188–190
  hemodynamic profile of, *187*
  left atrium effects, 188
  murmurs associated with, 189–190
  natural history of, 188–189, 189t
  open mitral commissurotomy for, 190
  opening snap associated with, *35*, 189
  pathology of, 186–187
  pathophysiology of, *187*, 187–188
  percutaneous balloon mitral valvuloplasty for,
      190
  pulmonary artery pressure in, 188
  pulmonary capillary wedge pressure increases
      associated with, 61
  radiographic findings, *47*, 50t, 190
  treatment of, 190
Mitral valve
  anatomy of, 5, *6*
  development of, 351–352
  myxomatous degeneration of, 191
  prolapse of, 195
  regurgitation of (*see* Mitral regurgitation)
  replacement of, 194–195
  stenosis of (*see* Mitral stenosis)
M-mode echocardiography, 50, *51*
Möbitz type I block, 272, *272*
Möbitz type II block, 273, *273*
Moderator band, 5
Monocyte chemoattractant protein 1, 118
Müller's sign, 200t
Multifocal atrial tachycardia, 282–284, *283*
Murmurs
  continuous, 40–41, 42t
  definition of, 36
  descriptive terms for, 36
  diastolic
    classification of, *40*
    early, 39, *40*, 42t
    grading of, 36
    hyperdynamic states that cause, 40
    mid to late, 39, *40*, 42t
  infective endocarditis, 206
  location of, 36
  maximum intensity locations for, *42*
  mechanisms of, 36
  in mitral stenosis, 189–190
  pitch of, 36
  shape of, 36

systolic
  classification of, 37, *37*
  grading of, 36
  late, 39, 42t
  pansystolic, 38–39, 42t, 193
  systolic ejection murmur, 37–38, *38*, 42t
  timing of, 36
Myocardial cells
  depolarization of, 257, *257*
  description of, 10–11
  gap junctions of, 255
  repolarization of, 257
Myocardial infarction
  angiotensin-converting enzyme inhibitors for,
      152–153
  β-blockers for, 151
  cell death mechanisms, *164*
  chest pain associated with, 168
  clinical features of, 170t
  complications of
    arrhythmias, 179–180
    conduction blocks, 180
    description of, 178–179
    Dressler syndrome, 182
    myocardial dysfunction, 180–181
    papillary muscle rupture, 181
    pericarditis, 182
    recurrent ischemia, 179
    right ventricular infarction, 181
    sinus bradycardia, 180
    thromboembolism, 182
    ventricular aneurysm, 182
    ventricular fibrillation, 179–180
    ventricular free wall rupture, 181
    ventricular septal rupture, 181–182
  definition of, 132t
  diagnosis of
    creatine kinase levels, 172
    echocardiography, 57t, 172
    electrocardiography
      QRS complex abnormalities, 95–98, *105*
      ST segment deviations, *99–100, 170–171*
    lactate dehydrogenase, 172
    serum markers, 170–172
    troponin levels, 171–172
  heart sounds, 169
  localization of, 96t
  non–Q-wave, 97, 99, 101, 167
  non-ST-segment elevation
    description of, 157, 162, 167
    electrocardiographic findings, *170*
    treatment of
      angiotensin-converting enzyme inhibitors, 178
      anti-ischemic agents, 174–175
      antithrombotic agents, 173–174
      β-blockers, 174–175
      calcium channel blockers, 175
      conservative vs. early invasive approaches, 175
      heparin, 174
      nitrates, 174
      statins, 178
      thienopyridines, 174
  nuclear imaging findings, 68t
  onset of, 161
  pain caused by, 168
  pathologic events associated with, *165*
  pericarditis after, 312–313, 316
  prevention of, 152–153

Q-wave, 97, *98,* 158, 167
risk stratification and management, 182–183
signs and symptoms of, 168, 168t
ST-segment elevation
  description of, 158, 167
  electrocardiographic findings, *171*
  treatment of
    angiotensin-converting enzyme inhibitors, 178
    antithrombotic agents, 177
    aspirin, 177
    β-blockers, 177
    description of, 175
    heparin, 177
    nitrates, 177–178
    percutaneous coronary interventions, 177
    statins, 178
    thrombolytic agents, 175–177, *176*
subendocardial, 163
transmural, 163, 166t
treatment of
  angiotensin-converting enzyme inhibitors, 178
  anti-ischemic agents, 174–175
  antithrombotic agents, 173–174, 177
  aspirin, 177
  β-blockers, 174–175, 177
  calcium channel blockers, 175
  conservative vs. early invasive approaches, 175
  description of, 175
  heparin, 174, 177
  nitrates, 174, 177–178
  percutaneous coronary interventions, 177
  statins, 178
  thienopyridines, 174
  thrombolytic agents, 175–177, *176*
ventricular remodeling after, 167
Myocardial ischemia (*see* Ischemic heart disease)
Myocardial oxygen supply and demand
  alterations in, 140
  description of, 131
  determinants of, *132,* 136–137
Myocarditis, viral, 237
Myocardium
  anatomy of, 2
  blood vessels of, 163
  coagulative necrosis of, 163
  contractility of, 136–137, 213–215, 214t
  edema of, 164
  hibernating, 68t, 141
  ischemia effects, 140
  metabolism, 68
  necrosis of, 169–170, 172
  perfusion, 65–67
  stunned, 140–141, 166
  viability assessments, 68
Myocytes (*see also* Cardiac cells)
  calcium levels in, 164
  contraction of, 23
  description of, 10
  destruction of, 224–225
  injured, 166
  loss of, 224–225
  potassium channels, 16
  refractory period of, 21, *21*
  relaxation of, 25
  repolarization of, 76–77, *77, 100*
Myofibrils, 10
Myoglobin, 172
Myomectomy, 249

Myopathy, 418
Myosin, 23

National Cholesterol Education Program, 124
Natriuretic peptides, 224
Neoplastic pericarditis, 313
Nephropathy, hypertension-induced, 303
Nernst potential, 13b
Nesiritide, 232, 379
Niacin, 417t, 419–420
Nifedipine, 152
Nitrates
  antianginal effects of, 387–388
  hemodynamic effects of, 387–388
  indications
    angina pectoris, 150–151, 174
    coronary artery disease, 151
    heart failure, 231
    myocardial infarction, 174
    ST-segment elevation myocardial infarction, 177–178
  mechanism of action, 387, *387*
  nitroglycerin (*see* Nitroglycerin)
  pharmacokinetics of, 388
  sites of action, *379*
  vascular smooth muscle effects, *387*
Nitric oxide
  actions of, 133, 134b–135b
  description of, 114
  platelet effects, 160–161
  relaxation effects of, 138
Nitric oxide synthase, 134b
Nitroglycerin
  intravenous, 388
  sublingual
    angina pectoris managed using, 144, 150, 174
    description of, 134b
    hemodynamic effects, 387
    pharmacokinetics of, 388
  transdermal, 388
Nonbacterial thrombotic endocarditis, 204
Non-ST-segment elevation myocardial infarction
  description of, 157, 162, 167
  electrocardiographic findings, *170*
  treatment of
    angiotensin-converting enzyme inhibitors, 178
    anti-ischemic agents, 174–175
    antithrombotic agents, 173–174
    β-blockers, 174–175
    calcium channel blockers, 175
    conservative vs. early invasive approaches, 175
    heparin, 174
    nitrates, 174
    statins, 178
    thienopyridines, 174
Nontuberculous bacterial pericarditis, 312
Norepinephrine, 376t, 377–378
Nuclear imaging
  angina pectoris evaluations, 147
  characteristics of, 72t
  description of, 64
  ischemic heart disease evaluations, 147
  myocardial assessments
    metabolism, 68
    perfusion, 65–67
  pharmacologic agents, 66
  positron emission tomography, 68, 72t

Nuclear imaging *(continued)*
  radioisotopes, 65–66
  radionuclide ventriculography, 67–68 *67*, 72t
  stress studies, 66

Occlusive arterial diseases
  acute arterial occlusion, 335–336
  peripheral arterial disease *(see* Peripheral arterial disease)
  vasculitis syndromes
    characteristics of, 336t
    description of, 336
    giant cell arteritis, 336t, 337
    polyarteritis nodosa, 336t, 336–337
    Takayasu's arteritis, 336t, 337
    thromboangiitis obliterans, 336t, 337–338
Ohm's law, 137
Open mitral commissurotomy, 190
Orthopnea, 226
Ostium primum atrial septal defect, 356
Ostium secundum
  atrial septal defect, 356, *356*
  definition of, 349
Overdrive suppression, 255–257

Pacemaker
  electronic, 266
  latent
    automaticity of, 259
    definition of, 255
  native, 255
  permanent, 266
Pacemaker cells
  action potential of, *254*
  anatomic connections, 257–258
  description of, 20, 253
  electrical coupling of, 257
  membrane potential of, 255
  repolarization phase of, 255
  sinoatrial node, 254
  voltage-gated, *258*
Pacemaker current
  alterations in, 255, *256*
  definition of, 20, 254
Pacing, 234, 249
Pansystolic murmurs, 38–39
Papillary muscles
  anatomy of, *4*, 5
  rupture of, 181
Papilledema, 304
Paradoxical embolism, 335
Paradoxical splitting, *32*, 33–34
Parietal pericardium, 1, *2f*, 311
Paroxysmal nocturnal dyspnea, 226–227
Paroxysmal supraventricular tachycardia
  characteristics of, 278–279
  class IV antiarrhythmic drugs for, 403
  Wolff-Parkinson-White syndrome and, 281
Patent ductus arteriosus
  incidence of, 359–360
  laboratory studies, 361
  pathophysiology of, 360
  physical examination, 361
  risk factors, 359–360
  symptoms of, 360–361
  treatment of, 361
Peptic ulcer disease, 145t
Percutaneous balloon mitral valvuloplasty, 190
Percutaneous coronary interventions

angina pectoris treated using, 153, 155t
ischemic heart disease treated using, 153, 155t
ST-segment elevation myocardial infarction treated using, 177
Percutaneous transluminal coronary angioplasty, 153
Perfusion pressure, 133
Pericardial effusion
  clinical features of, 317, 317t
  diagnostic studies of, 317
  echocardiographic evaluations, *56*
  etiology of, 316
  pathophysiology of, 316–317
  treatment of, 318
Pericardial friction rub, 169, 314
Pericardial knock, 36
Pericardiocentesis, 320
Pericarditis
  chest pain associated with, 145t
  clinical features of, 314, 314t
  connective tissue disease-related, 313
  constrictive
    cardiac catheterization evaluations, 322–323
    clinical features of, 322
    diagnostic approach, 322–323
    etiology of, 320–321
    pathogenesis of, 320–321
    pathology of, 321
    pathophysiology of, *319*, 321–322
    treatment of, 323
  corticosteroids for, 315
  description of, 311
  diagnostic approach, 314–315
  differential diagnosis, 169t
  drug-induced, 313, 313t
  echocardiographic evaluations, 55–56, 315
  electrocardiographic findings, 315, *315*
  etiology of, 312–313
  hemorrhagic, 314
  idiopathic, 312, 315
  leukocyte role in, 314
  myocardial infarction-related, 182, 312–313, 316
  nontuberculous bacterial, 312
  pathogenesis of, 313–314
  pathology of, 314
  postpericardiotomy, 313
  purulent, 316
  radiation-induced, 313
  serofibrinous, 314
  serous, 314
  suppurative, 314
  systemic lupus erythematosus and, 313
  treatment of, 315–316
  tuberculous, 312
  uremic, 313
  viral, 312, 314
Pericardium
  anatomy of, 1, *2f*, 311
  functions of, 311
  parietal, 311
  visceral, 311
  volume-pressure relationship in, *316*
Peripheral α-adrenergic receptor antagonists, 390–391, 391t
Peripheral arterial disease
  claudication associated with, 333, *334*
  clinical presentation of, 333–334
  description of, 332
  diagnosis of, 333–334
  etiology of, 332–333

exercise capacity reductions, 332
ischemic ulcers caused by, 334, *334*
pathogenesis of, 332–333
physical examination findings, 334
treatment of, 335
Peripheral edema, 227
Peripheral pruning, *48*, 49
Peripheral vascular disease
    definition of, 325
    occlusive arterial diseases (*see* Occlusive arterial
        diseases)
    Raynaud's phenomenon, 338–339, *339*
Peripheral vascular resistance, 293
Peroxisomal proliferation activating receptor-α, 124
Phenoxybenzamine, 391, 391t
Phentermine, 201b
Phentolamine, 391, 391t
Pheochromocytoma, 299
Phosphodiesterase inhibitors, 232, 378t
Phospholamban, 25
Phospholipase A$_2$, 410
Physiologic splitting, 31, *32*
Plaque, atherosclerotic
    cellular debris in, 119–120
    characteristics of, 119–120, *120*
    complications of, 120–121, 121t
    description of, 111
    fatty streak transition into, 118–119, *119*
    foam cells, 118–120
    formation of, 160
    renovascular hypertension caused by, 298
    rupture of, 121, *122*, 160–161
    schematic diagram of, *114*
Plasmin, 175
Plateau, 19
Platelet(s)
    activation of, 161, 410, *410*
    aggregation of, 139–140, 161, 409
    antiplatelet drugs effect, 410–411
    endogenous inhibition of, 159–160
    endothelial cells and, interactions between, *139*
    functions of, 409
    nitric oxide effects, 160–161
    substances released from, 409
    vasoconstricting actions of, 139
Platelet-derived growth factor, 119–120
Pleural effusion, 47, 49, *49*
Pneumonia, 169t
Pneumothorax, 169t
Poiseuille's law, 137, 332
Polyarteritis nodosa, 336t, 336–337
Positron emission tomography, 68, 72t
Posterior descending artery, 8, *9*
Posteroanterior radiographs
    cardiac silhouette, 46
    description of, 45, *46*
Postpericardiotomy pericarditis, 313
Postphlebitic syndrome, 341
Potassium-sparing diuretics, 406t, 408–409
PR interval
    description of, 88, 88t
    in first-degree atrioventricular block, 272
Pravastatin, 417t
Prazosin, 390–391, 391t
Preganglionic parasympathetic fibers, 7
Preganglionic sympathetic neurons, 7
Preload
    alterations in, 216–217, *217*
    definition of, 214t

description of, 212–214
reduction methods, 235
Pressure-volume loops, 215–218, *220*
Primary aldosteronism, 299
Prinzmetal's angina (*see* Angina pectoris,
        variant)
Proarrhythmic effect, 394
Procainamide, 313, 397
Propafenone, 399
Prostacyclin, 135, 159
Prosthetic heart valves
    description of, 53, 202
    failure of, 203
    infective endocarditis risks, 203–204
    types of, 202–203
Protein C, 158
Protein S, 158–159
Pseudoaneurysm, 181, 326
Pulmonary artery, 47, *48*
Pulmonary artery pressure
    cardiac catheterization measurements of, 60,
        60t
    in mitral stenosis, 188
Pulmonary artery wedge pressure, 60t, 60–61, *61*
Pulmonary blood flow, 49
Pulmonary capillary wedge pressure, 61
Pulmonary edema, 234–235
Pulmonary embolism, 169t, 225, 341, *342*
Pulmonary hypertension, radiographic findings,
        48
Pulmonary valve
    anatomy of, 5
    development of, 351–352
    regurgitation of, 39, 202
    stenosis of
        characteristics of, 202
        clinical features of, 363, *363*
        heart sounds associated with, 364
        laboratory studies, 364
        pathophysiology of, 363
        physical examination, 364
        radiographic findings, 50t, 364
        symptoms of, 363–364
        systolic ejection murmur caused by, 38
        treatment of, 364
Pulmonary vascular resistance
    calculation of, 62
    disorders that affect, 60
    perinatal, 358
    postnatal changes, 354–355, 360
Pulmonary vasculature, 47, 49, *49*, 354
Pulmonary venous pressure, 47
Pulse pressure, 199, 200t
Pulsus alternans, 228
Pulsus paradoxus, 318–319
Purkinje fibers, 7
Purulent pericarditis, 316
PVR (*see* Pulmonary vascular resistance)

QRS interval, 88, 88t
QT interval, 88, 88t
Quadruple rhythm, 35–36
Quincke's sign, 200t
Quinidine, 396–397

Radiation-induced pericarditis, 313
Radiography
    cardiac silhouette, 46–47
    characteristics of, 72t

Radiography *(continued)*
  frontal view, 45, *46*
  indications
    aortic regurgitation, 200
    aortic stenosis, 362
    atrial septal defect, 357
    coarctation of the aorta, 365
    constrictive pericarditis, 322
    dilated cardiomyopathy, 241
    Eisenmenger syndrome, 369
    mitral stenosis, 190
    patent ductus arteriosus, 361
    pericardial effusion, 317
    pulmonic stenosis, 364
    restrictive cardiomyopathy, 250
    tetralogy of Fallot, 367
    transposition of the great arteries, 368
    ventricular septal defect, 359
  lateral view, 45–46, *46*
  posteroanterior view
    cardiac silhouette, 46
    description of, 45, *46*
  principles of, 45
Radionuclide ventriculography, 67–68, *67*, 72t
Raynaud's phenomenon, 338–339, *339*
Reactive oxygen species, 114
Reentry
  antiarrhythmic drugs for, 394
  atrioventricular nodal, *280*
  interruption of, 267
  mechanisms of, 261–262, *263*
Renal insufficiency, 381
Renal parenchymal disease, 298
Renin-angiotensin-aldosterone system
  drug interactions, 381t
  heart failure-related compensatory response, 223
  inhibition of, 232
  schematic diagram of, *297, 380*
Renovascular hypertension, 298
Repolarization
  delayed afterdepolarizations, 261
  description of, 19, 76–77, *77, 100*
Reserpine, 390
Resting potential, 16–18, *17*
Resting state, 14, 75
Restrictive cardiomyopathy
  anatomic findings, *238*
  characteristics of, 237, 249, 251t
  clinical findings of, 250
  diagnostic studies, 250–251
  echocardiographic findings, 57t
  pathophysiology of, 250, *250*
  physical examination findings, 250
  treatment of, 251
  types of, 250t
Retinopathy, hypertensive, 303–304
Rheumatic fever, 185–186, 186t
Right atrium
  anatomy of, 2, 4, *4*
  pressure measurements, 58, *58*, 60t
Right bundle branch, 7
Right bundle branch block
  description of, 33
  electrocardiographic findings, 92–93, *94*
  QRS complex abnormalities associated with, 92–93, *94*
Right ventricle
  anatomy of, 4–5, 220
  failure of, 220–221

  infarction of, 181
  pressure measurements, *58,* 59, 59b, 60t
Right ventricular heave, 228
Ryanodine receptors, 23, *24*

S_1 *(see* First heart sound)
S_2 *(see* Second heart sound)
Sarcolemma, 11
Sarcomere, *10*
Sarcoplasmic reticulum, 11, *11*, 25
Second heart sound
  abnormalities of, 33
  in atrial septal defect, 357
  characteristics of, 41t
  description of, 29–30
  production of, 31
  splitting of, 31–34, *32*, 362
Secondary aldosteronism, 300
Second-degree atrioventricular block, *272*, 272–273
Semilunar valves, 351
Septum primum, 349, *350*
Septum secundum, 349
Serofibrinous pericarditis, 314
Serous pericarditis, 314
Sick sinus syndrome, *270*, 270–271
Silent ischemia
  characteristics of, 143
  definition of, 132t
Simvastatin, 417t
Single photon emission computed tomography, 65, *65*, 72t
Sinoatrial nodal artery, 8, *9*
Sinoatrial node
  anatomy of, 6, 7
  automaticity alterations, 258–259
  cells of, 20
  digitalis effects, 373t
  overdrive suppression of, 270
  pacemaker cells of, 254
  suppression of, 259
Sinus bradycardia
  benign, 269
  definition of, 86, 269
  etiology of, 269
  management of, 269
  myocardial infarction-related, 180
Sinus rhythm, 86
Sinus tachycardia
  characteristics of, 274
  definition of, 86
  electrocardiographic findings, 274, *275*
  in heart failure, 228
  myocardial infarction-related, 180
Sinus venosus, 348
Smoking
  atherosclerosis and, 126
  hypertension and, 306
Smooth muscle cells, vascular
  atherosclerotic role of, 118–119
  description of, 113
Sodium nitroprusside, 134b, 383t, 383–384, *384*
Sotalol, 402
Spironolactone, 233, 406t, 408
Splitting of second heart sound
  fixed, *32*, 33
  paradoxical, *32*, 33–34
  physiologic, 31, *32*
  wide, *32*, 33

Stable angina
  causes of, 142
  coronary angiography evaluations, 148–149
  definition of, 132t
  diagnostic studies for, 145–149
  differential diagnosis, 144–145, 145t
  electrocardiographic findings, 145–146
  exercise echocardiography evaluations, 148
  exercise stress test for, 146–147
  history-taking findings, 143–145
  natural history of, 149, 149t
  nitroglycerin for, 144
  nuclear studies for, 147
  oxygen supply inadequacies associated with, 142
  pathophysiologic findings, *141*
  physical examination findings, 145, *146*
  quality of, 143–144
  risk factors, 144
  signs and symptoms of, 143–144
  treatment of, 149–150, 150t
Staphylococcus aureus endocarditis, 204
Statins, 124–126, 125t, 152, 178 (*see also* HMG CoA
      reductase inhibitors)
"Steal" phenomenon, 66–67
Stents, 153
Stethoscopes, 30, *30*
Streptokinase, 175
Stress echocardiography
  description of, 55
  ischemic heart disease evaluations, 148
Stress tests
  angina pectoris evaluations using, 146–147
  pharmacologic, 148
Stroke volume
  afterload, 214, 214t
  contractility, 214t, 214–215
  definition of, 214t
  preload, 213–214, 214t
ST-segment elevation myocardial infarction
  description of, 158, 167
  electrocardiographic findings, *171*
  treatment of
    angiotensin-converting enzyme inhibitors, 178
    antithrombotic agents, 177
    aspirin, 177
    β-blockers, 177
    description of, 175
    heparin, 177
    nitrates, 177–178
    percutaneous coronary interventions, 177
    statins, 178
    thrombolytic agents, 175–177, *176*
Stunned myocardium, 140–141, 166
Subacute bacterial endocarditis, 204
Subclavian artery, 3
Subendocardial infarcts, 163
Sudden death
  hypertrophic cardiomyopathy and, 247, 249
  implantable cardioverter defibrillators for, 267–268
Summation gallop, 36
Superficial thrombophlebitis, 345
Superior vena cava, 2–3
Superoxide anion, 114
Superoxide dismutase, 114
Suppurative pericarditis, 314
Supraventricular arrhythmias, 180, 287
SVR (*see* Systemic vascular resistance)
Sympatholytic agents, 308

Sympathomimetic agents
  definition of, 375
  dobutamine, 376t, 377
  dopamine, 375–377, 376t
  epinephrine, 376t, 377
  isoproterenol, 376t, 377–378
  norepinephrine, 376t, 377
Syncope, 247
Syndrome X, 143
Systemic lupus erythematosus-related pericarditis,
      313
Systemic vascular resistance, 62
Systole
  blood flow during, 133
  description of, 29–30, *30*
Systolic dysfunction
  description of, 166
  heart failure caused by, 218–219
  hypertension and, 302
  treatment of, 233
Systolic murmurs
  classification of, 37, *37*
  grading of, 36
  late, 39, 42t
  pansystolic, 38–39, 42t
  systolic ejection murmur, 37–38, *38*, 42t

T cells, 118, 160
T tubules, 11, *11*
Tachyarrhythmias
  atrial fibrillation
    cardioversion for, 278
    definition of, 277
    electrocardiographic findings, *277*
    in heart failure, 233
    in hypertrophic cardiomyopathy, 248–249
    mechanism of, 277
    mitral stenosis effects, 188
    myocardial infarction-related, 180
    treatment of, 277–278
  atrial flutter, 276–277
  atrial premature beats, 180, 274, *275*
  definition of, 274
  differential diagnosis, *275*
  heart failure secondary to, 225
  impulse formation and conduction alterations,
      254
  mechanisms of, 265t
  tachycardia
    atrioventricular nodal reentrant, 279–281
    atrioventricular reentrant, 281
    concealed accessory pathway, 283
    ectopic atrial, 284
    multifocal atrial, 282–284, *283*
    paroxysmal supraventricular, 278–279
    sinus, 274, *275*
    ventricular, 285–286
    wide complex, 287t, 287–288
  treatment of
    cardioversion, 267
    catheter ablation, 268
    defibrillation, 267
    implantable cardioverter defibrillators, 267–268
    pharmacologic, 266–267
    vagotonic maneuvers, 267
  types of, 270t
Tachypnea, 227, 234
Takayasu's arteritis, 336t, 337

Technetium-99m sestamibi, 65–66
Technetium-99m tetrofosmin, 65
TEE (*see* Transesophageal echocardiography)
Terazosin, 390–391, 391t
Tetralogy of Fallot, 366–367
Thallium-201, 65–66
Thebesian veins, 8
Thiazide diuretics, 230–231, 406t, 407–408
Thienopyridines, 174, 412–413
Third heart sound, 35
Third-degree atrioventricular block, *273,* 273–274
Threshold potential, 19
Thrombin, 158, 161
Thromboangiitis obliterans, 336t, 337–338, *338*
Thrombocytopenia, heparin-induced, 414
Thromboembolism, 182, 335
Thrombolytic therapy
  blood flow restoration using, 176
  contraindications, 176
  ST-segment elevation myocardial infarction treated
       using, 175–177, *176*
  studies of, 177
  types of, 175
Thrombomodulin, 158–159
Thrombophlebitis, superficial, 345
Thrombosis
  antithrombotic agents, 158–160, 173–174
  consequences of, *162*
  deep venous (*see* Deep venous thrombosis)
  formation of, 161, 409
  partially occlusive, 157
  pathogenesis of, *160,* 160–162
  significance of, 161–162, *162*
Thromboxane A$_2$, 409–411
Ticlopidine, 412–413
Tirofiban, 413
Tissue factor pathway inhibitor, 159
Tissue plasminogen activator, 159, 175, 177
Titin, 23
Tobacco smoking, 126
Tocainide, 398
Torsades de pointes, 286, *286*
Torsemide, 406t, 407
Total peripheral resistance, 221–222
Trabeculae carneae, 4, *4*
Transesophageal echocardiography, 51, 53–54, *53–54,*
       72t
Transmembrane potential, 12, 14
Transmural infarcts, 163, 166t
Transposition of the great arteries, 367–369
Transthoracic echocardiography, 50–51, *52,* 72t,
       206
Transverse tubular system, 11, *11*
Traube's sign, 200t
Triamterene, 406t, 409
Tricuspid regurgitation
  characteristics of, 39, 202
  in heart failure, 228
Tricuspid valve
  anatomy of, 4, *4*
  development of, 351–352
  insufficiency of, 64t
  opening of, 34
  stenosis of, 58, 202
Triggered activity
  description of, 260–261
  treatment of, 267, 394
Triglycerides, 116b
Tropomyosin, 23–24

Troponins
  definition of, 171
  description of, 23
  I, 171
  myocardial infarction diagnosed using, 171–172
  myocardial necrosis detection by, 172
  T, 171
Truncus arteriosus, 348
Tuberculous pericarditis, 312
Tumor necrosis factor-α, 113
Two-dimensional echocardiography
  description of, 50, *52*

Unfractionated heparin, 414
Unidirectional block, 262
Unstable angina
  characteristics of, 142
  clinical features of, 170t
  clinical presentation of, 167–168
  complications of, 178–179
  definition of, 132t
  diagnosis of, 169–170
  pathophysiologic findings, *141*
  treatment of
    anti-ischemic agents, 174–175
    antithrombotic agents, 173–174
    β-blockers, 174–175
    calcium channel blockers, 175
    conservative vs. early invasive approaches, 175
    heparin, 174
    nitrates, 174
    thienopyridines, 174
Uremic pericarditis, 313

Valsalva maneuver, 247–248
Valvular heart disease
  aortic regurgitation (*see* Aortic regurgitation)
  aortic stenosis (*see* Aortic stenosis)
  diet drugs and, 201b
  mitral regurgitation (*see* Mitral regurgitation)
  mitral stenosis (*see* Mitral stenosis)
  mitral valve prolapse, 195
  pulmonic regurgitation, 39, 202
  pulmonic stenosis, 202
  tricuspid regurgitation, 39, 202
  tricuspid stenosis, 58, 202
Variant angina
  characteristics of, 142–143
  definition of, 132t
  pathophysiologic findings, *141*
Varicose veins, 340–341
Vascular cell adhesion molecule, 118
Vascular endothelial growth factor, 335
Vascular smooth muscle
  calcium channel blockers effect, 385
  nitrates effect, *387*
Vascular smooth muscle cells
  atherosclerotic role of, 118–119
  description of, 113
Vasculitis syndromes
  characteristics of, 336t
  description of, 336
  giant cell arteritis, 336t, 337
  polyarteritis nodosa, 336t, 336–337
  Takayasu's arteritis, 336t, 337
  thromboangiitis obliterans, 336t, 337–338
Vasoconstriction
  description of, 134b–135b, 136
  inappropriate, 139

platelets, 139
torsional stress caused by, 161
Vasodilatation
    antithrombotic effects, 159
    coronary arteries, 137
Vasodilators
    angiotensin II receptor blockers (*see* Angiotensin II
        receptor blockers)
    angiotensin-converting enzyme inhibitors (*see*
        Angiotensin-converting enzyme inhibitors)
    bradykinin, 379
    description of, 133–135, 134b, 138
    diazoxide, 383t, 385
    direct-acting, 382–385, 383t
    fenoldopam, 383t, 384–385
    heart failure treated using, 231–232
    hydralazine, 308, 313, 382–383, 383t
    hypertension treated using, 308
    indications, 379
    mechanism of action, 378–379
    minoxidil, 308, 383, 383t
    nesiritide, 232, 379
    nitrates (*see* Nitrates)
    sites of action, *379*
    sodium nitroprusside, 134b, 383t, 383–384, *384*
Veins
    anatomy of, 339–340
    description of, 339
    varicose, 340–341
Venography, 343, *344*
Venous compression duplex ultrasonography, 343
Venous insufficiency, *334*
Venous thrombosis (*see* Deep venous thrombosis)
Ventricles of heart
    contraction, 29
    contraction of, 29
    depolarization, 81–85, *83–84*, 89
    description of, 1–2
    dilated cardiomyopathy effects, 239–240
    "gallop" of, 35
    heart failure-related compensatory responses, 224
    left
        anatomy of, 5, *6*
        aneurysm of, 182
        depolarization of, 94
        diastolic dysfunction, 166, 182
        dilatation of, 199
        dilated cardiomyopathy effects, 239–240
        enlargement of, 191, 193
        hypertrophy of, 302
        outflow tract obstruction, in hypertrophic
            cardiomyopathy, 246, *246*
    nuclear imaging assessments, 68t
    outflow tract
        obstruction of, in hypertrophic cardiomyopathy,
            246, *246*
        septation of, 350–351
    remodeling of, 167, 224

right
    anatomy of, 4–5, 220
    failure of, 220–221
    infarction of, 181
    pressure measurements, *58*, 59, 59b, 60t
    septal rupture, 181–182
    septation of, 350–351
    two-dimensional echocardiography assessments,
        54, *55*
    wall stress, 136, 214, 224
Ventricular ectopy, 180
Ventricular fibrillation
    characteristics of, 286–287, *287*
    myocardial infarction-related, 179–180
Ventricular hypertrophy
    compensatory, 224
    eccentric, 224
    hypertension and, 302
    in hypertrophic cardiomyopathy, 244, *245*
    left, 92
    QRS complex abnormalities associated with, 91–92,
        93, *107*, *109*
    radiographic findings, 46
    right, 91–92, *93*
    wall stress effects, 136, 224
Ventricular preexcitation syndrome, 281–283
Ventricular premature beats, *284*, 284–285
Ventricular septal defect
    clinical features of, 358, *358*
    incidence of, 358
    laboratory studies, 359
    left-to-right shunting associated with, 359
    pansystolic murmurs caused by, 39
    pathophysiology of, 358–359
    physical examination, 359
    symptoms of, 359
    treatment of, 359
Ventricular tachycardia, 285–286
Verapamil, 152, 386–387
Very-low-density lipoproteins
    atherosclerosis risks and, 124
    characteristics of, 115t, 117b
    niacin effects, 419
Viral myocarditis, 237
Visceral pericardium, 1
Voltage-sensitive gating, 14

Warfarin, 344, 415–416
Wavy microfibers, 164
Wenckebach block, 272, *272*
Wide complex tachycardias, 287t, 287–288
Wide splitting, *32*, 33
Wolff-Parkinson-White syndrome, *281–282*,
    281–283

X-rays (*see* Radiography)

Yellow-softening, 166